D1482859

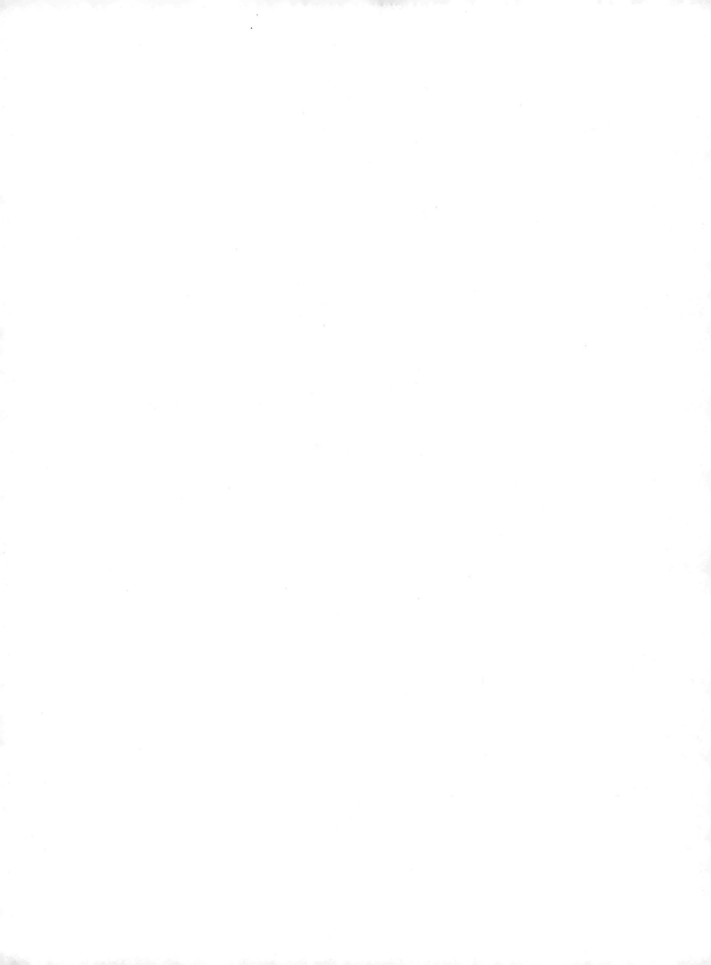

CONTEMPORARY ENDOCRINOLOGY

Series Editor:
P. Michael Conn, PhD
Oregon Health & Science University
Beaverton, OR

For other titles published in this series, go to
www.springer.com/series/7680

Michael Freemark

Editor

PEDIATRIC OBESITY

Etiology, Pathogenesis, and Treatment

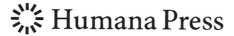 Humana Press

Editor
Michael Freemark
Robert C. and Veronica Atkins Professor of Pediatrics
Division of Pediatric Endocrinology and Diabetes
Duke University
DUMC Box 102820
Durham, NC 27710, USA
freem001@mc.duke.edu

ISBN 978-1-60327-873-7   e-ISBN 978-1-60327-874-4
DOI 10.1007/978-1-60327-874-4
Springer New York Dordrecht Heidelberg London

Library of Congress Control Number: 2010930709

Printed on acid-free paper

Humana Press is part of Springer Science+Business Media (www.springer.com)

Tell me what kind of food you eat, and I will tell you what kind of man you are.

– Jean-Anthelme Brillat-Savarin, *The Physiology of Taste,* 1825

To lengthen thy life, lessen thy meals.

– Benjamin Franklin, *Poor Richard's Almanack,* 1737

PREFACE

Our generation bears witness to striking increases in childhood obesity and its co-morbidities including type 2 diabetes, hypertension, dyslipidemia, sleep apnea, and fatty liver disease. Despite a wealth of investigation, there is considerable controversy regarding the etiology of childhood obesity and the optimal approaches for prevention and treatment.

This book has a number of features that should make it a unique resource for those who care for obese children and their families. First, the perspective is international in scope; the distinguished authors are drawn from Europe, Canada, and Israel as well as the United States. Second, the discussion of etiology and pathogenesis is far-reaching and includes an analysis of historical and sociocultural as well as biochemical, metabolic, neuroendocrinologic, and genetic determinants. Third, the short- and long-term complications of childhood obesity are reviewed in depth. Fourth, there is a detailed and lively discussion of therapeutic approaches including lifestyle counselling, pharmacotherapy, and bariatric surgery, followed by a thoughtful assessment of the biological and sociocultural challenges to success. Finally, the roles of globalization and governmental policy in the worldwide spread of childhood obesity are explored and implications for social action are discussed.

I conclude many of the chapters with one or more comments and questions raised during my editorial review. The authors' responses highlight some of the problems that we continue to face in understanding and coping with obesity and metabolic disorders in children.

For making this work possible I thank my wife Anne Slifkin, my soul mate, sounding board, and source of inspiration.

Michael Freemark

CONTENTS

Contributors

ANNA ALISI • *"Bambino Gesù" Children's Hospital and Research Institute, Rome, Italy*

SILVA A. ARSLANIAN • *Division of Pediatric Endocrinology, Metabolism and Diabetes Mellitus, Children's Hospital of Pittsburgh, Pittsburgh, PA 15224, USA; Division of Weight Management and Wellness, Children's Hospital of Pittsburgh, Pittsburgh, PA 15213, USA*

KELLY D. BROWNELL • *Department of Psychology and Public Health, Rudd Center for Food Policy and Obesity, Yale University, New Haven, CT 06520-8369, USA*

ANNA CALI • *Department of Pediatrics, Yale School of Medicine, New Haven, CT, USA*

SONIA CAPRIO • *Department of Pediatrics, Yale School of Medicine, New Haven, CT, USA*

MICHELLE CHRISTIAN • *Department of Sociology, Duke University, Durham, NC 27708-0088, USA*

DANA DABELEA • *Department of Epidemiology, Colorado School of Public Health, University of Colorado Denver, Denver, CO, USA*

ERIC J. DEMARIA • *Department of Surgery, Duke University Medical Center, Durham, NC 27710, USA*

CEM DEMIRCI • *Division of Pediatric Endocrinology, Metabolism and Diabetes Mellitus, Children's Hospital of Pittsburgh, Pittsburgh, PA 15201, USA*

RITA DEVITO • *"Bambino Gesù" Children's Hospital and Research Institute, Rome, Italy*

ALON ELIAKIM • *Department of Pediatrics, Sackler School of Medicine, Child Health and Sports Center, Meir Medical Center, Tel-Aviv University, Kfar-Saba, Israel*

CSABA FEKETE • *Department of Endocrine Neurobiology, Institute of Experimental Medicine, Hungarian Academy of Sciences, Budapest 1083, Hungary; Division of Endocrinology, Diabetes, Metabolism and Molecular Medicine, Tufts Medical Medical Center, Boston, MA, USA*

STEPHEN FRANKS • *Imperial College London, Institute of Reproductive and Developmental Biology, Hammersmith Hospital, London W2 0NN, UK*

MICHAEL FREEMARK • *Division of Pediatric Endocrinology and Diabetes, Duke University Medical Center, Durham, NC 27710, USA*

PHILIPPE FROGUEL • *CNRS UMR 8090, Institute of Biology, Pasteur Institute, Lille, France; Genomic Medicine, Hammersmith Hospital, Imperial College London, London, UK*

GARY GEREFFI • *Department of Sociology, Center on Globalization, Governance & Competitiveness, Duke University, Durham, NC 27708-0088, USA*

SAMUEL S. GIDDING • *Nemours Cardiac Center, Alfred I DuPont Hospital for Children, Wilmington, DE 19803, USA*

JOEL GITTELSOHN • *Bloomberg School of Public Health, Center for Human Nutrition, Johns Hopkins University, Baltimore, MD 21205-2179, USA*

CHARLES J. GLUECK • *Cholesterol Center, Jewish Hospital of Cincinnati, Cincinnati, OH 45229, USA*

NAILA GOLDENBERG • *Cholesterol Center, Jewish Hospital of Cincinnati, Cincinnati, OH 45229, USA*

JAIME HAIDET • *Division of Pediatric Endocrinology, Metabolism and Diabetes Mellitus, Children's Hospital of Pittsburgh, Pittsburgh, PA 15201, USA*

ANDREA M. HAQQ • *Division of Pediatric Endocrinology, Department of Pediatrics, University of Alberta, Edmonton, AB, Canada T6G 2J3*

JOHANNES HEBEBRAND • *Department of Child and Adolescent Psychiatry and Psychotherapy, LVR-Klinikum Essen, University of Duisburg-Essen, 45147 Essen, Germany*

DAVID C. HENDERSON • *Freedom Trail Clinic, Harvard Medical School, Massachusetts General Hospital, Boston, MA 02114, USA*

ANKE HINNEY • *Department of Child and Adolescent Psychiatry and Psychotherapy, LVR-Klinikum Essen, University of Duisburg-Essen, 45147 Essen, Germany*

JOANNA HOLSTEN • *School of Nursing, University of Pennsylvania, Philadelphia, PA, USA*

TRACY E. HUNLEY • *Division of Pediatric Nephrology, Monroe Carell Jr. Children's Hospital at Vanderbilt, Vanderbilt University School of Medicine, Nashville, TN, USA*

SUSAN JEBB • *Medical Research Council Collaborative Centre for Human Nutrition Research, Cambridge, UK*

JALINI JOHARATNAM • *Imperial College London, Institute of Reproductive and Developmental Biology, Hammersmith Hospital, London W2 0NN, UK*

LAURA JOHNSON • *Department of Epidemiology and Public Health, Cancer Research UK Health Behaviour Research Centre, University College London, London, UK*

VALENTINA KON • *Division of Pediatric Nephrology, Monroe Carell Jr. Children's Hospital at Vanderbilt, Vanderbilt University School of Medicine, Nashville, TN, USA*

SHIRIKI KUMANYIKA • *Center for Clinical Epidemiology and Biostatistics, University of Pennsylvania School of Medicine, Philadelphia, PA 19104-6021, USA*

LORRAINE LANNINGHAM-FOSTER • *Food Science and Human Nutrition, Iowa State University, Ames, IA 50011, USA*

RONALD M. LECHAN • *Division of Endocrinology, Diabetes and Metabolism, and Department of Neuroscience, Tufts Medical Center, and Tufts University School of Medicine, Boston, MA, USA*

JAMES A. LEVINE • *Endocrine Research Unit, Mayo Clinic, Rochester, MN 5590, USA*

ROBERT H. LUSTIG • *Division of Pediatric Endocrinology, Department of Pediatrics, University of California, San Francisco, CA 94143, USA*

MELANIA MANCO • *"Bambino Gesù" Children's Hospital and Research Institute, Rome, Italy*

ELIZABETH J. MAYER-DAVIS • *Department of Nutrition and Department of Medicine, Gillings School of Global Public Health and School of Medicine, School of Public Health and School of Medicine, University of North Carolina at Chapel Hill, Chapel Hill, NC 27599-7461, USA*

BRIAN W. MCCRINDLE • *Division of Cardiology, Department of Pediatrics, Labatt Family Heart Centre, The Hospital for Sick Children, University of Toronto, Toronto, ON, Canada M5G 1X8*

HENRY C. MCGILL • *Southwest Foundation for Biomedical Research, San Antonio, TX 78245-0549, USA*

C. ALEX MCMAHAN • *University of Texas Health Science Center, San Antonio, TX 78229-3900, USA*

DAVID MEYRE • *CNRS UMR 8090, Institute of Biology, Pasteur Institute, Lille, France*

JOHN A. MORRISON • *Division of Cardiology, Cincinnati Children's Hospital Medical Center, Cincinnati, OH 45229, USA*

DAN NEMET • *Department of Pediatrics, Sackler School of Medicine, Child Health and Sports Center, Meir Medical Center, Tel-Aviv University, Kfar-Saba, Israel*

VALERIO NOBILI • *"Bambino Gesù" Children's Hospital and Research Institute, Rome, Italy*

KEN K. ONG • *MRC Epidemiology Unit, Institute of Metabolic Science, Addenbrooke's Hospital, Box 285, Cambridge CB2 0QQ, UK*

ELIZABETH PROUT PARKS • *The Children's Hospital of Philadelphia, Philadelphia, PA, USA*

SOHYUN PARK • *Bloomberg School of Public Health, Center for Human Nutrition, Johns Hopkins University, Baltimore, MD 21205-2179, USA*

BARRY POPKIN • *UNC Interdisciplinary Obesity Program, School of Public Health, Carolina Population Center, University of North Carolina at Chapel Hill, Chapel Hill, NC 27516-3997, USA*

MARLENE B. SCHWARTZ • *Department of Psychology, Senior Research Scientist, Rudd Center for Food Policy and Obesity, Yale University, New Haven, CT 06520-8369, USA*

LAUREN SHIN • *Rush University Medical Center, Chicago, IL 60612, USA; Clinical Instructor of Psychiatry, Scott Nolan Center, Maryville Academy, Des Plaines, IL 60016, USA*

MUHAMMAD UMAR • *Cholesterol Center, Jewish Hospital of Cincinnati, Cincinnati, OH 45229, USA*

ANNA VANNUCCI • *Washington University School of Medicine, St. Louis, MO 63110, USA*

STIJN VERHULST • *Department of Pediatrics, University of Antwerp, Wilrijk 2610, Belgium*

PING WANG • *Cholesterol Center, Jewish Hospital of Cincinnati, Cincinnati, OH 45229, USA*

RAM WEISS • *Department of Human Metabolism and Nutrition, Department of Pediatrics, Hadassah – Hebrew University School of Medicine, Jerusalem, Israel*

EMILY K. WHITE • *Washington University School of Medicine, St. Louis, MO 63110, USA*

DENISE E. WILFLEY • *Pediatrics and Psychology, Department of Psychiatry, Washington University School of Medicine, St. Louis, MO 63110, USA*

KATHERINE J. WOJCIK • *Department of Nutrition, Gillings School of Global Public Health and School of Medicine, University of North Carolina at Chapel Hill, Chapel Hill, NC 27599-7461, USA*

BASIL M. YURCISIN • *Department of Surgery, Duke University Medical Center, Durham, NC 27710, USA*

I THE OBESITY EPIDEMIC: A GLOBAL PERSPECTIVE

1 Global Dynamics in Childhood Obesity: Reflections on a Life of Work in the Field

Barry Popkin

CONTENTS

Key Words: Global, malnutrition, income, sugar, oil, meat, supermarkets

INTRODUCTION

One of the more profound shifts in the last two decades has been the marked increase in child obesity in countries across the globe – rich and poor, urban and rural. The nature of this shift to a world that is fat needs to be understood very broadly, but the obesity engine is driven by local and well as national and international forces. In this chapter, I attempt to lay out the broad outlines of the shifts in obesity among school-age children and adolescents. I do not address the issues of preschoolers because there is currently a lack of reliable data in this age group.

After presenting an overview of global shifts, I examine some of the major trends in dietary and activity patterns; the analysis is based on limited in-depth measurements of dietary patterns and trends from a few countries with an overlay of cross-national comparisons. I draw extensively on a range of books and articles that I have written on this topic but present in a few cases new or updated information when available *(1)*. As much as possible, I rely on nationally representative or nationally sampled surveys and direct measurements of weight and height.

GLOBAL PATTERNS AND TRENDS

When I lived in India in the 1960s and traveled and worked in lower- and middle-income areas, the developing world (then termed the Third World) was dominated by hunger and malnutrition. But these problems were not confined to impoverished countries; my initial work in the USA related to feeding low-income children and their families through programs such as the Food Stamp Program and School

From: *Contemporary Endocrinology: Pediatric Obesity: Etiology, Pathogenesis, and Treatment*
Edited by: M. Freemark, DOI 10.1007/978-1-60327-874-4_1,
© Springer Science+Business Media, LLC 2010

Feeding Programs. It was only when I worked with a Presidential Select Panel for the Promotion of Child Health during the Carter era that I recognized that obesity was emerging as a worldwide concern *(2,3)*.

In this regard, moderate- and upper-income countries have led the way. One very useful study followed Danish schoolchildren from a national sample for 50 years (1930–1983). This study showed a slow increase in child and adolescent overweight from the 1930s to 1950s, a plateau period until the 1960s, and a steep increase thereafter *(4)*. Likewise, my research team and colleagues from Brazil have shown remarkable rates of increase in overweight and obesity status among adults, children, and teens globally; in other words, the percentage of adults and children in the USA, Europe, and Australia who become overweight and obese each year has increased since 1994. In Brazil the annual rate of change in the prevalence of child obesity doubled between 1990 and 2006.

However, in the past 20 years, obesity has also burst forth in the lower-income countries of Asia, the Middle East, Africa, and Central and South America. For example, 5–15% of adult women in the poorest countries of sub-Saharan Africa are overweight *(5)*. In 38 lower-income countries, more women are overweight than are underweight. Comparable data show similar trends in children in the few countries studied (e.g., Mexico, China, Brazil) *(6–11)*. Russia is the anomaly in which an increase in adult obesity is not mirrored by an increase in childhood obesity.

Comparative Levels of Childhood Obesity

Elsewhere I have published a comparison of the shifts in prevalence of adult, child, and adolescent overweight *(9,12)*. I use for this work the International Obesity Task Force (IOTF) cutoffs for child and adolescent obesity as they link better with those of NCHS-CDC and really do not show major differences in trends *(13)*.

Figure 1 shows the prevalence of overweight plus obesity in adults and children as measured by BMI.

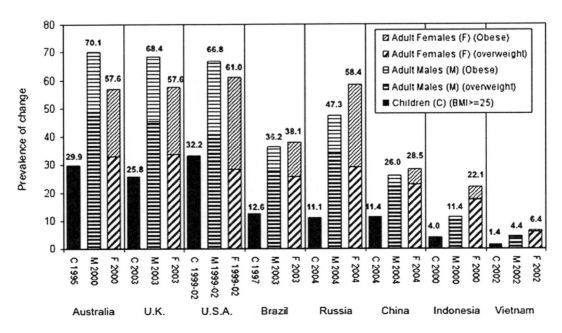

Fig. 1. The prevalence of overweight plus obesity (BMI > 25) children aged 6–17.9 and overweight and obese for adults aged 18 and older *(12,* p. 61*)*.

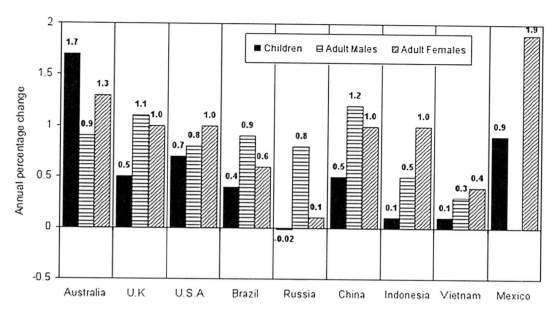

Fig. 2. Annual absolute change in the prevalence of overweight and obesity in seven countries from 1985/1995 to 1995/2006 (BMI ≥ 25.0 for adults; IOTF equivalent for children) *(12*, p. 61*)*.

Figure 2 shows the rates of increase in overweight and obesity in adults and children over time. The rate of increase for children is not as rapid as the rate for adults but nonetheless is very high *(9)*. About 0.5% of all children in most high- and moderate-income countries have become overweight or obese each year. Thus since 2006, approximately 9 million children and 30 million adults in these moderate- and low-income countries became overweight each year. These estimates, while not precise, approximate the global rates of change and total numbers per year of new overweight children and adults.

Rich vs. Poor Sectors of Society

In the USA and other developed countries, poor people are more likely to be overweight than upper-income people; they are also more likely to develop metabolic complications of obesity including diabetes and cardiovascular disease *(14–19)*. However, the inverse relationship between income and obesity found among adults is not clearly replicated in children *(20,21)*. Moreover, studies in China between 1991 and 2004 *(11)* reveal that it is higher-income children and those living in urban areas that have both the highest prevalence and the greatest annual and relative rates of increase in obesity. This likely reflects recent changes in diet and energy expenditure fostered by globalization and rapid urbanization.

WHY THE BROAD SHIFT IN ENERGY BALANCE?

The Sweetening of Child Diets

While there are a number of key global shifts during the last generation, a major one that stands out is the increasing sweetness of what children eat and drink. Intake of caloric sweeteners has expanded across the globe *(22)*. This is particularly the case for beverages. For instance, in the USA in the 1960s and 1970s more than two-thirds of caloric sweeteners came from food and one-third from liquids; the ratio has reversed in the past few years *(23)*. While the amount of sugar added to food has not

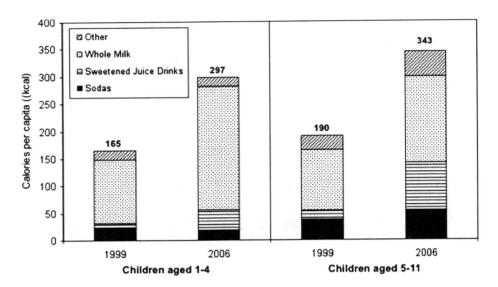

Fig. 3. Daily beverage consumption trends of Mexican children, 1999–2006. Note: Sweetened juice drinks include 100% fruit juice with sugar added and agua fresca (water, juice, sugar). Sodas include carbonated and noncarbonated sugar bottled beverages. Source: Barquera et al. *(25)*.

declined, the level of caloric beverage intake has exploded. This is the case in the USA, Australia, and South Africa. In Mexico, the intake of calories from beverages has doubled between 1999 and 2006 (see Fig. 3) *(24–29)*.

Large Increases in Edible Oil

The use of vegetable oils has increased in the past 20 years in lower-income countries and in the past half-century in higher-income countries. What is especially interesting to understand is that it is the poorest countries with the most rapid increases in use of fats *(1,30,31)*. Since vegetable oils are inexpensive, adding oil to a food product by frying is a remarkably efficient way to add calories and taste. In China, this has equated to a striking increase in the proportion of calories from fried foods (replacing steamed and boiled foods) and with the increasing use of oil in stir-frying and other cooking techniques. This is true in other Asian countries and in many other poor countries as well; cheap vegetable oils have increased the intake of fats among the world's poor to a level previously found only in wealthier countries *(31)*. In a country such as China, the average adult consumes more than 300 calories a day from vegetable oil alone (Fig. 4). Similarly, adults in Malaysia, all other Southeast Asian countries, and the Middle East consume equal or higher amounts of vegetable oil. This increase in oil-calorie intake has helped to fuel the rise in obesity worldwide.

Increased Intake of Animal Source Foods (Dairy, Beef, Pork, Poultry, Fish, and Eggs)

In 2002, the per capita intake of milk in developed countries was 202 kg in 2002; the relevant level in lower-income countries was 46 kg. Comparative red meat intakes were 78 and 28 kg/capita, respectively *(32)*. Over the last decade, there have been marked increases in the intake of animal food products in the developing world, led by China and India *(33)*. This is the case for red meats as well as dairy products, white meats, and processed meats. The high saturated fat content of red meat and whole fat dairy products may have also contributed to population weight gain.

Year	1989	1997	2006
Poorest (lowest income tertile)	11.8	26.5	30.8
Middle income tertile	15	29.7	30.9
Richest (highest income tertile)	17.4	31.3	30.9
Average for total adult population	14.8	28.9	30.9
% of all calories per capita from edible oil	4.9	11.2	12.4

Fig. 4. Edible oil consumption still rising in China (grams per day per capita). Source: China Health and Nutrition Survey for adults aged 20–45 *(57)*.

Marked Shifts in Patterns of Eating

Snacking is a relatively new phenomenon in the global diet. In the USA, the most marked change for children aside from the shift to caloric beverages is that of snacking. Snacks now represent nearly a quarter of an average American child's energy intake *(34–37)*. We have much less systematic data in this regard in other countries. Nevertheless a recent study in China shows rapid expansion of the processed food sector and an increase in the prevalence of snacking in adults as well as children (Fig. 5) *(38)*. As food companies explore new markets, I expect that the rapid growth of snacking in the USA will be replicated in Central and South America, the Middle East, and Asia. Certainly this is occurring in Europe already *(39–43)*.

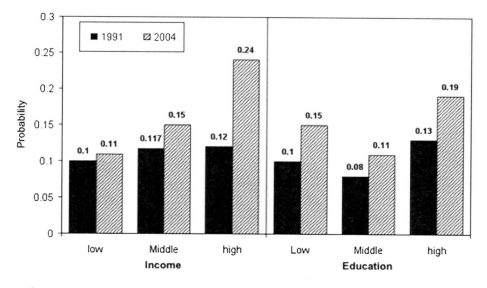

Fig. 5. The predicted probability of snacking behavior in China, 1991 and 2004. Source: CHNS 1991 and 2004; adjusted for socio-demographic factors *(57, p. 123)*.

A much bigger phenomenon with unclear impact on obesity is the shift to eating away-from-home and purchasing prepared food for home consumption. Much of the research has documented the dramatic shift in food expenditures to eating away and the potential adverse effects of fast food consumption on weight and related metabolic consequences *(44–48)*. As we have shown in one study of child diets across four countries, there is enormous heterogeneity in the patterns of food consumption away-from-home *(49)*. For instance in that study we found that Filipino and US children consumed very large proportions of total energy away-from-home while Russian and Chinese children did not.

Lastly, as noted previously, there is a large shift to consuming more fried foods both at home and away-from-home and fewer steamed and baked foods. We noted this emerging trend in China *(38)*.

Concurrent Shifts in Physical Activity

While there is extensive research across the globe on the increase of inactivity among children, particularly related to TV use, gaming, or computer use, clear overall patterns and trends in total child activity are few and far between *(50–53)*. Furthermore, few of these have been linked with shifts in weight *(54–58)*.

We know that energy expenditure matters; most interventions to prevent obesity in the preschool and schoolage period address this. Unfortunately, large trials in the USA and elsewhere to increase physical activity among children have been only marginally successful *(59–63)*. However, long-term monitoring of trends in overall activity is rare and much of the focus remains on means to decrease sedentary behavior *(64)*. Elsewhere I discuss in more depth the vast shifts in activity across all phases of life – work and school, travel to both, work inside the household, and leisure activity *(1)*.

UNDERLYING CHANGES

Major societal shifts affect how we eat, drink, and move. Clearly the globe has been urbanized; most countries have major urban centers, and many aspects of modern urban life are now found even in many small towns and villages (e.g., Cable TV, access to the Internet, roads linking them to more modernized shopping and marketing). In the same vein, globalization has brought vast shifts in access to modern food systems in terms of food shopping and away-from-home eating as well as wide exposure to food ads. Elsewhere I have presented in-depth some of the ways that globalization has affected the lives of individuals in the low- and middle-income world; these include ready access to modern supermarkets, rapid transmission of all the technologies that affect physical activity, and exposure to modern media *(1,12,65)*.

Global access to supermarkets is a cornerstone of changes in food distribution (see also Chapter 30 by Christian and Gereffi, this volume). We do not know exactly how the introduction of the Wal-Marts, Carrefour's, Aholds, and many other global supermarkets is affecting dietary intake patterns in low-income countries, but we are sure that the changes are mixed – some good and some bad. In the USA, changes in food distribution have followed a similar but more gradual course; we began with traditional supermarkets but have witnessed a sharp increase (to 40.3%) in the relative share controlled by Wal-Marts and other mass merchandisers. The trend is toward increased dominance of the mass merchandisers *(66)*.

In the lower-income world, the effects of this change are much more profound. Fresh (farmer, "wet") markets and small stores are disappearing, replaced increasingly by multinational, regional, and local large supermarkets – usually part of larger chains like Carrefour or Wal-Mart or in countries such as South Africa and China by local chains that mimic Wal-Mart. China has all the global and huge local chains, whereas a smaller country like South Africa has its own domestically developed chain expanding across the urban areas of sub-Saharan Africa. Increasingly, large mega stores are found. In Latin America, supermarkets' share of all retail food sales increased from 15% in 1990 to 60% by 2000 *(67–69)*. For comparison, 80% of retail food sales in the USA in 2000 occurred in supermarkets. In one decade, the role of supermarkets in Latin America has expanded to be the equivalent of about a half-century of expansion in the USA. Supermarket use has spread across both large and small countries, from capital cities to rural villages, and from upper- and middle-class families to working-class families *(70)*. This same process is also occurring at varying rates and at different stages in Asia,

Eastern Europe, and Africa. The chains function to cut costs and improve efficiencies, and as major purchasers can bargain for lower prices and other economies with suppliers. Nevertheless, they provide access to a wide array of inexpensive, calorically dense, packaged foods that may promote weight gain in low-income as well as high-income populations.

Consider India, where the bulk of retail outlets are still neighborhood shops. Carrefour, Wal-Mart, and others are spending billions to break into this market. From various reports, the India mass retailer market appears to be growing by at least $27 billion/year – a size bigger than the Gross National Product of half of the countries in the world *(71)*. But the growing middle class of India want these changes, want to shop more easily in air-conditioned comfort, and want many of the benefits in choice and variety that come from being part of a global food conglomerate *(71)*.

BRIEF SUMMARY

The shifts in obesity and related dietary and physical activity patterns across the globe during the past two decades have been remarkable. The rate of increase in obesity has accelerated, particularly for children and adolescents. The large-scale shifts in intake of calorically sweetened beverages, fried foods, and animal food products are striking, accompanied by powerful changes in patterns of eating. Concurrent trends toward reduced physical activity and increased sedentary behaviour have led to dramatic shifts in energy balance. The worldwide increases in intake of caloric sweeteners (particularly sweetened beverages) and the increased snacking and food consumption away-from-home are serious causes for concern.

REFERENCES

1. Popkin BM. The world is fat – the fads, trends, policies, and products that are fattening the human race. New York, NY: Avery-Penguin Group; 2008.
2. Popkin B, Akin J, Haines P, Macdonald MM, Spicer DS. Nutrition program options for maternal and child health. Madison, WI: Institute for Research on Poverty; 1980.
3. U.S. Department of Health and Human Services. Better health for our children: a national strategy report of the select panel for the promotion of child health to the United States Congress and the Secretary of Health and Human Services. Washington, DC: U.S. Government Printing Office; 1981.
4. Bua J, Olsen LW, Sorensen TIA. Secular trends in childhood obesity in Denmark during 50 years in relation to economic growth. Obesity. 2007;15(4):977–85.
5. Mendez MA, Monteiro CA, Popkin BM. Overweight exceeds underweight among women in most developing countries. Am J Clin Nutr. 2005;81(3):714–21.
6. Rivera J, Barquera S, Campirano F, Campos I, Safdie M, Tovar V. Epidemiological and nutritional transition in Mexico: rapid increase of non-communicable chronic diseases and obesity. Public Health Nutr. 2002;14(44):113–22.
7. Rivera JA, Barquera S, Gonzalez-Cossio T, Olaiz G, Sepulveda J. Nutrition transition in Mexico and in other Latin American countries. Nutr Rev. 2004;62(7 Pt 2):S149–57.
8. Monteiro PO, Victora CG. Rapid growth in infancy and childhood and obesity in later life – a systematic review. Obes Rev. 2005;6(2):143–54.
9. Popkin BM, Wolney C, Ningqi H, Carlos M. Is there a lag globally in overweight trends for children as compared to adults? Obesity. 2006;14:1846–53.
10. Wang Y, Monteiro C, Popkin BM. Trends of obesity and underweight in older children and adolescents in the United States, Brazil, China, and Russia. Am J Clin Nutr. 2002;75(6):971–7.
11. Dearth-Wesley T, Wang H, Popkin BM. Obesity dynamics in China: The poor are catching up. Eur J Clin Nutr. 2007;18:1–6.
12. Popkin BM. Understanding Global Nutrition Dynamics as a step toward controlling cancer morbidity and mortality. Nat Rev Cancer. 2007;247:61–7.
13. Cole TJ, Bellizz MC, Flegal KM, Dietz WH. Establishing a standard definition for child overweight and obesity worldwide: international survey. BMJ. 2000;320(7244):1240–43.
14. Sobal J, Stunkard AJ. Socioeconomic status and obesity: a review of the literature. Psychol Bull. 1989;105(2):260–75.

15. Davis SK, Winkleby MA, Farquhar JW. Increasing disparity in knowledge of cardiovascular disease risk factors and risk-reduction strategies by socioeconomic status: implications for policymakers. Am J Prev Med. 1995;11(5):318–23.

16. Kaufman JS, Cooper RS, McGee DL. Socioeconomic status and health in blacks and whites: the problem of residual confounding and the resiliency of race. Epidemiology. 1997;8(6):621–8.

17. Gordon-Larsen P, Nelson MC, Page P, Popkin BM. Inequality in the built environment underlies key health disparities in physical activity and obesity. Pediatrics. 2006;117(2):417–24.

18. Neumark-Sztainer D, Croll J, Story M, Hannan PJ, French SA, Perry C. Ethnic/racial differences in weight-related concerns and behaviors among adolescent girls and boys: findings from Project EAT. J Psychosom Res. 2002;53(5): 963–74.

19. Wang Y, Beydoun MA. The obesity epidemic in the United States–gender, age, socioeconomic, racial/ethnic, and geographic characteristics: a systematic review and meta-regression analysis. Epidemiol Rev. 2007;29:6–28.

20. Gordon-Larsen P, Adair LS, Popkin BM. The relationship of ethnicity, socioeconomic factors, and overweight in US adolescents. Obes Res. 2003;11(1):121–9.

21. Wang Y. Cross-national comparison of childhood obesity: the epidemic and the relationship between obesity and socioeconomic status. Int J Epidemiol. 2001;30(5):1129–36.

22. Popkin BM, Nielsen SJ. The sweetening of the world's diet. Obes Res. 2003;11(11):1325–32.

23. Duffey KJ, Popkin BM. High-fructose corn syrup: is this what's for dinner? Am J Clin Nutr. 2008;88(6):1722S–32S.

24. Steyn NP, Myburgh NG, Nel JH. Evidence to support a food-based dietary guideline on sugar consumption in South Africa. Bull World Health Organ. 2003;81(8):599–608.

25. Barquera S, Hernández L, Tolentino ML, et al. Energy from beverages is on the rise among Mexican adolescents and adults. J Nutr. 2008;138:2456–61.

26. Rivera JA, Muñoz-Hernández O, Rosas-Peralta M, Aguilar-Salinas CA, Popkin BM, Willett WC. Consumo de bebidas para una vida saludable: recomendaciones para la población (Beverage consumption for a healthy life: recommendations for the Mexican population). Salud Publica Mex. 2008;50(2):173–95.

27. Nielsen SJ, Popkin BM. Changes in beverage intake between 1977 and 2001. Am J Prev Med. 2004;27(3):205–10.

28. Rajeshwari R, Yang S-J, Nicklas TA, Berenson GS. Secular trends in children's sweetened-beverage consumption (1973 to 1994): The Bogalusa Heart Study. J Am Diet Assoc. 2005;105(2):208–14.

29. Sanigorski AM, Bell AC, Swinburn BA. Association of key foods and beverages with obesity in Australian schoolchildren. Public Health Nutr. 2007;10(2):152–7.

30. Drewnowski A, Popkin BM. The nutrition transition: new trends in the global diet. Nutr Rev. 1997;55(2):31–43.

31. Popkin B, Drewnowski A. Dietary fats and the nutrition transition: New trends in the global diet. Nutr Rev. 1997;55: 31–43.

32. Food and Agricultural Organization of the United Nations. Livestock's long shadow: environmental issues and options. Rome: Food and Agricultural Organization United Nations; 2007.

33. Delgado CL. A food revolution: rising consumption of meat and milk in developing countries. J Nutr. 2003;133(11 Suppl 2):3907S–10S.

34. Jahns L, Siega-Riz AM, Popkin BM. The increasing prevalence of snacking among US children from 1977 to 1996. J Pediatr. 2001;138(4):493–8.

35. Nielsen SJ, Siega-Riz AM, Popkin BM. Trends in food locations and sources among adolescents and young adults. Prev Med. 2002;35(2):107–13.

36. Nielsen SJ, Siega-Riz AM, Popkin BM. Trends in energy intake in U.S. between 1977 and 1996: similar shifts seen across age groups. Obes Res. 2002;10(5):370–8.

37. Zizza C, Siega-Riz AM, Popkin BM. Significant increase in young adults' snacking between 1977–1978 and 1994–1996 represents a cause for concern! Prev Med. 2001;32(4):303–10.

38. Wang Z, Zhai F, Shufa D, Popkin BM. Dynamic shifts in Chinese eating behaviors. Asia Pac J Clin Nutr. 2008;17: 123–30.

39. Kerr MA, Rennie KL, McCaffrey TA, Wallace JM, Hannon-Fletcher MP, Livingstone MB. Snacking patterns among adolescents: a comparison of type, frequency and portion size between Britain in 1997 and Northern Ireland in 2005. Br J Nutr. 2009;101(1):122–31.

40. Lloyd-Williams F, Mwatsama M, Ireland R, Capewell S. Small changes in snacking behaviour: the potential impact on CVD mortality. Public Health Nutr. 2008;12(6):1–6.

41. Alm A, Fahraeus C, Wendt LK, Koch G, Andersson-Gare B, Birkhed D. Body adiposity status in teenagers and snacking habits in early childhood in relation to approximal caries at 15 years of age. Int J Paediatr Dent. 2008;18(3):189–96.

42. Astrup A, Bovy MW, Nackenhorst K, Popova AE. Food for thought or thought for food?–a stakeholder dialogue around the role of the snacking industry in addressing the obesity epidemic. Obes Rev. 2006;7(3):303–12.

43. Erlanson-Albertsson C, Zetterstrom R. The global obesity epidemic: snacking and obesity may start with free meals during infant feeding. Acta Paediatr. 2005;94(11):1523–31.

44. Duffey KJ, Gordon-Larsen P, Jacobs DR Jr, Williams OD, Popkin BM. Differential associations of fast food and restaurant food consumption with 3-y change in body mass index: the Coronary Artery Risk Development in Young Adults Study. Am J Clin Nutr. 2007;85(1):201–8.

45. Nelson MC, Gordon-Larsen P, North KE, Adair LS. Body mass index gain, fast food, and physical activity: effects of shared environments over time. Obesity (Silver Spring). 2006;14(4):701–9.

46. Prentice AM, Jebb SA. Fast foods, energy density and obesity: a possible mechanistic link. Obes Rev. 2003;4(4):187–94.

47. Stender S, Dyerberg J, Astrup A. Fast food: unfriendly and unhealthy. Int J Obes. 2007;31:887–90.

48. French SA, Story M, Neumark-Sztainer D, Fulkerson JA, Hannan P. Fast food restaurant use among adolescents: associations with nutrient intake, food choices and behavioral and psychosocial variables. Int J Obes. 2001;25(12):1823–33.

49. Adair LS, Popkin BM. Are child eating patterns being transformed globally? Obes Res. 2005;13(7):1281–99.

50. Must A, Tybor DJ. Physical activity and sedentary behavior: a review of longitudinal studies of weight and adiposity in youth. Int J Obes (Lond). 2005;29(Suppl 2):S84–96.

51. Marshall SJ, Biddle SJ, Gorely T, Cameron N, Murdey I. Relationships between media use, body fatness and physical activity in children and youth: a meta-analysis. Int J Obes Relat Metab Disord. 2004;28(10):1238–46.

52. Boreham C, Robson PJ, Gallagher AM, Cran GW, Savage JM, Murray LJ. Tracking of physical activity, fitness, body composition and diet from adolescence to young adulthood: the Young Hearts Project, Northern Ireland. Int J Behav Nutr Phys Act. 2004;1(1):14.

53. Trost SG, Sirard JR, Dowda M, Pfeiffer KA, Pate RR. Physical activity in overweight and nonoverweight preschool children. Int J Obes Relat Metab Disord. 2003;27(7):834–9.

54. Tudor-Locke C, Ainsworth BE, Adair LS, Popkin BM. Physical activity in Filipino youth: the Cebu Longitudinal Health and Nutrition Survey. Int J Obes Relat Metab Disord. 2003;27(2):181–90.

55. Tudor-Locke C, Ainsworth BE, Adair LS, Popkin BM. Objective physical activity of Filipino youth stratified for commuting mode to school. Med Sci Sports Exerc. 2003;35(3):465–71.

56. Tudor-Locke C, Ainsworth BE, Adair LS, Du S, Popkin BM. Physical activity and inactivity in Chinese school-aged youth: the China Health and Nutrition Survey. Int J Obes Relat Metab Disord. 2003;27(9):1093–99.

57. Tudor-Locke C, Neff LJ, Ainsworth BE, Addy CL, Popkin BM. Omission of active commuting to school and the prevalence of children's health-related physical activity levels: the Russian Longitudinal Monitoring Study. Child Care Health Dev. 2002;28(6):507–12.

58. Tudor-Locke C, Ainsworth BE, Popkin BM. Active commuting to school: an overlooked source of childrens' physical activity? Sports Med. 2001;31(5):309–13.

59. Stevens J, Story M, Ring K, et al. The impact of the Pathways intervention on psychosocial variables related to diet and physical activity in American Indian schoolchildren. Prev Med. 2003;37(6 Pt 2):S70–9.

60. Caballero B, Clay T, Davis SM, et al. Pathways: a school-based, randomized controlled trial for the prevention of obesity in American Indian schoolchildren. Am J Clin Nutr. 2003;78(5):1030–8.

61. Stevens J, Murray DM, Baggett CD, et al. Objectively assessed associations between physical activity and body composition in middle-school girls: the Trial of Activity for Adolescent Girls. Am J Epidemiol. 2007;166(11):1298–305.

62. Webber LS, Catellier DJ, Lytle LA, et al. Promoting physical activity in middle school girls: Trial of Activity for Adolescent Girls. Am J Prev Med. 2008;34(3):173–84.

63. Young DR, Steckler A, Cohen S, et al. Process evaluation results from a school- and community-linked intervention: the Trial of Activity for Adolescent Girls (TAAG). Health Educ Res. 2008;23(6):976–86.

64. Food and Nutrition Board. Preventing childhood obesity: health in the balance. Washington, DC: National Academy Press; 2004.

65. Popkin BM. Technology, transport, globalization and the nutrition transition. Food Policy. 2006;31:554–69.

66. Trager J. The food chronology: a food lover's compendium of events and anecdotes, from prehistory to the present. New York, NY: Owl Books; 1997.

67. Reardon T, Berdegué J. The rapid rise of supermarkets in Latin America: challenges and opportunities for development. Dev Policy Rev. 2002;20:371–88.

68. Reardon T, Timmer P, Berdegue J. The rapid rise of supermarkets in developing countries: induced organizational, institutional, and technological change in agrifood systems. Electron J Agric Dev Econ. 2004;1(2):168–83.

69. Reardon T, Timmer CP, Barrett CB, Berdegue JA. The rise of supermarkets in Africa, Asia, and Latin America. Am J Agric Econ. 2003;85:1140–6.

70. Hu D, Reardon T, Rozelle S, Timmer P, Wang H. The emergence of supermarkets with Chinese characteristics: challenges and opportunities for China's agricultural development. Dev Policy Rev. 2004;22:557–86.

71. Wax E. In India, a retail revolution takes hold: small vendors feel squeeze of chaines. Washington Post. 23 May 2007;Financial:D.1.

II | THE NEUROENDOCRINE PERSPECTIVE: THE CONTROL OF APPETITE AND ENERGY EXPENDITURE

2 The Neuroendocrine Control of Energy Balance

Robert H. Lustig

CONTENTS

Key Words: Leptin, hypothalamus, vagus, reward, stress, ghrelin, insulin, endocannabinoids, sympathetic nervous system, amygdala

INTRODUCTION

When discussing the causes of obesity, it is easy to point fingers at the individual. "Gluttony" and "sloth" after all are two of the seven "deadly sins." Obese adults and their children are assumed to have "free choice" with regard to food intake and energy expenditure and are therefore "responsible" for their metabolic "fates" *(1)*. But no child chooses to become obese; indeed the quality of life of an obese child is similar to that of children receiving cancer chemotherapy *(2)*. Furthermore, the striking increases in obesity prevalence in 2- to 5-year-old children *(3)* suggest that there are other explanations for the obesity epidemic. Here I explore the biochemical determinants that control energy balance and argue that difficulties in achieving and/or maintaining weight loss reflect the potency of central reinforcement systems, the effects of stress, and the resilience of the body's adaptive responses.

The discovery of leptin in 1994 *(4)* revealed a complex neuroendocrine axis regulating energy balance. Much of what we know about energy balance is derived from studies of animal models, but clinical studies provide invaluable insights.

From: *Contemporary Endocrinology: Pediatric Obesity: Etiology, Pathogenesis, and Treatment*
Edited by: M. Freemark, DOI 10.1007/978-1-60327-874-4_2,
© Springer Science+Business Media, LLC 2010

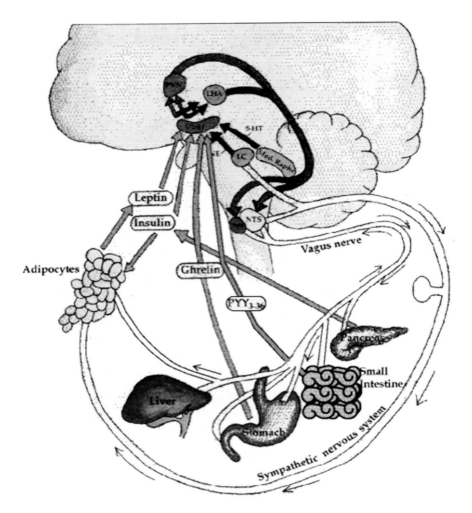

Fig. 1. The homeostatic pathway of energy balance. Afferent (*blue*), central (*black*), and efferent (*white*) pathways
are delineated. The hormones insulin, leptin, ghrelin, and peptide $YY_{(3-36)}$ (PYY_{3-36}) provide afferent information
to the ventromedial hypothalamus regarding short-term energy metabolism and energy sufficiency. From there, the
ventromedial hypothalamus elicits anorexigenic (α-melanocyte-stimulating hormone, cocaine–amphetamine-regulated
transcript) and orexigenic (neuropeptide Y, agouti-related protein) signals to the melanocortin-4 receptor in the paraventricular nucleus and lateral hypothalamic area. These lead to efferent output via the locus coeruleus and the nucleus
tractus solitarius, which activate the sympathetic nervous system, causing the adipocyte to undergo lipolysis; or the
dorsal motor nucleus of the vagus, which activates the vagus nerve to store energy, both by increasing pancreatic insulin
secretion and (in rodents) by increasing adipose tissue sensitivity to insulin. 5-HT, serotonin (5-hydroxytryptamine);
DMV, dorsal motor nucleus of the vagus; LC, locus coeruleus; LHA, lateral hypothalamic area; NE, norepinephrine;
NTS, nucleus tractus solitarius; PVN, paraventricular nucleus; VMH, ventromedial hypothalamus. From Lustig *(21)*.
(Courtesy of Nature Publishing Group, with permission.)

The neuroendocrine axis is composed of three arms (Fig. 1). The first is the *afferent arm*, which
conveys peripheral information on hunger and peripheral metabolism (in the form of hormonal and
neural inputs) to the hypothalamus. The second is a *central processing unit*, consisting of various areas
within the hypothalamus. These include (a) the ventromedial hypothalamus (VMH; consisting of the
ventromedial (VMN) and arcuate (ARC) nuclei), which integrates afferent peripheral signals as well as
other central stimuli, and (b) the paraventricular nuclei (PVN) and lateral hypothalamic area (LHA),

which serve as a gated neurotransmitter system to alter neural signals for changes in feeding and energy expenditure. Other brain areas serve as neuromodulators of this system. The third component is an *efferent arm* of autonomic effectors with origins in the locus coeruleus (LC) and dorsal motor nucleus of the vagus (DMV), which regulate energy intake, expenditure, and storage *(5,6)*. Anatomic disruptions or genetic or metabolic alterations of either the afferent, central processing, or efferent arms can alter energy intake or expenditure, leading to either obesity or cachexia.

There are three primary stimuli to eat: *hunger, reward,* and *stress.* While each of these internal phenomena infer altered behavior, each is actually mediated through a complex cascade of biochemicals that perturb the negative feedback pathway of energy balance and "drive" food intake in stereotypical patterns.

COMPONENTS OF THE AFFERENT SYSTEM

Alimentary Afferents That Promote Hunger

The afferent vagus: The vagus nerve is the primary neural connection between the brain and the gut. The afferent vagus nerve conveys information regarding mechanical stretch of the stomach and duodenum and feelings of gastric fullness to the nucleus tractus solitarius (NTS) *(7)*. Of note, the effects of alimentary neuropeptides (below) on hunger and satiety are obviated by concomitant vagotomy, implicating the afferent vagus as the primary mediator of alimentary energy balance signals *(8–10)*.

Ghrelin: Ghrelin, an octanoylated 28-amino acid peptide, was discovered serendipitously during a search for the endogenous ligand of the growth hormone secretagogue receptor (GHS-R) *(11)*. Ghrelin induces GH release through stimulation of the pituitary GHS-R. The endogenous secretion of ghrelin from the stomach is high during fasting and decreased by nutrient administration; volumetric stretching of the stomach wall has no effect. In addition to interacting with pituitary GHS receptors, ghrelin binds to the GHS-R in the VMH and thereby increases hunger, food intake, and fat deposition *(12,13)*. Ghrelin also increases the respiratory quotient (RQ) in rats, suggesting a reduction of fat oxidation. Ghrelin appears to link the lipolytic effect of GH with hunger signals and is probably important in the acute response to fasting. In humans, ghrelin levels rise with increasing subjective hunger and peak at the time of voluntary food consumption *(14)*, suggesting that ghrelin acts on the VMH to trigger meal initiation. Ghrelin infusion increases food intake in humans *(15)*. However, plasma ghrelin levels are low in most obese individuals and increase with fasting *(16)*, suggesting that ghrelin is a response to, rather than a cause of, obesity. The Prader–Willi syndrome, an obesity disorder associated with hyperghrelinemia, may be a unique exception (see Chapter 4 by Haqq, this volume).

Alimentary Afferents That Promote Satiety

Peptide YY$_{3-36}$ (PYY$_{3-36}$): PYY$_{3-36}$ is a gastrointestinal signal to control meal volume *(17)*. This peptide fragment is secreted by intestinal L-cells following exposure to nutrients; PYY crosses the blood–brain barrier and binds to the Y$_2$ receptor in the VMH. Activation of this receptor reduces neuropeptide Y (NPY) mRNA in neurons of the orexigenic arm of the central processing unit (below). In non-obese humans, infusion of PYY$_{3-36}$ during a 12-h period decreased the total volume of food ingested from 2,200 to 1,500 k/cal but had no effect on food ingested during the next 12-h interval *(17)*. Although the pharmacology of this peptide is being elucidated, and agonists are being developed, its specific role in obesity is not yet known.

Glucagon-like peptide-1 (GLP-1): Those same intestinal L-cells produce GLP-1 through posttranslational processing of the preproglucagon molecule. Two equipotent forms of GLP-1 are generated: a glycine-extended form GLP-1$_{7-37}$ and the amidated peptide GLP-1$_{7-36}$ amide *(18)*. GLP-1 acts on the stomach to inhibit gastric emptying; this increases the time available for absorption of a meal. GLP-1 also activates its receptor on β-cells to stimulate cAMP production, protein

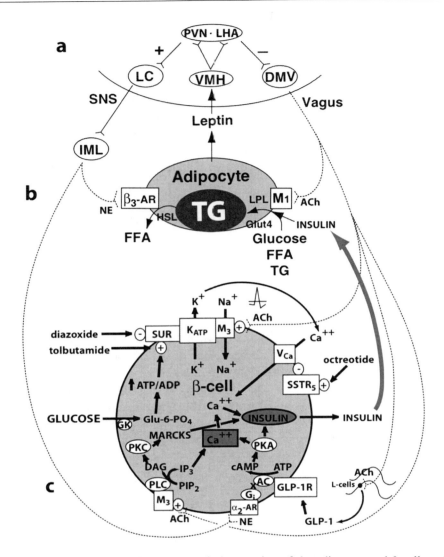

Fig. 2. Central regulation of leptin signaling, autonomic innervation of the adipocyte and β-cell, and the starvation response. (**a**) The arcuate nucleus transduces the peripheral leptin signal as one of sufficiency or deficiency. In leptin sufficiency, efferents from the hypothalamus synapse in the locus coeruleus, which stimulates the sympathetic nervous system. In leptin deficiency or resistance, efferents from the hypothalamus stimulate the dorsal motor nucleus of the vagus. (**b**) Autonomic innervation and hormonal stimulation of white adipose tissue. In leptin sufficiency, norepinephrine binds to the β₃-adrenergic receptor, which stimulates hormone-sensitive lipase, promoting lipolysis of stored triglyceride into free fatty acids. In leptin deficiency or resistance, vagal acetylcholine increases adipose tissue insulin sensitivity (documented only in rats to date), promotes uptake of glucose and free fatty acids for lipogenesis, and promotes triglyceride uptake through activation of lipoprotein lipase. (**c**) Autonomic innervation and hormonal stimulation of the β-cell. Glucose entering the cell is converted to glucose-6-phosphate by the enzyme glucokinase, generating ATP, which closes an ATP-dependent potassium channel, resulting in cell depolarization. A voltage-gated calcium channel opens, allowing for intracellular calcium influx, which activates neurosecretory mechanisms leading to insulin vesicular exocytosis. In leptin sufficiency, norepinephrine binds to α₂-adrenoceptors on the β-cell membrane to stimulate inhibitory G proteins, decrease adenyl cyclase and its product cAMP, and thereby reduce protein kinase A levels and insulin release. In leptin deficiency or resistance, the vagus stimulates insulin secretion *(105)*. Octreotide binds to a somatostatin receptor on the β-cell, which is coupled to the voltage-gated calcium channel, limiting calcium influx and the amount of insulin released in response to glucose (reprinted with kind permission of Springer Science and Business media). α₂-AR, α₂-adrenergic receptor; β₃-AR, β₃-adrenergic receptor; AC, adenyl cyclase;

kinase A activation, and insulin secretion (Fig. 2) and thereby improves glucose tolerance in patients with type 2 diabetes. GLP-1 also stimulates β-cell replication and increases β-cell mass (19). Lastly, GLP-1 reduces food intake by reducing gastric emptying and corticotropin-releasing hormone (CRH) signaling in the PVN and increasing leptin signaling in the VMH (20).

Cholecystokinin (CCK): CCK is an 8-amino acid gut peptide released in response to a caloric load. It circulates and binds to CCK_A receptors in the pylorus, vagus nerve, NTS, and area postrema (7) to promote satiety.

Metabolic Afferents Controlling Energy Balance

Leptin: The balance of energy intake and expenditure is normally regulated very tightly (within 0.15% per year) by the hormone leptin. Leptin is a 167-amino acid hormone produced by white adipocytes. Leptin's primary neuroendocrine role is to mediate information about the size of peripheral adipocyte energy stores to the VMH (4,21). As such, it is a prerequisite signal to the VMH for the initiation of high-energy processes such as puberty and pregnancy (22,23). Leptin reduces food intake and increases the activity of the sympathetic nervous system (SNS) (24). Conversely, low leptin levels infer diminished energy stores, which impact on the VMH to increase food intake and reduce energy expenditure. Serum leptin concentrations drop precipitously (and to a greater degree than fat mass) during short-term fasting (25,26), and it seems likely that leptin functions more as a peripheral signal to the hypothalamus of inadequate caloric intake than as a hunger or satiety signal per se (27).

In the fed state, circulating levels of leptin correlate with percent body fat (28,29). Leptin production by adipocytes is stimulated by insulin and glucocorticoids (30,31) and inhibited by β-adrenergic stimulation (27). Programming of relative leptin concentrations by early caloric intake may be one mechanism that links early overnutrition with later obesity (32).

Leptin binds to its receptor (a member of the Class 1 cytokine receptor superfamily) on target VMH neurons. There are four receptor isoforms formed by differential splicing: ObRa, an isoform with a shortened intracellular domain, which may function as a transporter; ObRb, the intact full-length receptor; ObRc, also with a short intracellular domain; and ObRe, which lacks an intracellular domain and functions as a soluble receptor (33).

As leptin binds to its VMH receptor, three neuronal signals are transduced. The first is opening of an ATP-sensitive potassium channel, which hyperpolarizes the neuron and decreases its firing rate (34). The second is the activation of a cytoplasmic Janus kinase 2 (JAK2), which phosphorylates a tyrosine moiety on proteins of a family called signal transduction and transcription (STAT-3) (35). The phosphorylated STAT-3 translocates to the nucleus, where it promotes leptin-dependent gene transcription (36). Third, leptin activates the insulin receptor substrate 2/phosphatidylinositol-3-kinase (IRS2/PI3K) second messenger system in ARC neurons, which increases neurotransmission of the central anorexigenic signaling pathway (37).

Fig. 2. (continued) ACh, acetylcholine; DAG, diacylglycerol; DMV, dorsal motor nucleus of the vagus; FFA, free fatty acids; G_i, inhibitory G protein; GK, glucokinase; GLP-1, glucagon-like peptide-1; GLP-1R, GLP-1 receptor; Glu-6-PO_4, glucose-6-phosphate; Glut4, glucose transporter-4; HSL, hormone-sensitive lipase; IML, intermediolateral cell column; IP_3, inositol triphosphate; LC, locus coeruleus; LHA, lateral hypothalamic area; LPL, lipoprotein lipase; MARCKS, myristoylated alanine-rich protein kinase C substrate; NE, norepinephrine; PIP_2, phosphatidylinositol pyrophosphate; PKA, protein kinase A; PKC, protein kinase C; PLC, phospholipase C; PVN, paraventricular nucleus; $SSTR_5$, somatostatin-5 receptor; TG, triglyceride; V_{Ca}, voltage-gated calcium channel; VMH, ventromedial hypothalamus; SUR, sufonylurea receptor. From Lustig (21). (Courtesy of Nature Publishing Group, with permission.)

Insulin: Insulin plays a critical role in energy balance *(38)*. In peripheral tissues it promotes glycogenesis, muscle protein synthesis, and fat storage and regulates the production and action of neuroendocrine modulators of nutrient uptake and metabolism. But insulin is also transported across the blood–brain barrier and binds to receptors in a subpopulation of VMH neurons *(39,40)*, suggesting that it acts centrally to regulate food intake. Indeed in animals, acute and chronic intracerebroventricular insulin infusions decrease feeding behavior and induce satiety *(41–43)*. The data on acute and chronic peripheral insulin infusions are less clear. Studies of overinsulinized diabetic rats demonstrate increased caloric intake (in order to prevent subacute hypoglycemia) and the development of peripheral insulin resistance *(44,45)*. Chronic peripheral insulin infusions in experimental animals decrease hepatic and skeletal muscle glucose uptake by reducing Glut4 expression but do not alter adipose tissue glucose uptake *(46,47)*. One human study injecting short-term insulin peripherally during meals did not demonstrate an effect on satiety *(48)*. Insulin acutely activates the insulin receptor substrate 2/phosphatidylinositol-3-kinase (IRS2/PI3K) second messenger system in arcuate nucleus (ARC) neurons *(49)*, which increases neurotransmission of the central anorexigenic signaling pathway (see below). The importance of CNS insulin action was underscored by the phenotype of a brain (neuron)-specific insulin receptor knockout (NIRKO) mouse, which cannot transduce a CNS insulin signal *(50)*. NIRKO mice become hyperphagic, obese, and infertile with age and have high peripheral insulin levels. These findings suggest that peripheral insulin mediates a satiety signal in the VMH to help control energy balance *(51)*. Various knockouts of the insulin signal transduction pathway that reduce insulin signaling lead to an obese phenotype *(52,53)*, while those that increase insulin signaling lead to a lean phenotype *(54,55)*.

CENTRAL PROCESSING

Peripheral afferent (neural and hormonal) signals reaching VMH neurons are integrated by a gated neural circuit designed to control both energy intake and expenditure (Fig. 2). This circuit consists of two arms: the anorexigenic arm, which contains neurons expressing the co-localized peptides proopiomelanocortin (POMC) and cocaine/amphetamine-regulated transcript (CART), and the orexigenic arm, which contains neurons with the co-localized peptides neuropeptide Y (NPY) and agouti-related protein (AgRP). Ghrelin receptor immunoreactivity co-localizes with NPY and AgRP neurons, while insulin and leptin receptors are located on both POMC/CART and NPY/AgRP neurons in the VMH *(56)*, suggesting divergent regulation of each arm. These two arms compete for occupancy of melanocortin receptors (MCRs; either MC_3R or MC_4R) in the PVN and LHA.

Anorexigenesis, POMC/α-MSH, and CART

POMC is differentially cleaved in different tissues and neurons. The ligand α-melanocyte-stimulating hormone (α-MSH) is the primary product involved in anorexigenesis. Both overfeeding and peripheral leptin infusion induce the synthesis of POMC and α-MSH within the ARC *(57)*. α-MSH induces anorexia by binding to melanocortin receptors within the PVN or LHA. CART is a hypothalamic neuropeptide induced by leptin and reduced by fasting. Intrahypothalamic infusion blocks appetite, while antagonism of endogenous CART increases caloric intake *(58)*.

Orexigenesis, NPY, and AgRP

NPY and AgRP co-localize to a different set of neurons within the ARC, immediately adjacent to those expressing POMC/CART *(59)*. NPY has numerous functions within the hypothalamus, including initiation of feeding, puberty, and regulation of gonadotropin secretion and adrenal responsiveness *(60,61)*. NPY is the primary orexigenic peptide. ICV infusion of NPY in rats causes hyperphagia, energy storage, and obesity *(62,63)*. These actions are mediated through Y_1 and Y_5 receptors. Fasting and weight loss increase NPY expression in the ARC, accounting for increased hunger, while PYY_{3-36} (through Y_2 receptors) and leptin decrease NPY mRNA *(17,64)*.

AgRP is the human homolog of the protein agouti, which is present in abundance in the yellow $(A^y$-a) mouse *(65)*. This protein is an endogenous competitive antagonist of all melanocortin receptors (MCR), accounting for the yellow color in these mice. In the presence of large amounts of AgRP at the synaptic cleft in the PVN, α-MSH cannot bind to the MC_4R to induce satiety *(66)*.

Other Neuroendocrine Modulators of Energy Balance

Norepinephrine (NE): NE neurons in the locus coeruleus synapse on VMH neurons to regulate food intake *(67)*. The actions of NE on food intake seem paradoxical, as intrahypothalamic NE infusions stimulate food intake through effects on central α_2- and β-adrenergic receptors *(68)*, whereas central infusion of α_1-agonists markedly reduces food intake *(69)*.

Serotonin (5-HT): Five lines of evidence impicate a role for 5-HT in the perception of satiety: (1) Injection of 5-HT into the hypothalamus increases satiety, particularly with respect to carbohydrate *(70)*; (2) central administration of 5-HT_{2c} receptor agonists increases satiety, while antagonists induce feeding *(71)*; (3) administration of selective 5-HT reuptake inhibitors induces early satiety *(72)*; (4) leptin increases 5-HT turnover *(73)*; and (5) the 5-HT_{2c}R-KO mouse exhibits increased food intake and body weight *(74)*. The role of 5-HT in the transduction of the satiety signal may have both central and peripheral components, as intestinal 5-HT secreted into the bloodstream during a meal may impact GI neuronal function and muscle tone while binding to 5-HT receptors in the NTS (see earlier) to promote satiety *(75)*.

Melanin-concentrating hormone (MCH): MCH is a 17-amino acid peptide expressed in the zona incerta and LHA. MCH neurons synapse on neurons in the forebrain and the locus coeruleus. MCH appears to be important in behavioral responses to food such as anxiety and aggression *(76)*. Expression of the peptide is upregulated in *ob/ob* mice. MCH knockout mice are hypophagic and lean *(77)*, while transgenic MCH-overexpressing mice develop obesity and insulin resistance *(78)*. ICV administration of MCH stimulates food intake, similar to that seen with NPY administration *(79)*.

Orexins A and B: These 33- and 28-amino acid peptides, respectively, have been implicated in both energy balance and autonomic function in mice *(80)*. Orexin knockout mice develop narcolepsy, hypophagia, and obesity *(81)*, suggesting that orexins bridge the gap between the afferent and efferent energy balance systems *(82)*. Orexins in the LHA stimulate neuropeptide Y (NPY) release, which may account for their induction of food intake; they also increase corticotropin-releasing factor (CRF) and sympathetic nervous system (SNS) output to promote wakefulness, energy expenditure, learning and memory, and the hedonic reward system (see later) *(83)*. Conversely, orexin neurons in the perifornical and dorsomedial hypothalamus regulate arousal and the response to stress.

Endocannabinoids (ECs): It has long been known that marijuana and its major constituent tetrahydrocannabinol stimulate food intake. Recently, endogenous ECs and the CB_1 receptor have been linked to energy balance and the metabolic syndrome *(84)*. The CB_1 receptor is expressed in corticotropin-releasing factor (CRH) neurons in the PVN, in CART neurons in the VMN, and in MCH- and orexin-positive neurons in the LHA and perifornical region. Fasting and feeding are associated with high and low levels of ECs in the hypothalamus, respectively. CB_1 receptor knockout mice have increased CRH and reduced CART expression. Hypothalamic EC levels are increased in leptin-deficient *ob/ob* mice; intravenous leptin reduces EC levels, indicating that a direct negative control is exerted by leptin on the EC system. Glucocorticoids increase food intake in part by stimulating EC synthesis and secretion, while leptin blocks this effect *(85)*. Finally, the presence of CB_1 receptors on afferent vagal neurons suggests that endocannabinoids may be involved in mediating satiety signals originating in the gut.

Melanocortin Receptors (MCR) and Central Neural Integration

The human MC_4R localizes to chromosome 2 and is a 7-transmembrane G-coupled receptor, encoded by an intronless 1 kB gene. The binding of hypothalamic α-MSH to the MC_4R in the PVN and LHA results in a state of satiety, whereas ICV administration of MC_4R antagonists stimulates feeding. These observations suggest that the MC_4R transduces satiety information on caloric sufficiency. The role of the MC_4R in human obesity is well known; in some studies, 2.5–5% of morbidly obese adults had heterozygous mutations in the MC_4R (86). In the MC_3R knockout mouse, a different phenotype is seen. These animals are obese but hypophagic and have increased body fat relative to lean body mass. They gain weight on either low- or high-fat chow and do not change caloric oxidation in response to changes in dietary fat content. These findings suggest a defect in energy expenditure (87). The role of the MC_3R in human obesity is less clear. Functional variants of the MC_3R have been noted in certain populations (88,89). One hypothesis is that the MC_4R modulates energy intake, while the MC_3R modulates energy expenditure (90).

THE EFFERENT SYSTEM

The MCRs in the PVN and LHA transduce signals emanating from the VMH in order to modulate activity of the sympathetic nervous system (SNS), which promotes energy expenditure, and the efferent vagus, which promotes energy storage (Fig. 2).

The Sympathetic Nervous System (SNS) and Energy Expenditure

Anorexigenic pressure increases energy expenditure through activation of the SNS (91). For instance, leptin administration to *ob/ob* mice increases brown adipose tissue thermogenesis, renovascular activity, and spontaneous motor activity; all are associated with increased energy expenditure and facilitate weight loss (92). Similarly, insulin administration acutely increases SNS activity in normal rats and in humans (93,94).

The SNS increases energy expenditure by activating lipolysis in white and brown adipose tissue and promoting energy utilization in skeletal and cardiac muscle. Binding of catecholamines to muscle $β_2$-adrenergic receptors (95) stimulates glycogenolysis, myocardial energy expenditure, and increases in glucose and fatty acid oxidation and increases protein synthesis (96,97). Binding to $β_3$-adrenergic receptors in white and brown adipose tissue increases cAMP, which activates protein kinase A (PKA) (98). In white adipose PKA activates hormone-sensitive lipase, which generates ATP from hydrolysis of triglyceride. In brown fat PKA phosphorylates CREB, which induces expression of PGC-1α. PGC-1α in turn binds to the uncoupling protein-1 (UCP-1) promoter and increases its expression (99,100).

UCP1 is an inner membrane mitochondrial protein that uncouples proton entry from ATP synthesis (101); therefore, UCP1 expression dissipates energy as heat and thereby reduces the energy efficiency of brown fat. UCP1 is induced by FFAs derived from triglyceride breakdown; FFAs released from adipocytes are transported to the liver, where they are utilized for energy through ketogenesis. Lipolysis reduces leptin expression; thus a negative feedback loop is achieved between leptin and the SNS (Fig. 2).

The Efferent Vagus and Energy Storage

In response to declining levels of leptin and/or persistent orexigenic pressure, the LHA and PVN send efferent projections residing in the medial longitudinal fasciculus to the dorsal motor nucleus of the vagus nerve (DMV), activating the efferent vagus *(102)*. The efferent vagus opposes the SNS by promoting energy storage in four ways: (a) it reduces myocardial oxygen consumption by reducing heart rate; (b) it increases nutrient absorption by promoting GI peristalsis and pyloric opening; (c) it increases insulin sensitivity by potentiating the uptake of glucose and FFA into adipose tissue; and (d) it increases postprandial insulin secretion, which increases fat deposition *(103–106)*.

Retrograde tracing of white adipose tissue reveals a wealth of efferents originating at the DMV *(106)*. These efferents synapse on M_1 muscarinic receptors, which increase insulin sensitivity. Denervation of white adipose tissue reduces glucose and FFA uptake and increases HSL expression. Thus, vagal modulation of the adipocyte augments storage of both glucose and FFAs by improving adipose insulin sensitivity and reducing triglyceride breakdown *(107)* (Fig. 2).

The DMV also sends efferent projections to the β-cells of the pancreas *(108)*. This pathway is responsible for the "cephalic" or preabsorptive phase of insulin secretion, which is glucose independent and can be blocked by atropine *(109)*. Overactive vagal neurotransmission increases insulin secretion from β-cells in response to an oral glucose load through three distinct but overlapping mechanisms (Fig. 2; see the Chapter 26 on Hypothalamic Obesity for full discussion): (1) the muscarinic activation of a sodium channel, resulting in increased β-cell depolarization; (2) the muscarinic activation of β-cell phospholipases which hydrolyze intracellular phosphatidylinositol to diacylglycerol (DAG) and inositol triphosphate (IP_3), inducing insulin vesicular exocytosis; and (3) the stimulation of GLP-1 from intestinal L-cells, which activates protein kinase A and increases insulin exocytosis. Vagal induction of insulin secretion promotes lipogenesis through increased expression of Glut 4, acetyl-CoA carboxylase, fatty acid synthase, and lipoprotein lipase *(110,111)*.

THE HEDONIC PATHWAY OF FOOD REWARD

Hypothalamic feedback systems are modulated by a "hedonic pathway" that mediates the pleasurable and motivational responses to food. The hedonic pathway comprises the ventral tegmental area (VTA) and the nucleus accumbens (NA), with inputs from various components of the limbic system including the striatum, amygdala, hypothalamus, and hippocampus. Food intake is a readout of the hedonic pathway; administration of morphine to the NA increases food intake in a dose-dependent fashion *(112)*. Functional suppression of the hedonic pathway curtails food intake when energy stores are replete; dysfunction or continuous activation of the hedonic pathway can increase food intake and promote excessive weight gain.

The VTA appears to mediate feeding on the basis of palatability rather than energy need. The dopaminergic projection from the VTA to the NA mediates the motivating, rewarding, and reinforcing properties of various stimuli, such as food and addictive drugs. Leptin and insulin receptors are expressed in the VTA, and both hormones have been implicated in modulating rewarding responses to food and other pleasurable stimuli *(113)*. For instance, fasting and food restriction (when insulin and leptin levels are low) increase the addictive properties of drugs of abuse, while central leptin administration can reverse these effects *(114)*. Food deprivation in rodents increases addictive behavior and the pleasurable responses to a food reward, as measured by dopamine release and dopamine receptor signaling *(115)*. Conversely, insulin increases expression and activity of the dopamine transporter, which clears and removes dopamine from the synapse; thus acute insulin exposure blunts the reward of food *(116)*. Furthermore, insulin appears to inhibit the ability of VTA agonists (e.g., opioids) to increase intake of sucrose *(117)*. Finally, insulin blocks the ability of rats to form a conditioned place preference association to a palatable food *(118)*.

The role of the hedonic pathway in human obesity is not yet elucidated, but can be surmised. Dopamine D_2 receptor abundance is inversely related to BMI; the depression of dopaminergic activity in obese subjects might trigger a "reward-seeking" increase in food intake that promotes further weight gain. This may explain in part the higher risk of obesity in patients taking drugs that block D_2 receptors (e.g., antipsychotics *(119)*). Alternatively, the down-regulation of dopaminergic activity in obese subjects may be an adaptive response to prior weight gain. Under normal circumstances, leptin and insulin signal adipose and nutrient sufficiency to the VTA, suppressing dopamine neurotransmission and the reward of food *(113)*. However, these negative feedback loops are blocked in states of insulin and leptin resistance that characterize obesity *(120)*.

Positron emission tomography suggests that hunger and satiety neuronal circuits in the VMH connect with other regions of the limbic system *(121)* that control primal emotions, reproductive activity, and survival instinct; a primal "reward" or pleasure response might explain ingestive behavior in the absence of hunger, a common finding in obese children and adults. It has been argued that much of the impasse in efforts to both treat and prevent obesity stems from the intrinsic difficulty of overriding instinct with reason *(122)*.

THE AMYGDALA AND THE STRESS PATHWAY OF FOOD INTAKE

The VMH and VTA-NA mediate satiety when energy stores are replete, but appear to be overridden by amygdala activation and the concomitant stress response associated with insulin resistance *(123)*. Stress hormones such as the glucocorticoids are essential for the full expression of obesity in rodents and humans and may explain the disruptive role that stress plays in weight regulation *(124)*.

Stress and glucocorticoids are integral in promoting the constellation of features characteristic of the metabolic syndrome. Studies of adrenalectomized (ADX) rats supplemented with corticosterone demonstrate that exogenous fat intake is directly proportional to circulating corticosterone concentrations *(125,126)*. In intact rats, corticosterone stimulates intake of high-fat food; likewise, cortisol administration increases food intake in humans *(127)*. Human research shows increased caloric intake of "comfort foods" (i.e., those with high energy density) after acute stress *(128)*. Moreover, several studies in children have observed relationships between stress and unhealthy dietary practices, including increased snacking and an elevated risk of weight gain during adolescence and adulthood *(129,130)*.

NPY and catecholamines co-localize in sympathetic neurons in the peripheral nervous system as well as the central nervous system. In response to chronic stress, peripheral neurons express more NPY, which stimulates endothelial cell (angiogenesis) and preadipocyte proliferation, differentiation, and adipogenesis by activating Y2 receptors in visceral adipose tissue. This causes abdominal obesity, inflammation, hyperlipidemia, hyperinsulinemia, glucose intolerance, hepatic steatosis, and hypertension, reproducing the features of the human metabolic syndrome. Conversely, local intra-fat Y2R antagonists or adenoviral Y2R knock-down reverses or prevents fat accumulation and metabolic complications *(131)*. This suggests that acute stress causes lipolysis and weight loss, but chronic stress "hijacks" the SNS, increasing NPY expression to cause visceral fat accumulation and metabolic dysfunction.

NEGATIVE FEEDBACK OF ENERGY BALANCE – THE RESPONSE TO CALORIC DEPRIVATION

The response to caloric deprivation serves as a model for understanding the regulation of energy balance and the adaptation to weight loss. Everyone appears to have a "personal leptin threshold," probably genetically determined, above which the brain interprets a state of energy sufficiency *(132)*. The leptin-replete fed state is characterized by increased physical activity, decreased appetite, and feelings of well-being. In response to caloric restriction, leptin levels decline even before weight loss is manifest *(25,26)*. This is interpreted by the VMH as starvation. Gastric secretion of ghrelin increases; this stimulates pituitary GH release, which promotes lipolysis to provide energy substrate for catabolism. Ghrelin also stimulates the expression of NPY/AgRP, which antagonizes α-MSH/CART and reduces MC_4R occupancy. The resultant lack of anorexigenic pressure on the MC_4R increases feeding behavior, reduces fat oxidation, and promotes fat deposition. Fat storage is facilitated by increases in insulin sensitivity.

Total and resting energy expenditure decline in an attempt to conserve energy *(133)*; the fall in leptin reduces plasma T3 levels, and UCP1 levels in adipose tissue decline *(134)* as a result of decreased SNS activity *(135)*. Yet, in spite of decreased SNS tone at the adipocyte, there is an obligate lipolysis due to insulin suppression and upregulation of hormone-sensitive lipase. Lipolysis is necessary to maintain energy delivery to the musculature and brain in the form of liver-derived ketone bodies.

Under conditions of fasting or caloric deprivation, vagal tone is increased. Together with the fall in T3 levels, this slows the heart rate and reduces myocardial oxygen consumption. Heightened vagal tone also increases β-cell insulin secretion and adipose insulin sensitivity; in sum, these effects promote increased energy fat storage *(135)*. The effects of fasting revert once caloric sufficiency is re-established and leptin levels rise.

Thus the adaptive/compensatory response to fasting or caloric deprivation is designed to re-establish homeostasis and recover lost weight by inducing food intake and reducing energy expenditure; this explains the great difficulty that most obese people have in achieving or maintaining long-term weight loss.

LEPTIN RESISTANCE

Most obese children have high leptin levels but do not have receptor mutations, manifesting what is commonly referred to as "leptin resistance." Leptin resistance prevents exogenous leptin administration from promoting weight loss *(136)*. The response to most weight loss regimens plateaus rapidly due to the rapid fall of peripheral leptin levels below a personal "leptin threshold" *(137)*, which is likely genetically determined. Leptin decline causes the VMH to sense a reduction in peripheral energy stores. This fosters a decrease in REE to conserve energy, analogous to the starvation response described earlier *(133)* but occurring at elevated leptin levels.

The cause of leptin resistance in obesity is likely multifactorial. First, leptin crosses the blood–brain barrier via a saturable transporter, which limits the amount of leptin reaching its receptor in the VMH *(138,139)*. Second, activation of the leptin receptor induces intraneuronal expression of suppressor of cytokine signaling-3 (SOCS-3), which limits leptin signal transduction *(54)*. Finally, hypertriglyceridemia limits access of peripheral leptin to the VMH *(140)* and interferes with leptin signal transduction upstream of STAT-3, its primary second messenger *(141)*. Thus, factors that induce hypertriglyceridemia, such as dietary fructose and insulin resistance, tend to promote leptin resistance *(21)*.

Two clinical paradigms have been shown to improve leptin sensitivity. After weight loss through caloric restriction, exogenous administration of leptin can then increase REE back to baseline and permit further weight loss *(142,143)*. This suggests that weight loss itself improves leptin sensitivity. Second, suppression of insulin correlates with improvement in leptin sensitivity and promotes weight loss *(144)*, suggesting that hyperinsulinemia promotes leptin resistance by interfering with leptin signal transduction in the VMH and VTA *(145)*. Indeed, insulin reduction strategies may be effective in promoting weight loss in obese children by improving leptin sensitivity *(146)*. This has led to the hypothesis that chronic hyperinsulinemia functions to block leptin signal transduction at the VMH and VTA, which turns a negative feedback cycle into a vicious feedforward cycle (Fig. 3) *(147)*. However, this hypothesis remains to be proven.

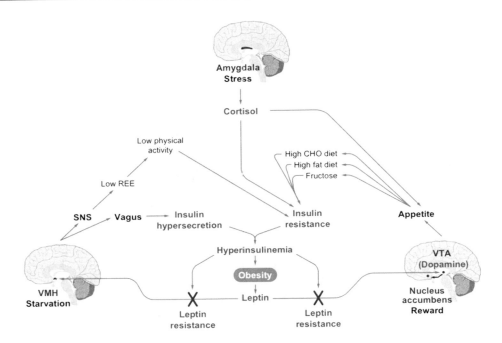

Fig. 3. The "limbic triangle." Three areas of the CNS conspire to drive food intake and reduce physical activity, resulting in persistent weight gain. The ventromedial hypothalamus (VMH) transduces the leptin signal from adipocytes to reduce energy intake and increase energy expenditure; however, hyperinsulinemia inhibits leptin signaling, promoting the "starvation response." The ventral tegmental area (VTA) transduces the leptin signal to reduce dopamine neurotransmission to the nucleus accumbens (NA) to reduce palatable food intake; however, insulin resistance and leptin resistance increase dopamine neurotransmission and promote the "reward" of food. The amygdala transduces fear and stress, resulting in increased cortisol, which also drives energy-rich food intake and promotes insulin resistance, further interfering with leptin signaling at the other two CNS sites. Thus, interference with any of the negative feedback aspects of the "limbic triangle" transforms it into a positive feedback loop, promoting continued weight gain and obesity. From Mietus-Snyder and Lustig (147). (Courtesy of Annual Reviews, with permission.)

SUMMARY

It is clear that childhood obesity is not just the outcome of "gluttony" and "sloth." Rather, genetic and environmental factors alter the neurohormonal milieu, driving the propensity for both increased energy storage and decreased energy expenditure. When this feedback pathway is perturbed, it becomes a feedforward pathway, with resultant weight gain and worsening leptin resistance. The biochemistry of energy balance and the psychology and sociology of food intake have thereby converged to create an obesity epidemic with serious personal and public health ramifications.

REFERENCES

1. Mello MM. Obesity – personal choice or public health issue? Nat Clin Pract Endocrinol Metab. 2008;4:2–3.
2. Schwimmer JB, Burwinkle TM, Varni JW. Health-related quality of life of severely obese children and adolescents. J Am Med Assoc. 2003;289:1813–19.
3. Ogden CL, Carroll MD, Flegal KM. High body mass index for age among US children and adolescents, 2003–2006. J Am Med Assoc. 2008;299:2401–5.
4. Zhang Y, Proenca R, Maffei M, Barone M, Leopold L, Friedman JM. Positional cloning of the mouse obese gene and its human homologue. Nature. 1994;393:372–425.
5. Druce MR, Small CJ, Bloom SR. Minireview: gut peptides regulating satiety. Endocrinology. 2004;145:2660–65.
6. Morton GJ, Cummings DE, Baskin DG, Barsh GS, Schwartz MW. Central nervous system control of food intake and body weight. Nature. 2006;443:289–95.

7. Hellstrom PM, Geliebter A, Naslund E, Schmidt PT, Yahav EK, Hashim SA, Yeomans MR. Peripheral and central signals in the control of eating in normal, obese and binge-eating human subjects. Br J Nutr. 2004;92:S47–57.

8. Date Y, Murakami N, Toshinai K, Matsukura S, Niijima A, Matsuo H, Kangawa K, Nakazato M. The role of the gastric afferent vagal nerve in ghrelin-induced feeding and growth hormone secretion in rats. Gastroenterology. 2002;123:1120–28.

9. Bi S, Moran TH. Actions of CCK in the control of food intake and body weight: lessons from the CCK-A receptor deficient OLETF rat. Neuropeptides. 2002;36:171–81.

10. Abbott CR, Monteiro M, Small CJ, Sajedi A, Smith KL, Parkinson JRC, Ghatei MA, Bloom SR. The inhibitory effects of peripheral administration of peptide YY3–36 and glucagon-like peptide-1 on food intake are attenuated by ablation of the vagal–brainstem–hypothalamic pathway. Brain Res. 2005;1044:127–31.

11. Kojima M, Hosoda H, Date Y, Nakazato M, Matsuo H, Kangawa K. Ghrelin is a growth-hormone-releasing acylated peptide from stomach. Nature. 1999;402:656–60.

12. Kamegai J, Tamura H, Shimizu T, Ishii S, Sugihara H, Wakabayashi I. Central effect of ghrelin, an endogenous growth hormone secretagogue, on hypothalamic peptide gene expression. Endocrinology. 2000;141:4797–800.

13. Tschöp M, Smiley DL, Heiman ML. Ghrelin induces adiposity in rodents. Nature. 2000;407:908–13.

14. Cummings DE, Purnell JQ, Frayo RS, Schmidova K, Wisse BF, Weigle DS. A preprandial rise in plasma ghrelin levels suggests a role in meal initiation in humans. Diabetes. 2001;50:1714–19.

15. Druce MR, Neary NM, Small CJ, Milton J, Monteiro M, Patterson M, Ghatei MA, Bloom SR. Subcutaneous administration of ghrelin stimulates energy intake in healthy lean human volunteers. Int J Obes. 2006;30:293–96.

16. Cummings DE, Weigle DS, Frayo RS, Breen PA, Ma MK, Dellinger EP, Purnell JQ. Plasma ghrelin levels after diet-induced weight loss or gastric bypass surgery. N Engl J Med. 2002;346:1623–30.

17. Batterham RL, Cowley MA, Small CJ, Herzog H, Cohen MA, Dakin CL, Wren AM, Brynes AE, Low MJ, Ghatel MA, Cone RD, Bloom SR. Gut hormone $PYY_{3–36}$ physiologically inhibits food intake. Nature. 2002;418:650–54.

18. Kiefer TJ, Habener JF. The glucagon-like peptides. Endocr Rev. 1999;20:876–913.

19. Drucker DJ. Biologic actions and therapeutic potential of the proglucagon-derived peptides. Nat Clin Pract Endocrinol Metab. 2005;1:22–31.

20. Gotoh K, Fukagawa K, Fukagawa T, Noguchi H, Kakuma T, Sakata T, Yoshimatsu H. Glucagon-like peptide-1, corticotropin-releasing hormone, and hypothalamic neuronal histamine interact in the leptin-signaling pathway to regulate feeding behavior. FASEB J. 2005;19:1131–33.

21. Lustig RH. Childhood obesity: behavioral aberration or biochemical drive? Reinterpreting the First Law of Thermodynamics. Nat Clin Pract Endocrinol Metab. 2006;2:447–58.

22. Chehab FF, Mounzih K, Lu R, Lim ME. Early onset of reproductive function in normal female mice treated with leptin. Science. 1997;275:88–90.

23. Mantzoros CS, Flier JS, Rogol AD. A longitudinal assessment of hormonal and physical alterations during normal puberty in boys. Rising leptin levels may signal the onset of puberty. J Clin Endocrinol Metab. 1997;82:1066–70.

24. Mark AL, Rahmouni K, Correia M, Haynes WG. A leptin-sympathetic-leptin feedback loop: potential implications for regulation of arterial pressure and body fat. Acta Physiol Scand. 2003;177:345–49.

25. Boden G, Chen X, Mozzoli M, Ryan I. Effect of fasting on serum leptin in normal human subjects. J Clin Endocrinol Metabol. 1996;81:454–58.

26. Keim NL, Stern JS, Havel PJ. Relation between circulating leptin concentrations and appetite during a prolonged, moderate energy deficit in women. Am J Clin Nutr. 1998;68:794–801.

27. Flier JS. What's in a name? In search of leptin's physiologic role. J Clin Endocrinol Metab. 1998;83:1407–13.

28. Hassink SG, Sheslow DV, de Lancy E, Opentanova I, Considine RV, Caro JF. Serum leptin in children with obesity: relationship to gender and development. Pediatrics. 1996;98:201–3.

29. Guven S, El-Bershawi A, Sonnenberg GE, Wilson CR, Hoffman RG, Krakower GR, Kissebah AH. Plasma leptin and insulin levels in weight-reduced obese women with normal body mass index: relationships with body composition and insulin. Diabetes. 1999;48:347–52.

30. Barr VA, Malide D, Zarnowski MJ, Taylor SI, Cushman SW. Insulin stimulates both leptin secretion and production by white adipose tissue. Endocrinology. 1997;138:4463–72.

31. Kolaczynski JW, Nyce MR, Considine RV, Boden G, Nolan JJ, Henry R, Mudaliar SR, Olefsky J, Caro JF. Acute and chronic effects of insulin on leptin production in humans: studies in vivo and in vitro. Diabetes. 1996;45:699–701.

32. Singhal A, Farooqi IS, O'Rahilly S, Cole TJ, Fewtrell M, Lucas A. Early nutrition and leptin concentrations later in life. Am J Clin Nutr. 2002;75:993–99.

33. Lee GH, Proenca R, Montez JM, Carroll KM, Darvishzadeh JG, Lee JI, Friedman JM. Abnormal splicing of the leptin receptor in diabetic mice. Nature. 1996;379:632–35.

34. Spanswick D, Smith MA, Groppi VE, Logan SD, Ashford ML. Leptin inhibits hypothalamic neurons by activation of ATP-sensitive potassium channels. Nature. 1997;390:521–25.

35. Kishimoto T, Taga T, Akira S. Cytokine signal transduction. Cell. 1994;76:252–62.

36. Banks AS, Davis SM, Bates SJ, Myers MG. Activation of downstream signals by the long form of the leptin receptor. J Biol Chem. 2000;275:14563–72.

37. Niswender KD, Schwartz MW. Insulin and leptin revisited: adiposity signals with overlapping physiological and intracellular signaling capabilities. Front Neuroendocrinol. 2003;24:1–10.

38. Porte D, Baskin DG, Schwartz MW. Insulin signaling in the central nervous system: a critical role in metabolic homeostasis and disease from C. elegans to humans. Diabetes. 2005;54:1264–76.

39. Baskin DG, Wilcox BJ, Figlewicz DP, Dorsa DM. Insulin and insulin-like growth factors in the CNS. Trends Neurosci. 1988;11:107–11.

40. Baura GD, Foster DM, Porte D, Kahn SE, Bergman RN, Cobelli C, Schwartz MW. Saturable transport of insulin from plasma into the central nervous system of dogs in vivo: a mechanism for regulated insulin delivery to the brain. J Clin Investig. 1993;92:1824–30.

41. VanderWeele DA. Insulin is a prandial satiety hormone. Physiol Behav. 1994;56:619–22.

42. McGowan MK, Andrews KM, Grossman SP. Role of intrahypothalamic insulin in circadian patterns of food intake, activity, and body temperature. Behav Neurosci. 1992;106:380–85.

43. Woods SC, Lotter EC, McKay LD, Porte D. Chronic intracerebroventricular infusion of insulin reduces food intake and body weight of baboons. Nature. 1979;282:503–5.

44. Abusrewil SS, Savage DL. Obesity and diabetic control. Arch Dis Child. 1989;64:1313–15.

45. VanderWeele DA. Insulin and satiety from feeding in pancreatic-normal and diabetic rats. Physiol Behav. 1993;54:477–85.

46. Assimacopoulos-Jeannet F, Brichard S, Rencurel F, Cusin I, Jeanrenaud B. In vivo effects of hyperinsulinemia on lipogenic enzymes and glucose transporter expression in rat liver and adipose tissues. Metabolism. 1995;44(2):228–33.

47. Cusin I, Terrettaz J, Rohner-Jeanrenaud F, Zarjevski N, Assimacopoulos-Jeannet F, Jeanrenaud B. Hyperinsulinemia increases the amount of GLUT4 mRNA in white adipose tissue and decreases that of muscles: a clue for increased fat depot and insulin resistance. Endocrinology. 1990;127:3246–48.

48. Woo R, Kissileff HR, Pi-Sunyer FX. Elevated post-prandial insulin levels do not induce satiety in normal-weight humans. Am J Physiol. 1984;247:R776–87.

49. Niswender KD, Morton GJ, Stearns WH, Rhodes CJ, Myers MG, Schwartz MW. Intracellular signalling. Key enzyme in leptin-induced anorexia. Nature. 2001;413:794–795.

50. Brüning JC, Gautam D, Burks DJ, Gillette J, Schubert M, Orban PC, Klein R, Krone W, Müller-Wieland D, Kahn CR. Role of brain insulin receptor in control of body weight and reproduction. Science. 2000;289:2122–25.

51. Schwartz MW, Figlewicz DP, Baskin DG, Woods SC, Porte D. Insulin and the central regulation of energy balance: Update 1994. Endocr Rev. 1994;2:109–13.

52. Lin X, Taguchi A, Park S, Kushner JA, Li F, Li Y, White MF. Dysregulation of insulin receptor substrate 2 in β-cells and brain causes obesity and diabetes. J Clin Investig. 2004;114:908–16.

53. Plum L, Ma X, Hampel B, Balthasar N, Coppari R, Munzberg H, Shanabrough M, Burdakov D, Rother E, Janoschek R, Alber J, Belgardt BF, Koch L, Seibler J, Schwenk F, Fekete C, Suzuki A, Mak TW, Krone W, Horvath TL, Ashcroft FM, Bruning JC. Enhanced PIP(3) signaling in POMC neurons causes K(ATP) channel activation and leads to diet-sensitive obesity. J Clin Invest. 2006;116:1886–901.

54. Bjorkbaek C, Elmquist JK, Frantz JD, Shoelson SE, Flier JS. Identification of SOCS-3 as a potential mediator of central leptin resistance. Mol Cell. 1998;1:619–25.

55. Bence KK, Delibegovic M, Xue B, Gorgun CZ, Hotamisligil GS, Neel BG, Kahn BB. Neuronal PTP1B regulates body weight, adiposity, and leptin action. Nat Med. 2006;12:917–24.

56. Elmquist JK, Ahima RS, Elias CF, Flier JS, Saper CB. Leptin activates distinct projections from the dorsomedial and ventromedial hypothalamic nuclei. Proc Natl Acad Sci USA. 1998;95:741–46.

57. Thornton JE, Cheung CC, Clifton DK, Steiner RA. Regulation of hypothalamic proopiomelanocortin mRNA by leptin in ob/ob mice. Endocrinology. 1997;138:5063–66.

58. Kristensen P, Judge ME, Thim L, Ribel U, Christjansen KN, Wulff BS, Clausen JT, Jensen PB, Madsen OD, Vrang N, Larsen PJ, Hastrup S. Hypothalamic CART is a new anorectic peptide regulated by leptin. Nature. 1998;393:72–76.

59. Broberger C, Johansen J, Johasson C, Schalling M, Hokfelt T. The neuropeptide Y/agouti gene related protein (AGRP) brain circuitry in normal, anorectic, and monosodium glutamate-treated mice. Proc Natl Acad Sci USA. 1998;95:15043–48.

60. Liebowitz SF. Brain peptides and obesity: pharmacologic treatment. Obes Res. 1995;3:573S–89S.

61. Kalra SP, Kalra PS. Nutritional infertility: the role of the interconnected hypothalamic neuropeptide Y-galanin-opioid network. Front Neuroendocrinol. 1996;17:371–401.

62. Beck B, Stricker-Krongard A, Nicolas JP, Burlet C. Chronic and continuous intracerebroventricular infusion of neuropeptide Y in Long-Evans rats mimics the feeding behavior of obese Zucker rats. Int J Obes. 1992;16:295–302.

63. Stephens TW, Basinski M, Bristow PK, Bue-Valleskey JM, Burgett SG, Craft L, Hale J, Hoffmann J, Hsiung HM, Kriaciunas A. The role of neuropeptide Y in the antiobesity action of the obese gene product. Nature. 1995;377:530–34.

64. Broberger C, Landry M, Wong H, Walsh JN, Hokfelt T. Subtypes of the Y_1 and Y_2 of the neuropeptide Y receptor are respectively expressed in pro-opiomelanocortin and neuropeptide Y-containing neurons of the rat hypothalamic arcuate nucleus. Neuroendocrinology. 1997;66:393–408.

65. Shutter JR, Graham M, Kinsey AC, Scully S, Luthy R, Stark KL. Hypothalamic expression of ART, a novel gene related to agouti, is up-regulated in obese and diabetic mutant mice. Genes Dev. 1997;7:454–67.

66. Graham M, Shutter JR, Sarmiento U, Sarosi I, Stark KL. Overexpression of Agrt leads to obesity in transgenic mice. Nat Genet. 1997;17:273–274.

67. Wellman PJ. Modulation of eating by central catecholamine systems. Curr Drug Targets. 2005;6:191–99.

68. Leibowitz S, Roosin P, Rosenn M. Chronic norepinephrine injection into the hypothalamic paraventricular nucleus produces hyperphagia and increased body weight in the rat. Pharmacol Biochem Behav. 1984;21:801–8.

69. Wellman PJ, Davies BT. Reversal of cirazoline-induced and phenylpropanolamine-induced anorexia by the alpha-1-receptor antagonist prazosin. Pharmacol Biochem Behav. 1992;42:97–100.

70. Liebowitz SF, Alexander JT, Cheung WK, Weiss GF. Effects of serotonin and the serotonin blocker metergoline on meal patterns and macronutrient selection. Pharmacol Biochem Behav. 1993;45:185–94.

71. Wong DT, Reid LR, Threlkeld PG. Suppression of food intake in rats by fluoxetine: comparison of enantiomers and effects of serotonin antagonists. Pharmacol Biochem Behav. 1988;31:475–79.

72. Garattini S, Bizzi A, Caccia S, Mennini T. Progress report on the anorectic effects of dexfenfluramine, fluoxetine, and sertraline. Int J Obes. 1992;16:S43–50.

73. Calapai G, Corica F, Corsonello A, Saubetin L, DiRosa M, Campo GM, Buemi M, Mauro VN, Caputi AP. Leptin increases serotonin turnover by inhibition of nitric oxide synthesis. J Clin Investig. 1999;104:975–82.

74. Nonogaki K, Strack AM, Dallman MF, Tecott LH. Leptin-independent hyperphagia and type 2 diabetes in mice with a mutated serotonin 5-HT$_{2c}$ receptor gene. Nat Med. 1998;4:1152–56.

75. Simansky KJ. Serotonergic control of the organization of feeding and satiety. Behav Brain Res. 1996;73:37–42.

76. Pissios P, Bradley RL, Maratos-Flier E. Expanding the scales: the multiple roles of MCH in regulating energy balance and other biological functions. Endocr Rev. 2006;27:606–20.

77. Shimada M, Tritos NA, Lowell BB, Flier JS, Maratos-Flier E. Mice lacking melanin-concentrating hormone receptor are hypophagic and lean. Nature. 1998;396:670–74.

78. Ludwig DS, Tritos NA, Mastaitis JW, Kulkarni R, Kokkotou E, Elmquist J, Lowell B, Flier JS, Maratos-Flier E. Melanin-concentrating hormone overexpression in transgenic mice leads to obesity and insulin resistance. J Clin Investig. 2001;107:379–86.

79. Gomori A, Ishihara A, Ito M, Mashiko S, Matsushita H, Yumoto M, Tanaka T, Tokita S, Moriya M, Iwaasa H, Kanatani A. Chronic intracerebroventricular infusion of MCH causes obesity in mice. Am J Physiol. 2003;284:E583–8.

80. Taylor MM, Samson WK. The other side of the orexins: endocrine and metabolic actions. Am J Physiol. 2003;284:E13–7.

81. Hara J, Beuckmann CT, Nambu T, Willie JT, Chemelli RM, Sinton CM, Sugiyama F, Yagami K, Goto K, Yanigasawa M, Sakurai T. Genetic ablation of orexin neurons in mice results in narcolepsy, hypophagia, and obesity. Neuron. 2001;30:345–54.

82. Harris GC, Aston-Jones G. Arousal and reward: a dichotomy in orexin function. Trends Neurosci. 2006;29:571–77.

83. Mieda M, Yanigasawa M. Sleep, feeding, and neuropeptides: roles of orexins and orexin receptors. Curr Opin Neurobiol. 2002;12:339–46.

84. Pagotto U, Marsicano G, Cota D, Lutz B, Pasquali R. The emerging role of the endocannabinoid system in endocrine regulation and energy balance. Endocr Rev. 2006;27:73–100.

85. Malcher-Lopes R, Di S, Marcheselli VS, Weng FJ, Stuart CT, Bazan NG, Tasker JG. Opposing crosstalk between leptin and glucocorticoids rapidly modulates synaptic excitation via endocannabinoid release. J Neurosci. 2006;26:6643–50.

86. Ranadive S, Vaisse C. Lessons from extreme human obesity: monogenetic disorders. Endocrinol Metab Clin North Am. 2008;37:733–51.

87. Chen AS, Marsh DJ, Trumbauer ME, Frazier EG, Guan XM, Yu H, Rosenblum CI, Vongs A, Feng Y, Cao L, Metzger JM, Strack AM, Camacho RE, Mellin TN, Nunes CN, Min W, Fisher J, Gopal-Truter S, MacIntyre DE, Chen HY, Van der Ploeg LH. Inactivation of the mouse melanocortin-3 receptor results in increased fat mass and reduced lean body mass. Nat Genet. 2000;26:97–102.

88. Li WD, Joo EJ, Furlong EB, et al. Melanocortin 3 receptor (MC3R) gene variants in extremely obese women. Int J Obes. 2000;24:206–10.

89. Mencarelli M, Walker GE, Maestrini S, Alberti L, Verti B, Brunani A, Petroni ML, Tagliaferri M, Liuzzi A, Di Blasio AM. Sporadic mutations in melanocortin receptor 3 in morbid obese individuals. Eur J Hum Genet. 2008;16:581–86.

90. Butler AA, Cone RD. The melanocortin receptors: lessons from knockout models. Neuropeptides. 2002;36:77–84.

91. Rahmouni K, Haynes WG, Morgan DA, Mark AL. Role of melanocortin-4 receptors in mediating renal sympathoactivation to leptin and insulin J. Neurosciences. 2003;23:5998–6004.

92. Collins S, Kuhn CM, Petro AE, Swick AG, Chrunyk BA, Surwit RS. Role of leptin in fat regulation. Nature. 1996;380:677.

93. Muntzel M, Morgan DA, Mark AL, Johnson AK. Intracerebroventricular insulin produces non-uniform regional increases in sympathetic nerve activity. Am J Physiol. 1994;267:R1350–5.

94. Vollenweider L, Tappy L, Owlya R, Jequier E, Nicod P, Scherrer U. Insulin-induced sympathetic activation and vasodilation in skeletal muscle. Effects of insulin resistance in lean subjects. Diabetes. 1995;44:641–45.

95. Blaak EE, Saris WH, van Baak MA. Adrenoceptor subtypes mediating catecholamine-induced thermogenesis in man. Int J Obes. 1993;17:S78–81.

96. Viguerie N, Clement K, Barbe P, Courtine M, Benis A, Larrouy D, Hanczar B, Pelloux V, Poitou C, Khalfallah Y, Barsh GS, Thalamas C, Zucker JD, Langin D. In vivo epinephrine-mediated regulation of gene express in human skeletal muscle. J Clin Endocrinol Metabol. 2004;89:2000–14.

97. Navegantes LC, Migliorini RH, do Carmo Kettelhut I. Adrenergic control of protein metabolism in skeletal muscle. Curr Opin Clin Nutr Metab Care. 2002;5:281–6.

98. Susulic VS, Frederich RC, Lawitts J, Tozzo E, Kahn BB, Harper ME, Himms-Hagen J, Flier JS, Lowell BB. Targeted disruption of the beta 3-adrenergic receptor gene. J Biol Chem. 1995;270:29483–92.

99. Boss O, Bachman E, Vidal-Puig A, Zhang CY, Peroni O, Lowell BB. Role of the β_3-adrenergic receptor and/or a putative β_3-adrenergic receptor on the expression of uncoupling proteins and peroxisome proliferator-activated receptor-γ coactivator-1. Biochem Biophys Res Commun. 1999;261:870–76.

100. Lowell BB, Spiegelman BM. Towards a molecular understanding of adaptive thermogenesis. Nature. 2000;404:652–60.

101. Klingenberg M, Huang SG. Structure and function of the uncoupling protein from brown adipose tissue. Biochem Biophys Acta. 1999;1415:271–96.

102. Powley TL, Laughton W. Neural pathways involved in the hypothalamic integration of autonomic responses. Diabetologia. 1981;20:378–87.

103. Peles E, Goldstein DS, Akselrod S, Nitzan H, Azaria M, Almog S, Dolphin D, Halkin H, Modan M. Interrelationships among measures of autonomic activity and cardiovascular risk factors during orthostasis and the oral glucose tolerance test. Clin Auton Res. 1995;5:271–8.

104. Rohner-Jeanrenaud F, Jeanrenaud B. Involvement of the cholinergic system in insulin and glucagon oversecretion of genetic preobesity. Endocrinology. 1985;116:830–4.

105. Lustig RH. Autonomic dysfunction of the β-cell and the pathogenesis of obesity. Rev Endocr Metab Dis. 2003;4:23–32.

106. Kreier F, Fliers E, Voshol PJ, Van Eden CG, Havekes LM, Kalsbeek A, Van Heijningen CL, Sluiter AA, Mettenleiter TC, Romijn JA, Sauerwein HP, Buijs RM. Selective parasympathetic innervation of subcutaneous and intra-abdominal fat-functional implications. J Clin Investig. 2002;110:1243–50.

107. Boden G, Hoeldtke RD. Nerves, fat, and insulin resistance. N Engl J Med. 2003;349:1966–7.

108. D'Alessio DA, Kieffer TJ, Taborsky GJ, Havel PJ. Activation of the parasympathetic nervous system is necessary for normal meal induced-insulin secretion in rhesus macaques. J Clin Endocrinol Metab. 2001;86:1253–9.

109. Ahren B, Holst JJ. The cephalic insulin response to meal ingestion in humans is dependent on both cholinergic and noncholingergic mechanisms and is important for postprandial glycemia. Diabetes. 2001;50:1030–8.

110. Marin P, Russeffé-Scrive A, Smith J, Bjorntorp P. Glucose uptake in human adipose tissue. Metabolism. 1988;36:1154–64.

111. Ramsay TG. Fat cells. Endocrinol Metab Clin North Am. 1996;25:847–70.

112. Kelley AE, Bakshi VP, Haber SN, Steininger TL, Will MJ, Zhang M. Opioid modulation of taste hedonics within the ventral striatum. Physiol Behav. 2002;76:365–77.

113. Hommel JD, Trinko R, Sears RM, Georgescu D, Liu ZW, Gao XB, Thurmon JJ, Marinelli M, DiLeone RJ. Leptin receptor signaling in midbrain dopamine neurons regulates feeding. Neuron. 2006;51:801–10.

114. Shalev U, Yap J, Shaham Y. Leptin attenuates food deprivation-induced relapse to heroin seeking. J Neurosci. 2001;21:RC129:121–5.

115. Carr KD, Tsimberg Y, Berman Y, Yamamoto N. Evidence of increased dopamine receptor signaling in food-restricted rats. Neuroscience. 2003;119:1157–67.

116. Figlewicz DP, Szot P, Chavez M, Woods SC, Veith RC. Intraventricular insulin increases dopaminergic transporter mRNA in rat VTA/substantia nigra. Brain Res. 1994;644:331–4.

117. Sipols AJ, Bayer J, Bennett R, Figlewicz DP. Intraventricular insulin decreases kappa opioid-mediated sucrose intake in rats. Peptides. 2002;23:2181–7.

118. Figlewicz DP. Adiposity signals and food reward: expanding the CNS roles of insulin and leptin. Am J Phyisol Regul Integr Comp Physiol. 2003;284:R882–92.

119. Volkow ND, Wise RA. How can drug addiction help us understand obesity? Nat. Neurosciences. 2005;8:555–60.

120. Figlewicz DP, MacDonald Naleid A, Sipols AJ. Modulation of food reward by adiposity signals. Physiol Behav. 2007;91:473–78.

121. Tataranni PA, Gautier JF, Chen K, Uecker A, Bandy D, Salbe AD, Pratley RE, Lawson M, Reiman EM, Ravussin E. Neuroanatomical correlates of hunger and satiation in humans using positron emission tomography. Proc Natl Acad Sci USA. 1999;96:4569–74.

122. Peters JC, Wyatt HR, Donahoo WT, Hill JO. From instinct to intellect: the challenge of maintaining healthy weight in the modern world. Obes Res. 2002;3:69–74.

123. Black PH. The inflammatory consequences of psychologic stress: relationship to insulin resistance, obesity, atherosclerosis and diabetes mellitus, type II. Med Hypotheses. 2006;67:879–91.

124. Dallman MF, Pecoraro NC, La Fleur SE. Chronic stress and comfort foods: self-medication and abdominal obesity. Brain Behav Immun. 2005;19:275–80.

125. La Fleur SE, Akana SF, Manalo SL, Dallman MF. Interaction between corticosterone and insulin in obesity: regulation of lard intake and fat stores. Endocrinology. 2004;145:2174–85.

126. Dallman MF, Pecoraro N, Akana SF, La Fleur SE, Gomez F, Houshyar H, Bell ME, Bhatnagar S, Laugero KD, Manalo S. Chronic stress and obesity: a new view of "comfort food". Proc Natl Acad Sci USA. 2003;100:11696–701.

127. Tataranni PA, Larson DE, Snitker S, Young JB, Flatt JP, Ravussin E. Effects of glucocorticoids on energy metabolism and food intake in humans. Am J Physiol. 1996;271:E317–25.

128. Adam TC, Epel ES. Stress, eating, and the reward system. Physiol Behav. 2007;91:449–58.

129. Oliver G, Wardle J. Perceived effects of stress on food choice. Physiol Behav. 1999;66:511–5.

130. Roemmich JN, Wright SM, Epstein LH. Dietary restraint and stress-induced snacking in youth. Obes Res. 2002;10:1120–6.

131. Kuo LE, Kitlinska JB, Tilan JU, Li L, Baker SB, Johnson MD, Lee EW, Burnett MS, Fricke ST, Kvetnansky R, Herzog H, Zukowska Z. Neuropeptide Y acts directly in the periphery on fat tissue and mediates stress-induced obesity and metabolic syndrome. Nat Med. 2007;13:803–11.

132. Leibel RL. The role of leptin in the control of body weight. Nutr Rev. 2002;60:S15–9.

133. Leibel RL, Rosenbaum M, Hirsch J. Changes in energy expenditure resulting from altered body weight. N Engl J Med. 1995;332:621–8.

134. Champigny O, Ricquier D. Effects of fasting and refeeding on the level of uncoupling protein mRNA in rat brown adipose tissue: evidence for diet-induced and cold-induced responses. J Nutr. 1990;120:1730–6.

135. Aronne LJ, Mackintosh R, Rosenbaum M, Leibel RL, Hirsch J. Autonomic nervous system activity in weight gain and weight loss. Am J Physiol. 1995;269:R222–5.

136. Heymsfield SB, Greenberg AS, Fujioka K, Dixon RM, Kushner R, Hunt T, Lubina JA, Patane J, Self B, Hunt P, McCamish M. Recombinant leptin for weight loss in obese and lean adults: a randomized, controlled, dose-escalation trial. J Am Med Assoc. 1999;282:1568–75.

137. Rosenbaum M, Nicolson M, Hirsch J, Murphy E, Chu F, Leibel RL. Effects of weight change on plasma leptin concentrations and energy expenditure. J Clin Endocrinol Metab. 1997;82:3647–54.

138. Caro JF, Kolaczynski JW, Nyce MR, Ohannesian JP, Opentanova I, Goldman WH, Lynn RB, Zhang PL, Sinha MK, Considine RV. Decreased cerebrospinal fluid/serum leptin ratio in obesity: a possible mechanism for leptin resistance. Lancet. 1996;348:159–61.

139. Banks WA, Kastin AJ, Huang W, Jaspan JB, Maness LM. Leptin enters the brain by a saturable system independent of insulin. Peptides. 1996;17:305–11.

140. Banks WA, Coon AB, Robinson SM, Moinuddin A, Shultz JM, Nakaoke R, Morley JE. Triglycerides induce leptin resistance at the blood-brain barrier. Diabetes. 2004;53:1253–60.

141. El-Haschimi K, Pierroz DD, Hileman SM, Bjorbaek C, Flier JS. Two defects contribute to hypothalamic leptin resistance in mice with diet-induced obesity. J Clin Investig. 2000;105:1827–32.

142. Rosenbaum M, Murphy EM, Heymsfield SB, Matthews DE, Leibel RL. Low dose leptin administration reverses effects of sustained weight reduction on energy expenditure and circulating concentrations of thyroid hormones. J Clin Endocrinol Metab. 2002;87:2391–4.

143. Rosenbaum M, Goldsmith R, Bloomfield D, Magnano A, Weimer L, Heymsfield S, Gallagher D, Mayer L, Murphy E, Leibel RL. Low-dose leptin reverses skeletal muscle, autonomic, and neuroendocrine adaptations to maintenance of reduced weight. J Clin Invest. 2005;115:3579–86.

144. Lustig RH, Sen S, Soberman JE, Velasquez-Mieyer PA. Obesity, leptin resistance, and the effects of insulin suppression. Int J Obes. 2004;28:1344–8.

145. Isganaitis E, Lustig RH. Fast food, central nervous system insulin resistance, and obesity. Arterioscler Thromb Vasc Biol. 2005;25:2451–62.
146. Lustig RH, Mietus-Snyder ML, Bacchetti P, Lazar AA, Velasquez-Mieyer PA, Christensen ML. Insulin dynamics predict BMI and z-score response to insulin suppression or sensitization pharmacotherapy in obese children. J Pediatr. 2006;148:23–9.
147. Mietus-Snyder ML, Lustig RH. Childhood obesity: adrift in the "limbic triangle". Annu Rev Med. 2008;59:119–34.

III THE GENETICS OF CHILDHOOD OBESITY

3 Monogenic Obesity

David Meyre and Philippe Froguel

Key Words: Leptin, melanocortin, POMC, prohormone convertase, SIM1, BDNF

INTRODUCTION

Obesity is increasing dramatically worldwide and is projected to affect 1.12 billion people by 2030 *(1)*. The epidemic of obesity is attributed to recent changes in the environment (easy access to high-energy palatable food, combined with a decreased physical activity), whereas individual differences in obesity risk are attributed to genetic differences between individuals: the heritability of body mass index (BMI) has been estimated to approximate 70% in adults and is even higher (77%) for younger people raised in an increasingly obesogenic environment *(2)*. The prevalence of obesity (defined by a BMI $\geq$ 30 kg/m^2) in the United States increased by 24% between 2000 and 2005; the prevalence of morbid obesity (BMI $\geq$ 40 kg/m^2) and super obesity (BMI $\geq$ 50 kg/m^2) increased by 50 and 75%, respectively, during the same period *(3)*. These data clearly indicate that the current environment acts as a "catalyst" to reveal subjects with higher genetic susceptibility to obesity.

Whereas the key role of heredity in obesity was established from 1986 with seminal twin studies by Stunkard and colleagues *(4)*, the first discovery of a gene involved in human obesity came more recently, with the discovery of mutations in the leptin gene in 1997 *(5)*. Since then, seven additional genes have been linked to human monogenic obesity, illuminating the alteration of central control of food intake as a major causative mechanism leading to obesity (Fig. 1). The recent harvest of polygenic genes influencing obesity and corpulence has confirmed the importance of neuronal influence on food intake regulation in body weight regulation *(6)*. Here we review the main advances in the elucidation of monogenic forms of human obesity and offer a specific focus on the future directions of research in the genetic dissection of obesity single gene disorders.

From: *Contemporary Endocrinology: Pediatric Obesity: Etiology, Pathogenesis, and Treatment*
Edited by: M. Freemark, DOI 10.1007/978-1-60327-874-4_3,
© Springer Science+Business Media, LLC 2010

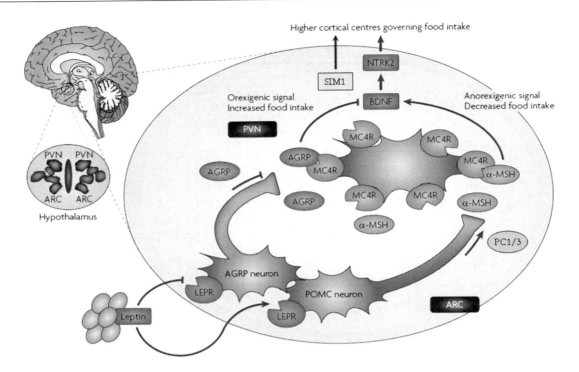

Fig. 1. The leptin–melanocortin pathway (Modified from Walley et al., Nat Rev Genet 2009, with the permission of Nat Rev Genet). The melanocortin 4 receptor (MC4R) is highly expressed in the paraventricular nucleus (PVN) of the hypothalamus, where it has a key role in the control of appetite. Leptin released from adipose tissue binds to leptin receptors (LEPR) on agouti-related protein (AGRP)-producing neurons and proopiomelanocortin (POMC)-producing neurons in the arcuate nucleus (ARC) of the hypothalamus. Leptin binding inhibits AGRP production and stimulates the production of POMC, which undergoes post-translational modification by prohormone convertase 1/3 (PC1/3) to generate a range of peptides, including alpha-, beta-, gamma-melanocyte-stimulating hormone (MSH). AGRP and alpha-MSH compete for MC4R–AGRP binding suppresses MC4R activity and alpha-MSH binding stimulates MC4R activity. Decreased receptor activity generates an orexigenic signal, whereas increased receptor activity generates an anorexigenic signal. Signals from MC4R govern food intake through secondary effector neurons that lead to higher cortical centres, a process that involves single-minded homologue 1 (SIM1), brain-derived neurotrophic factor (BDNF), and neurotrophic tyrosine kinase receptor type 2 (NTRK2; also known as tropomyosin-related kinase B, TRKB).

MONOGENIC OBESITY CAUSED BY MUTATIONS IN THE LEPTIN/MELANOCORTIN PATHWAY

1-Leptin and Leptin Receptor Deficiency

Leptin is a cytokine secreted by adipocytes in proportion to body's fat content. It binds to receptors in two different specific populations of neurons (neuropeptide Y/agouti-related peptide-expressing neurons and proopiomelanocortin/cocaine and amphetamine-related transcript-expressing neurons) of the arcuate nucleus of the hypothalamus. The key role of leptin and its receptor in energy metabolism was first demonstrated by the successful positional cloning of two mouse models of obesity (the *ob/ob* and *db/db* mice). These seminal studies were rapidly followed by the analysis of candidate genes in obese patients, which led to the identification of pathogenic mutations in both leptin (*LEP*) and its receptor (*LEPR*) in extreme forms of early-onset obesity *(5,7)*.

Thus far, 13 patients of Turkish, Pakistani, and Egyptian origin have been found to have *congenital leptin deficiency*. They are all homozygous carriers of a frameshift (deltaG133) or two missense (R105Y and N103K) mutations in the *LEP* gene, resulting in very low circulating leptin levels.

The first patients with *congenital leptin receptor deficiency* were three sisters from a consanguineous Algerian pedigree who had a homozygous G→A mutation in the splice donor site of exon 16 that results in a truncated leptin receptor lacking both the transmembrane and the intracellular domains *(7)*. The prevalence of patients with pathogenic *LEPR* mutations (homozygous/compound heterozygous) was 2.7% in a highly consanguineous cohort of 300 severely obese children *(8)*. Frameshift or nonsense mutations result in the loss of all isoforms of the leptin receptor, whereas missense mutations affect only the extracellular domain of the receptor *(8)*.

Subjects with *congenital leptin deficiency* exhibit normal weight at birth but gain weight rapidly in the early postnatal period. Leptin deficiency is associated with marked hyperphagia, impaired satiety, and excessive fat deposition in the trunk and limbs *(5)*. Complete leptin deficiency is also associated with hypothalamic hypothyroidism (low free T4 and mildly elevated serum TSH) and hypogonadotropic hypogonadism, with delayed or absent pubertal progression. Linear growth and serum IGF-1 are normal but final height is reduced because of the absence of a pubertal growth spurt. Children with leptin deficiency have altered T-cell number and function and suffer high rates of childhood morbidity and mortality from infectious disease *(9)*.

Leptin-deficient patients can be treated with daily injections of recombinant human leptin, which reverses the obesity and associated phenotypic abnormalities *(10,11)*. Leptin administration dramatically reduces food intake through the modulation of neural activation in key striatal regions, suggesting that the hormone acts centrally to diminish the perception of food reward and to enhance the response to satiety signals during food consumption *(12)*. Leptin administration is also associated with decreased food preference for carbohydrates *(13)*. Long-term (4 years) leptin administration also confers sustained beneficial effects on fat mass, hyperinsulinemia, and hyperlipidemia. Appropriately timed pubertal development and restoration of T-cell responsiveness are also observed, allowing the withdrawal of T4 treatment *(14)*. Leptin replacement in patients with congenital leptin deficiency is proposed to increase grey matter concentration in the anterior cingulate gyrus, the inferior parietal lobule, and the cerebellum *(15)* and to induce changes in rates of development in many neurocognitive domains *(16)*.

Heterozygous carriers of deleterious mutations in LEP have a partial leptin deficiency associated with an overweight or obese phenotype (85%) *(17)*. Peripheral leptin supplementation was shown to induce significant weight loss in the subgroup of subjects with low levels of leptin *(18)*, suggesting that leptin administration may be warranted in subjects with partial leptin deficiency to reduce their propensity to develop obesity.

Patients with *congenital leptin receptor deficiency* consume three times the amount of energy eaten by controls in a test meal, and they all become severely obese during childhood *(8)*. They present alterations in immune function and frequent childhood infections of the respiratory tract associated with high rates of premature death. They also manifest delayed puberty due to hypogonadotropic hypogonadism, and some are hypothyroid *(7)*. However, their clinical features are usually less severe (mean BMIz +5.1) than those of subjects with congenital homozygous leptin deficiency (mean BMIz +6.8), and hypothyroidism is less common *(8)*. Importantly, serum leptin levels in patients with leptin receptor mutations (36–365 ng/ml at age 4–18 years) were not significantly different than those in comparably obese subjects with no apparent mutations of the leptin receptor *(8)*. Interestingly, the body fat content is higher in *heterozygous carriers of LEPR mutations* than in their wild-type relatives *(8)*. Leptin treatment is ineffective.

2-Proopiomelanocortin (POMC) Deficiency

POMC/CART neurons are activated by leptin (Fig. 1). In contrast to CART, there is clear evidence that POMC peptides play critical roles in feeding behaviour. POMC is processed by prohormone convertases 1/3 and 2 into five biologically active proteins: adrenocorticotropic hormone (ACTH), alpha-, beta-, and gamma-melanocyte-stimulating hormone (MSH), and beta-endorphin. Mouse models with disruption of both alleles of the *POMC* gene are characterized by obesity, defective adrenal development, and altered pigmentation (19,20). Krude and colleagues provided the first description of human obesity associated with congenital deficiency of all *POMC* gene products (21). To date, six patients carrying either homozygous or compound heterozygous *POMC* mutations have been reported. Patients with complete POMC deficiency present in early life with hypoadrenalism secondary to ACTH deficiency, leading to hypoglycaemia, jaundice, and in one case neonatal death associated with severe liver cholestasis. Treatment with glucocorticoids reverses hypocortisolemia in these patients, but they develop severe early-onset obesity associated with hyperphagia.

As a result of the lack of ligand for melanocortin 1 receptors, POMC-deficient patients of European ancestry have pale skin and red hair (21). However, two subjects of Turkish or Algerian origin had normal hair and skin pigmentation despite congenital POMC deficiency (22,23). Chemical analysis of hair pigment revealed an increased production of both pheomelanin and eumelanin, but these subtle pigmentary features were not distinguishable during a clinical examination (23). This observation is concordant with a polygenic control of hair and skin pigmentation (24) and suggests that the molecular screening of POMC can be considered in patients with early-onset adrenal insufficiency and obesity, even in the presence of normal pigmentation.

A Turkish pedigree including 1 homozygous and 12 heterozygous carriers of the C6906del mutation of POMC was recently reported (22). The mutation was predicted to lead to the loss of all POMC-derived products. Interestingly, 11 of 12 heterozygous carriers were obese or overweight, strongly suggesting that loss of one copy of the POMC gene predisposes to obesity (22).

Heterozygosity for a variety of mutations in the region encoding alpha-MSH (25) or beta-MSH (26,27) is also associated with a high risk of obesity. A missense mutation (R236G) disrupting the dibasic cleavage site between beta-MSH and beta-endorphin resulted in a fusion protein that binds to the melanocortin 4 receptor (MC4R) but has reduced ability to activate it (28). This mutation was fourfold more prevalent in subjects with early-onset obesity than in lean controls (28).

3-Proprotein Convertase 1 Deficiency

Prohormone convertase 1/3 (*PCSK1*) represents the major processing enzyme of prohormones involved in the regulated secretory pathway. This enzyme converts prohormones (like proinsulin, proglucagon, or pro-POMC) into functional hormones that regulate central and/or peripheral energy metabolism. To date, three patients with monogenic forms of human obesity due to *PCSK1* deficiency have been described (29–31). Complete *PCSK1* deficiency due to compound heterozygous or homozygous mutations leads to early-onset obesity (29–31), hyperphagia (31), reactive hypoglycemia (29,30), and an increased ratio of proinsuiln to insulin (29–31). In addition, PC1/3 mutations are associated with an enteropathy with diarrhea, suggesting that enteroendocrine cell expression of PC1/3 is essential for the normal absorptive function of the human small intestine (30,31). Family members who are heterozygous for PC1/3 mutations are clinically unaffected and not obese (29–31). In contrast mice heterozygous for a *PCSK1* mutation are characterized by an intermediate phenotype (32): N222D-heterozygous mice had increased body fat content compared to wild-type mice.

4-Melanocortin 4 Receptor Deficiency

Of the five melanocortin receptors, only the melanocortin 4 receptor has been described as pivotal in the control of energy balance in rodents. The melanocortin 4 receptor is a seven transmembrane-spanning α-helices protein of the class A, G-protein-coupled receptors that include rhodopsin and the adrenergic receptors. Targeted disruption of the melanocortin-4 receptor results in an allelic dosage-dependent obesity phenotype in mice *(33)*.

The first cases of human obesity caused by heterozygous *MC4R* mutations were identified in 1998 *(34,35)*. Since then, more than 100 mutations in the coding sequence of *MC4R* have been reported to cause familial forms of obesity. The prevalence of *MC4R* pathogenic mutations has been reported to be as high as 5.8% in a cohort of children with extreme obesity and consanguinity *(36)*, but more commonly approximates 2% in more general obesity cohorts of European origin *(37,38)*. In contrast, pathogenic mutations are found in only 0.1% of the European general population *(39,40)*. Indeed, the penetrance of obesity in heterozygous mutated individuals is not complete and non-obese mutation carriers have been occasionally described *(37,41,42)*. Modifying factors like gender or generational environment have been proposed to modulate substantially the obesity phenotype associated with partial *MC4R* deficiency *(37,43)*. In contrast, homozygous or compound heterozygous pathogenic mutations lead to an obligatory severe obesity phenotype *(36,37,44)*. Co-dominance is therefore the most likely pattern of inheritance in case of *MC4R* deficiency *(36,37)*.

MC4R deficiency is associated with early-onset hyperphagia (often in the first year of life) and subsequent rapid increase in fat mass during childhood *(36)*. However, hyperphagia and body fat accumulation are also observed in adulthood (mean BMIz homozygotes +4.8–5.0, heterozygotes +2.8) *(8,37)*. Body fat mass averages 42 and 50%, respectively, in heterozygotes and homozygotes. Accelerated linear growth and tall stature are apparent within the first year of life, possibly due to exaggerated secretion of insulin associated with early-onset severe obesity; serum IGF-1 is normal *(36)*. Bone density is increased approximately 1.5 SD. Serum and urinary cortisol and serum lipids are normal and the leptin levels correlate with fat mass. Gonadotropin secretion and pubertal development are also appropriate for age. *MC4R* deficiency is paradoxically associated with lower systolic and diastolic blood pressure (melanocortinergic signalling modulates the control of blood pressure through an insulin-independent mechanism) *(45)*.

Up to 80% of pathogenic mutations in *MC4R* cause an intracellular retention of the abnormal receptor, but mutations affecting only agonist/antagonist-binding affinity or even causing constitutive receptor activation have also been reported *(46–48)*. Most *MC4R* mutations are more likely to result in obesity through haplo-insufficiency *(47)* with the exception of the D90N mutation, which has a dominant-negative effect due to abnormal receptor dimerization *(49)*.

MC4R-deficient obese children treated with exercise counselling and behavioural and nutritional therapy initially lose weight but fail to maintain weight loss after discontinuation of treatment *(50)*. No specific treatment currently exists to reverse the *MC4R* deficiency-associated obesity phenotype. Nevertheless, small-molecule MC4R agonists might provide a personalized treatment for *MC4R*-deficient patients *(51)*. Interestingly, a recent case report suggests that early diagnosis of MC4R deficiency followed up by lifestyle intervention may prevent the development of obesity *(52)*.

II-MONOGENIC OBESITY WITH NEUROLOGICAL FEATURES

1-Brain-Derived Neurotrophic Factor and Its Receptor TrkB

Brain-derived neurotrophic factor (BDNF) and its receptor tropomyosin-related kinase B (TrkB) are involved in proliferation, survival, and differentiation of neurons during development and postnatal synaptic plasticity in the central nervous system, especially in hypothalamic neurons; BDNF is expressed at high levels in the ventromedial hypothalamus, where it is regulated by nutritional state and MC4R signalling. Partial deficiency of BDNF or TrkB in mice increases food intake and fat deposition *(53–55)*. In addition, BDNF haplo-insufficiency induces abnormalities in behavioural and locomotor activity *(53,54)*.

Human BDNF haplo-insufficiency was first described in a 8-year-old girl who harboured a de novo chromosomal inversion, 46,XX,inv(11)(p13p15.3), which is the region encompassing *BDNF*. Clinical phenotypes included hyperphagia, severe obesity, impaired cognitive function, and hyperactivity *(56)*. Hyperphagia and obesity are also observed in a subgroup of patients with the WAGR syndrome (the main clinical features are Wilms' tumor, aniridia, genitourinary anomalies, and mental retardation). This syndrome is due to heterozygous, variably sized deletions on chromosome 11p14.1, in the vicinity of the *BDNF* gene. Han and colleagues demonstrated that 58% of the 11p heterozygous deletions they analyzed included the *BDNF* gene. These caused a 50% reduction in serum BDNF concentrations. In patients with the WAGR syndrome and *BDNF* deletions, 100% were obese; in contrast, the rate of obesity was 20% in those without *BDNF* deletions, which corresponds to the obesity prevalence in the United States *(57)*. A child with severe obesity, hyperactivity, and impairments in short-term memory, learning, and nociception was found to be a de novo carrier of a *NTRK2* (the gene coding for TrkB) missense mutation (Y722C) that markedly impaired receptor autophosphorylation and signalling to MAP kinase *(58,59)*.

2-Single-Minded 1 Transcription Factor

SIM1, the mammalian homologue of *Drosophila sim,* is a transcription factor playing a major role in neuronal differentiation of the paraventricular nucleus of the hypothalamus, a critical brain region for food intake regulation. Mice haplo-insufficient for *Sim1* develop hyperphagia and early-onset obesity *(60)*. Holder and colleagues described a de novo balanced translocation disrupting *SIM1* in a patient with hyperphagia and severe obesity *(61)*. Additional evidence of a role of *SIM1* haplo-insufficiency in human obesity was provided by the finding of rare non-synonymous *SIM1* mutations in severely obese patients (6/379) in comparison with lean subjects (0/378) *(62)*. Patients with obesity and a Prader–Willi-like (PWL) syndrome harbour interstitial deletions in the 6q16 region that contains *SIM1*gene *(63)*. The critical region for 6q PWL syndrome encompasses about 10 genes or gene prediction apart from *SIM1 (63)*, but recent data have more specifically linked SIM1 haplo-insufficiency with the PWL syndrome *(64)*.

III-A CONTINUUM BETWEEN MONOGENIC AND POLYGENIC OBESITY?

Up till now, eight genes (*LEP, LEPR, MC4R, POMC, PCSK1, BDNF, NTRK2,* and *SIM1*) have been convincingly linked to human monogenic obesity. In addition, the recent wave of genome-wide association studies (GWAS) has increased our knowledge of the polygenic background of more common forms of obesity *(65)*. A striking observation from GWAS is the existence of a partially overlapping continuum between monogenic and polygenic forms of obesity. At least five genes causing monogenic obesity also increase the risk for polygenic obesity. They are *MC4R (66,67)*, *POMC (68)*, *PCSK1 (69)*, *BDNF (70)*, and *SIM1 (71)*. The case of *MC4R*, a "three-headed" Cerberus obesity gene, is really illustrative from this point of view. Whereas loss-of-function mutations in the *MC4R* gene are the commonest cause of monogenic forms of obesity *(36)*, the two infrequent gain-of-function V103I and I251L coding non-synonymous polymorphisms have been associated with protection against obesity *(66)*. Furthermore, a SNP located 188 kb downstream of the *MC4R*-coding sequence has been consistently associated with a modest increase in the risk for obesity *(67)* and an altered eating behaviour pattern *(72)*.

CONCLUSIONS AND PERSPECTIVES

Candidate gene approaches based on information from obesity mouse models have shown that defects in eight genes involved in the neuronal differentiation of the paraventricular nucleus and in the leptin/melanocortin pathway lead to monogenic forms of early-onset severe obesity with hyperphagia as a key feature (Fig. 1). Elucidation of these genes delineates obesity as an inherited disorder of central regulation of food intake (73). Recent progress in the elucidation of polygenic predisposition to obesity also points to a key role of the central nervous system in body weight regulation (65). This is not totally surprising, since food intake-related parameters are heritable (74) and are strongly correlated to body mass index (75).

It remains for us to establish the proportion of "random" obese patients from different ethnic backgrounds who carry rare pathogenic mutations in these eight genes. The presence of specific features in some of these obese subjects (such as a low level of circulating leptin despite severe obesity, a susceptibility to infections, intestinal dysfunction, reactive hypoglycaemia, red hair and pale skin, adrenal insufficiency) can guide our approach to gene sequencing (Fig. 2).

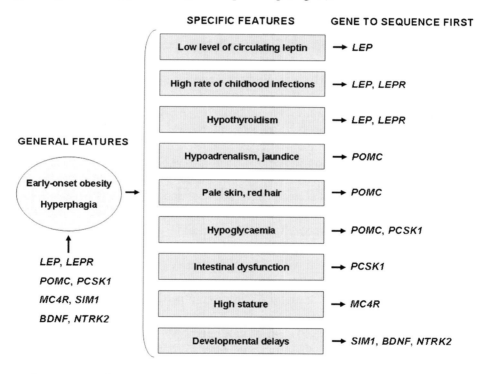

Fig. 2. Monogenic gene screening strategies during clinical examination. Early-onset obesity and hyperphagia are general features of monogenic obesity. Specific features can be useful to prioritize which gene can be sequenced first.

The most effective preventive strategy may be stringent restriction of food access restriction for monogenic mutation carriers. This will require the training and active participation of the parents and the identification of critical environmental components (physical activity, rural/urban environment, physical activity, dietary profile, tobacco consumption, family structure, socioeconomic status, social network, and gender) that modulate the penetrance of obesity associated with pathogenic mutations. Beyond the eight currently known genes, the high occurrence of Mendelian patterns of inheritance observed in multigenerational pedigrees with extreme obesity suggests that many monogenic cases remain to be elucidated (76).

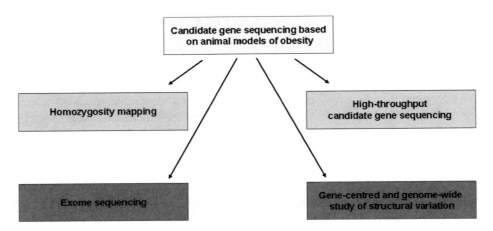

Fig. 3. Past and ongoing strategies for the identification of novel obesity single gene disorders.

Several innovative strategies may shortly lead to a more exhaustive picture of monogenic obesity (Fig. 3). High-resolution homozygosity mapping in large consanguineous pedigrees is a powerful approach to discover novel obesity loci with a recessive mode of inheritance, as recently exemplified in syndromic forms of obesity *(77)*. High-throughput gene resequencing strategies are now available with the new generation of sequencers (Illumina/Solexa Genome Analyzer, Roche SOLID) and can be used in different situations: candidate gene approach *(78)* (e.g. 103 genes are associated with a frank obesity phenotype in mouse models of obesity and represent valuable candidate genes for mutation screening in extremely obese humans); genes identified from genome-wide association studies for BMI and obesity; and resequencing in regions of homozygosity *(79)* or regions with evidence of linkage in multiple independent samples *(80)*. Exome capture and parallel sequencing strategies in carefully selected unrelated cases and controls have proven successful for gene identification *(81)* and this approach should be successfully extended in the future to pedigrees with extreme obesity and a Mendelian pattern of inheritance. Almost 20% of the heritable variation in gene expression has been attributed to structural variation (e.g. copy number variations) *(82)*. Recently, a 45 kb deletion in the *NEGR1* gene region has been associated with polygenic obesity risk *(83)*. Structural variation has been recently linked to Mendelian disorders *(84)*; gene-centred (e.g. the currently identified monogenic obesity genes) or genome-wide studies of structural variation in pedigrees may help to identify additional Mendelian obesity genes.

Although we are aware that the elucidation of monogenic forms of obesity is only a first step in a better prevention and management of this epidemic disease; it should provide novel hypotheses and bio-markers that should help us to translate to the era of genomic personalized medicine.

REFERENCES

1. Olshansky SJ, Passaro DJ, Hershow RC, et al. A potential decline in life expectancy in the United States in the 21st century. N Engl J Med. 17 Mar 2005;352(11):1138–45.
2. Wardle J, Carnell S, Haworth CM, Plomin R. Evidence for a strong genetic influence on childhood adiposity despite the force of the obesogenic environment. Am J Clin Nutr. Feb 2008;87(2):398–404.
3. Sturm R. Increases in morbid obesity in the USA: 2000–2005. Publ Health. Jul 2007;121(7):492–96.
4. Stunkard AJ, Foch TT, Hrubec Z. A twin study of human obesity. J Am Med Assoc. 4 Jul 1986;256(1):51–54.
5. Montague CT, Farooqi IS, Whitehead JP, et al. Congenital leptin deficiency is associated with severe early-onset obesity in humans. Nature. 1997;387(6636):903–8.
6. Hofker M, Wijmenga C. A supersized list of obesity genes. Nat Genet. Feb 2009;41(2):139–140.
7. Clement K, Vaisse C, Lahlou N, et al. A mutation in the human leptin receptor gene causes obesity and pituitary dysfunction. Nature. 1998;392(6674):398–401.

8. Farooqi IS, Wangensteen T, Collins S, et al. Clinical and molecular genetic spectrum of congenital deficiency of the leptin receptor. N Engl J Med. 18 Jan 2007;356(3):237–47.

9. Ozata M, Ozdemir IC, Licinio J. Human leptin deficiency caused by a missense mutation: multiple endocrine defects, decreased sympathetic tone, and immune system dysfunction indicate new targets for leptin action, greater central than peripheral resistance to the effects of leptin, and spontaneous correction of leptin-mediated defects. J Clin Endocrinol Metab. Oct 1999;84(10):3686–95.

10. Farooqi IS, Matarese G, Lord GM, et al. Beneficial effects of leptin on obesity, T cell hyporesponsiveness, and neuroendocrine/metabolic dysfunction of human congenital leptin deficiency. J Clin Invest. Oct 2002;110(8):1093–103.

11. Licinio J, Caglayan S, Ozata M, et al. Phenotypic effects of leptin replacement on morbid obesity, diabetes mellitus, hypogonadism, and behavior in leptin-deficient adults. Proc Natl Acad Sci USA. 30 Mar 2004;101(13):4531–36.

12. Farooqi IS, Bullmore E, Keogh J, Gillard J, O'Rahilly S, Fletcher PC. Leptin regulates striatal regions and human eating behavior. Science. 7 Sept 2007;317(5843):1355.

13. Licinio J, Ribeiro L, Busnello JV, et al. Effects of leptin replacement on macro- and micronutrient preferences. Int J Obes (Lond). Dec 2007;31(12):1859–63.

14. Gibson WT, Farooqi IS, Moreau M, et al. Congenital leptin deficiency due to homozygosity for the Delta133G mutation: report of another case and evaluation of response to four years of leptin therapy. J Clin Endocrinol Metab. Oct 2004;89(10):4821–26.

15. Matochik JA, London ED, Yildiz BO, et al. Effect of leptin replacement on brain structure in genetically leptin-deficient adults. J Clin Endocrinol Metab. May 2005;90(5):2851–54.

16. Paz-Filho GJ, Babikian T, Asarnow R, et al. Leptin replacement improves cognitive development. PLoS ONE. 2008;3(8):e3098.

17. Farooqi IS, Keogh JM, Kamath S, et al. Partial leptin deficiency and human adiposity. Nature. 1 Nov 2001;414(6859):34–35.

18. Heymsfield SB, Greenberg AS, Fujioka K, et al. Recombinant leptin for weight loss in obese and lean adults: a randomized, controlled, dose-escalation trial. J Am Med Assoc. 27 Oct 1999;282(16):1568–75.

19. Yaswen L, Diehl N, Brennan MB, Hochgeschwender U. Obesity in the mouse model of pro-opiomelanocortin deficiency responds to peripheral melanocortin. Nat Med. Sept 1999;5(9):1066–70.

20. Challis BG, Coll AP, Yeo GS, et al. Mice lacking pro-opiomelanocortin are sensitive to high-fat feeding but respond normally to the acute anorectic effects of peptide-YY(3–36). Proc Natl Acad Sci USA. 30 Mar 2004;101(13):4695–700.

21. Krude H, Biebermann H, Luck W, Horn R, Brabant G, Gruters A. Severe early-onset obesity, adrenal insufficiency and red hair pigmentation caused by POMC mutations in humans. Nat Genet. 1998;19(2):155–57.

22. Farooqi IS, Drop S, Clements A, et al. Heterozygosity for a POMC-null mutation and increased obesity risk in humans. Diabetes. Sep 2006;55(9):2549–53.

23. Clement K, Dubern B, Mencarelli M, et al. Unexpected endocrine features and normal pigmentation in a young adult patient carrying a novel homozygous mutation in the POMC gene. J Clin Endocrinol Metab. Dec 2008;93(12):4955–62.

24. Sulem P, Gudbjartsson DF, Stacey SN, et al. Two newly identified genetic determinants of pigmentation in Europeans. Nat Genet. Jul 2008;40(7):835–37.

25. Dubern B, Lubrano-Berthelier C, Mencarelli M, et al. Mutational analysis of the pro-opiomelanocortin gene in French obese children led to the identification of a novel deleterious heterozygous mutation located in the alpha-melanocyte stimulating hormone domain. Pediatr Res. Feb 2008;63(2):211–16.

26. Lee YS, Challis BG, Thompson DA, et al. A POMC variant implicates beta-melanocyte-stimulating hormone in the control of human energy balance. Cell Metab. Feb 2006;3(2):135–40.

27. Biebermann H, Castaneda TR, van Landeghem F, et al. A role for beta-melanocyte-stimulating hormone in human body-weight regulation. Cell Metab. Feb 2006;3(2):141–46.

28. Challis BG, Pritchard LE, Creemers JW, et al. A missense mutation disrupting a dibasic prohormone processing site in pro-opiomelanocortin (POMC) increases susceptibility to early-onset obesity through a novel molecular mechanism. Hum Mol Genet. 15 Aug 2002;11(17):1997–2004.

29. Jackson RS, Creemers JW, Ohagi S, et al. Obesity and impaired prohormone processing associated with mutations in the human prohormone convertase 1 gene. Nat Genet. 1997;16(3):303–6.

30. Jackson RS, Creemers JW, Farooqi IS, et al. Small-intestinal dysfunction accompanies the complex endocrinopathy of human proprotein convertase 1 deficiency. J Clin Invest. Nov 2003;112(10):1550–60.

31. Farooqi IS, Volders K, Stanhope R, et al. Hyperphagia and early-onset obesity due to a novel homozygous missense mutation in prohormone convertase 1/3. J Clin Endocrinol Metab. Sep 2007;92(9):3369–73.

32. Lloyd DJ, Bohan S, Gekakis N. Obesity, hyperphagia and increased metabolic efficiency in Pc1 mutant mice. Hum Mol Genet. 1 Jun 2006;15(11):1884–93.

33. Huszar D, Lynch CA, Fairchild-Huntress V, et al. Targeted disruption of the melanocortin-4 receptor results in obesity in mice. Cell. 10 Jan 1997;88(1):131–41.

34. Vaisse C, Clement K, Guy-Grand B, Froguel P. A frameshift mutation in human MC4R is associated with a dominant form of obesity. Nat Genet. 1998;20(2):113–114.

35. Yeo GS, Farooqi IS, Aminian S, Halsall DJ, Stanhope RG, O'Rahilly S. A frameshift mutation in MC4R associated with dominantly inherited human obesity. Nat Genet. Oct 1998;20(2):111–112.

36. Farooqi IS, Keogh JM, Yeo GS, Lank EJ, Cheetham T, O'Rahilly S. Clinical spectrum of obesity and mutations in the melanocortin 4 receptor gene. N Engl J Med. 2003;348(12):1085–95.

37. Stutzmann F, Tan K, Vatin V, et al. Prevalence of melanocortin-4 receptor deficiency in Europeans and their age-dependent penetrance in multigenerational pedigrees. Diabetes. Sep 2008;57(9):2511–18.

38. Calton MA, Ersoy BA, Zhang S, et al. Association of functionally significant Melanocortin-4 but not Melanocortin-3 receptor mutations with severe adult obesity in a large North American case-control study. Hum Mol Genet. 15 Mar 2009;18(6):1140–47.

39. Hinney A, Bettecken T, Tarnow P, et al. Prevalence, spectrum, and functional characterization of melanocortin-4 receptor gene mutations in a representative population-based sample and obese adults from Germany. J Clin Endocrinol Metab. May 2006;91(5):1761–69.

40. Alharbi KK, Spanakis E, Tan K, et al. Prevalence and functionality of paucimorphic and private MC4R mutations in a large, unselected European British population, scanned by meltMADGE. Hum Mutat. Mar 2007;28(3):294–302.

41. Vaisse C, Clement K, Durand E, Hercberg S, Guy-Grand B, Froguel P. Melanocortin-4 receptor mutations are a frequent and heterogeneous cause of morbid obesity. J Clin Invest. 2000;106(2):253–62.

42. Farooqi IS, Yeo GS, Keogh JM, et al. Dominant and recessive inheritance of morbid obesity associated with melanocortin 4 receptor deficiency. J Clin Invest. Jul 2000;106(2):271–79.

43. Dempfle A, Hinney A, Heinzel-Gutenbrunner M, et al. Large quantitative effect of melanocortin-4 receptor gene mutations on body mass index. J Med Genet. Oct 2004;41(10):795–800.

44. Lubrano-Berthelier C, Le Stunff C, Bougneres P, Vaisse C. A homozygous null mutation delineates the role of the melanocortin-4 receptor in humans. J Clin Endocrinol Metab. May 2004;89(5):2028–32.

45. Greenfield JR, Miller JW, Keogh JM, et al. Modulation of blood pressure by central melanocortinergic pathways. N Engl J Med. 1 Jan 2009;360(1):44–52.

46. Lubrano-Berthelier C, Durand E, Dubern B, et al. Intracellular retention is a common characteristic of childhood obesity-associated MC4R mutations. Hum Mol Genet. 2003;12(2):145–53.

47. Yeo GS, Lank EJ, Farooqi IS, Keogh J, Challis BG, O'Rahilly S. Mutations in the human melanocortin-4 receptor gene associated with severe familial obesity disrupts receptor function through multiple molecular mechanisms. Hum Mol Genet. 1 Mar 2003;12(5):561–74.

48. Xiang Z, Litherland SA, Sorensen NB, et al. Pharmacological characterization of 40 human melanocortin-4 receptor polymorphisms with the endogenous proopiomelanocortin-derived agonists and the agouti-related protein (AGRP) antagonist. Biochemistry. 13 Jun 2006;45(23):7277–88.

49. Biebermann H, Krude H, Elsner A, Chubanov V, Gudermann T, Gruters A. Autosomal-dominant mode of inheritance of a melanocortin-4 receptor mutation in a patient with severe early-onset obesity is due to a dominant-negative effect caused by receptor dimerization. Diabetes. Dec 2003;52(12):2984–88.

50. Reinehr T, Hebebrand J, Friedel S, et al. Lifestyle intervention in obese children with variations in the melanocortin 4 receptor gene. Obesity (Silver Spring). Feb 2009;17(2):382–89.

51. Wikberg JE, Mutulis F. Targeting melanocortin receptors: an approach to treat weight disorders and sexual dysfunction. Nat Rev Drug Discov. 2008;7(4):307–23.

52. Melchior C, Kiess W, Dittrich K, Schulz A, Schoneberg T, Korner A. Slim despite a genetic predisposition for obesity–influence of environmental factors as chance? A case report. Dtsch Med Wochenschr. May 2009;134(20):1047–50.

53. Lyons WE, Mamounas LA, Ricaurte GA, et al. Brain-derived neurotrophic factor-deficient mice develop aggressiveness and hyperphagia in conjunction with brain serotonergic abnormalities. Proc Natl Acad Sci USA. 21 Dec 1999;96(26):15239–44.

54. Kernie SG, Liebl DJ, Parada LF. BDNF regulates eating behavior and locomotor activity in mice. EMBO J. 15 Mar 2000;19(6):1290–300.

55. Xu B, Goulding EH, Zang K, et al. Brain-derived neurotrophic factor regulates energy balance downstream of melanocortin-4 receptor. Nat Neurosci. Jul 2003;6(7):736–42.

56. Gray J, Yeo GS, Cox JJ, et al. Hyperphagia, severe obesity, impaired cognitive function, and hyperactivity associated with functional loss of one copy of the brain-derived neurotrophic factor (BDNF) gene. Diabetes. Dec 2006;55(12):3366–71.

57. Han JC, Liu QR, Jones M, et al. Brain-derived neurotrophic factor and obesity in the WAGR syndrome. N Engl J Med. 28 Aug 2008;359(9):918–27.

58. Yeo GS, Connie Hung CC, Rochford J, et al. A de novo mutation affecting human TrkB associated with severe obesity and developmental delay. Nat Neurosci. Nov 2004;7(11):1187–89.

59. Gray J, Yeo G, Hung C, et al. Functional characterization of human NTRK2 mutations identified in patients with severe early-onset obesity. Int J Obes (Lond). Feb 2007;31(2):359–64.

60. Michaud JL, Boucher F, Melnyk A, et al. Sim1 haploinsufficiency causes hyperphagia, obesity and reduction of the paraventricular nucleus of the hypothalamus. Hum Mol Genet. 2001;10(14):1465–73.

61. Holder JL Jr, Butte NF, Zinn AR. Profound obesity associated with a balanced translocation that disrupts the SIM1 gene. Hum Mol Genet. 2000;9(1):101–8.

62. Ahituv N, Kavaslar N, Schackwitz W, et al. Medical sequencing at the extremes of human body mass. Am J Hum Genet. Apr 2007;80(4):779–91.

63. Bonaglia MC, Ciccone R, Gimelli G, et al. Detailed phenotype-genotype study in five patients with chromosome 6q16 deletion: narrowing the critical region for Prader-Willi-like phenotype. Eur J Hum Genet. Dec 2008;16(12):1443–49.

64. Stutzmann F, Ghoussaini M, Couturier C, et al. Haplo-insufficiency of the SIM1 gene is related with Mendelian obesity and a Prader-Willi-like syndrome. EASD Meeting, Vienna, Austria, September 29–October 2. 2009.

65. Walley AJ, Asher JE, Froguel P. The genetic contribution to non-syndromic human obesity. Nat Rev Genet. Jul 2009;10(7):431–42.

66. Stutzmann F, Vatin V, Cauchi S, et al. Non-synonymous polymorphisms in melanocortin-4 receptor protect against obesity: the two facets of a Janus obesity gene. Hum Mol Genet. 1 Aug 2007;16(15):1837–44.

67. Loos RJ, Lindgren CM, Li S, et al. Common variants near MC4R are associated with fat mass, weight and risk of obesity. Nat Genet. Jun 2008;40(6):768–75.

68. Baker M, Gaukrodger N, Mayosi BM, et al. Association between common polymorphisms of the proopiomelanocortin gene and body fat distribution: a family study. Diabetes. Aug 2005;54(8):2492–96.

69. Benzinou M, Creemers JW, Choquet H, et al. Common nonsynonymous variants in PCSK1 confer risk of obesity. Nat Genet. Aug 2008;40(8):943–45.

70. Thorleifsson G, Walters GB, Gudbjartsson DF, et al. Genome-wide association yields new sequence variants at seven loci that associate with measures of obesity. Nat Genet. Jan 2009;41(1):18–24.

71. Traurig M, Mack J, Hanson RL, et al. Common variation in SIM1 is reproducibly associated with BMI in Pima Indians. Diabetes. Jul 2009;58(7):1682–89.

72. Stutzmann F, Cauchi S, Durand E, et al. Common genetic variation near MC4R is associated with eating behaviour patterns in European populations. Int J Obes (Lond). 2009;33(3):373–78. Epub 2009 Jan 20.

73. O'Rahilly S, Farooqi IS. Human obesity as a heritable disorder of the central control of energy balance. Int J Obes (Lond). Dec 2008;32(Suppl 7):S55–S61.

74. Wardle J, Carnell S. Appetite is a Heritable Phenotype Associated with Adiposity. Ann Behav Med. 2009;Epub 3 Sept 2009.

75. Fricker J, Fumeron F, Clair D, Apfelbaum M. A positive correlation between energy intake and body mass index in a population of 1312 overweight subjects. Int J Obes. 1989;13(5):673–81.

76. Stone S, Abkevich V, Hunt SC, et al. A major predisposition locus for severe obesity, at 4p15-p14. Am J Hum Genet. 2002;70:1459–68.

77. Harville HM, Held S, Diaz-Font A, et al. Identification of 11 Novel Mutations in 8 BBS Genes by High-Resolution Homozygosity Mapping. J Med Genet. Apr 2010;47(4):262–7.

78. Nejentsev S, Walker N, Riches D, Egholm M, Todd JA. Rare variants of IFIH1, a gene implicated in antiviral responses, protect against type 1 diabetes. Science. 17 Apr 2009;324(5925):387–89.

79. Reversade B, Escande-Beillard N, Dimopoulou A, et al. Mutations in PYCR1 cause cutis laxa with progeroid features. Nat Genet. Sep 2009;41(9):1016–21.

80. Kremer H, Cremers FP. Positional cloning of deafness genes. Methods Mol Biol. 2009;493:215–38.

81. Ng SB, Buckingham KJ, Lee C, et al. Exome sequencing identifies the cause of a Mendelian disorder. Nat Genet. 2010;42(1):30–35. Epub 13 Nov 2009.

82. Stranger BE, Forrest MS, Dunning M, et al. Relative impact of nucleotide and copy number variation on gene expression phenotypes. Science. 9 Feb 2007;315(5813):848–53.

83. Willer CJ, Speliotes EK, Loos RJ, et al. Six new loci associated with body mass index highlight a neuronal influence on body weight regulation. Nat Genet. Jan 2009;41(1):25–34.

84. Balikova I, Martens K, Melotte C, et al. Autosomal-dominant microtia linked to five tandem copies of a copy-number-variable region at chromosome 4p16. Am J Hum Genet. Jan 2008;82(1):181–87.

4 Syndromic Obesity

Andrea M. Haqq

CONTENTS

Key Words: Prader–Willi Syndrome, Albright's hereditary osteodystrophy (AHO), Bardet–Biedl, Alstrom, SIM1, BDNF

OVERVIEW

It is well established that genetic mutations or chromosomal abnormalities can lead to obesity. The term "syndromic obesity" is used to describe obese children and adults with mental retardation, dysmorphic features, organ-specific abnormalities, hyperphagia, and/or other signs of hypothalamic dysfunction *(1,2)*. Obesity syndromes may be inherited in either an autosomal or an X-linked pattern.

This chapter focuses on two of the most common obesity syndromes, Prader–Willi syndrome and Albright hereditary osteodystrophy, and highlights other obesity syndromes (Bardet–Biedl and Alstrom syndrome) whose pathogenesis has now been linked to dysfunction of the primary cilium. Finally, focus is given to three genes, *SIM1, BDNF*, and *TRKB*, all implicated in the development and neuronal plasticity of hypothalamic neurons (see Table 1).

PRADER–WILLI SYNDROME (PWS)

Overview: Prader–Willi syndrome (PWS) was originally described by Andrea Prader, Alexis Labhart, and Heinrich Willi in 1956 *(3)*. It is one of the most commonly recognized genetic obesity syndromes *(4)*.

From: *Contemporary Endocrinology: Pediatric Obesity: Etiology, Pathogenesis, and Treatment*
Edited by: M. Freemark, DOI 10.1007/978-1-60327-874-4_4,
© Springer Science+Business Media, LLC 2010

Table 1
Summary

	Overview	Incidence/ prevalence	Clinical features	Etiology	Diagnostic considerations	Treatment and future research
Prader–Willi syndrome (PWS)	Originally described in 1956 Common genetic obesity syndrome	Incidence of 1 in 10,000 to 1 in 15,000 live births	Characteristic facies, small hands and feet, hypopigmentation Hypotonia and FTT in newborn Short stature, hyperphagia, obesity, hypogonadism, delayed motor/cognitive development, sleep disturbances and behavior abnormalities in childhood	Lack of expression of paternally derived genes on chromosome 15q11-q13 Deletion (~70%), uniparental disomy (~20–30%), or imprinting center defect (~5%)	Consider in infant with hypotonia and FTT or obese child with short stature and hypogonadism All forms of PWS are detected by methylation analysis	Appropriate use and dosage of rhGH therapy Possible central adrenal insufficiency Regulation of ghrelin and design of specific ghrelin antagonists Understanding abnormalities leading to the abnormal partitioning of body fat in PWS Understanding autonomic nervous system function in PWS Understanding branched chain amino acid and fatty acid metabolic changes in PWS

Albright hereditary osteodystrophy (AHO)	Originally described in 1942	Incidence is approximately 1:20,000 individuals	Short stature, round face, obesity, brachydactyly, subcutaneous calcification, dental and sensorineural abnormalities Generalized hormonal resistance to PTH, TSH, GHRH, and gonadotropins Biochemical functional hypoparathyroidism (low Ca, high phosphate but with increased PTH levels) Pseudo-pseudohypopara-thyroidism is AHO phenotype with normocalcemia and no hormonal resistance	Heterozygous inactivating mutations in the GNAS1 gene on chromosome 20q13.3 Mutations can result in impaired expression of $G_s\alpha$ mRNA or dysfunctional $G_s\alpha$ proteins Genomic imprinting of GNAS1 explains variable phenotypes	Consider in cases of functional hypoparathyroidism (low Ca, high phosphate, with increased PTH levels), obesity, round face, brachydactyly, and mental retardation Hypomagnesemia and vitamin D deficiency should be ruled out	Treat with oral calcium supplements and 1,25-dihydroxyvitamin D Monitor blood chemistries and urine calcium excretion to avoid hypercalciuria

(Continued)

Table 1
(continued)

	Overview	Incidence/ prevalence	Clinical features	Etiology	Diagnostic considerations	Treatment and future research
Bardet–Biedel syndrome (BBS)	Originally described in 1866	Rare Prevalence is 1 in 13,500 to 1 in 125,000 Depends on geographic region	Progressive rod–cone dystrophy Obesity in first year of life Post-axial polydactyly Primary hypogonadism GU and renal abnormalities	Rare recessive, genetically heterogeneous condition 12 genes (BBS1–12) implicated Defect in primary cilia and intraflagellar transport	Diagnosis often delayed until vision deteriorates Major cause of mortality is renal disease Association with renal cell carcinoma may warrant monitoring	Treatment of renal disease includes dialysis or transplantation Further studies needed to understand and identify key defective pathways
Alstrom syndrome (ALMS)	Rare multiorgan disorder first described in 1959	Prevalence of <1:100,000 ~450 cases described	Progressive rod–cone dystrophy leading to juvenile blindness Sensorineural hearing loss Early-onset childhood obesity Diabetes Adult short stature Mortality due to cardiac failure secondary to dilated cardiomyopathy or renal failure	ALMS1 gene on chromosome 2p13 Eighty different ALMS1 mutations reported Defect in centrosomes or basal bodies of cilia	Clinical features manifest during teen years Often confused with other diagnoses Presence of dilated cardiomyopathy and early hearing loss and absence of digit abnormalities distinguish from BBS	No treatment that will cure ALMS or delay disease progression Management of photophobia Close cardiac monitoring May require insulin or metformin

SIM1 deletion syndrome	Originally described in 2000	Five individuals reported in the literature	Similar phenotype to PWS – hypotonia, obesity, hyperphagia, developmental delay, almond-shaped eyes, strabismus, thin upper lip, hypogonadism, short extremities. Cardiac and neurological abnormalities distinguish SIM1 from PWS	SIM1 is a member of the basic helix-loop-helix period aryl hydrocarbon receptor family. Expressed in the supraoptic and paraventricular nuclei of the hypothalamus. SIM1 gene may function downstream of the MC4R to control energy balance	Consider SIM1 deletion syndrome in patients with PWS-like features but a normal PWS testing. Most patients with SIM1 deletion have a 6q16.2 deletion	Further studies are needed to examine the relationship between common variants of SIM1 and body weight gain
BDNF and tropomyosin-related kinase B (TrkB)	First described in 2006	Rare	Hyperphagia, morbid obesity, and complex neurobehavioral phenotype including impaired cognition, memory, and nociception	BDNF acting through TrkB receptor regulates the development, differentiation, and survival of neurons. BDNF haploinsufficiency in mice or humans leads to morbid obesity and hyperphagia	Consider BDNF or TrkB deficiency in patients with morbid obesity and hyperphagia	Further research needed to understand the role of BDNF, and its receptor, TrkB, in the regulation of energy balance in humans

Incidence: PWS occurs in both sexes and all races with a frequency of approximately 1 in 10,000 to 1 in 15,000 live births *(4)*.

Clinical Features: A characteristic facial appearance is noted in PWS, including narrow bifrontal diameter, almond-shaped palpebral fissures, and down-turned mouth with a thin upper lip. Small, narrow hands with a straight ulnar border and tapering fingers and short, broad feet are typical in Caucasians with this disorder *(4)*. One-third of patients with PWS are also fairer (lighter skin, hair, and eye color) than other members of their family. Newborns with PWS have hypotonia, poor suck, decreased arousal, and failure to thrive and often require tube feedings for several weeks to months. This period is followed by progressive obesity by 1–6 years of age, insatiable appetite, short stature secondary to deficient growth hormone (GH) secretion, further delayed motor and cognitive development, behavioral difficulties, and sleep disturbances. A recent report showed that as many as 60% of PWS patients have an insufficient ACTH response to metyrapone, consistent with central adrenal insufficiency *(5)*. Autonomic nervous system dysfunction is thought to be responsible for these individuals' thick, viscous saliva, high pain threshold, skin picking, and high threshold for vomiting *(6)*. Additional common features include strabismus and scoliosis and/or kyphosis.

Etiology: PWS is due to lack of expression of paternally derived genes on chromosome 15q11-q13 *(7)*. The genes within this region of the chromosome are imprinted: imprinted genes are modified by methylation or histone acetylation in different ways depending on the gender of the parent from whom they were inherited. The majority of PWS cases (~70%) are due to deletions spanning 4–4.5 Mb of the paternal 15q11-q13. The next most common cause of PWS is maternal uniparental disomy (UPD) (20–30%), which is due to maternal meiotic nondisjunction followed by mitotic loss of a single paternal chromosome 15 postzygotically. PWS caused by deletions or UPD does not recur in sibs. Additionally, two types of imprinting defects occur in ~5% of cases; in one case there is a submicroscopic deletion of a genetic element called the imprinting center (IC): in the other case, there is an abnormal imprint but no detectable mutation *(8,9)*. There is an up to 50% risk of recurrence in these latter cases and prenatal diagnosis may be possible. In general, those individuals with UPD or IC defects have a milder phenotype than those with deletions *(4)*.

The exact gene(s) responsible for PWS is not known. However, the *SNURF-SNRPN* gene is one major candidate gene that may play a role in causing PWS. This gene locus is very complex, spanning ~465 kb and consisting of >148 exons, which can undergo alternative splicing *(10)*. Several additional paternally expressed imprinted genes have been identified in 15q11-q13 including NDN (encoding NECDIN protein) and MAGEL2 and MKRN3 (Makorin 3) *(11–13)*. Recently, additional genes and transcripts have been identified in this region, but their involvement in the etiology of PWS is unknown. Except for the function of NDN in neural differentiation and survival, the function of these genes is poorly understood. One recent report describes gene expression studies of a novel translocation t(4;15)(q27;q11.2) associated with Prader–Willi syndrome and concludes that the snoRNA, PWCR1/HBII-85, may be the cause of PWS in this individual *(14)*. The function of known snoRNAs is to guide $2'$-O-ribose methylation of mainly ribosomal RNA; however, this novel imprinted snoRNA has no known target. It is postulated that snoRNAs might be involved in the posttranscriptional regulation of a gene responsible for PWS.

Diagnostic Considerations: A diagnosis of PWS should be considered in infants with hypotonia and failure to thrive at birth and developmental delays, mild cognitive impairment, early childhood-onset obesity, hypogonadism with genital hypoplasia, short stature, and behavior disorders in early childhood. All three forms of PWS are detected by methylation analysis. If the methylation pattern is abnormal (signifying one parent of origin), then fluorescence in situ hybridization (FISH) can be used to confirm a deletion and/or microsatellite probes may be used to verify maternal UPD. Note that high-resolution chromosome analysis alone is insufficient because false positives and false negatives have occurred with this method without FISH. Finally, an abnormal methylation pattern in the presence of normal FISH and uniparental disomy studies suggests an imprinting center mutation. Analysis for mutations in the imprinting center can be performed in a few select research laboratories on a research basis only.

Treatment and Future Research: The use of growth hormone (GH) in PWS is now FDA approved. GH treatment of PWS infants and children has been shown in randomized trials to exert favorable effects on growth, body mass index, body composition, and motor and cognitive development (15–17). Growth velocity is increased in childhood and final height augmented (18). GH reduces fat mass, increases lean body mass and bone mineral density, and increases resting energy expenditure (REE), with improved fatty acid oxidation (18–23). Improvements in physical strength, respiratory muscle hypotonia, and peripheral chemoreceptor sensitivity to carbon dioxide have also been reported (18,19,23). One study has also reported a trend toward improvement in overall sleep quality, including reduction in the number of hypopnea and apnea events with administration of GH (23). Further studies investigating the optimal dosage of growth hormone and use of growth hormone in children and adults with PWS are needed.

Controversy continues about whether growth hormone treatment causes an excess of mortality beyond that expected from PWS alone. There have been a total of approximately 28 cases of sudden death in PWS children undergoing treatment with GH (24,25). These sudden deaths have been concentrated in young children with a history of respiratory obstruction/infection or severe obesity (26–28) and have occurred early in the course of GH therapy. The exact cause of these sudden deaths has not been determined. Possibilities include impaired ventilatory responsiveness to hypercapnea and hypoxia, increased lymphoid tissue or tonsillar hyperplasia, and adrenal insufficiency. Alternatively, there is no true increased mortality above the baseline expected from the PWS diagnosis alone. Indeed, other studies suggest that GH increases ventilation responsiveness to carbon dioxide and improves sleep quality in children with PWS (23). Until studies definitively address these issues, a pre-treatment airway and sleep evaluation is recommended prior to, and possibly during, GH therapy. Finally, GH treatment should be initiated by experienced centers and the dose of GH adjusted to maintain insulin-like growth factor-I (IGF-I) levels in the normal range. Children receiving GH therapy should be monitored for potential side effects including glucose intolerance and worsening scoliosis.

Recent advances in the pathogenesis of PWS (detailed later) will foster the development of new therapeutic approaches for the control of hyperphagia and weight gain in this disorder.

1. Children and adults with PWS have high fasting and post-prandial levels of total ghrelin, an orexigenic peptide produced in the stomach. In contrast, total ghrelin levels are suppressed in children and adults with "exogenous" obesity or with obesity caused by mutations in leptin or the melanocortin-4 receptor (29–31). Young PWS infants, who have not yet developed hyperphagia or obesity, have median fasting total ghrelin levels similar to age- and sex-matched controls. However, a subset (33%) of young PWS is already hyperghrelinemic (32). The high circulating concentrations of ghrelin may be critical for the pathogenesis of weight gain in PWS because ghrelin stimulates appetite and weight gain in rodents and human adults. Octreotide treatment in children with PWS has been shown to decrease fasting ghrelin concentrations, but does not alter body weight (33–35). Octreotide, however, is a nonspecific inhibitor of ghrelin and, therefore, might have affected levels of additional weight-regulating neuropeptides. It will be important to develop future strategies that employ *specific* ghrelin antagonists, leading to sustained ghrelin suppression and weight loss in this population.

2. PWS individuals demonstrate abnormal partitioning of body fat and lean mass. Whole-body magnetic resonance imaging (MRI) has found PWS adults to have a greater fat mass relative to fat-free mass, but significantly less visceral adiposity compared to controls (36,37). Our group has also demonstrated higher total and high molecular weight adiponectin concentrations and increased ratios of HMW/total adiponectin and higher insulin sensitivity in PWS children compared to BMI-matched controls (38). The lack of visceral fat and the relative hyperadiponectinemia may protect PWS individuals against

metabolic complications of obesity such as insulin resistance, type 2 diabetes, and hypertriglyceridemia *(36)*. Future studies are needed to understand the abnormalities which lead to abnormal partitioning of body fat in PWS and its metabolic consequences.

3. Several features of PWS including abnormal temperature regulation, altered sleep control (excessive daytime somnolence and a primary abnormality of the circadian rhythm of rapid eye movement sleep), increased pain tolerance, decreased salivation and hypopigmentation suggest abnormalities in the autonomic nervous system (ANS). However, the evidence for ANS dysfunction is inconclusive. One study reported diminished parasympathetic nervous system function based on findings of higher resting pulse rates and lesser increases in diastolic blood pressure upon standing *(6)*. However, when controlling for body mass index (BMI), other studies report no differences in ANS function (control of heart rate and blood pressure) in PWS subjects *(39)*. Interestingly, necdin-null mice have abnormal outgrowth of sympathetic neurons predominantly from the superior cervical ganglion (the most rostral of the paravertebral sympathetic ganglions innervating the pupil, lacrimal and salivary glands, and cerebrum). Therefore, future studies examining the autonomic system in PWS will likely lead to further understanding of the autonomic nervous system's contribution to the control of energy homeostasis in PWS.

4. Finally, some preliminary evidence also points to alterations in fatty acid and branched chain amino acid metabolism in individuals with PWS (Haqq, unpublished). Future studies are needed to explore the roles of specific metabolites in the pathogenesis of obesity and insulin resistance in PWS.

ALBRIGHT HEREDITARY OSTEODYSTROPHY

Overview: Albright's hereditary osteodystrophy (AHO) was first described in 1942 in a child with short stocky build, round face, short metacarpals and metatarsals, and numerous areas of soft tissue calcification. These patients were hypocalcemic and hyperphosphatemic despite high serum levels of parathyroid hormone (PTH), and there was no calcemic or phosphaturic response after administration of parathyroid extract *(40)*. Thus, the disorder is associated with (variable) resistance of target organs (bone and kidney) to the actions of PTH (psuedohypoparathyroidism).

Incidence: The incidence of AHO is approximately 1:20,000 individuals.

Clinical Features: Subjects with pseudohypoparathyroidism type 1a (PHP type 1a) have a generalized form of hormonal resistance (resistance to PTH, thyroid stimulating hormone (TSH), growth hormone-releasing hormone, and gonadotropins) and a constellation of developmental defects that is referred to as AHO. This AHO phenotype includes short stature, round face, obesity, brachydactyly, and subcutaneous calcification. In some individuals, dental and sensorineural abnormalities have also been reported. Primary hypothyroidism (due to TSH resistance), GH deficiency (secondary to GHRH resistance), and hypogonadism (due to gonadotropin resistance) are common *(41)*. Hypocalcemia associated with PTH resistance can in some cases lead to nervous excitability, cramps, tetany, hyperreflexia, convulsions, and tetanic crisis. Some individuals with AHO are normocalcemic and lack hormone resistance; these cases are termed pseudo-pseudohypoparathyroidism *(42)*. Both isolated AHO and PHP type 1a can occur in the same family and are due to a functional tissue deficiency of $G_s\alpha$. Generalized obesity develops in 50–65% of AHO patients *(43)*. The etiology of the obesity is not clear; however, it is possible that loss of signaling from various G-protein-coupled receptors such as the melanocortin 4 receptor might lead to hyperphagia.

Etiology: Heterozygous inactivating mutations in the *GNAS1* gene on chromosome 20q13.3 form the basis for $G_s\alpha$ deficiency of patients with AHO, an autosomal dominant disorder *(44)*. The *GNAS1* gene consists of 13 exons and 3 alternate initial exons with different promoters allowing for formation of 4 different isoforms via alternative splicing *(45)*. Some mutations result in impaired expression of $G_s\alpha$ mRNA, while others result in dysfunctional $G_s\alpha$ proteins. Several lines of evidence suggest that genomic imprinting of *GNAS1* explains the variable phenotypes that occur with identical *GNAS1* gene defects. First, PHP type Ia and pseudo-PHP frequently occur in the same family, but not in the same generation. Second, nearly all cases of maternal transmission of $G_s\alpha$ deficiency lead to PHP type 1a, whereas paternal transmission of the same mutation leads to pseudo-PHP *(46,47)*; this suggests that variable AHO phenotypes originate from differential tissue-specific genomic imprinting.

Diagnostic Considerations: A diagnosis of AHO should be considered in an individual with functional hypoparathyroidism (hypocalcemia and hyperphosphatemia) and increased PTH concentrations or in those with clinical features of AHO such as obesity, round face, brachydactyly, or mental retardation. Hypomagnesemia and vitamin D deficiency should be ruled out as these states can mimic the biochemical features of AHO. Synthetic PTH (1–34) peptide is available and various protocols exist for diagnosis of AHO based on intravenous infusion of PTH and measurement of resulting urine cAMP, phosphorus, and creatinine concentrations. *GNAS1* gene analysis is also available through various commercial laboratories.

Treatment and Future Research: Treatment with oral calcium supplements and 1,25-dihydroxyvitamin D is needed to normalize calcium, phosphate, and PTH levels and thereby prevent hyperparathyroid bone disease. Blood chemistries and urine calcium excretion should be monitored at least yearly to avoid hypercalciuria. Although a number of defects in *GNAS1* are responsible for AHO, the molecular mechanisms underlying hormone resistance and imprinting defects remain incompletely understood. Further characterization of novel *GNAS1* defects will likely further our knowledge of this disorder, and additional characterization of the obese phenotype of AHO will likely aid in our understanding of the molecular mechanisms of body weight regulation.

BARDET–BIEDEL SYNDROME (BBS)

Overview: Four affected siblings with retinal dystrophy, obesity, and cognitive impairment were first described in 1866 by Laurence and Moon. The three males in this cohort also had small external genitalia and an abnormal gait *(48)*. A similar phenotype including polydactyly was then described by Bardet and Biedl *(49,50)*.

Incidence: BBS is rare; the prevalence ranges from 1 in 125,000–160,000 in Europe *(51,52)* to 1 in 13,500 in the Bedouin of Kuwait *(53)* and 1 in 17,500 in Newfoundland, Canada *(54)*.

Clinical Features: BBS is characterized by five primary features including progressive rod–cone dystrophy (93% prevalence), obesity (72%), post-axial polydactyly (extra digits) (69%), primary hypogonadism (98%), and genitourinary tract malformations and progressive renal dysfunction (24%). Additional secondary features include cognitive impairment (50%), speech delay (54%), behavior abnormalities (33%), hearing loss (21%), ataxia/imbalance (40%), type 2 diabetes (6%), and, occasionally, congenital heart disease (7%) *(54,55)*. Polycystic kidney disease and complications of obesity (type 2 diabetes, hypertension, and hypercholesterolemia) are the leading causes of premature death in BBS *(55)*. The obesity of BBS manifests as rapid progressive weight gain and hyperphagia in the first year of life and has been associated with reduced physical activity compared to obese controls; no differences in resting metabolic rate or body composition are reported *(56)*.

Etiology: BBS is a genetically heterogeneous condition inherited in a recessive manner. Little evidence of genotype–phenotype correlation is observed. In 2003, Ansley and colleagues were the first to propose that BBS was caused by a defect at the basal body of ciliated cells *(57)*. Thus far, 12 genes have been implicated in the etiology of BBS *(55)*. BBS 1, 2, 4, 5, 6, and 8 localize to the basal body and pericentriolar region; BBS 6, 10, and 12 are likely chaperones that facilitate protein folding and account for one-third of cases. BBS 3 (a member of the Ras superfamily of small GTP-binding proteins) and BBS 11 (an E3 ubiquitin ligase) encode known proteins *(58–65)* (see Table 1). BBS is probably caused by a defect in primary cilia and the intraflagellar transport (IFT) process. Although not proven, the renal abnormalities seen in BBS are thought to be secondary to disordered cilia function. This is supported by features of the oakridge polycystic kidney disease mouse mutant (or^{pkd})

which exhibits dilated proximal tubules and cysts and has short and malformed cilia *(66)*; the mutation in this mouse maps to a gene encoding polaris, a protein required for assembly of renal cilia. Ciliary defects in hypothalamic neurons may impair trafficking of leptin receptors and thereby reduce leptin signal transduction; in theory, this would facilitate the development of obesity in BBS *(67)*.

Diagnostic Considerations: The diagnosis of BBS is often delayed until visual deterioration manifests; night blindness typically emerges around 8 years of age, followed by loss of peripheral vision and blindness by 15 years of age *(55)*. Renal disease remains a major cause of mortality in BBS. Additionally, an excess of early-onset renal cell carcinomas in obligate carriers of BBS mutations suggests that BBS patients need to be carefully monitored for development of malignancies *(68)*. The majority of adults have obesity complicated by hypertension, type 2 diabetes mellitus, and dyslipidemia.

Treatment and Future Research: Chronic renal dialysis or transplantation is the only successful mode of managing renal disease in most patients. Further studies examining long-term outcomes after renal transplantation are needed. The precise role of BBS proteins in renal pathogenesis also needs to be further delineated. Additionally, the cilium is now understood to control many key developmental signaling cascades. For example, defects in ciliogenesis have now been implicated in effects on Sonic Hedgehog (Shh) signaling *(69)*. Further studies that lead to understanding of possible defective Shh signaling in the limb bud of BBS patients as a cause of their polydactyly are also needed. The etiology of the disordered satiety and obesity seen in BBS is not fully understood at this time. It is possible that BBS proteins function in ciliated hypothalamic neurons that integrate nutrient information to control energy homeostasis. In support of this theory, Davenport and colleagues recently showed that deletion of cilia from pro-opiomelanocortin (POMC)-expressing hypothalamic neurons led to obesity in mice *(70)*. It is important to identify these key defective pathways in BBS so that more effective therapeutic alternatives can be offered to patients in the future.

ALSTROM SYNDROME (AS)

Overview: Alstrom syndrome (AS), a rare autosomal recessive multiorgan disorder, was first described in 1959 *(71)*.

Incidence: AS has an estimated prevalence of <1:100,000 *(72)*. Approximately 450 cases have been described since first reported *(73)*.

Clinical Features: AS exhibits much phenotypic variability, even within families. Some characteristic features include progressive rod–cone dystrophy beginning in infancy and leading to juvenile blindness (90% by age 16 years), sensorineural hearing loss (89%; mean age of 5 years), early-onset childhood obesity (nearly 100%), and adult short stature (due to early rapid growth and early fusion of growth plates) *(74)*. Most patients have normal intelligence, although delayed fine and gross motor and language development is described in some *(73)*. Endocrinologic manifestations include hyperinsulinemia (92%) and acanthosis nigricans (68%), diabetes mellitus (median age of onset of 16 years; 82%), hypertriglyceridemia (nearly 100%), infertility (hypergonadotropic hypogonadism; 77%), increased androgen production and hirsutism in females, primary hypothyroidism, growth hormone deficiency, and bone-skeletal abnormalities *(73,74)*. In younger patients, mortality is primarily due to cardiac failure secondary to dilated cardiomyopathy *(72)*. In older subjects, renal failure is the most common cause of death *(73)*. Fibrosis in multiple organs has been reported.

Etiology: The *ALMS1* gene on chromosome 2p13 was identified by two independent research groups in 2002. *ALMS1* encodes a 4,169 amino acid protein which includes a large 47 amino acid tandem-repeat domain *(75,76)*. The function of the ALMS protein remains unknown. However, it is expressed ubiquitously throughout all organ tissues and is thought to be involved in the function of centrosomes or basal bodies *(77)*. In support of this theory, *ALMS1* knockout mice recapitulate many features of the human syndrome including obesity, hyperinsulinemia, hypogonadism, retinal degeneration, and renal dysfunction and demonstrate abnormal ciliary structure; this phenotype is rescued by a prematurely truncated N-terminal fragment of ALMS1 *(77,78)*. To date, approximately 80 different ALMS1 mutations, located primarily in exons 8, 10, and 16, have been implicated in AS *(79)*. The majority of mutations described are nonsense or frameshift abnormalities that are predicted to cause premature protein truncation; studies to date suggest no strong genotype–phenotype correlation *(79)*.

Diagnostic Considerations: Diagnosis can be challenging in young children as many of the characteristic clinical features (type 2 diabetes mellitus and hepatic, pulmonary, and renal dysfunction) do not manifest until the teenage years. Alstrom syndrome is often confused with other diagnoses early on. For example, photophobia in infancy might be misclassified as Leber congenital amaurosis or achromatopsia, and childhood obesity and type 2 DM often lead to an incorrect diagnosis of Bardet–Biedl syndrome (BBS). The presence of dilated cardiomyopathy, early hearing loss, and absence of digit abnormalities are often helpful in distinguishing between BBS and Alstrom syndrome. A diagnosis of Alstrom syndrome is proven when two *ALMS1* mutations (one from each parent) are identified in a patient. However, lack of genetic confirmation does not exclude this diagnosis and repeated clinical monitoring of these individuals is recommended.

Treatment and Future Research: Currently there is no treatment that will cure Alstrom syndrome or delay or reverse the progression of disease. Management of photophobia in young children with red-tinted glasses is helpful to alleviate distress with bright lights. Total vision loss should be anticipated and early development of Braille or other non-visual language skills is very important. Monitoring of cardiac function with echocardiography is essential in all patients; treatment with angiotensin-converting enzyme (ACE) inhibitors is indicated in those with cardiomyopathy. Weight management and exercise are important in managing the metabolic disorders in AS. Many patients eventually require insulin sensitizers (metformin and/or thiazolidinediones) or insulin therapy. Hormonal replacement with thyroxine and/or testosterone is useful when indicated. The benefits and risks of use of growth hormone therapy in AS are not fully understood at this time; thus, GH treatment is still considered investigational. Further elucidation of the function of ALMS1 will provide insight into the pathogenesis of AS and other common forms of obesity, diabetes, and retinal disease.

SIM1 DELETION SYNDROME

Overview: Human SIM1 (Single-minded) deletion syndrome caused by a de novo balanced translocation between chromosomes 1p22.1 and 6q16.2 in a young girl with early-onset obesity, hyperphagia, and increased linear growth was first described by Holder and colleagues in 2000 *(80)*.

Incidence: Five individuals with SIM1 deletion syndrome have been reported in the literature.

Clinical Features: Subjects with SIM1 deletions exhibit features in common with Prader–Willi syndrome including hypotonia, obesity, hyperphagia, developmental delay, almond-shaped eyes, strabismus, thin upper lip, hypogonadism, and short extremities. However, patients with SIM1 deletions may have additional findings including increased linear growth and cardiac (bicuspid aortic valve, aortic stenosis, right branch block) and neurological abnormalities (polygyria, leukomalacia, Arnold–Chiari malformation, seizures, and hearing loss).

Etiology: SIM1 is a mammalian homolog of the *Drosophila* transcription factor, Single-minded, a member of the basic helix-loop-helix period aryl hydrocarbon receptor family of proteins. Homozygous deletion of *Drosophila* Single-minded results in failure of formation of midline central nervous system structures *(81)*. The majority of patients with SIM1 deletion syndrome have a 6q16.2 deletion. In 2000, Holder et al. described a patient with profound obesity with a balanced translocation between chromosomes 1p22.1 and 6q16.2 which disrupted the SIM1 gene *(82)*. A mouse model of heterozygous SIM1 deletion also exhibits early-onset obesity with hyperphagia, increased linear growth, hyperinsulinemia, hyperleptinemia, normal energy expenditure, and a decreased number of neurons in the paraventricular nucleus (PVN) *(83)*. Further studies now show that the *Sim1* gene is expressed in the supraoptic (SON) and paraventricular nuclei (PVN) of the hypothalamus, both important areas involved in the regulation of body weight *(84)*. More recent studies show that SIM1 is required for terminal differentiation of the neurons in the PVN and SON nuclei of the hypothalamus and suggest that SIM1 might function downstream of the melanocortin-4 receptor to control energy balance *(85)*.

Diagnostic Considerations: Deletion of the 6q16.2 region and SIM1 gene deletion should be sought in patients who exhibit Prader–Willi syndrome-like features, but have a normal cytogenetic study of the 15q11-q12 region.

Treatment and Future Research: Several genome-wide scans in various populations have shown strong linkage of loci on chromosome 6q with obesity and type 2 diabetes-related traits *(86,87)*. One association study with common single-nucleotide polymorphisms (SNPs) in the *SIM1* gene was performed in two population-based cohorts, and mutations in SIM1 were not commonly found in these individuals with early-onset obesity; an association between P352T/A371V haplotype and BMI in males and in females homozygous for the P352T/A371V haplotype was found *(88)*. However, further studies to examine the relationship between common variants of SIM1 and body weight gain are needed.

BDNF AND TROPOMYOSIN-RELATED KINASE B

Overview: An 8-year-old girl with severe early-onset obesity, hyperactivity, impaired cognition, memory, and nociception due to haploinsufficiency of brain-derived neurotrophic factor (BDNF) was described in 2006 *(89)*. This child had a de novo chromosomal inversion 46, XX, inv(11)(p13p15.3), a region encompassing the BDNF gene, and reduced serum concentrations of BDNF. Another report described an obese, hyperphagic tall child with impairment in memory, cognition, and nociception with a heterozygous missense mutation in the neurotrophin receptor TrkB, the receptor of BDNF *(90)*. Interestingly, among persons with Wilms' tumor, aniridia, genitourinary anomalies, and mental retardation (WAGR) syndrome, BDNF haploinsufficiency is associated with lower serum BDNF concentrations and childhood-onset obesity *(91)*.

Incidence: Mutations in BDNF and TrkB are rare genetic causes of human obesity.

Clinical Features: BDNF or TrkB haploinsufficiency leads to hyperphagia, morbid obesity, and a complex neurobehavioral phenotype including impaired cognition, memory, and nociception.

Etiology: Acting through its receptor, tropomyosin-related kinase B (TrkB), BDNF regulates the development, differentiation, and survival of neurons *(92)*. BDNF is implicated in energy homeostasis; BDNF expression is reduced by fasting, and BDNF administration causes weight loss in wild-type mice via reduction in food intake *(93)*. BDNF haploinsufficiency in mice leads to hyperphagia and obesity and has been implicated in memory and various behavioral abnormalities *(94)*.

Diagnostic Considerations: BDNF or TrkB deficiency should be considered in individuals with early-onset morbid obesity and hyperphagia.

Treatment and Future Research: There is some evidence that BDNF-expressing neurons might lie downstream of melanocortin 4 (MC4) neuronal pathways, since BDNF mRNA levels are reduced in the ventromedial hypothalamus of MC4R knockout mice and levels are restored by administration of an MC4R agonist, MT-II *(93)*. Further research should elucidate the role of BDNF and its receptor, TrkB, in regulation of energy balance in humans. Data by Pelleymounter and colleagues provide evidence that BDNF might induce appetite suppression and weight loss via increases in hypothalamic 5-HIAA/5-HT *(95)*. It is possible that BDNF influences energy balance via effects on development of the hypothalamus or through modulation of synaptic plasticity in hypothalamic feeding circuits.

Understanding BDNF and TrkB's role in regulation of body weight will likely lead to novel therapeutic approaches for the treatment of human obesity.

CONCLUSIONS

Currently the obesity associated with these syndromes is managed by caloric restriction. The genetics involved in these syndromes is complex and multiple genes within a pathway can lead to the same clinical phenotype. In order to develop future effective and innovative obesity treatments, it will be imperative to further unravel the molecular defects leading to these various syndromic obese conditions.

ACKNOWLEDGMENTS

This work was supported by NIH grant 1K23-RR-021979 to AMH. I thank Dr. Seth Marks for his helpful editorial comments.

Editor's Comment

- One condition that can be confused with other syndromes associated with early-onset obesity (see also Chapter 3 by Meyre and Froguel) is the so-called *ROHHAD or ROHHADNET syndrome* (Ize-Ludlow et al., 2007; Bougneres et al., 2008). It is a complex multisystem disorder associated with rapid onset of hyperphagia and obesity at 1.5–4.3 years of age and progressive accumulation of fat in the face, trunk, and breasts. Interestingly, height velocity declines, suggesting a diagnosis of Cushing's syndrome. Yet there is neither plethora nor striae and the diurnal rhythm of plasma cortisol, the 24 h urine free cortisol levels, and the response to high-dose dexamethasone are normal. Plasma IGF-1 levels are low in some patients, and there is variable hyperprolactinemia and TSH dysregulation. Leptin levels are comparable to those of age-matched children with similar BMI. Gonadotropin levels are low and puberty is delayed or absent. Hypernatremia without classic diabetes insipidus occurs in one-half of subjects. Major associated problems include developmental delay, seizures, autonomic dysregulation (temperature instability, papillary dysfunction, and GI dysmotility), and central hypoventilation, which may lead to cardiopulmonary arrest. Ganglioneuromas of the adrenal and posterior mediastinum develop in at least one-half of patients; urine catecholamines, VMA, HVA, and plasma adrenal steroid levels are normal, and resection of the tumors in two patients caused no change in phenotype or biochemical parameters. The etiology of the ROHHAD syndrome is unclear. Phox 2 mutations in patients with congenital central hypoventilation and hypothalamic dysfunction may be associated with neural tumors but not with obesity.

Bougnéres P, Pantalone L, Linglart A, Rothenbühler A, Le Stunff C. Endocrine manifestations of the rapid-onset obesity with hypoventilation, hypothalamic, autonomic dysregulation, and neural tumor syndrome in childhood. J Clin Endocrinol Metab. 2008 Oct;93(10):3971–80. Epub 2008 Jul 15.

Ize-Ludlow D, Gray JA, Sperling MA, Berry-Kravis EM, Milunsky JM, Farooqi IS, Rand CM, Weese-Mayer DE. Rapid-onset obesity with hypothalamic dysfunction, hypoventilation, and autonomic dysregulation presenting in childhood. Pediatrics. 2007 Jul;120(1):e179–88.

REFERENCES

1. Bell CG, Walley AJ, Froguel P. The genetics of human obesity. Nat Rev Genet. 2005;6(3):221–34.
2. Farooqi IS, O'Rahilly S. Monogenic obesity in humans. Annu Rev Med. 2005;56:443–58.

3. Prader A, Labhart A, Willi H. Ein Syndrom von Adipositas, Kleinwuchs, Kryptorchismus und Oligophrenie nach myotoniertigem Zustand im Neugeborenalter. Schweiz Med Wochenschr. 1956;86:1260–1.

4. Cassidy SB, Dykens E, Williams CA. Prader-Willi and Angelman syndromes: sister imprinted disorders. Am J Med Genet. 2000;97(2):136–46.

5. de Lind van Wijngaarden RF, Otten BJ, Festen DA, Joosten KF, de Jong FH, Sweep FC, Hokken-Koelega AC. High prevalence of central adrenal insufficiency in patients with Prader-Willi syndrome. J Clin Endocrinol Metab. 2008;93(5):1649–54.

6. DiMario FJ Jr, Dunham B, Burleson JA, Moskovitz J, Cassidy SB. An evaluation of autonomic nervous system function in patients with Prader-Willi syndrome. Pediatrics. 1994;93(1):76–81.

7. Nicholls RD, Knepper JL. Genome organization, function, and imprinting in Prader-Willi and Angelman syndromes. Annu Rev Genomics Hum Genet. 2001;2:153–75.

8. Nicholls RD, Saitoh S, Horsthemke B. Imprinting in Prader-Willi and Angelman syndromes. Trends Genet. 1998;14(5):194–200.

9. Ohta T, Gray TA, Rogan PK, Buiting K, Gabriel JM, Saitoh S, Muralidhar B, Bilienska B, Krajewska-Walasek M, Driscoll DJ, Horsthemke B, Butler MG, Nicholls RD. Imprinting-mutation mechanisms in Prader-Willi syndrome. Am J Hum Genet. 1999;64(2):397–413.

10. Runte M, Huttenhofer A, Gross S, Kiefmann M, Horsthemke B, Buiting K. The IC-SNURF-SNRPN transcript serves as a host for multiple small nucleolar RNA species and as an antisense RNA for UBE3A. Hum Mol Genet. 2001;10(23):2687–700.

11. Niinobe M, Koyama K, Yoshikawa K. Cellular and subcellular localization of necdin in fetal and adult mouse brain. Dev Neurosci. 2000;22(4):310–19.

12. Muscatelli F, Abrous DN, Massacrier A, Boccaccio I, Le Moal M, Cau P, Cremer H. Disruption of the mouse Necdin gene results in hypothalamic and behavioral alterations reminiscent of the human Prader-Willi syndrome. Hum Mol Genet. 2000;9(20):3101–10.

13. Lee S, Kozlov S, Hernandez L, Chamberlain SJ, Brannan CI, Stewart CL, Wevrick R. Expression and imprinting of MAGEL2 suggest a role in Prader-Willi syndrome and the homologous murine imprinting phenotype. Hum Mol Genet. 2000;9(12):1813–19.

14. Gallagher RC, Pils B, Albalwi M, Francke U. Evidence for the role of PWCR1/HBII-85 C/D box small nucleolar RNAs in Prader-Willi syndrome. Am J Hum Genet. 2002;71(3):669–78.

15. Festen DA, Wevers M, Lindgren AC, Bohm B, Otten BJ, Wit JM, Duivenvoorden HJ, Hokken-Koelega AC. Mental and motor development before and during growth hormone treatment in infants and toddlers with Prader-Willi syndrome. Clin Endocrinol (Oxf). 2008;68(6):919–25.

16. Festen DA, de Lind van Wijngaarden R, van Eekelen M, Otten BJ, Wit JM, Duivenvoorden HJ, Hokken-Koelega AC. Randomized controlled GH trial: effects on anthropometry, body composition and body proportions in a large group of children with Prader-Willi syndrome. Clin Endocrinol (Oxf). 2008;69(3):443–51.

17. Myers SE, Whitman BY, Carrel AL, Moerchen V, Bekx MT, Allen DB. Two years of growth hormone therapy in young children with Prader-Willi syndrome: physical and neurodevelopmental benefits. Am J Med Genet A. 2007;143(5):443–48.

18. Carrel AL, Myers SE, Whitman BY, Allen DB. Benefits of long-term GH therapy in Prader-Willi syndrome: a 4-year study. J Clin Endocrinol Metab. 2002;87(4):1581–85.

19. Carrel AL, Myers SE, Whitman BY, Allen DB. Growth hormone improves body composition, fat utilization, physical strength and agility, and growth in Prader-Willi syndrome: A controlled study. J Pediatr. 1999;134(2):215–21.

20. Eiholzer U, l'Allemand D. Growth hormone normalises height, prediction of final height and hand length in children with Prader-Willi syndrome after 4 years of therapy. Horm Res. 2000;53(4):185–92.

21. Myers SE, Carrel AL, Whitman BY, Allen DB. Sustained benefit after 2 years of growth hormone on body composition, fat utilization, physical strength and agility, and growth in Prader-Willi syndrome. J Pediatr. 2000;137(1):42–49.

22. Carrel AL, Myers SE, Whitman BY, Allen DB. Sustained benefits of growth hormone on body composition, fat utilization, physical strength and agility, and growth in Prader-Willi syndrome are dose-dependent. J Pediatr Endocrinol Metab. 2001;14(8):1097–105.

23. Haqq AM, Stadler DD, Jackson RH, Rosenfeld RG, Purnell JQ, LaFranchi SH. Effects of growth hormone on pulmonary function, sleep quality, behavior, cognition, growth velocity, body composition, and resting energy expenditure in Prader-Willi syndrome. J Clin Endocrinol Metab. 2003;88(5):2206–12.

24. Bakker B, Maneatis T, Lippe B. Sudden death in Prader-Willi syndrome: brief review of five additional cases. Concerning the article by U. Eiholzer et al.: Deaths in children with Prader-Willi syndrome. A contribution to the debate about the safety of growth hormone treatment in children with PWS (Horm Res 2005;63:33–39). Horm Res. 2007;67(4):203–4.

25. Tauber M, Diene G, Molinas C, Hebert M. Review of 64 cases of death in children with Prader-Willi syndrome (PWS). Am J Med Genet A. 2008;146(7):881–87.

26. Schrander-Stumpel CT, Curfs LM, Sastrowijoto P, Cassidy SB, Schrander JJ, Fryns JP. Prader-Willi syndrome: causes of death in an international series of 27 cases. Am J Med Genet A. 2004;124(4):333–38.

27. Vogels A, Van Den Ende J, Keymolen K, Mortier G, Devriendt K, Legius E, Fryns JP. Minimum prevalence, birth incidence and cause of death for Prader-Willi syndrome in Flanders. Eur J Hum Genet. 2004;12(3):238–40.

28. Van Vliet G, Deal CL, Crock PA, Robitaille Y, Oligny LL. Sudden death in growth hormone-treated children with Prader-Willi syndrome. J Pediatr. 2004;144(1):129–31.

29. Cummings DE, Clement K, Purnell JQ, Vaisse C, Foster KE, Frayo RS, Schwartz MW, Basdevant A, Weigle DS. Elevated plasma ghrelin levels in Prader-Willi syndrome. Nat Med. 2002;8(7):643–644.

30. DelParigi A, Tschop M, Heiman ML, Salbe AD, Vozarova B, Sell SM, Bunt JC, Tataranni PA. High Circulating Ghrelin: A Potential Cause for Hyperphagia and Obesity in Prader-Willi Syndrome. J Clin Endocrinol Metab. 2002;87(12): 5461–64.

31. Haqq AM, Farooqi IS, O'Rahilly S, Stadler DD, Rosenfeld RG, Pratt KL, LaFranchi SH, Purnell JQ. Serum ghrelin levels are inversely correlated with body mass index, age, and insulin concentrations in normal children and are markedly increased in Prader-Willi syndrome. J Clin Endocrinol Metab. 2003;88(1):174–78.

32. Haqq AM, Grambow SC, Muehlbauer M, Newgard CB, Svetkey LP, Carrel AL, Yanovski JA, Purnell JQ, Freemark M. Ghrelin concentrations in Prader-Willi syndrome (PWS) infants and children: changes during development. Clin Endocrinol (Oxf). 2008;69(6):911–20.

33. Haqq AM, Stadler DD, Rosenfeld RG, Pratt KL, Weigle DS, Frayo RS, LaFranchi SH, Cummings DE, Purnell JQ. Circulating ghrelin levels are suppressed by meals and octreotide therapy in children with Prader-Willi syndrome. J Clin Endocrinol Metab. 2003;88(8):3573–76.

34. Tan TM, Vanderpump M, Khoo B, Patterson M, Ghatei MA, Goldstone AP. Somatostatin infusion lowers plasma ghrelin without reducing appetite in adults with Prader-Willi syndrome. J Clin Endocrinol Metab. 2004;89(8):4162–65.

35. De Waele K, Ishkanian SL, Bogarin R, Miranda CA, Ghatei MA, Bloom SR, Pacaud D, Chanoine JP. Long-acting octreotide treatment causes a sustained decrease in ghrelin concentrations but does not affect weight, behaviour and appetite in subjects with Prader-Willi syndrome. Eur J Endocrinol. 2008;159(4):381–88.

36. Goldstone AP, Thomas EL, Brynes AE, Bell JD, Frost G, Saeed N, Hajnal JV, Howard JK, Holland A, Bloom SR. Visceral adipose tissue and metabolic complications of obesity are reduced in Prader-Willi syndrome female adults: evidence for novel influences on body fat distribution. J Clin Endocrinol Metab. 2001;86(9):4330–38.

37. Goldstone AP, Brynes AE, Thomas EL, Bell JD, Frost G, Holland A, Ghatei MA, Bloom SR. Resting metabolic rate, plasma leptin concentrations, leptin receptor expression, and adipose tissue measured by whole-body magnetic resonance imaging in women with Prader-Willi syndrome. Am J Clin Nutr. 2002;75(3):468–75.

38. Haqq AM, Muehlbauer M, Svetkey LP, Newgard CB, Purnell JQ, Grambow SC, Freemark MS. Altered distribution of adiponectin isoforms in children with Prader-Willi syndrome (PWS): association with insulin sensitivity and circulating satiety peptide hormones. Clin Endocrinol (Oxf). 2007;67(6):944–51.

39. Wade CK, De Meersman RE, Angulo M, Lieberman JS, Downey JA. Prader-Willi syndrome fails to alter cardiac autonomic modulation. Clin Auton Res. 2000;10(4):203–6.

40. Albright F, Burnett C, Smith P, Parson W. Pseudohypoparathyroidism: an example of Seabright-Bantam syndrome. Endocrinology. 1942;30:922–32.

41. Levine MA, Germain-Lee E, Jan de Beur S. Genetic basis for resistance to parathyroid hormone. Horm Res. 2003;60: 87–95. See also Germain-Lee EL. Short stature, obesity, and growth hormone deficiency in pseudohypoparathyroidism type 1a. Pediatr Endocrinol Rev 2006;3(Suppl 2):318–27.

42. Albright F, Forbes A, Henneman P. Pseudopseudohypoparathyroidism. Trans Assoc Am Physicians. 1952;65:337–50.

43. Ong KK, Amin R, Dunger DB. Pseudohypoparathyroidism – another monogenic obesity syndrome. Clin Endocrinol (Oxf). 2000;52(3):389–91.

44. Miric A, Vechio JD, Levine MA. Heterogeneous mutations in the gene encoding the alpha-subunit of the stimulatory G protein of adenylyl cyclase in Albright hereditary osteodystrophy. J Clin Endocrinol Metab. 1993;76(6): 1560–68.

45. Weinstein LS, Liu J, Sakamoto A, Xie T, Chen M. Minireview: GNAS: Normal and Abnormal Functions. Endocrinology. 2004;145(12):5459–64.

46. Nakamoto JM, Sandstrom AT, Brickman AS, Christenson RA, Van Dop C. Pseudohypoparathyroidism type Ia from maternal but not paternal transmission of a Gsalpha gene mutation. Am J Med Genet. 1998;77(4):261–67.

47. Davies SJ, Hughes HE. Imprinting in Albright's hereditary osteodystrophy. J Med Genet. 1993;30(2):101–3.

48. Laurence JZ, Moon RC. Four cases of retinitis pigmentosa occurring in the same family, and accompanied by general imperfections of development. Ophthalmol Rev. 1866;2:32–41.

49. Bardet G. Sur un syndrome d'obesite congenitale avec plydactylie et retinite pigmentaire (contribution a l'etude des formes cliniques de l'obesite hypophysaire). These de Paris (Le Grand). 1920;470:107.

50. Biedl A. Ein Geschwister mit adiposogenitaler Dystrophie. Dtsch Med Wochenschr. 1922;48:1630.

51. Beales PL, Warner AM, Hitman GA, Thakker R, Flinter FA. Bardet-Biedl syndrome: a molecular and phenotypic study of 18 families. J Med Genet. 1997;34(2):92–98.

52. Klein D, Ammann F. The syndrome of Laurence-Moon-Bardet-Biedl and allied diseases in Switzerland: Clinical, genetic and epidemiological studies. J Neurol Sci. 1969;9(3):479–513.

53. Farag TI, Teebi AS. High incidence of Bardet Biedl syndrome among the Bedouin. Clin Genet. 1989;36(6):463–4.

54. Green JS, Parfrey PS, Harnett JD, Farid NR, Cramer BC, Johnson G, Heath O, McManamon PJ, O'Leary E, Pryse-Phillips W. The cardinal manifestations of Bardet-Biedl syndrome, a form of Laurence-Moon-Biedl syndrome. N Engl J Med. 1989;321(15):1002–9.

55. Beales PL, Elcioglu N, Woolf AS, Parker D, Flinter FA. New criteria for improved diagnosis of Bardet-Biedl syndrome: results of a population survey. J Med Genet. 1999;36(6):437–46.

56. Grace C, Beales P, Summerbell C, Jebb SA, Wright A, Parker D, Kopelman P. Energy metabolism in Bardet-Biedl syndrome. Int J Obes Relat Metab Disord. 2003;27(11):1319–24.

57. Ansley SJ, Badano JL, Blacque OE, Hill J, Hoskins BE, Leitch CC, Chul Kim J, Ross AJ, Eichers ER, Teslovich TM, Mah AK, Johnsen RC, Cavender JC, Alan Lewis R, Leroux MR, Beales PL, Katsanis N. Basal body dysfunction is a likely cause of pleiotropic Bardet-Biedl syndrome. Nature. 2003;425(6958):628–33.

58. Kulaga HM, Leitch CC, Eichers ER, Badano JL, Lesemann A, Hoskins BE, Lupski JR, Beales PL, Reed RR, Katsanis N. Loss of BBS proteins causes anosmia in humans and defects in olfactory cilia structure and function in the mouse. Nat Genet. 2004;36(9):994–98.

59. Nishimura DY, Fath M, Mullins RF, Searby C, Andrews M, Davis R, Andorf JL, Mykytyn K, Swiderski RE, Yang B, Carmi R, Stone EM, Sheffield VC. Bbs2-null mice have neurosensory deficits, a defect in social dominance, and retinopathy associated with mislocalization of rhodopsin. Proc Natl Acad Sci USA. 2004;101(47):16588–93.

60. Kim JC, Ou YY, Badano JL, Esmail MA, Leitch CC, Fiedrich E, Beales PL, Archibald JM, Katsanis N, Rattner JB, Leroux MR. MKKS/BBS6, a divergent chaperonin-like protein linked to the obesity disorder Bardet-Biedl syndrome, is a novel centrosomal component required for cytokinesis. J Cell Sci. 2005;118(Pt 5):1007–20.

61. Blacque OE, Reardon MJ, Li C, McCarthy J, Mahjoub MR, Ansley SJ, Badano JL, Mah AK, Beales PL, Davidson WS, Johnsen RC, Audeh M, Plasterk RH, Baillie DL, Katsanis N, Quarmby LM, Wicks SR, Leroux MR. Loss of C. elegans BBS-7 and BBS-8 protein function results in cilia defects and compromised intraflagellar transport. Genes Dev. 2004;18(13):1630–42.

62. Nishimura DY, Swiderski RE, Searby CC, Berg EM, Ferguson AL, Hennekam R, Merin S, Weleber RG, Biesecker LG, Stone EM, Sheffield VC. Comparative genomics and gene expression analysis identifies BBS9, a new Bardet-Biedl syndrome gene. Am J Hum Genet. 2005;77(6):1021–33.

63. Stoetzel C, Laurier V, Davis EE, Muller J, Rix S, Badano JL, Leitch CC, Salem N, Chouery E, Corbani S, Jalk N, Vicaire S, Sarda P, Hamel C, Lacombe D, Holder M, Odent S, Holder S, Brooks AS, Elcioglu NH, Silva ED, Rossillion B, Sigaudy S, de Ravel TJL, Alan Lewis R, Leheup B, Verloes A, Amati-Bonneau P, Megarbane A, Poch O, Bonneau D, Beales PL, Mandel J-L, Katsanis N, Dollfus H. BBS10 encodes a vertebrate-specific chaperonin-like protein and is a major BBS locus. Nat Genet. 2006;38(5):521–24.

64. Chiang AP, Beck JS, Yen H-J, Tayeh MK, Scheetz TE, Swiderski RE, Nishimura DY, Braun TA, Kim K-YA, Huang J, Elbedour K, Carmi R, Slusarski DC, Casavant TL, Stone EM, Sheffield VC. Homozygosity mapping with SNP arrays identifies TRIM32, an E3 ubiquitin ligase, as a Bardetâ–Biedl syndrome gene (BBS11). Proc Natl Acad Sci USA. 2006;103(16):6287–92.

65. Stoetzel C, Muller J, Laurier V, Davis EE, Zaghloul NA, Vicaire S, Jacquelin C, Plewniak F, Leitch CC, Sarda P, Hamel C, de Ravel TJL, Lewis RA, Friederich E, Thibault C, Danse J-M, Verloes A, Bonneau D, Katsanis N, Poch O, Mandel J-L, Dollfus H. Identification of a Novel BBS Gene (BBS12) Highlights the Major Role of a Vertebrate-Specific Branch of Chaperonin-Related Proteins in Bardet-Biedl Syndrome. Am J Hum Genet. 2007;80(1):1–11.

66. Yoder BK, Tousson A, Millican L, Wu JH, Bugg CE Jr, Schafer JA, Balkovetz DF. Polaris, a protein disrupted in orpk mutant mice, is required for assembly of renal cilium. Am J Physiol Renal Physiol. 2002;282(3):F541–F52.

67. Seo S, Guo DF, Bugge K, Morgan DA, Rahmouni K, Sheffield VC. Requirement of Bardet-Biedl syndrome proteins for leptin receptor signaling. Hum Mol Genet. 2009;18(7):1323–31.

68. Beales PL, Reid HA, Griffiths MH, Maher ER, Flinter FA, Woolf AS. Renal cancer and malformations in relatives of patients with Bardet-Biedl syndrome. Nephrol Dial Transplant. 2000;15(12):1977–85.

69. Park TJ, Haigo SL, Wallingford JB. Ciliogenesis defects in embryos lacking inturned or fuzzy function are associated with failure of planar cell polarity and Hedgehog signaling. Nat Genet. 2006;38(3):303–11.

70. Davenport JR, Watts AJ, Roper VC, Croyle MJ, van Groen T, Wyss JM, Nagy TR, Kesterson RA, Yoder BK. Disruption of intraflagellar transport in adult mice leads to obesity and slow-onset cystic kidney disease. Curr Biol. 2007;17(18):1586–94.

71. Alstrom C, Hallgren B, Nilsson L, Asander H. Retinal degeneration combined with obesity, diabetes mellitus and neurogenous deafness: a specific syndrome (not hitherto described) distinct from the Laurence-Moon-Bardet-Biedl syndrome: a clinical, endocrinological and genetic examination based on a large pedigree. Acta Psychiatr Neurol Scand. 1959;129:1–35.

72. Minton JA, Owen KR, Ricketts CJ, Crabtree N, Shaikh G, Ehtisham S, Porter JR, Carey C, Hodge D, Paisey R, Walker M, Barrett TG. Syndromic obesity and diabetes: changes in body composition with age and mutation analysis of ALMS1 in 12 United Kingdom kindreds with Alstrom syndrome. J Clin Endocrinol Metab. 2006;91(8):3110–16.

73. Marshall JD, Beck S, Maffei P, Naggert JK. Alstrom syndrome. Eur J Hum Genet. 2007;15(12):1193–202.

74. Marshall JD, Ludman MD, Shea SE, Salisbury SR, Willi SM, LaRoche RG, Nishina PM. Genealogy, natural history, and phenotype of Alstrom syndrome in a large Acadian kindred and three additional families. Am J Med Genet. 1997;73(2):150–61.

75. Hearn T, Renforth GL, Spalluto C, Hanley NA, Piper K, Brickwood S, White C, Connolly V, Taylor JFN, Russell-Eggitt I, Bonneau D, Walker M, Wilson DI. Mutation of ALMS1, a large gene with a tandem repeat encoding 47 amino acids, causes Alstrom syndrome. Nat Genet. 2002;31(1):79–83.

76. Collin GB, Marshall JD, Ikeda A, So WV, Russell-Eggitt I, Maffei P, Beck S, Boerkoel CF, Sicolo N, Martin M, Nishina PM, Naggert JK. Mutations in ALMS1 cause obesity, type 2 diabetes and neurosensory degeneration in Alstrom syndrome. Nat Genet. 2002;31(1):74–78.

77. Hearn T, Spalluto C, Phillips VJ, Renforth GL, Copin N, Hanley NA, Wilson DI. Subcellular localization of ALMS1 supports involvement of centrosome and basal body dysfunction in the pathogenesis of obesity, insulin resistance, and type 2 diabetes. Diabetes. 2005;54(5):1581–87.

78. Collin GB, Cyr E, Bronson R, Marshall JD, Gifford EJ, Hicks W, Murray SA, Zheng QY, Smith RS, Nishina PM, Naggert JK. Alms1-disrupted mice recapitulate human Alstrom syndrome. Hum Mol Genet. 2005;14(16):2323–33.

79. Marshall JD, Hinman EG, Collin GB, Beck S, Cerqueira R, Maffei P, Milan G, Zhang W, Wilson DI, Hearn T, Tavares P, Vettor R, Veronese C, Martin M, So WV, Nishina PM, Naggert JK. Spectrum of ALMS1 variants and evaluation of genotype-phenotype correlations in Alstrom syndrome. Hum Mutat. 2007;28(11):1114–23.

80. Bonora E. Relationship between regional fat distribution and insulin resistance. Int J Obes Relat Metab Disord. 2000;24:S32.

81. Nambu JR, Franks RG, Hu S, Crews ST. The single-minded gene of Drosophila is required for the expression of genes important for the development of CNS midline cells. Cell. 1990;63(1):63–75.

82. Holder JL Jr, Butte NF, Zinn AR. Profound obesity associated with a balanced translocation that disrupts the SIM1 gene. Hum Mol Genet. 2000;9(1):101–8.

83. Michaud JL, Boucher F, Melnyk A, Gauthier F, Goshu E, Levy E, Mitchell GA, Himms-Hagen J, Fan CM. Sim1 haploinsufficiency causes hyperphagia, obesity and reduction of the paraventricular nucleus of the hypothalamus. Hum Mol Genet. 2001;10(14):1465–73.

84. Michaud JL, Rosenquist T, May NR, Fan CM. Development of neuroendocrine lineages requires the bHLH-PAS transcription factor SIM1. Genes Dev. 1998;12(20):3264–75.

85. Kublaoui BM, Holder JL Jr, Tolson KP, Gemelli T, Zinn AR. SIM1 overexpression partially rescues agouti yellow and diet-induced obesity by normalizing food intake. Endocrinology. 2006;147(10):4542–9.

86. Meyre D, Lecoeur C, Delplanque J, Francke S, Vatin V, Durand E, Weill J, Dina C, Froguel P. A genome-wide scan for childhood obesity-associated traits in French families shows significant linkage on chromosome 6q22.31-q23.2. Diabetes. 2004;53(3):803–11.

87. Duggirala R, Blangero J, Almasy L, Arya R, Dyer TD, Williams KL, Leach RJ, O'Connell P, Stern MP. A major locus for fasting insulin concentrations and insulin resistance on chromosome 6q with strong pleiotropic effects on obesity-related phenotypes in nondiabetic Mexican Americans. Am J Hum Genet. 2001;68(5):1149–64.

88. Hung C-CC, Luan J, Sims M, Keogh JM, Hall C, Wareham NJ, O'Rahilly S, Farooqi IS. Studies of the SIM1 gene in relation to human obesity and obesity-related traits. Int J Obes. 2006;31(3):429–34.

89. Gray J, Yeo GS, Cox JJ, Morton J, Adlam AL, Keogh JM, Yanovski JA, El Gharbawy A, Han JC, Tung YC, Hodges JR, Raymond FL, O'Rahilly S, Farooqi IS. Hyperphagia, severe obesity, impaired cognitive function, and hyperactivity associated with functional loss of one copy of the brain-derived neurotrophic factor (BDNF) gene. Diabetes. 2006;55(12):3366–71.

90. Yeo GS, Connie Hung CC, Rochford J, Keogh J, Gray J, Sivaramakrishnan S, O'Rahilly S, Farooqi IS. A de novo mutation affecting human TrkB associated with severe obesity and developmental delay. Nat Neurosci. 2004;7(11):1187–9.

91. Han JC, Liu QR, Jones M, Levinn RL, Menzie CM, Jefferson-George KS, Adler-Wailes DC, Sanford EL, Lacbawan FL, Uhl GR, Rennert OM, Yanovski JA. Brain-derived neurotrophic factor and obesity in the WAGR syndrome. N Engl J Med. 2008;359(9):918–27.

92. Tapia-Arancibia L, Rage F, Givalois L, Arancibia S. Physiology of BDNF: focus on hypothalamic function. Front Neuroendocrinol. 2004;25(2):77–107.

93. Xu B, Goulding EH, Zang K, Cepoi D, Cone RD, Jones KR, Tecott LH, Reichardt LF. Brain-derived neurotrophic factor regulates energy balance downstream of melanocortin-4 receptor. Nat Neurosci. 2003;6(7):736–42.

94. Kernie SG, Liebl DJ, Parada LF. BDNF regulates eating behavior and locomotor activity in mice. EMBO J. 2000;19(6):1290–300.

95. Pelleymounter MA, Cullen MJ, Wellman CL. Characteristics of BDNF-induced weight loss. Exp Neurol. 1995;131(2):229–38.

5 Polygenic Obesity

Anke Hinney and Johannes Hebebrand

CONTENTS

Key Words: Candidate gene, genome-wide association, melanocortin, insulin-induced gene 2 (INSIG2), FTO (fat mass and obesity-associated gene)

INTRODUCTION

A small number of major genes for human obesity have been identified by molecular genetic analyses; the responsible mutations are rare and are therefore only of minor clinical importance. The genetic mechanisms involved in the predisposition to obesity in most affected people are more likely polygenic *(1,2)*; detection of the first such polygenes has just recently been initiated. Each single polygene makes only a small contribution, in the magnitude of a few hundred grams or less, to the development of obesity. A number of such predisposing gene variants (alleles) should be found in most obese subjects; however, the same alleles would, although at a lower frequency, also be found in normal weight and even lean individuals. Evidently, these alleles can only be identified and validated as obesity risk alleles by statistical analyses *(2)*. Currently, combined genome-wide association (GWAS) analyses on more than 100,000 population-based individuals are under way. Functional in vitro and in vivo studies will ensue and lead to a better understanding of the molecular genetic mechanisms involved in body weight regulation. Prevention and therapeutic approaches will presumably benefit from this knowledge.

From: *Contemporary Endocrinology: Pediatric Obesity: Etiology, Pathogenesis, and Treatment*
Edited by: M. Freemark, DOI 10.1007/978-1-60327-874-4_5,
© Springer Science+Business Media, LLC 2010

POLYGENES FOR BODY WEIGHT

The term polygene is used for a gene known to harbor inter-individual sequence variation and to account for a fraction of the variation of a specific quantitative trait. Each polygene contains one allele predisposing to higher and the other to lower body weight. It is presumed that more than 100 polygenes play a role in body weight regulation. Based on the thrifty genotype hypothesis (3), those alleles that predispose to a higher body weight are hypothesized to be more common than alleles giving rise to lower body weight. This is because, in evolutionary terms, it was important to both survive and reproduce during periods of food scarcity; as a consequence, mutations enabling a more efficient storage of energy became common in both animals and humans. Obesity is the result of the interaction of several or many of these polygenic variants and their combined interaction with environmental factors. Inter-individual heterogeneity is most likely pronounced and implies that the specific set of polygenes predisposing to obesity in any one individual is unlikely to be the same in another randomly selected obese subject (1).

In contrast to most of the initially detected genetic influences on obesity, which are conferred by a single gene with either a recessive or a dominant mode of inheritance, polygenic effects are small. Polygenic obesity can only ensue if an individual harbors many such variants and lives in an obesogenic environment. Associations between genetic variants and obesity could have implications for diagnosis and risk prediction, prevention, and treatment. So far, 17 gene variants with small but replicable effects on body weight have been identified and validated (4).

CANDIDATE GENE ANALYSIS AND GENOME-WIDE APPROACHES

Two major approaches have been used for the detection of genes involved in body weight regulation.

Candidate gene analyses: Genes considered "candidates" for BMI variance are analyzed because prior research (biochemical, physiological, and/or clinical) implicates their roles in central or peripheral pathways controlling energy intake and expenditure. Pharmacological findings or the location of a gene within a linkage region can also entail its classification as a candidate gene. A large number of association studies for obesity involving cases and controls or, less frequently, families comprising one or more affected children and both parents have been performed. For a limited number of genes, meta-analyses are available.

Genome-wide approaches: Genome-wide linkage studies aim to identify chromosomal regions harboring one (or more) genes relevant for the respective phenotype. For candidate gene analyses, those regions underlying linkage peaks are narrowed down by fine mapping. Over 40 microsatellite-based genome-wide linkage scans have been performed for obesity. As in other complex disorders, the success of linkage studies has been very limited. Interestingly, the region on chromosome 16 harboring the currently most relevant polygene, the 'fat mass and obesity-associated' gene (*FTO*), proved to be the strongest but nevertheless nonsignificant signal in a meta-analysis of 37 genome-wide linkage studies comprising data on more than 31,000 individuals from over 10,000 families (5). This most likely indicates that the effect sizes of genes influencing obesity are small and additionally suggests substantial genetic heterogeneity and variable dependence on environmental factors.

Genome-wide association studies (GWAS) have far greater power to detect polygenes (6). Current advances in DNA chip technology have made high-density single nucleotide polymorphism (SNP)-based GWAS feasible and led recently to the identification of a number of confirmed genes for different disorders (http://www.genome.gov/26525384). Within a brief period of time, they have revolutionized the molecular genetic analyses of complex disorders.

MELANOCORTIN-4 RECEPTOR GENE (MC4R)

The melanocortin-4 receptor gene (*MC4R*) has been a focus of intense investigation in obesity research. Reduced melanocortinergic tone leads to obesity. More than 130 different infrequent non-synonymous, nonsense, and frameshift *MC4R* mutations have been described thus far; most of these mutations were identified in (extremely) obese individuals (*7–11*). In vitro assays showed that most of these mutations lead to total or partial loss of MCR4 function. Among *extremely* obese individuals, combined frequencies for all functionally relevant mutations range from 2 to 5%.

Interestingly, *MC4R* can also be considered a polygene. The minor alleles of two *MC4R* polymorphisms (Val103Ile, Ile251Leu) are negatively associated with obesity (*12–15*). Large study groups had to be screened to detect these polymorphisms because they are relatively uncommon and have small effect sizes.

Val103Ile polymorphism. Heterozygosity for the 103Ile variant (Val103Ile) of MC4R is found in 2–9% of people (*12*). A family-based association test (TDT; (*16*)) in 520 trios (ascertained via a young obese offspring) revealed a reduced transmission of the Ile103 variant. A subsequent meta-analysis, comprising a total of 7,713 individuals (3,631 obese cases and 4,082 controls), confirmed the negative association of the Ile103 variant with obesity (odds ratio 0.69; 95% confidence interval 0.59–0.99). An effect estimate of –0.48 kg/m^2 was calculated for Ile103 carriers, which is approximately equivalent to a reduction of 1.5 kg in a 1.8 m tall individual (*12*). The negative association of 103Ile with obesity was subsequently confirmed in a single large epidemiological study group of approximately 8,000 individuals (*13*). Recently, two additional meta-analyses, encompassing a total of up to 29,563 individuals, also have confirmed the initial finding (*15*).

A recent study showed that the Ile103 polymorphism increased the response to agouti-related peptide, which impairs melanocortin signaling and increases food intake, and reduced the response to proopiomelanocortin-derived agonists, which increase melanocortin signaling and reduce food intake (*17*). Hence, the polymorphism is associated with increased MC4R function, which could explain its weight-reducing effect.

Ile251Leu polymorphism. Heterozygosity for the Ile251Leu variant of MC4R is found in 0.41–1.21% of people. Its contribution to obesity was analyzed in 16,797 individuals of European origin. In eight of nine studies, a consistent negative association of the 251Leu variant with both childhood and adult extreme obesity (odds ratios 0.25–0.76) was detected; the variant was also associated with reduced BMI in population-based samples. A meta-analysis provided strong evidence of the obesity protective effect of MC4R-251Leu (odds ratio 0.52) (*14*).

rs17782313 downstream of MC4R. Recently, a large-scale international cooperation encompassing DNA samples of over 90,000 individuals detected a SNP in the vicinity of the *MC4R* by a genome-wide association study (GWAS; (*18*)). Initially, GWAS data from seven studies (a total of 16,876 Europeans) have been analyzed jointly. The second strongest association signal, after *FTO* (see below), mapped 188 kb downstream of the *MC4R* (rs17782313). The location of rs17782313 suggests that its effect on weight regulation may be mediated through effects on *MC4R* expression and may be exerted in concert with variations in *FTO* (*18*). The association result was confirmed in an additional 60,352 adults and 5,988 children and 660 nuclear German families encompassing one or more obese offspring and both parents. Among the adults, each copy of the rs17782313 obesity risk allele (C) was associated with a difference in BMI of ~0.22 kg/m^2. A copy of the allele resulted in 8 and 12% increased risks for overweight and obesity, respectively. Interestingly, a copy of the C-allele also resulted in a higher mean height (0.21 cm), suggesting that this SNP (or the functionally relevant SNP(s) in linkage disequilibrium) influences overall adult size.

The association of the rs17782313 SNP with obesity was recently confirmed in a GWAS comprising a total of more than 150,000 individuals (see (*4*)). Interestingly, genotyping of nearly 6,000 children of the Avon Longitudinal Study of Children and Parents revealed that the effect of the C-allele was not detectable in children prior to age 7. However, in children aged 7–11, the effect size of a copy of the C-allele was twice the amount observed in adults; no effect was observed for body height. The effect on weight was disproportionately due to fat mass.

INSULIN-INDUCED GENE 2 (INSIG2)

A total of 694 individuals from 288 families of the Framingham Heart Study were screened by a dense, whole-genome scan (100k Affymetrix). In both children and adults, homozygosity for a common SNP (rs7566605) in the vicinity of the insulin-induced gene 2 (*INSIG2*) was found to be associated with obesity. Confirmation of the initial finding was shown in four of five separate samples comprising individuals of Western European ancestry, African-Americans, and German children and adolescents, respectively. Approximately 10% of the subjects harbored the CC-genotype that, according to this study, predisposes to obesity *(19)*.

Several attempts to replicate the *INSIG2* finding have been or are currently being undertaken. Both confirmations *(20)* and negative findings *(21–23)* have been reported. Currently, data are being compiled for a large-scale meta-analysis, which in the near future will help to determine if *INSIG2* is an obesity polygene. However, *INSIG2* was not detected in any of the GWAS for obesity or body weight regulation either from large population-based samples or meta-analyses or in case–control approaches on individuals at the extremes of the body weight distribution *(24–26)*.

FAT MASS AND OBESITY-ASSOCIATED GENE (FTO)

FTO was first identified in GWAS for type 2 diabetes mellitus (T2DM; *(27,28)*). By adjustment for BMI, Frayling et al. *(27)* found that its association with T2DM was actually due to the higher BMI of diabetic cases in comparison to non-diabetic controls. Confirmation of the BMI effect was obtained in 13 study groups comprising 38,759 adults. A meta-analysis showed that the A-allele of the variant rs9939609 (intron 1 of *FTO*) was associated with a 31% increased risk for developing obesity. The 16% of adults who were homozygous for the risk allele weighed on average about 3 kg more and had a 1.67-fold increased odds for obesity when compared to individuals without risk allele.

Variations in *FTO* were also detected in the first GWAS for early-onset obesity, which was performed in 487 extremely obese German children and adolescents and 442 lean controls (case–control study). Because only individuals at the opposite ends of the BMI distribution were included, this study was well powered to detect obesity polygenes despite the comparatively small sample size. Six intronic SNPs in *FTO* showed the strongest evidence for association with obesity (best SNP: rs1121980, odds ratios for obesity for heterozygosity and homozygosity for the T-allele were 1.67 and 2.76, respectively; *(29)*). Eleven SNPs (including two *FTO* SNPs) were subsequently genotyped in 644 independent obesity families based on at least one young obese index patient. The association with early-onset obesity was confirmed only for the two *FTO* SNPs (rs9939609 and rs1121980).

FTO rs9939609 was genotyped in a total of 17,508 middle-aged Danes. Again, the A-allele was associated with overweight and obesity. Obesity-related quantitative traits such as body weight, waist circumference, fat mass, and fasting serum leptin levels were significantly increased in A-allele carriers. There was an interaction between the *FTO* rs9939609 genotype and physical activity; physically inactive homozygous risk A-allele carriers had an increased BMI (1.95 ± 0.3 kg/m^2) compared with homozygotes for the T-allele. Low physical activity thus seemingly accentuates the effect of *FTO* rs9939609 on body fat accumulation *(30)*.

The obesity risk variant of *FTO* at rs8050136 was associated with a reduced insulin effect on beta activity measured by magnetoencephalography, which implicates a lower cerebrocortical response to insulin. Since the *FTO* gene is expressed in hypothalamic centers controlling appetite (see below), this might be a mechanism by which variation in *FTO* contributes to the pathogenesis of obesity *(31)*. Wåhlén et al. *(32)* suggested that *FTO* may also play a role in fat cell lipolysis, providing a functional link to body weight regulation.

Detailed computational analysis of the sequence and predicted structure of the protein encoded by *FTO* has been performed. Human FTO is apparently a member of the non-heme dioxygenase (Fe(II)- and 2-oxoglutarate-dependent dioxygenases) superfamily *(33,34)*. Both 2-oxoglutarate and iron should therefore be important for FTO function *(34)*.

Very recently, the first individuals with a non-synonymous mutation (Arg316Gln) leading to inactivation of FTO were described *(35)*. The subjects were members of a large Palestinian Arab consanguineous multiplex family. All affected individuals had postnatal growth retardation, microcephaly, severe psychomotor delay, functional brain deficits, and characteristic facial dysmorphic features. Structural brain malformations, cardiac defects, genital anomalies, and cleft palate were described in some of the affected individuals. Death occurred at 1–30 months of age; it was caused by intercurrent infection or unidentified causes.

The mutation in this family localizes to an evolutionarily conserved region of FTO and leads to inactivation of its enzymatic activity. Functional data further implied that FTO is essential for normal development of the cardiovascular and central nervous systems in humans. Detailed anthropometric data were unfortunately not available on unaffected family members. However, none of the heterozygous parents were obese; nor did they show any of the clinical features detectable in homozygotes. It was speculated that carriers of loss-of-function mutations in *FTO* might be relatively resistant to develop obesity *(35)*.

A series of studies evaluated the functional role of FTO. Recombinant murine Fto catalyzes the Fe(II)- and 2OG-dependent demethylation of 3-methylthymine in single-stranded DNA. Concomitantly succinate, formaldehyde, and carbon dioxide are produced. Fto localizes to the nucleus in transfected cells, which is consistent with a potential role in nucleic acid demethylation. In wild-type mice, *Fto* mRNA is most abundant in the brain, particularly in hypothalamic nuclei governing energy balance. In fasted mice *Fto* mRNA levels in the arcuate nucleus were reduced by approximately 60%. Future studies will identify the physiologically relevant FTO substrates and determine how nucleic acid methylation status is linked to an elevated fat mass *(33)*. Recently it was shown that complete (homozygous knockout) loss of *Fto* in mice leads to postnatal growth retardation and a significant reduction in adipose tissue and lean body mass. The leanness of *Fto*-deficient mice results from increased energy expenditure and systemic sympathetic activation despite decreased spontaneous locomotor activity and relative hyperphagia. *Fto* expression in heterozygous *Fto*± mice was reduced; this led to reduced weight gain after 12 weeks. These observations suggest that the effects of *Fto* on energy homeostasis are mediated, at least in part, through the control of energy expenditure *(36)*.

In summary, complete *Fto* disruption leads to growth failure, with reductions in adipose tissue and lean body mass. These effects appear to be mediated, at least in part, through central-dependent increases in energy expenditure. Heterozygosity for *FTO* mutations may protect against obesity. The association of obesity with intronic polymorphisms in *FTO* suggests that the polymorphisms may increase FTO activity.

MORE POLYGENES IDENTIFIED IN RECENT GENOME-WIDE ASSOCIATION STUDIES

In 2009 three groups reported novel obesity genes with small effect sizes *(24–26)*; more than 150,000 individuals were analyzed in total.

A meta-analysis of 15 GWAS for body weight regulation ($n = 32,387$) was performed by the Genetic Investigation of ANthropometric Traits (GIANT) consortium based on approximately 2.4 million genotyped or imputed SNPs. The top 35 signals were followed up in 14 additional cohorts ($n = 59,082$). A strong confirmation was detected for *FTO* and *MC4R*. Additionally, six novel loci were identified near or within the following candidate genes: *TMEM18* (transmembrane protein 18), *KCTD15* (potassium channel tetramerization domain), *GNPDA2* (glucosamine-6-phosphate deaminase 2), *SH2B1* (SH2B adaptor protein 1), *MTCH2* (mitochondrial carrier 2), and *NEGR1* (neuronal growth regulator 1; a 45 kb deletion copy number variation is the candidate variant). Several of these presumptive 'obesity' genes are highly expressed and/or known to play a role in the function of the central nervous system. The effect of the variants on BMI ranged from 0.06 to 0.33 kg/m^2 per allele, which corresponds to 173–954 g of weight per allele in adults who measure ~170 cm in height. Together, the six newly discovered loci account for 0.40%, and in combination with *FTO* and *MC4R* a total of 0.84%, of BMI variance in otherwise normal individuals. The combined impact of these loci on BMI was also estimated: Individuals with 13 or more obesity predisposing alleles across eight loci were on average 1.46 kg/m^2 (equivalent to 3.7–4.7 kg for an adult 160–180 cm in height) heavier than individuals with less than 3 of these alleles *(24)*.

Another GWAS was performed in 25,344 Icelandic, 2,998 Dutch, 1,890 European American, and 1,160 African-American subjects and combined with results published by the Diabetes Genetics Initiative (DGI) based on 3,024 Scandinavians. A total of 19 regions comprising 43 variants were selected for follow-up in 5,586 Danish individuals. The results were compared with results of the obesity GWAS of the GIANT consortium (see above; *(24)*). In 11 chromosomal regions a total of 29 variants reached a genome-wide significance threshold of $p < 1.6 \times 10^{-7}$. In addition to variants at seven loci that had previously not been associated with obesity, both *FTO* and *MC4R* were reconfirmed; furthermore, the two obesity candidate genes *BDNF* and *SH2B1* were reidentified *(25)*.

The third GWAS on 1,380 Europeans with early-onset or late-onset morbid obesity and 1,416 age-matched normal weight controls revealed 38 markers showing strong association. These were further evaluated in 14,186 European subjects *(26)*. In addition to *FTO* and *MC4R*, significant association with obesity was detected for three new risk loci within the endosomal/lysosomal Niemann–Pick C1 gene (*NPC1*), near the transcription factor c-MAF gene (*MAF*) and near the phosphotriesterase-related gene (*PTER*). Additionally, candidate genes were analyzed in the GWAS data set. Interestingly, the association with Val103Ile of the *MC4R* was, among other genes, confirmed. Most of these results were replicated in independent approaches *(37,38)*.

CONCLUSIONS AND PERSPECTIVES

Initially, molecular genetic studies led to the identification of a small number of major genes for human obesity. The relevant mutations have a profound influence on the development of excess body weight, but they are rare and therefore only of minor clinical importance. The majority of confirmed genes involved in the predisposition to obesity are of polygenic nature. The contribution of any single polygene to the development of obesity is small; detection and confirmation of such variants require screening of thousands of individuals.

In 2007 a variation in exon 1 of *FTO* was shown to be associated with obesity. Within a short period of time it became evident that *FTO* represents a major polygene in populations of European, African, and Asian descent. Clinical and experimental observations confirm its importance in energy homeostasis. Sixteen other polygenes for body weight regulation have been reported. The 103Ile variant (minor allele) of the *MC4R* is of interest as it confers protection from obesity. Other *MCR4* variants also contribute to obesity risk. Thus, genetic variation of genes expressed in the CNS plays a prominent role in BMI variation. This is not surprising, given the role of the brain in behavior and energy balance.

If genetic variation accounts for 50–70% of the variance in human BMI, we have far to go; only 1–2% of BMI variance is explained by the currently known polygenes. Realistically, we might assume that the currently detected variants represent the tip of the iceberg; effect sizes of variants detected in the future may be even smaller. Obviously, sample sizes have to be very large to detect these signals and to confirm them independently. If BMI heritability results from the effect of hundreds of alleles, many of which account for less than 50 g, we would have substantial genetic heterogeneity among obese individuals. Assuming this scenario, simplistic ideas of genotype–phenotype correlations would have to be dismissed.

In light of the low BMI variance explained by the polygenes detected in recent GWAS, we can speculate that infrequent alleles with stronger effect sizes, not readily detected in GWAS, may explain a larger part of the variance of BMI. Another disconcerting idea pertains to genotype–environment interactions. These may be rather specific, based on the genotype of an individual. While formal genetic studies have taught us that non-additive factors play a prominent role in BMI heritability estimates, the currently known variants seemingly act in an additive manner only. Future analysis of genetic factors involved in body weight regulation will substantiate our understanding of the mechanisms leading to obesity and hopefully lead to improved therapeutic approaches.

ACKNOWLEDGMENTS

This work was supported by grants from the Bundesministerium für Bildung und Forschung (NGFNplus 01GS0820), the Deutsche Forschungsgemeinschaft (HE 1446/4-1), and the European Union (FP6 LSHMCT-2003-503041).

Editor's Questions and Authors' Response

- **BMI heritability appears to result from the effects of hundreds of alleles with small effects, and there is substantial genetic heterogeneity among obese individuals. Moreover, recent investigations suggest that epigenetic effects on a number of imprinted genes are likely to play important roles in disease risk (Kong et al., 2009). Given this complexity of regulation, is it likely that future genetic analysis of parents or young people will be able to predict reliably the risk of childhood or adult obesity?**

- The predictive value of the detected obesity alleles varies between monogenic gene and polygenic effects. The effect sizes (and thus the explained part of the respective individual's body weight) are in the magnitude of 30–50 kg or more for the monogenic forms. The polygenic variants increase the body weight just by a few hundred grams to 1–2 kg. Hence, the predictive value of these genetic variants is quite different. If a lot of these variants are indeed detected in the future, prediction will potentially become feasible. However, we are currently far from being able to do so because the BMI variance that can be explained currently by polygenic variants is only about 1–2%. Thus, a lot of variance remains to be detected in order to explain the heritability estimates in the range of 0.5.

- **More to the point, would a straightforward but detailed family history provide as much or more predictive power?**

- The answer currently is yes (see above). However, the analysis of a family history cannot give hints to the involvement of specific genetic mechanisms. Hence, genetic tests could provide much more detailed data pertaining to pathways predisposing to obesity within the analyzed family. Currently, obese children and adolescents are in some cases being screened for MC4R mutations. We assume that the obesity of such individuals is largely due to their respective mutation.

Kong A, Steinthorsdottir V, Masson G, Thorleifsson G, Sulem P, Besenbacher S, Jonasdottir A, Sigurdsson A, Kristinsson KT, Jonasdottir A, Frigge ML, Gylfason A, Olason PI, Gudjonsson SA, Sverrisson S, Stacey SN, Sigurgeirsson B, Benediktsdottir KR, Sigurdsson H, Jonsson T, Benediktsson R, Olafsson JH, Johannsson OT, Hreidarsson AB, Sigurdsson G; DIAGRAM Consortium, Ferguson-Smith AC, Gudbjartsson DF, Thorsteinsdottir U, Stefansson K. Parental origin of sequence variants associated with complex diseases. Nature. 2009 Dec 17;462(7275):868–74.

REFERENCES

1. Walley AJ, Asher JE, Froguel P. The genetic contribution to non-syndromic human obesity. Nat Rev Genet. 2009;10:431–42.
2. Hinney A, Hebebrand J. Polygenic obesity in humans. Obes Facts. 2008;1:35–42.
3. Neel JV. Diabetes mellitus: "thrifty" genotype rendered detrimental by "progress"? Am J Hum Genet. 1962;14: 353–62.
4. Hinney A, Hebebrand J. Three at One Swoop!. Obes Facts. 2009;2:3–8.
5. Saunders CL, Chiodini BD, Sham P, et al. Meta-analysis of genome-wide linkage studies in BMI and obesity. Obesity (Silver Spring). 2007;15:2263–75.
6. Risch N, Merikangas K. The future of genetic studies of complex human diseases. Science. 1996;273:1516–7.
7. Farooqi IS, O'Rahilly S. Monogenic obesity in humans. Annu Rev Med. 2005;56:443–58.
8. Hinney A, Schmidt A, Nottebom K, et al. Several mutations in the melanocortin-4 receptor gene including a non-sense and a frameshift mutation associated with dominantly inherited obesity in humans. J Clin Endocrinol Metab. 1999;84:1483–86.
9. Hinney A, Hohmann S, Geller F, et al. Melanocortin-4 receptor gene: case-control study and transmission disequilibrium test confirm that functionally relevant mutations are compatible with a major gene effect for extreme obesity. J Clin Endocrinol Metab. 2003;88:4258–67.
10. Hinney A, Bettecken T, Tarnow P, et al. Prevalence, spectrum, and functional characterization of melanocortin-4 receptor gene mutations in a representative population based sample and obese adults from Germany. J Clin Endocrinol Metab. 2006;91:1761–9.
11. Lubrano-Berthelier C, Dubern B, Lacorte JM, et al. Melanocortin 4 receptor mutations in a large cohort of severely obese adults: prevalence, functional classification, genotype-phenotype relationship, and lack of association with binge eating. J Clin Endocrinol Metab. 2006;91:1811–8.
12. Geller F, Reichwald K, Dempfle A, et al. Melanocortin-4 receptor gene variant I103 is negatively associated with obesity. Am J Hum Genet. 2004;74:572–81.
13. Heid IM, Vollmert C, Hinney A, et al. Association of the 103I MC4R allele with decreased body mass in 7937 participants of two population based surveys. J Med Genet. 2005;42:e21.
14. Stutzmann F, Vatin V, Cauchi S, et al. Non-synonymous polymorphisms in melanocortin-4 receptor protect against obesity: the two facets of a Janus obesity gene. Hum Mol Genet. 2007;16:1837–44.
15. Young EH, Wareham NJ, Farooqi S, et al. The V103I polymorphism of the MC4R gene and obesity: population based studies and meta-analysis of 29 563 individuals. Int J Obes (Lond). 2007;31:1437–41.
16. Spielman RS, McGinnis RE, Ewens WJ. Transmission test for linkage disequilibrium: the insulin gene region and insulin-dependent diabetes mellitus (IDDM). Am J Hum Genet. 1993;52:506–16.
17. Xiang Z, Litherland SA, Sorensen NB, et al. Pharmacological characterization of 40 human melanocortin-4 receptor polymorphisms with the endogenous proopiomelanocortin-derived agonists and the agouti-related protein (AGRP) antagonist. Biochemistry. 2006;45:7277–88.
18. Loos RJF, Lindgren CM, Li S, et al. Common variants near *MC4R* are associated with fat mass, weight and risk of obesity. Nat Genet. 2008;40:768–75.
19. Herbert A, Gerry NP, McQueen MB, et al. A common genetic variant is associated with adult and childhood obesity. Science. 2006;312:279–83.
20. Lyon HN, Emilsson V, Hinney A, et al. The association of a SNP upstream of INSIG2 with body mass index is reproduced in several but not all cohorts. PLoS Genet. 2007;3:e61.
21. Dina C, Meyre D, Samson C, et al. Comment on 'A common genetic variant is associated with adult and childhood obesity'. Science. 2007;315:187.
22. Loos RJ, Barroso I, O'Rahilly S, et al. Comment on 'A common genetic variant is associated with adult and childhood obesity'. Science. 2007;315:187.

23. Rosskopf D, Bornhorst A, Rimmbach C, et al. Comment on 'A common genetic variant is associated with adult and childhood obesity'. Science. 2007;315:187.

24. Willer CJ, Speliotes EK, Loos RJ, et al. Six new loci associated with body mass index highlight a neuronal influence on body weight regulation. Nat Genet. 2009;41:25–34.

25. Thorleifsson G, Walters GB, Gudbjartsson DF, et al. Genome-wide association yields new sequence variants at seven loci that associate with measures of obesity. Nat Genet. 2009;41:18–24.

26. Meyre D, Delplanque J, Chèvre JC, et al. Genome-wide association study for early-onset and morbid adult obesity identifies three new risk loci in European populations. Nat Genet. 2009;41:157–59.

27. Frayling TM, Timpson NJ, Weedon MN, et al. A common variant in the FTO gene is associated with body mass index and predisposes to childhood and adult obesity. Science. 2007;316:889–94.

28. Scott LJ, Mohlke KL, Bonnycastle LL, et al. A genome-wide association study of type 2 diabetes in Finns detects multiple susceptibility variants. Science. 2007;316:1341–45.

29. Hinney A, Nguyen TT, Scherag A, et al. Genome Wide Association (GWA) study for early onset extreme obesity supports the role of fat mass and obesity associated gene (FTO) variants. PLoS ONE. 2007;2:e1361.

30. Andreasen CH, Stender-Petersen KL, Mogensen MS, et al. Low physical activity accentuates the effect of the FTO rs9939609 polymorphism on body fat accumulation. Diabetes. 2008;57:95–101.

31. Tschritter O, Preissl H, Yokoyama Y, et al. Variation in the FTO gene locus is associated with cerebrocortical insulin resistance in humans. Diabetologia. 2007;50:2602–3.

32. Wåhlén K, Sjölin E, Hoffstedt J. The common rs9939609 gene variant of the fat mass and obesity associated gene (FTO) is related to fat cell lipolysis. J Lipid Res. 2008;49:607–11.

33. Gerken T, Girard CA, Tung YC, et al. The obesity-associated FTO gene encodes a 2-oxoglutarate-dependent nucleic acid demethylase. Science. 2007;318:1469–72.

34. Sanchez-Pulido L, Andrade-Navarro MA. The FTO (fat mass and obesity associated) gene codes for a novel member of the non-heme dioxygenase superfamily. BMC Biochem. 2007;8:23.

35. Boissel S, Reish O, Proulx K, et al. Loss-of-function mutation in the dioxygenase-encoding FTO gene causes severe growth retardation and multiple malformations. Am J Hum Genet. 2009;85:106–11.

36. Fischer J, Koch L, Emmerling C, et al. Inactivation of the FTO gene protects from obesity. Nature. 2009;58:894–8.

37. Renström F, Payne F, Nordström A, et al. Replication and extension of genome-wide association study results for obesity in 4923 adults from northern Sweden. Hum Mol Genet. 2009;18:1489–596.

38. Zhao J, Bradfield JP, Li M, et al. The role of obesity-associated loci identified in genome-wide association studies in the determination of pediatric BMI. Obesity (Silver Spring). 2009;17(12):2254–7. Epub 28 May 2009.

6 Racial Differences in Childhood Obesity: Pathogenesis and Complications

Jaime Haidet, Cem Demirci, and Silva A. Arslanian

CONTENTS

Key Words: Race, ethnicity, insulin resistance, prediabetes, fat distribution, socioeconomic status, NAFLD, lipid, type 2 diabetes

INTRODUCTION

Race and ethnicity are terms used to categorize populations on the basis of shared characteristics. Race is traditionally used to categorize populations on the basis of shared biological characteristics such as skin color, other observable features, and the genetic determinants of such differences (*1*). Ethnicity is used to categorize individuals on the basis of cultural characteristics such as shared language, ancestry, religious traditions, dietary preferences, and history. Although ethnic groups can share a range of phenotypic characteristics due to shared ancestry, the term is typically used to highlight cultural and social characteristics instead of biological ones (*1*). Both race and ethnicity are frequently used interchangeably and are constantly evolving concepts, especially in the United States, making the task of comparing groups or following the same group over time quite challenging. There is an emerging number of Americans who describe their race as "mixed" or "other," and there are changes in ethnic self-identification across generations. Such emerging patterns make it difficult to assign

From: *Contemporary Endocrinology: Pediatric Obesity: Etiology, Pathogenesis, and Treatment*
Edited by: M. Freemark, DOI 10.1007/978-1-60327-874-4_6,
© Springer Science+Business Media, LLC 2010

individuals to invariant categories of race or ethnicity. Nevertheless, we continue to use the terms race and ethnicity because there is social importance given to these constructs, and because such classifications have revealed important biological differences in disease predisposition and complications as well as inequalities in access to health care (1).

Obesity is a worldwide problem affecting all ethnic and social groups; however, there are important racial differences in the prevalence as well as the health complications of obesity. Although childhood obesity is increasing in all ethnic and racial groups, there is a disproportionate rise among black Americans and Hispanic/Mexican Americans. The reasons are complex, involving interactions among genetic, biological, cultural, socioeconomic, environmental, and other influences (1,2). This chapter will focus primarily on the biological differences between black and white children in risk of obesity and its complications.

OBESITY AND RACE

Data from the National Health and Nutrition Examination Survey (NHANES) demonstrate that the prevalence of overweight in American youth has increased in all age and racial groups during each of the survey periods during the past 20 years. Between 1999 and 2004, the prevalence of "at risk of overweight" (BMI $\geq$ 85th percentile) or "overweight" (BMI $\geq$ 95th percentile) in youth ages 12–19 years has increased from 30 to 34.4% and 14.8 to 17.4%, respectively (3). However, the increases in childhood overweight were considerably greater in non-Hispanic blacks (13.4–23.6%) and Mexican Americans (13.8–23.4%) than in American whites; 25% of black girls (12–19 years) are now overweight compared with 15% of white girls of similar age (3). The trends are similar in younger children and adults. On the other hand, among a sample of preschool children drawn from 20 large US cities, the prevalence of obesity was 25.8% among Hispanics, 16.2% among blacks, and 14.8% among whites (4). These differences were not explained by racial/ethnic differences in socioeconomic indicators.

The National Heart, Lung, and Blood Institute Growth and Health Study shows that the racial divergence in adiposity begins during adolescence and relates temporally to puberty, with the prevalence increasing in blacks during pubertal maturation (5). Although the mechanisms responsible for these differences are not fully understood, environmental factors such as high energy intake (6), low-physical activity level (7), and sedentary behavior (e.g., increased television watching) have been reported in black vs. white girls. However, in adult women, racial differences in the prevalence of obesity persist after accounting for these environmental factors (8), suggesting that inherent metabolic/physiological differences exist between the two racial groups (9). Thus, unmodifiable and modifiable risk factors, together or independent of each other, could explain the racial disparity in obesity. Among the former would be genetic/biological/inherent factors predisposing to obesity, involving appetite regulation, energy expenditure, and metabolic alterations; among the latter would be environmental/behavioral/sociocultural factors conducive to a positive energy balance. While the former may not be amenable to therapy until such time that specific genetic alterations and their mechanism of action are identified and lead to specific pharmacogenomic therapies, the latter could be targeted to correct the racial disparity in childhood obesity and its consequences.

RACE AND GENETIC/BIOLOGICAL DIFFERENTIAL IN RISK OF OBESITY

Race, Obesity, and Genetics

Human adiposity is highly heritable, but only a few of the genes that predispose to obesity in most humans are known (see the chapters in Part III). Less well understood are race-specific genes that could modulate the risk of obesity in any group. Because the prevalence of higher obesity rates in minority populations persists even after adjusting for socioeconomic factors, genetic factors have been implicated to explain some of the differences.

To identify genetic loci influencing BMI, a pooled analysis of genome-wide admixture mapping scans was performed in 15,280 African-American adults from 14 epidemiologic studies *(10)*. After adjusting for age, sex, and study, BMI was analyzed both as a dichotomized and a continuous trait. The results revealed that a higher percentage of European ancestry correlated with lower BMI. In addition, in obese individuals there were two loci with increased African ancestry on chromosome X (Xq13.1 and Xq25) and one locus with increased European ancestry on chromosome 5 (5q13.3).

The 5q13.3 and Xq25 regions both contain genes that are known to be involved in appetite regulation; thus it is possible that genetic differences in the hormonal regulation of appetite and energy intake play a role in race-related differences in obesity. Ghrelin is a "hunger" peptide whose levels increase before meals and decrease postprandially *(11)*. Conversely, peptide YY (PYY) is a "satiety" hormone that is low preprandially and increases after meals *(11)*. Therefore, impaired regulation of ghrelin and PYY might lead to impaired hunger and/or satiety. We demonstrated that suppression of ghrelin following an oral glucose load was attenuated in black children relative to whites. Additionally, PYY levels were lower in blacks *(11)*. Thus, lesser suppression of ghrelin and lower levels of PYY after a meal could in theory promote subsequent food intake and thereby contribute to the higher risk of obesity in black youth. However, there are no epidemiological data or well-controlled studies that demonstrate differences in food intake between black and white children.

Other hormones and peptides likely contribute to obesity risk. A genome-wide association study in a racially and ethnically diverse sample of 24,722 adults from four cohorts observed no variation in the frequencies of the three insulin-induced gene 2 (*INSIG2*) single nucleotide polymorphism (SNP) genotypes between white, Hispanic, and black American obese adults and non-obese individuals *(12)*. Association analysis of the *FTO* gene with obesity in children of Caucasian and African ancestry revealed a common tagging SNP with some differences in allele frequencies *(13)*. In contrast, an association between obesity and a SNP of the *MC4R* locus in European American children was not found in African-American obese youth *(14)*. Thus, much work remains to be done to identify potential genetic differences which could explain the higher rates of obesity in minority children.

RACE, OBESITY, AND BIOLOGY

Hyperinsulinemia/Insulin Resistance

There are convincing epidemiological data that black children are hyperinsulinemic compared with their white peers. The Bogalusa Heart Study was the first to show that black children, 5–17-years-old, have higher insulin responses than their white counterparts during an oral glucose tolerance test (OGTT) *(15)*. In another study, the higher insulin levels in black children remained significant after controlling for adiposity differences *(16)*. In well-controlled patient-oriented research in which healthy black and white children were matched for age, puberty, total and visceral adiposity, and physical fitness (variables that impact insulin sensitivity and secretion), black children were found to have ~20% lower in vivo insulin sensitivity *(17)*. This was accompanied by ~150% higher first-phase insulin secretion in blacks, which was over and beyond the expected compensatory response to lower insulin sensitivity (Fig. 1).

Using genetic admixture analysis, others demonstrated that these differences in insulin sensitivity and secretion could be explained both on genetic and environmental bases *(19)*. In favor of the former is the observation that low adiponectin levels in black vs. white children may be a biological marker that predisposes them to a greater risk of insulin resistance *(18)*. Adiponectin is an adipocytokine that is exclusively expressed and secreted from adipose tissue. Its levels are low in obesity, states of

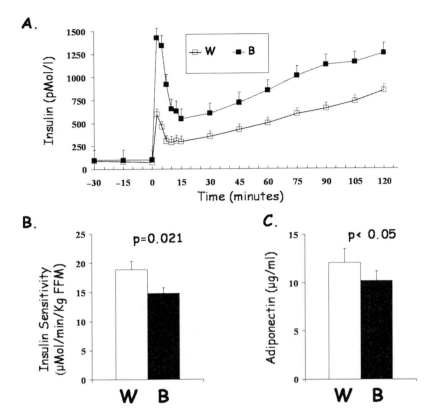

Fig. 1. (a) Insulin concentrations during a 2-h hyperglycemic clamp (225 mg/dl). (b) In vivo insulin sensitivity measured during a 40 mU/m^2/min hyperinsulinemic-euglycemic clamp. (c) Adiponectin levels, in black (B) and white (W) youth. Adapted with permission *(17,18)*.

insulin resistance, type 2 diabetes, and cardiovascular disease. The antidiabetogenic and antiatherogenic properties of adiponectin are evident early in life because hypoadiponectinemia is a strong and independent correlate of insulin resistance and β-cell dysfunction in youth. The low adiponectin level in black youth is independent of visceral adiposity. Moreover, the race-related difference in insulin sensitivity disappears after controlling for the lower adiponectin levels in blacks.

Lifestyle differences in dietary habits may also contribute to racial differences in insulin sensitivity. High-fat diets have been implicated in the pathogenesis of insulin resistance in adults. Correlation analysis reveals an inverse relationship between the higher fat/carbohydrate ratio in the diets of black children and insulin sensitivity *(17)*. Black children are reported to have high-fat intake in some but not all studies *(20)*. Low levels of physical activity and physical fitness might also play roles. However, in one study, neither physical activity nor fitness could explain the racial difference in insulin sensitivity *(21)*.

Even when black and white youth are matched for degree of insulin sensitivity, insulin levels and insulin secretion are higher in blacks *(22)*. Although the mechanisms responsible for the up-regulation of β-cell function in black youth are unknown, potential causes include dietary/lifestyle factors, genetic differences, and inherent differences in neuronal and/or metabolic signaling for insulin secretion. Increased dietary fat relative to carbohydrate was found to correlate positively with first-phase insulin levels in children *(17)*. On the other hand, genetic admixture was independently related to acute insulin response to glucose, indicating that hyperinsulinemia in black youth may have a genetic basis *(19)*.

Thus, much work remains to be done to decipher the underlying causes for race-related differences in insulinemia.

Lipid Metabolism

Irrespective of what causes the hyperinsulinemia in black youth, it is plausible that it plays a role in the increased risk of obesity in blacks. Hyperinsulinemia inhibits lipolysis and leads over time to progressive fat accretion under conditions of excess energy intake or diminished physical activity. Indeed, the rate of whole body lipolysis, measured by [^{2}H$_5$]glycerol stable isotope, was 40% lower in black vs. white healthy prepubertal children (Fig. 2) (23). This may constitute an early metabolic phenotype in blacks that may mediate fat trapping and susceptibility to obesity in a specific environmental context of energy excess. Thus, both genetics and environment together may play a pathophysiological role in the excess risk of development of obesity in blacks.

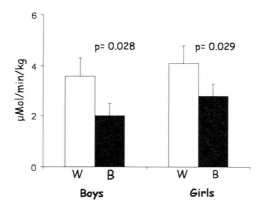

Fig. 2. Rates of total body lipolysis in black (B) and white (W) boys and girls. Adapted with permission (23). Copyright 2001, The Endocrine Society.

Debate continues in the literature as to whether or not hyperinsulinemia is a consequence or cause of obesity. In 1962, the so-called thrifty genotype hypothesis was proposed by Neel (24). Fundamental to this theory is the hypothesis that hyperinsulinemia precedes obesity, with a differential in insulin action on glucose vs. fat metabolism (23); the antilipolytic effect of insulin is increased and mobilization of stored fat is inhibited, leading to lipid storage. In favor of this theory, fasting insulin levels in 5- to 9-year-old Pima Indian children were associated with higher rates of weight gain during a 10-year follow-up period. In a cohort of black and white children, fasting insulin levels were positively associated with the rate of increase in fat mass (25).

Reduced postabsorptive fat oxidation also contributes to positive energy balance and, therefore, future weight gain and obesity (26). Puberty is associated with increased fat oxidation. However, the puberty-associated increase in fat oxidation is diminished in black girls compared with their white peers (9). In addition we and others have shown reduced resting metabolic rates in black vs. white youth (9). A two-year longitudinal study in 9- to 11-year-old black and white youth indicates that total daily energy expenditure, resting metabolic rate, and substrate oxidation are predictors of gain in body fatness (27). Collectively, these observations suggest that the lower metabolic rate and the reduced fat oxidation during puberty in black girls may predispose them to future weight gain and obesity in the context of an obesogenic environment. This metabolic phenotype could potentially explain the divergence in adiposity in black girls during adolescence (5).

Several factors influence resting substrate oxidation; these include genetic factors, the amount of adipose tissue, level of activity, caloric intake, and composition of diet *(28)*. However, the underlying mechanisms of racial differences in fat oxidation are still unclear. A single recent study in adults showed that the mass of metabolically active organs (e.g. brain, liver, heart, kidney, and spleen) was significantly smaller in blacks than in whites, and the racial difference in resting metabolic rate disappeared once the mass of these organs was accounted *(29)*. It is currently unknown whether this holds true in children. On the other hand, it is also plausible that higher inactivity levels and lower cardiorespiratory fitness in black vs. white children *(30)* may contribute to lower metabolic rate and fat oxidation.

It remains to be investigated whether the smaller mass of metabolically active organs, the lower fat oxidation, and the lower cardiorespiratory fitness are biologically/genetically driven, environmentally determined, or both. The skeletal muscles of obese or type 2 diabetic adults are characterized by fewer mitochondria, smaller mitochondrial size, and reduced mitochondrial oxidative capacity *(31)*; these findings suggest that there could be race-related biological differences in mitochondrial characteristics that underlie differences in fat oxidation, resting metabolic rate, and insulin sensitivity. In a study of young adult black and white men, we demonstrated race-related variations in skeletal muscle oxidative metabolism using ^{31}phosphorous nuclear magnetic resonance spectroscopy. The results suggested a lower proportion of type 1 oxidative fibers and a higher proportion of type 2 glycolytic fibers in blacks, which explained their lower peak oxygen consumption *(32)*. It remains to be determined if similar black vs. white differences in skeletal muscle oxidative metabolism are present early in childhood.

RACE, OBESITY, AND BODY FAT DISTRIBUTION

Racial differences in body composition and body fat topography are well documented in adults. When matched for BMI, waist/hip ratio, or total adiposity, black adults have less visceral adipose tissue than their white counterparts *(33)*. This racial dimorphism in visceral adipose tissue accumulation is evident in prepubertal children *(34)*, and over time the growth in visceral fat is greater in white children compared with blacks with a difference of $\sim 1.9 \pm 0.8$ cm^2/year *(35)*. We and others have shown that black obese adolescents have significantly less visceral fat, measured by CT, than white peers with similar BMI and total body adiposity *(36,37)*. Furthermore, for a given BMI, whites have higher waist circumferences than blacks. Additionally, for a given waist circumference, blacks have more subcutaneous adipose tissue than white peers, with the magnitude of the difference increasing with increasing waist circumference *(37)*. Such information is of importance, given that visceral obesity plays an important role in the metabolic complications of obesity including insulin resistance, hypertension, dyslipidemia, type 2 diabetes, nonalcoholic fatty liver disease, and the metabolic syndrome *(36,38)*. Thus, racial differences in body composition and body fat topography could result in race-related differences in obesity co-morbidities and the metabolic syndrome.

Our research shows that for similar degrees of BMI and total body adiposity, white obese adolescents have a more atherogenic lipid risk profile, because of increased visceral adiposity, than blacks. Conversely, blacks have a heightened diabetogenic risk *(36)*. Triglyceride levels are substantially lower in black children and adults than in whites, making the application of a uniform cutoff of triglycerides for the metabolic syndrome questionable. Thus, using BMI alone may be misleading when children of different racial groups are evaluated, and future studies are needed to develop race-specific anthropometric criteria for obesity-related co-morbidities and health outcomes *(37)*.

RACE AND ENVIRONMENTAL/SOCIOCULTURAL DIFFERENTIAL IN RISK OF OBESITY

Obesity and Socioeconomic Status (SES)

Socioeconomic status (SES) is a risk factor for obesity. There is an inverse association between SES and obesity prevalence in children which is independent of parental weight status. The higher prevalence of obesity in lower SES children is assumed to be due to greater exposure to risk factors for positive energy balance both within the home (e.g., sedentary lifestyles, energy-dense diet, and permissive parental-feeding styles) and in the local neighborhood (e.g., availability of fast foods, limited access to safe, and pleasant areas for physical activity) *(39,40)*. In environments that facilitate positive energy balance – as is likely to be true in lower SES environments – genetically susceptible individuals will show even higher weight gain.

Parental SES is associated inversely with childhood obesity among whites: 40% of poor white women and 34% of poor white men were obese in the 1999–2002 NHANES survey, compared with 23% of white women and 14% of men with family incomes greater than 400% of the poverty line. In contrast, higher SES does not appear to protect black children against obesity. In this group, childhood obesity is not associated significantly with parental income and education *(41)*. Nevertheless, obesity rates in whites vary inversely with educational status and are significantly higher in high school dropouts than in high school graduates and twice as high as those in college graduates *(42,43)*.

Obesity and Sociocultural Differences

Sociocultural factors play an important role in shaping body image and desirable weight and may contribute to racial/ethnic differences in obesity. Body image is a multidimensional concept thought to influence the desire to lose weight and the self-perception of body size *(44)*. Racial/ethnic differences in weight misperception have been reported; misperception among overweight people (that is belief among overweight people that they are healthy weight) was more common in blacks than in whites and more common in men than women *(45)*. In addition, several studies demonstrate black/white differences in consumption of regular soda, high-fat foods, and fast-food restaurant use, which could be culturally mediated, enhancing the risk of obesity in black children (Table 1) *(46,47)*. Limited evidence suggests that blacks are more consistently exposed to food promotion and distribution patterns that promote adverse health effects *(48)*. Thus, ethnic, cultural, environmental, and economic factors might enhance the inherent/genetic predisposition of black youth to obesity.

Table 1
Cultural Differences in Black Adolescents

Heavy black adolescents do not perceive themselves heavy

More black girls express a desire to be on the fat side

Black children have higher total fat and cholesterol intake

Black children prefer sweet taste in liquids

Black girls have higher total energy intake

Black children are physically less active

Black girls spent more time watching television

Black high school students have the highest consumption of sugar-sweetened beverages, high-fat foods, and the highest frequency of fast-food restaurant use

RACE AND CO-MORBIDITIES OF OBESITY

Numerous co-morbidities are associated with childhood obesity, which serves as a segway to adult morbidity and mortality (49). Here we provide information on race-related differences, mostly focusing on black vs. white children.

Race and Nonalcoholic Fatty Liver Disease

Nonalcoholic fatty liver disease (NAFLD) encompasses a wide range of liver damage, from simple steatosis to steatohepatitis, advanced fibrosis, and cirrhosis (50) and is the most common cause of pediatric liver disease (51). The prevalence of NAFLD increases with age and varies by race (52). NAFLD prevalence is lowest in blacks, followed by whites, then Asians (variability among the subgroups), and is highest in Hispanics (52,53). The odds of a Hispanic child having fatty liver is five times greater than that of a black child (52). The prevalence of cryptogenic cirrhosis is 3.1-fold higher in Hispanic Americans compared with European Americans and 3.9-fold lower in black Americans compared with European Americans (53,54). It is felt that NAFLD may play an under-recognized role in cryptogenic cirrhosis (53,55). The lower prevalence of NAFLD in blacks is counterintuitive given their increased risk for obesity and insulin resistance (51). However, it might be explained in part by the smaller visceral adipose tissue compartment and the lower triglyceride levels (see later).

Race and Lipids

Black–white differences in lipids and lipoproteins occur early in childhood and are clearly established by 9 years of age (56). Few studies have been carried out in neonates; these have not found significant differences between blacks and whites (56,57). By age 2, total serum cholesterol approaches young adult levels and further dynamic changes occur with sexual maturation, establishing adult patterns (56,57). During sexual maturation, the most striking difference occurs in white males, with progressive increases in the ratio of LDL-C to HDL-C (56). In both childhood and adolescence, blacks have lower triglyceride and higher HDL levels compared with whites (57). Increased prevalence of hypertriglyceridemia is also seen in Mexican Americans (1,58,59).

The elevated triglyceride level in whites has been related to an increased large VLDL subclass in comparison to blacks (60); however, racial differences in particle sizes may be attributed to levels of triglyceride and HDL cholesterol (61). Our research demonstrates that there are significant black/white differences in lipoprotein particle size and concentrations in childhood. However, after adjusting for visceral adiposity differences between black and white children, only VLDL size and concentration remain significantly favorable in blacks (62). Moreover, analysis of lipoprotein particle size and concentration across in vivo insulin sensitivity quartiles revealed that in both racial groups, the most insulin-resistant children had higher concentrations of small dense LDL, small HDL, large VLDL, and smaller LDL and HDL sizes than their more insulin-sensitive counterparts (62).

Race and Cardiovascular Disease

Though the repercussions of cardiovascular disease are not usually seen until adulthood, the initiation of cardiovascular disease occurs early in life and childhood risk factors are associated with adult cardiovascular disease (63). The fatty streak is the earliest lesion of atherosclerosis and has been found in aortas of children as young as 9 months of age and invariably after the age of 3 years (64). By the age of 20, raised lesions have already appeared in the coronary arteries and are implicated in clinical disease (57,65). In adolescence and early adulthood, blacks have more aortic fatty streaks than whites, with 1.5 times greater surface involvement; this cannot be attributed to antemortem cardiovascular risks (64–66) and is not as obvious in the coronary arteries (66). Interestingly, white adults have more extensive raised lesions in the aorta than blacks (65) and have significantly higher rates of coronary heart disease *(57)*. Thus the progression to advanced lesions from fatty streaks likely differs between races; the mechanisms are yet to be elucidated *(65)*.

Race and Prediabetes and Type 2 Diabetes (T2DM)

Based on population-based registries, the rates of type 1 diabetes are typically lower in black than white children *(67)*. On the other hand T2DM is disproportionately higher among blacks, Hispanics, American Indians, and Asians/South Pacific Islanders *(1,67–71)*. The earliest reports from pediatric diabetes clinics found that 68–100% of children with T2DM were black *(71–73)*. In the more recent SEARCH for Diabetes in Youth Population Study, T2DM in 10- to 19-year-olds varied by ethnicity: 33% of patients were black, 76% American Indian, 40% Asians/Pacific Islanders, 22% Hispanic youth, and 6% white *(74)*. The TODAY (Treatment Options for type 2 Diabetes in Adolescents and Youth) study found that 36% of adolescents with type 2 diabetes are black, 35% Hispanic, and 19% white *(75)*.

Reported rates of *prediabetes* [i.e., impaired fasting glucose (IFG) *and/or* impaired glucose tolerance (IGT)] in obese children vary tremendously, from 2 to 40%, depending on the population. Adolescent data from the NHANES 2005–2006 using fasting and 2-h glucose during an oral glucose tolerance test revealed unadjusted prevalence rates of IFG, IGT, and prediabetes of 13.1, 3.4, and 16.1%, respectively *(76)*. Blacks had lower rates than non-Hispanic whites and Mexican Americans (IFG: 9.7, 14.1, and 14.3%, respectively; IGT: 0.9, 3.7, and 3.5% respectively, prediabetes: 10.3, 17.2, and 16.9%, respectively). The IFG prevalence of 13.1% among US adolescents in 2005–2006 was ~87% higher than the 7% estimated from NHANES 1999–2000 (13% in Mexican Americans, 7% in whites, and 4.2% in blacks) *(77)*. The lower prevalence rate in blacks is surprising considering their increased risk of obesity and insulin resistance. However, the data included adolescents who were normal weight and overweight without separation for only obese adolescents of different racial groups. The results of the Studies to Treat or Prevent Pediatric Type 2 Diabetes (STOPP-T2D) revealed that the prevalence of IGT was 4.1% among overweight eighth graders in four middle schools *(78)*. In contrast to the NHANES findings, the prevalence rates of IGT were highest in Native Americans and Hispanics, followed by blacks and lowest in whites (7.3, 3.2, 1.3, and 0.9%, respectively). Prevalence of IFG was lowest in blacks (32.4%) and highest in Native Americans and Hispanics (~45%). In the Princeton School District of Cincinnati rates of IGT were much lower, detected among only 0.5% of 5th–12th graders and more in non-Hispanic whites than blacks or whites *(79)*. These highly variable estimates, whether overall or race specific, may stem from sampling and geographic variations.

Race and the Metabolic Syndrome

The prevalence of the metabolic syndrome varies depending on the definition used in the literature. Applying four different criteria to a well-characterized population of children, we demonstrated that the prevalence of the metabolic syndrome was significantly higher in overweight youth compared with non-overweight black and white youth *(80)*. The prevalence of metabolic syndrome was 31.3% in overweight black and 42.9% in overweight white youth, compared with 0.7% in non-overweight blacks and 2.8% in non-overweight whites. In overweight Hispanic children age 8–13 years, the prevalence of three or more features of the metabolic syndrome was 30% *(81)*. Path analyses of metabolic syndrome components in black and white children, adolescents, and adults revealed that path coefficients were generally greater in whites than blacks; this may account for the greater prevalence of metabolic syndrome in whites *(82)*. Importantly, individual components of the metabolic syndrome differ between races, especially abdominal adiposity and triglycerides (see previous sections for further details) *(83)*. Triglyceride levels increase significantly with enlarging waist circumference in whites but not in blacks (Fig. 3) *(84)*.

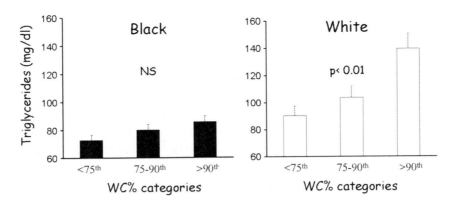

Fig. 3. Triglyceride concentrations according to waist circumference (WC) categories in black and white youth; NS, not significant. Adapted with permission *(84)*.

In a study by Weiss et al., the prevalence of metabolic syndrome was lower in blacks than whites when the groups were analyzed using the same criteria for lipid levels; however, when lipid thresholds specific to blacks were used in the analysis, the prevalence of metabolic syndrome in blacks was comparable to that in whites *(85)*. Independent of race, however, our research demonstrates that visceral obesity, insulin resistance, hyperinsulinemia, and hypoadiponectinemia are the common characteristics of youth with the metabolic syndrome *(80)*. Irrespective of race, the prevalence of large waist circumference, high triglycerides, low HDL, high blood pressure, and prediabetes is highest among youth in the lowest quartile of in vivo insulin sensitivity (Fig. 4). However, in white but not black children, the metabolic syndrome is associated with increased inflammatory markers (Fig. 5) *(83)*. The translation of such race-related differences remains to be determined based on long-term longitudinal outcome studies in different racial groups. Further research in childhood metabolic syndrome is needed not only to unify the definition of the syndrome, but also to test the validity of race-specific criteria.

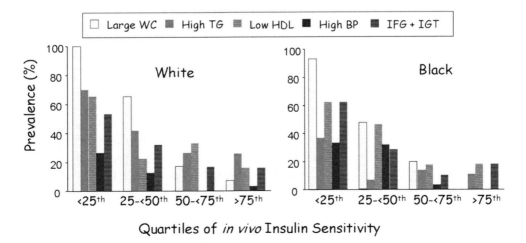

Fig. 4. The prevalence of the individual components of metabolic syndrome by quartiles of in vivo insulin sensitivity in black and white youth. (WC, waist circumference; TG, triglycerides; BP, blood pressure; IFG, impaired fasting glucose; IGT, impaired glucose tolerance.) Adapted with permission *(83)*.

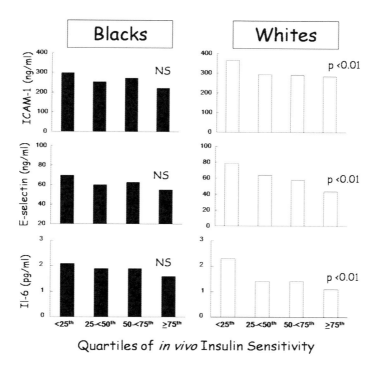

Fig. 5. Circulating biomarkers of endothelial dysfunction and IL-6 in black and white youth according to quartiles of insulin sensitivity. Adapted with permission *(83)*.

RACE AND THE TREATMENT OF OBESITY

Considering that racial differences (biological, environmental, or both) influence the risks of childhood obesity and its complications, it may seem intuitive that obesity treatments be individualized to specific racial/ethnic groups. Though guidelines exist for the treatment of obese children (see *(86)* and treatment sections of this book), there is currently no justification for recommending race-specific treatment *(1)*. Limited data suggest that white adolescents may have more weight loss with either metformin or the combination of sibutramine (an appetite suppressant that inhibits the reuptake of norepinephrine and serotonin) and behavioral therapy than black adolescents *(1)*. In adults, blacks lose less weight after gastric bypass surgery than whites but have comparable improvements in cardiovascular risk factors; these differences in weight loss post-gastric bypass may be related to differences in energy expenditure rather than dietary intake *(1)*. It is unclear whether these racial differences would be replicated in large randomized, controlled studies or whether they reflect the influence of genetics as opposed to cultural and environmental factors. In any case, providers caring for obese children must consider many factors when making treatment decisions, including differences in the perception of obesity, which may play a role in motivation; access to healthcare; availability and affordability of treatment for obesity (lack of insurance is more common in Hispanics than blacks and more common in blacks than whites); dietary preferences; and physical activity preferences *(1)*.

CLOSING REMARKS AND FUTURE DIRECTIONS

Increases in obesity in childhood and adulthood will result in major morbidity and mortality and will inflate health care costs at a time of severe financial deficits in the US economy. The medical profession and its allies may very well be able to advance research in the field of obesity, but what is needed to stop the epidemic of obesity is societal change. The latter will require major policy change, akin to the smoking campaign, combined with economic change and incentives and education. Racial/ethnic factors must be considered in the overall approach to prevention and treatment of childhood obesity.

ACKNOWLEDGMENTS

This work was supported by the United States Public Health Service grant RO1 HD27503 (SA), K24 HD01357 (SA), MO1 RR00084 (GCRC) and UL1 RR024153 (CTSA), T32 DK063686 (CD), and T32 DK007729 (JH).

Editor's Questions and Authors' Response

- **Do you think that differences in rates of pubertal maturation among ethnic groups could contribute to differential rates of obesity or co-morbidities?**

- No. Actually I believe that differences in adiposity are important determinants of the onset of puberty and its tempo. Differences in rates of pubertal maturation exist among ethnic groups with black girls tending to enter puberty and experience menarche about 1 year before white girls. Additionally, increased body mass index is associated with earlier sexual maturation. It is difficult to delineate cause and effect, especially with numerous confounding variables. Irrespective, however, divergence in adiposity begins during adolescence and relates temporally to puberty. In one of our studies we showed that lower increases in fat oxidation between prepubertal and pubertal black girls (puberty is characterized by higher rates of fat oxidation) could predispose them to faster weight gain compared with their white peers. The definitive answer to your question requires longitudinal studies to follow children from prepuberty to completion of puberty in different racial groups.

- **Do we have any data that compares the caloric intake or macronutrient composition of diets of the various ethnic groups?**

- Dietary intake trends are affected by many variables including socioeconomic status, education, environment, food availability, individual preference, and culture. In children and adolescents, the National Health and Nutrition Examination Surveys (NHANES) revealed no clear difference in overall energy intake among racial groups; however, the percentage of energy from total fat was highest among non-Hispanic blacks followed by Mexican Americans then non-Hispanic whites without significant difference in saturated fatty acids (Troiano et al., 2000). According to self-reported dietary recalls, Mexican American children aged 9 years ate higher than recommended fat servings and had higher percent energy from fat and saturated fat and their daily fruit and vegetable intake was half of that recommended by national guidelines (Trevino et al., 1999).

Trevino RP, et al. Diabetes risk factors in low-income Mexican-American children. Diabetes Care. 1999;22:202–7.
Troiano RP, et al. Energy and fat intakes of children and adolescents in the United States: data from the national health and nutrition examination surveys. Am J Clin Nutr. 2000;72(5 Suppl):1343S–53S.

REFERENCES

1. Caprio S, et al. Influence of race, ethnicity, and culture on childhood obesity: implications for prevention and treatment: a consensus statement of Shaping America's Health and the Obesity Society. Diabetes Care. 2008;31(11):2211–21.
2. Nesbitt SD, et al. Overweight as a risk factor in children: a focus on ethnicity. Ethn Dis. 2004;14(1):94–110.

3. Ogden CL, et al. Prevalence of overweight and obesity in the United States, 1999–2004. J Am Med Assoc. 2006;295(13):1549–55.

4. Whitaker RC, Orzol SM. Obesity among US urban preschool children: relationships to race, ethnicity, and socioeconomic status. Arch Pediatr Adolesc Med. 2006;160(6):578–84.

5. Kimm SY, et al. Racial divergence in adiposity during adolescence: The NHLBI Growth and Health Study. Pediatrics. 2001;107(3):E34.

6. Troiano RP, et al. Energy and fat intakes of children and adolescents in the united states: data from the national health and nutrition examination surveys. Am J Clin Nutr. 2000;72(5 Suppl):1343S–53S.

7. Kimm SY, et al. Decline in physical activity in black girls and white girls during adolescence. N Engl J Med. 2002;347(10):709–15.

8. Burke GL, et al. Differences in weight gain in relation to race, gender, age and education in young adults: the CARDIA Study. Coronary Artery Risk Development in Young Adults. Ethn Health. 1996;1(4):327–35.

9. Lee S, Arslanian SA. Fat oxidation in black and white youth: a metabolic phenotype potentially predisposing black girls to obesity. J Clin Endocrinol Metab. 2008;93(11):4547–51.

10. Egyud MR, et al. Use of weighted reference panels based on empirical estimates of ancestry for capturing untyped variation. Hum Genet. 2009;125(3):295–303.

11. Bacha F, Arslanian SA. Ghrelin and peptide YY in youth: are there race-related differences? J Clin Endocrinol Metab. 2006;91(8):3117–22.

12. Bressler J, et al. The INSIG2 rs7566605 genetic variant does not play a major role in obesity in a sample of 24,722 individuals from four cohorts. BMC Med Genet. 2009;10:56.

13. Grant SF, et al. Association analysis of the FTO gene with obesity in children of Caucasian and African ancestry reveals a common tagging SNP. PLoS ONE. 2008;3(3):e1746.

14. Grant SF, et al. Investigation of the Locus near MC4R with childhood obesity in Americans of European and African Ancestry. Obesity (Silver Spring). 2009;17(7):1461–65.

15. Svec F, et al. Black-white contrasts in insulin levels during pubertal development. The Bogalusa Heart Study. Diabetes. 1992;41(3):313–17.

16. Gutin B, et al. Relation of percentage of body fat and maximal aerobic capacity to risk factors for atherosclerosis and diabetes in black and white seven- to eleven-year-old children. J Pediatr. 1994;125(6 Pt 1):847–52.

17. Arslanian SA, et al. Hyperinsulinemia in African-American children: decreased insulin clearance and increased insulin secretion and its relationship to insulin sensitivity. Diabetes. 2002;51(10):3014–19.

19. Gower BA, et al. Using genetic admixture to explain racial differences in insulin-related phenotypes. Diabetes. 2003;52(4):1047–51.

18. Lee S, et al. Racial differences in adiponectin in youth: relationship to visceral fat and insulin sensitivity. Diabetes Care. 2006;29(1):51–56.

20. Lindquist CH, Gower BA, Goran MI. Role of dietary factors in ethnic differences in early risk of cardiovascular disease and type 2 diabetes. Am J Clin Nutr. 2000;71(3):725–32.

21. Ku CY, et al. Racial differences in insulin secretion and sensitivity in prepubertal children: role of physical fitness and physical activity. Obes Res. 2000;8(7):506–15.

22. Hannon TS, et al. Hyperinsulinemia in African-American adolescents compared with their American white peers despite similar insulin sensitivity: a reflection of upregulated beta-cell function? Diabetes Care. 2008;31(7):1445–47.

23. Danadian K, et al. Lipolysis in African-American children: is it a metabolic risk factor predisposing to obesity? J Clin Endocrinol Metab. 2001;86(7):3022–26.

24. Neel JV. Diabetes mellitus: a "thrifty" genotype rendered detrimental by "progress"? Am J Hum Genet. 1962;14:353–62.

25. Johnson MS, et al. Longitudinal changes in body fat in African American and Caucasian children: influence of fasting insulin and insulin sensitivity. J Clin Endocrinol Metab. 2001;86(7):3182–87.

26. Zurlo F, et al. Low ratio of fat to carbohydrate oxidation as predictor of weight gain: study of 24-h RQ. Am J Physiol. 1990;259(5 Pt 1):E650–7.

27. DeLany JP, et al. Energy expenditure and substrate oxidation predict changes in body fat in children. Am J Clin Nutr. 2006;84(4):862–70.

28. Schutz Y. Abnormalities of fuel utilization as predisposing to the development of obesity in humans. Obes Res. 1995;3(Suppl 2):173S–8S.

29. Gallagher D, et al. Small organs with a high metabolic rate explain lower resting energy expenditure in African American than in white adults. Am J Clin Nutr. 2006;83(5):1062–67.

30. Andreacci JL, et al. Comparison of maximal oxygen consumption between obese black and white adolescents. Pediatr Res. 2005;58(3):478–82.

31. Turner N, Heilbronn LK. Is mitochondrial dysfunction a cause of insulin resistance? Trends Endocrinol Metab. 2008;19(9):324–30.

32. Suminski RR, et al. Peak oxygen consumption and skeletal muscle bioenergetics in African-American and Caucasian men. Med Sci Sports Exerc. 2000;32(12):2059–66.

33. Hoffman DJ, et al. Comparison of visceral adipose tissue mass in adult African Americans and whites. Obes Res. 2005;13(1):66–74.

34. Goran MI, et al. Visceral fat in white and African American prepubertal children. Am J Clin Nutr. 1997;65(6):1703–8.

35. Huang TT, et al. Growth of visceral fat, subcutaneous abdominal fat, and total body fat in children. Obes Res. 2001;9(5):283–89.

36. Bacha F, et al. Obesity, regional fat distribution, and syndrome X in obese black versus white adolescents: race differential in diabetogenic and atherogenic risk factors. J Clin Endocrinol Metab. 2003;88(6):2534–40.

37. Lee S, et al. Race and gender differences in the relationships between anthropometrics and abdominal fat in youth. Obesity (Silver Spring). 2008;16(5):1066–71.

38. Taksali SE, et al. High visceral and low abdominal subcutaneous fat stores in the obese adolescent: a determinant of an adverse metabolic phenotype. Diabetes. 2008;57(2):367–71.

39. Shrewsbury V, Wardle J. Socioeconomic status and adiposity in childhood: a systematic review of cross-sectional studies 1990–2005. Obesity (Silver Spring). 2008;16(2):275–84.

40. Rosenkranz RR, Dzewaltowski DA. Model of the home food environment pertaining to childhood obesity. Nutr Rev. 2008;66(3):123–40.

41. Crawford PB, et al. Ethnic issues in the epidemiology of childhood obesity. Pediatr Clin North Am. 2001;48(4):855–78.

42. Mokdad AH, et al. Diabetes trends among American Indians and Alaska natives: 1990–1998. Diabetes Care. 2001;24(8):1508–9.

43. Mokdad AH, Bowman BA, Ford ES, Marks JS, Koplan JP. The continuing epidemic of obesity and diabetes in the United States. JAMA. 21 Sept 2001;286(10):1195–200. Full Text via CrossRef | View Record in Scopus | Cited By in Scopus (1185).

44. Dorsey RR, Eberhardt MS, Ogden CL. Racial/Ethnic differences in weight perception. Obesity (Silver Spring). 2009;17(4):790–95.

45. Paeratakul S, et al. Sex, race/ethnicity, socioeconomic status, and BMI in relation to self-perception of overweight. Obes Res. 2002;10(5):345–50.

46. Melnyk MG, Weinstein E. Preventing obesity in black women by targeting adolescents: a literature review. J Am Diet Assoc. 1994;94(5):536–40.

47. Arcan C, et al. Sociodemographic differences in selected eating practices among alternative high school students. J Am Diet Assoc. 2009;109(5):823–29.

48. Grier SA, Kumanyika SK. The context for choice: health implications of targeted food and beverage marketing to African Americans. Am J Public Health. 2008;98(9):1616–29.

49. Dietz WH. Health consequences of obesity in youth: childhood predictors of adult disease. Pediatrics. 1998;101(3 Pt 2):518–25.

50. Angulo P. Nonalcoholic fatty liver disease. N Engl J Med. 2002;346(16):1221–31.

51. Barshop NJ, et al. Review article: epidemiology, pathogenesis and potential treatments of paediatric non-alcoholic fatty liver disease. Aliment Pharmacol Ther. 2008;28(1):13–24.

52. Schwimmer JB, et al. Prevalence of fatty liver in children and adolescents. Pediatrics. 2006;118(4):1388–93.

53. Schwimmer JB, et al. Histopathology of pediatric nonalcoholic fatty liver disease. Hepatology. 2005;42(3):641–49.

54. Browning JD, et al. Ethnic differences in the prevalence of cryptogenic cirrhosis. Am J Gastroenterol. 2004;99(2):292–98.

55. Poonawala A, Nair SP, Thuluvath PJ. Prevalence of obesity and diabetes in patients with cryptogenic cirrhosis: a case-control study. Hepatology. 2000;32(4 Pt 1):689–92.

56. Berenson GS, et al. Risk factors in early life as predictors of adult heart disease: the Bogalusa Heart Study. Am J Med Sci. 1989;298(3):141–51.

57. Zoratti R. A review on ethnic differences in plasma triglycerides and high-density-lipoprotein cholesterol: is the lipid pattern the key factor for the low coronary heart disease rate in people of African origin? Eur J Epidemiol. 1998;14(1):9–21.

58. Jago R, et al. Prevalence of abnormal lipid and blood pressure values among an ethnically diverse population of eighth-grade adolescents and screening implications. Pediatrics. 2006;117(6):2065–73.

59. Duncan GE, Li SM, Zhou XH. Prevalence and trends of a metabolic syndrome phenotype among U.S. Adolescents, 1999–2000. Diabetes Care. 2004;27(10):2438–43.

60. Freedman DS, et al. Differences in the relation of obesity to serum triacylglycerol and VLDL subclass concentrations between black and white children: the Bogalusa Heart Study. Am J Clin Nutr. 2002;75(5):827–33.

61. Freedman DS, et al. Levels and correlates of LDL and VLDL particle sizes among children: the Bogalusa heart study. Atherosclerosis. 2000;152(2):441–49.

62. Burns SF, Lee SJ, Arslanian SA. In vivo insulin sensitivity and lipoprotein particle size and concentration in black and white children. Diabetes Care. 2009;32(11):2087–93. Epub 12 Aug 2009.

63. Frontini MG, et al. Usefulness of childhood non-high density lipoprotein cholesterol levels versus other lipoprotein measures in predicting adult subclinical atherosclerosis: the Bogalusa Heart Study. Pediatrics. 2008;121(5):924–29.

64. Holman RL, et al. The natural history of atherosclerosis: the early aortic lesions as seen in New Orleans in the middle of the 20th century. Am J Pathol. 1958;34(2):209–35.

65. Freedman DS, et al. Black-white differences in aortic fatty streaks in adolescence and early adulthood: the Bogalusa Heart Study. Circulation. 1988;77(4):856–64.

66. Tracy RE, et al. Histologic features of atherosclerosis and hypertension from autopsies of young individuals in a defined geographic population: the Bogalusa Heart Study. Atherosclerosis. 1995;116(2):163–79.

67. Gungor N, et al. Type 2 diabetes mellitus in youth: the complete picture to date. Pediatr Clin North Am. 2005;52(6):1579–609.

68. Type 2 diabetes in children and adolescents. American diabetes association. Diabetes Care. 2000;23(3):381–89.

69. Scott CR, et al. Characteristics of youth-onset noninsulin-dependent diabetes mellitus and insulin-dependent diabetes mellitus at diagnosis. Pediatrics. 1997;100(1):84–91.

70. Fagot-Campagna A, et al. Type 2 diabetes among North American children and adolescents: an epidemiologic review and a public health perspective. J Pediatr. 2000;136(5):664–72.

71. Dabelea D, et al. Type 2 diabetes mellitus in minority children and adolescents. An emerging problem. Endocrinol Metab Clin North Am. 1999;28(4):709–29.

72. Pinhas-Hamiel O, et al. Increased incidence of non-insulin-dependent diabetes mellitus among adolescents. J Pediatr. 1996;128(5 Pt 1):608–15.

73. Pihoker C, et al. Non-insulin dependent diabetes mellitus in African-American youths of Arkansas. Clin Pediatr (Phila). 1998;37(2):97–102.

74. Liese AD, et al. The burden of diabetes mellitus among US youth: prevalence estimates from the SEARCH for Diabetes in Youth Study. Pediatrics. 2006;118(4):1510–18.

75. White N, et al. Clinical characteristics and co-morbidities in a large cohort of youth with Type-2 Diabetes Mellitus (T2DM) screened for the treatment options for Type-2 Diabetes in adolescents and youth (TODAY) study. Diabetes. 2009;58:A70.

76. Li C, et al. Prevalence of pre-diabetes and its association with clustering of cardiometabolic risk factors and hyper-insulinemia among U.S. adolescents: National Health and Nutrition Examination Survey 2005–2006. Diabetes Care. 2009;32(2):342–47.

77. Williams DE, et al. Prevalence of impaired fasting glucose and its relationship with cardiovascular disease risk factors in US adolescents, 1999–2000. Pediatrics. 2005;116(5):1122–26.

78. Baranowski T, et al. Presence of diabetes risk factors in a large U.S. eighth-grade cohort. Diabetes Care. 2006;29(2): 212–17.

79. Dolan LM, et al. Frequency of abnormal carbohydrate metabolism and diabetes in a population-based screening of adolescents. J Pediatr. 2005;146(6):751–58.

80. Lee S, et al. Comparison of different definitions of pediatric metabolic syndrome: relation to abdominal adiposity, insulin resistance, adiponectin, and inflammatory biomarkers. J Pediatr. 2008;152(2):177–84.

81. Cruz ML, et al. The metabolic syndrome in overweight Hispanic youth and the role of insulin sensitivity. J Clin Endocrinol Metab. 2004;89(1):108–13.

82. Chen W, Srinivasan SR, Berenson GS. Path analysis of metabolic syndrome components in black versus white children, adolescents, and adults: the Bogalusa Heart Study. Ann Epidemiol. 2008;18(2):85–91.

83. Lee S, et al. Insulin resistance: link to the components of the metabolic syndrome and biomarkers of endothelial dysfunction in youth. Diabetes Care. 2007;30(8):2091–97.

84. Lee S, et al. Waist circumference, blood pressure, and lipid components of the metabolic syndrome. J Pediatr. 2006;149:809–16.

85. Weiss R, et al. Obesity and the metabolic syndrome in children and adolescents. N Engl J Med. 2004;350(23):2362–74.

86. Spear BA, et al. Recommendations for treatment of child and adolescent overweight and obesity. Pediatrics. 2007;120(Suppl 4):S254–88.

IV PRE- AND PERINATAL DETERMINANTS OF CHILDHOOD OBESITY

7 Maternal Determinants of Childhood Obesity: Weight Gain, Smoking, and Breastfeeding

Katherine J. Wojcik and Elizabeth J. Mayer-Davis

CONTENTS

Key Words: Maternal, pregnancy, weight gain, undernutrition, diet, sleep, smoking-child-obesity

INTRODUCTION

The mother's genetic background and her metabolic status and behavior before, during, and after pregnancy function as important determinants of obesity and related health outcomes in her child. A substantial body of research has explored the roles of maternal factors in childhood obesity-related outcomes; however, many questions remain as to how and when during development these factors exert their influence. Thus, priorities for either clinical or public health action to reduce the risk for childhood obesity are uncertain.

In this chapter, we discuss those maternal factors that appear to have the strongest influence on pediatric obesity: these include maternal weight status, breastfeeding, and smoking. Limited information on maternal dietary habits and physical activity is also presented. Some population sub-groups may be more strongly influenced by these maternal factors than others. For example, African-American girls are at substantially greater risk of becoming obese earlier in life (nearly one-third in 2003–2006 NHANES) than African-American boys or youth of other races and ethnicities. Compared to non-Hispanic white women, African-American women are at higher risk for being overweight at conception *(1)*, for developing gestational diabetes *(2)*, and are less likely to breastfeed their offspring *(3)*. Similarly, Hispanic boys appear to be at greater risk of early obesity (more than 20% in 2003–2006 NHANES) than boys of other races and ethnicities, and Hispanic women are more likely to

From: *Contemporary Endocrinology: Pediatric Obesity: Etiology, Pathogenesis, and Treatment*
Edited by: M. Freemark, DOI 10.1007/978-1-60327-874-4_7,
© Springer Science+Business Media, LLC 2010

be overweight at conception than their non-Hispanic white counterparts *(1)*. Considering that genes and environment can have powerful interactions, maternal factors may be particularly strong within population subgroups at increased risk.

Throughout our discussion, it will be noted when maternal factors related to socioeconomic status, race and ethnicity, and cultural influences may be acting in concert. However, socioeconomic status and related topics will be discussed at greater length in other chapters of this book.

MATERNAL WEIGHT STATUS

Obesity in children is associated with maternal overweight prior to, during, or after pregnancy. The potential public health impact of maternal weight status is quite high owing to the exceedingly high prevalence of overweight among women. Based on National Health and Nutrition Examination Survey (NHANES) 2003–2004 data, the most recent reports available from the Centers for Disease Control and Prevention (CDC) reveal that approximately 33% of all adult women (≥20 years) in the United States are obese and nearly 62% of all adult women are either overweight or obese *(4)*.

Pregravid Weight Status

One of the stronger predictors of childhood overweight is presence of overweight or obesity in the mother prior to pregnancy *(5)*. Maternal obesity may serve as a proxy for the child's genetic predisposition to obesity and/or for early fetal exposure to a biochemical environment altered by maternal overweight status.

Several studies have found pregravid obesity to be a consistently strong predictor of childhood obesity. For example, the odds ratios (ORs) of childhood obesity at 7 years of age were 1.38 with pregravid maternal overweight (BMI=26–29) and 2.56 with pregravid maternal obesity (BMI > 29); however, an interaction between maternal underweight status and maternal weight gain was also reported, as discussed later in this section *(6)*. In a study examining 2- to 14-year olds, the odds of obesity were 3.6 among children with mothers who were obese (BMI ≥ 30) prior to pregnancy compared to the referent group of children with non-obese mothers (BMI < 25) *(5)*. When the same analysis was stratified by age (2- to 6-year olds, 7- to 10-year olds, and 11- to 14-year olds), the most dramatic increase in odds (OR: 5.7) was observed in the 7- to 10-year-old group *(5)*. Among low income children, the odds ratios for obesity were 2.28 among 2-year olds, 3.06 among 3-year olds, and 3.07 among 4-year olds with obese mothers (BMI 30–39.9) compared to those with normal weight mothers (BMI 18.5–24.9) *(7)*.

The impact of maternal obesity may extend through early adulthood; indeed, pregravid BMI has been related to higher adult BMI by age 20 *(8)*. Yet conflicting evidence exists, as a recent study following children from birth to 5 years of age found that adjusting for prenatal factors including pregravid BMI accounted for some of the BMI Z-score differences in normal versus obese children; however, the effect was only observed until 24 months of age, having little or no further effect on BMI Z-score from 24 months to 5 years *(9)*.

The findings of this study are difficult to interpret, because maternal obesity is associated with births of large-for-gestational-age (LGA) babies, which is in turn a predictor of childhood obesity *(7,10–12)*. In an extensive review of maternal obesity, metabolism, and pregnancy outcomes conducted in 2006, obese women were more likely to have LGA/macrosomic infants *(11)*.

Does the father's weight function as a determinant of childhood weight gain? In one recent study, the odds of overweight in children at age 4.5 years were nearly two to three times higher in those with overweight or obese parents than in children with normal weight parents *(13)*. This effect was noted when maternal or paternal BMI was analyzed separately or in combination. Interestingly, same-sex parental BMI, mother–daughter or father–son, may also predict child obesity risk *(14)*.

In addition to maternal overweight or obesity, maternal underweight may also lead to child obesity if there is excess or inadequate gestational weight gain (see below) or rapid catch-up growth of the child during infancy and early childhood (see Chapter 8 by Ong, this volume) *(6,11)*.

Gestational Weight Gain

Excess gestational weight gain is associated with the birth of LGA infants (defined as birth weight ≥ 90th percentile for age) *(10,15)*. Regardless of the woman's weight status prior to pregnancy *(15)*, excess gestational weight gain may double the risk of macrosomia, although much of this effect may be attributable to gestational diabetes (GDM) status *(16,17)*. Key outcomes – high birth weight, LGA, and macrosomia – associated with excess gestational weight gain are, in turn, predictors of childhood obesity *(11,12,15,18,19)*. The impact of gestational weight gain may extend well into childhood, as suggested by the increase in odds of obesity at 7 years of age (OR: 1.48) in offspring of women with excess weight gain during pregnancy compared to women with recommended weight gain *(6)*. Despite the increasing body of evidence, a full understanding of the association of gestational weight gain with childhood obesity remains elusive due to complexities of gestational weight gain intertwined with issues of maternal obesity and GDM, which also have strong effects on the intrauterine environment, birth weight, and child obesity outcomes.

The impact of excess gestational weight gain may be most pronounced among underweight mothers. Maternal overweight and maternal obesity, compared to normal weight, each increased odds of childhood obesity at age 7 years (OR: 1.38 and 2.56, respectively), but a pronounced interaction (OR: 3.36) of *low maternal BMI with excess gestational weight gain* was reported when the model was adjusted for the child's sex, gestational age, first-born status, as well as the mother's race, maternal age, maternal prepregnancy BMI, smoking, and study site *(6)*.

The relationship between absolute gestational weight gain and higher birth weight is less clear among overweight and obese women than among normal weight women. This is because their pre-existing weight status confers an increased risk of fetal macrosomia and childhood obesity even in the absence of excess gestational weight gain; alternatively, their *relative* gestational weight gain is less than that of normal weight women who gain equivalent amounts of excess weight during pregnancy *(15,18,20,21)*.

Even when gestational weight gain in overweight women is comparable to that in normal weight women, the overweight women have significantly heavier offspring *(21)*. It is possible (though not established) that overweight/obese mothers, even in the absence of pre-existing diabetes or GDM, transport excess glucose and fatty acids to the fetus and thereby contribute to fetal fat deposition *(12)*.

New Guidelines for Pregnancy Weight Gain in Overweight and Obese Women

During the past two decades in the United States, the rise in obesity rates occurred in parallel with increases in adverse maternal health and birth outcomes. Understandably, concerns were raised regarding excess gestational weight gain, particularly among the growing number of overweight and obese women. Indeed, analysis of trends from the Pregnancy Risk Assessment Monitoring System (PRAMS) showed substantial excess in weight gain during pregnancy among those classified as either overweight or obese. Previously, the guidelines for maternal weight gain formulated by the Institute of Medicine (IOM) were designed primarily to reduce the risk of intrauterine growth retardation. However, given recent findings, an update was released in May 2009. The new guidelines recommended that obese women lower their targeted weight gain (see Table 1 based on the 2009 IOM guidelines). The new recommendations highlight the importance of prepregnancy weight and gestational weight gain as determinants of metabolic outcome in the mother, fetus, and growing child.

Table 1
Total Pregnancy Weight Gain Recommendations by BMI Status

Prepregnancy BMI	BMI[a]	Range of Recommended Total Weight Gain[b]
Underweight	<18.5	28–40
Normal weight	18.5–24.9	25–35
Overweight	25.0–29.9	15–25
Obese	≥30.0	11–20

[a]BMI calculation based on World Health Organization (WHO) standards
[b]Expressed in pounds (lbs)

Effects of Maternal Undernutrition

Maternal undernutrition, manifested as low prepregnancy BMI, inadequate gestational weight gain, or both, may negatively impact birth weight. The Dutch famine of 1944–1945 is an example of the relationship between inadequate maternal nutrition and its relationship to later obesity in the offspring. The timing of nutrient restriction was found to have important effects on birth weight and subsequent adiposity. Short-term nutrient restriction in the second and third trimesters resulted in lower mean birth weight (22). In contrast, nutrient restriction in early pregnancy resulted in higher mean infant birth weights when compared to infants of unexposed mothers (23). If early trimester nutrient restriction increases birth weight, and high birth weight increases the risk of childhood obesity, then nutrient restriction early in pregnancy may contribute to the development of obesity in childhood.

More commonly, however, inadequate gestational weight gain results in small-for-gestational-age (SGA) or low-birth-weight (LBW) infants. Interestingly, low birth weight may be a risk factor for rapid weight gain in the first 5 months of life, which in turn may also increase childhood obesity risk. Rapid catch-up growth from age 1–7 years has also been linked to adult BMI (8). The pathogenesis of childhood obesity and metabolic dysfunction in growth retarded infants is discussed in detail in Chapter 8 by Ong.

Postnatal Maternal Weight Status

It has been reported that women gaining the most weight while pregnant also experience increased postpartum weight retention (24). Excess gestational weight gain has also been associated with long-term obesity in the mother (25). This may predispose the mother to metabolic dysfunction or gestational diabetes in subsequent pregnancies, creating a vicious cycle that sustains the obesity epidemic. Thus, the failure to shed excess gestational weight gain could impact both future maternal BMI status and future offspring risk.

SMOKING

The relationship between maternal smoking and adverse outcomes such as intrauterine growth restriction, LBW, and SGA has been established through much research over the past four decades (26–28). More recently, researchers have explored the relationship between smoking and childhood obesity. In one study, maternal smoking in early pregnancy was found to increase significantly the odds of obesity in 5-year-old children (OR: 5.04) compared with children whose mothers were either former smokers or never smokers during early pregnancy *(29)*. Other studies showed that maternal smoking during pregnancy significantly increased odds of BMI ≥ 95th percentile at 4.5 years (OR: 1.8) *(13)*. Similar risks were noted at age 9–10 years (OR: 2.56) *(29)*. Meta-analyses support the hypothesis that maternal smoking is related to increased risk of early childhood overweight and obesity *(30,31)*.

The vast majority of research to date collectively points in the same direction: that smoking increases risks of LBW and SGA, that LBW and SGA infants experience rapid postnatal catch-up growth with greater adiposity, and that each of these outcomes is associated with increased odds of childhood obesity. As noted by Oken et al., studies that reported the amount of maternal smoking in relation to childhood obesity provided evidence of a dose–response *(30)*; the prevalence of childhood obesity and the mean BMI and skinfold thickness at 5 years of age *(32,33)* correlated with the number of cigarettes smoked by the mother per day.

A recent study by McCowan et al. examined the effects of smoking cessation on gestational length and birth weight *(26)*. Among women who stopped smoking prior to 15 weeks of gestation, there was no increase in spontaneous preterm births or the number of children born SGA relative to non-smoking mothers. However, among women who continued to smoke, there was threefold increase in the number of preterm births and a 76% increase in the number of children born SGA.

The public health implications here are clear. Health professionals should continue to promote smoking cessation, particularly among women as a part of early prenatal care.

BREASTFEEDING

Breastfeeding is the optimal form of nutrition for infants; however, evidence to support its role in the prevention of childhood obesity remains controversial. Maternal behaviors that modulate the relationship between infant consumption of breast milk, duration of breastfeeding, and risk of childhood obesity are complex, and studies often fail to control effectively for confounding factors. Indeed, factors that may be considered confounders by some may be considered mediators by others. These include the rate and timing of weight gain in infancy in response to early feeding practices, and the co-occurrence of other health-promoting habits by the mother or the overall family. It has been therefore difficult to determine if breastfeeding per se reduces the risks or severity of childhood obesity.

Nevertheless, meta-analyses largely support the hypothesis that breastfeeding reduces the odds of childhood obesity *(34–38)*. This is true if children who are breastfed exclusively are compared to formula-fed children (OR: 0.66) *(37)* or if children who were breastfed at any time are compared with non-breastfed subjects (OR: 0.78) *(38)*. A recent meta-analysis showed a protective effect of breastfeeding among the larger studies (>1,500 participants) despite evidence for publication bias *(38)*.

Strong evidence for dose–response protection against development of child obesity with increased duration of breastfeeding is described in Harder's meta-analysis. Odds ratios were 0.81, 0.76, 0.67, and 0.68 for periods of breastfeeding ranging from 1 to 3 months, 4 to 6 months, 7 to 9 months, and >9 months, respectively. However, in most cases significant effects were not observed until children were breastfed for at least 3–6 months *(5,37,39–42)*, and at least one study reported an unexpected increased risk with breastfeeding duration <1 month compared to infants who never breastfed (OR: 1.36) *(37)*. Another study reported that when formula was used with breastfeeding, a significant dose–response effect was not seen until 26 weeks *(40)*.

Since there are obvious ethical concerns in conducting randomized controlled trials (RCTs) of breastfeeding among infants, observational studies are the primary source of information. However, one study was conducted as a breastfeeding promotion intervention using RCT methods *(43)*. Researchers found no protective effect for breastfeeding compared to formula feeding, but the results should be interpreted with caution due to several methodological limitations. The study was conducted in a Belarusian population with very low obesity prevalence, the duration of breastfeeding did not exceed 3 months in the intervention group, and only 43% were breastfed exclusively.

If breastfeeding protects against childhood obesity, breastfeeding may also have beneficial effects on obesity-related health outcomes in childhood. From a case–control study, youth with type 2 diabetes were substantially less likely to have been breastfed as infants compared to their non-diabetic counterparts (unadjusted OR for the association of breastfeeding (ever versus never) and T2DM, 0.26) (37). Results were similar for non-Hispanic white, African-American, and Hispanic youth. The OR after adjusting for 12 potential confounders was 0.43 (37). When current BMI Z-score was added to the model, the OR was attenuated (OR: 0.82), suggesting possible mediation of the protective effect of breastfeeding through current childhood weight status (37).

Exactly how breastfeeding confers protection, if any, is not well understood. Rapid weight gain in the first 4 months of life is associated with childhood obesity (44), and breastfeeding has been associated with slower weight gain during the first 12 months of life (45). Since bisphenol-A (BPA) has been implicated in the development of obesity through its role as an endocrine disruptor (46), another possible mechanism is that exposure to endocrine disruptors through use of baby bottles containing BPA could be higher among formula-fed versus breastfed babies.

As discussed earlier, maternal prepregnancy overweight or obese status has been associated with an increased risk of childhood obesity. Due to the high energy cost of producing milk, breastfeeding may facilitate return to prepregnancy weight following delivery (47). Therefore, the decision to breastfeed can play a role in determining the mother's future weight status, possibly influencing future offspring risk.

A variety of factors, including socioeconomic status and race/ethnicity, may influence the decision to breastfeed. Low maternal education or low income status was associated with lower rates of breastfeeding, and African-American infants were reported to have lower rates of breastfeeding compared to all other race/ethnicities. Some evidence of differential effects of breastfeeding has emerged, as studies of children whose mothers were white, black, or Hispanic reported that protection from childhood obesity was conferred only among children of white mothers (40,41). The reasons for this remain unclear.

MATERNAL DIETARY HABITS AND PHYSICAL ACTIVITY

Interacting with breastfeeding are the physical activity and dietary habits of the mother. They are important contributors to the environment in which a child is raised. Maternal dietary habits will directly influence breast milk fat and protein content (47), and physical activity has the ability to indirectly influence breast milk nutrient content via its effects on energy balance and weight status. Maintaining a healthier weight and balanced dietary habits can lead to the production of breast milk containing a higher proportion of medium chain triglycerides (MCTs). Milk contains a higher proportion of MCTs when mammary tissue synthesizes fatty acids (48) rather than incorporating fatty acids released into blood from maternal fat stores; the latter are composed primarily of longer chain fatty acids and require bile for transport across intestinal cells. Infants have immature digestive systems and MCTs do not require bile acids for intestinal absorption; this is clearly advantageous in ensuring that the infant can meet caloric needs during the early and critical periods of development.

As a child transitions to solid foods, the dietary habits and activity patterns of the mother are likely to exert even more influence. Maternal dietary choices not only will affect the selection of foods available to the child but also will provide a means through which the child will watch and learn eating behaviors that may not be directly related to basic energy balance cues, such as satiety. Maternal activity patterns, including television viewing *(49)*, will shape the child's daily lifestyle. Maternal dietary and physical activity habits thus seem likely to be critical in the development of childhood obesity, yet a strong body of evidence examining their roles simply does not exist.

What has been studied are the roles played by parental education, income, and social environments, such as home and daycare, in modeling healthy behaviors and habits. Adolescents with mothers having graduate or professional degrees had lower odds of being very inactive (OR: 0.61) compared to adolescents with mothers having less education *(50)* and are less likely to be obese.

There is evidence showing that parental and peer modeling is crucial to early childhood development of healthy eating behaviors. Extensive research in this area has been conducted by Birch and colleagues. Among 3- to 5-year-old children, the strongest fat preferences and the highest fat intakes were observed among those with heavier parents *(51)*. In another study, children showing dislike for a particular vegetable began choosing the non-preferred vegetable when placed into an environment where peers were actively choosing and consuming the non-preferred vegetable *(52)*. In young children, food preferences increase with familiarity, and Birch notes that current "availability of energy dense foods...provides an eating environment that fosters food preferences inconsistent with dietary guidelines, which can promote excess weight gain and obesity" *(53)*. Promotion of balanced dietary habits and increasing physical activity among children through a combination of parental and social context will remain important factors in reducing the alarming rates of overweight and obesity currently observed in developed countries.

OTHER INFLUENCES

Some interesting factors related in general to maternal lifestyle, such as the child's sleep duration, television watching, and computer screen time, have recently emerged as potential determinants of childhood obesity.

Short sleep duration has been associated with obesity via its association with a reduction in leptin and an increase in ghrelin, which may lead to hormonal disregulation of appetite and satiety controls *(54)* (see also the Chapter 17 by Verhulst, this volume). In a study to identify early-life risk factors associated with childhood obesity in the United Kingdom, short sleep duration (<10.5 h compared to >12 h at age 3) and *television watching* (>8 h/week at age 3) were associated with obesity at age 7 (OR: 1.45 and 1.55, respectively) *(55)*. A recent meta-analysis examining short sleep duration and risk of obesity in children found an OR of 1.89 for short sleep duration (defined as either <10 or <10.5 h except in one study which used <8 h to classify short sleep duration) *(56)*.

Since low-wage jobs usually involve long hours and a work schedule that may change week to week, maternal lifestyle as modified by low *socioeconomic status (SES)* may inhibit the establishment of both the mother's and the child's regular sleep patterns, adversely affecting the quality and duration of sleep. It must, however, be noted that the inverse correlation between sleep duration and obesity prevalence does not necessarily imply causation; no studies have shown that increasing sleep duration can reduce body weight.

The *birth weight of the mother and her early weight gain in childhood* were recently reported as predictive for next generation (her offspring's) birth weight as well as obesity risk *(57)*. Another study found that *grandparental obesity* may influence childhood obesity independent of parental obesity status *(58)*. Among children with normal weight parents, prevalence of childhood overweight was similarly elevated if the grandparents were obese (prevalence 17.4%, $p < 0.0001$) or if the grandparents had missing BMI status (16.9%, $p < 0.0001$) *(58)*. These findings suggest that genetic factors exert a powerful influence on childhood weight gain.

SUMMARY

Maternal weight status, whether prepregnancy or postpartum, appears to be the strongest indicator of risk for childhood obesity. However, the offspring of underweight women gaining in excess of the IOM pregnancy weight gain guidelines also experienced a marked increase in risk of childhood obesity. Maternal weight is modifiable through increased physical activity and balanced dietary habits, but research associating maternal physical activity patterns with childhood risk of obesity is lacking. The evidence for breastfeeding remains inconclusive, but the available data suggest a modest benefit for protection against development of childhood obesity. Future studies must account fully for confounding factors such as maternal behavior, family habits/environment, and genetic inheritance.

Children inherently rely on adults to model appropriate behaviors. Hence, it is imperative that we gain a better understanding of high-risk factors through more research and translate that information into targeted public health interventions to empower parents and children alike to stop the obesity epidemic and improve the quality of life for generations to come.

Editor's Question and Authors' Response

- **The research you (and others in this volume) cite makes it clear that the critical factors controlling the risk of childhood obesity include the family history and the mother's general health, metabolic status, drug use (smoking), and approach to infant feeding. Family history is immutable but the various other maternal factors should be modifiable if addressed effectively long before pregnancy is even contemplated. This argues for a targeted approach to improve the health and metabolic status of teenage girls, particularly those from high-risk families. Do you agree?**

- "Absolutely! A two-tiered approach could be considered in which nutrition and physical activity education and programs are readily available to all youth as the first tier, with a second tier established to target girls from high-risk families. Current research is exploring a variety of multi-level approaches that will inform such programs to maximize effectiveness and sustainability to reduce overweight and obesity which should, in turn, improve health outcomes for both mothers and their offspring."

REFERENCES

1. CDC. Differences in prevalence of obesity among black, white, and hispanic adults – United States, 2006–2008. MMWR. 2009;58(27):740.

2. Dabelea D, Snell-Bergeon JK, Hartsfield CL, Bischoff KJ, Hamman RF, McDuffie RS. Increasing prevalence of gestational diabetes mellitus (GDM) over time and by birth cohort kaiser permanente of colorado GDM screening program A table elsewhere in this issue shows conventional and systeme international (SI) units and conversion factors for many substances. Diabetes Care. 2005;28(3):579–84.

3. Li R, Darling N, Maurice E, Barker L, Grummer-Strawn LM. Breastfeeding rates in the United States by characteristics of the child, mother, or family: the 2002 national immunization survey. Pediatrics. 2005;115(1):e31–7.

4. Ogden CL, Carroll MD, Curtin LR, McDowell MA, Tabak CJ, Flegal KM. Prevalence of overweight and obesity in the United States, 1999–2004. J Am Med Assoc. 2006;295(13):1549–55.

5. Li C, Kaur H, Choi WS, Huang TTK, Lee RE, Ahluwalia JS. Additive interactions of maternal prepregnancy BMI and breast-feeding on childhood overweight. Obes Res. 2005;13(2):362–71.

6. Wrotniak BH, Shults J, Butts S, Stettler N. Gestational weight gain and risk of overweight in the offspring at age 7 y in a multicenter, multiethnic cohort study. Am J Clin Nutr. 2008;87(6):1818.

7. Whitaker RC. Predicting preschooler obesity at birth: the role of maternal obesity in early pregnancy. Pediatrics. 2004;114(1):e29–36.

8. Terry MB, Wei Y, Esserman D. Maternal, birth, and early-life influences on adult body size in women. Am J Epidemiol. 2007;166(1):5–13.

9. Kain J, Corvalán C, Lera L, Galván M, Uauy R. Accelerated growth in early life and obesity in preschool Chilean children. Obesity. 2009;17(8):1603–8.

10. Shapiro C, Sutija V, Bush J. Effect of maternal weight gain on infant birth weight. J Perinat Med. 2000;28(6):428–31.

11. King JC. Maternal obesity, metabolism, and pregnancy outcomes. Annu Rev Nutr. 2006;26:271–91.

12. Catalano PM. Management of obesity in pregnancy. Obstet Gynecol. 2007;109(2 Pt 1):419–33.

13. Dubois L, Girard M. Early determinants of overweight at 4.5 years in a population-based longitudinal study. Int J Obes. 2006;30(4):610–17.

14. Perez-Pastor E, Metcalf B, Hosking J, Jeffery A, Voss L, Wilkin T. Assortative weight gain in mother–daughter and father–son pairs: an emerging source of childhood obesity. Longitudinal study of trios (EarlyBird 43). Int J Obes. 2009;33:727–35.

15. Crane JMG, White J, Murphy P. The effect of gestational weight gain by body mass index on maternal and neonatal outcomes. J Obstet Gynaecol Can. 2009;31(1):28–35.

16. Hillier TA, Pedula KL, Vesco KK, et al. Excess gestational weight gain: modifying fetal macrosomia risk associated with maternal glucose. Obstet Gynecol. 2008;112(5):1007–14.

17. Kabali C, Werler M. Pre-pregnant body mass index, weight gain and the risk of delivering large babies among non-diabetic mothers. Int J Gynecol Obstet. 2007;97(2):100–4.

18. Viswanathan M, Siega-Riz AM, Moos M, et al. Outcomes of maternal weight gain. Evid Rep Technol Assess. 2008;168:290–302.

19. Martorell R, Stein AD, Schroeder DG. Early nutrition and later adiposity 1. J Nutr. 2001;131(3):874–80.

20. Rode L, Hegaard HK, Kjaergaard H, Møller LF, Tabor A, Ottesen B. Association between maternal weight gain and birth weight. Obstet Gynecol. 2007;109(6):1309.

21. Mitchell M, Lerner E. A comparison of pregnancy outcome in overweight and normal weight women. J Am Coll Nutr. 1989;8(6):617–24.

22. Smith CA. Effects of maternal undernutrition upon the newborn infant in holland (1944–1945). J Pediatr. 1947;30(3):229–43.

23. Lumey LH, Stein AD, Ravelli AC. Timing of prenatal starvation in women and birth weight in their first and second born offspring: the Dutch famine birth cohort study. Eur J Obstet Gynecol Reprod Biol. 1995;61(1):23–30.

24. Olson C, Strawderman M, Hinton P, Pearson T. Gestational weight gain and postpartum behaviors associated with weight change from early pregnancy to 1 y postpartum. Int J Obes. 2003;27(1):117–27.

25. Rooney BL, Schauberger CW. Excess pregnancy weight gain and long-term obesity: one decade later. Obstet Gynecol. 2002;100(2):245.

26. McCowan LME, Dekker GA, Chan E, et al. Spontaneous preterm birth and small for gestational age infants in women who stop smoking early in pregnancy: Prospective Cohort study. BMJ. 2009;338:b1081.

27. Butler N, Goldstein H, Ross E. Cigarette smoking in pregnancy: its influence on birth weight and perinatal mortality. BMJ. 1972;2(5806):127.

28. MacMahon B, Alpert M, Salber EJ. Infant weight and parental smoking habits 1. Am J Epidemiol. 1965;82(3):247–61.

29. Suzuki K, Ando D, Sato M, Tanaka T, Kondo N, Yamagata Z. The association between maternal smoking during pregnancy and childhood obesity persists to the age of 9–10 years. J Epidemiol. 2009;19(3):136–42.

30. Oken E, Levitan E, Gillman M. Maternal smoking during pregnancy and child overweight: systematic review and meta-analysis. Int J Obes (Lond). 2008;32(2):201–10. Epub 27 Nov 2007.

31. Ino T. A meta-analysis of association between maternal smoking during pregnancy and offspring obesity. Pediatr Int. 2010;52(1):94–9. Epub 27 Apr 2009.

32. Wideroe M, Vik T, Jacobsen G, Bakketeig LS. Does maternal smoking during pregnancy cause childhood overweight? Paediatr Perinat Epidemiol. 2003;17(2):171.

33. Von Kries R, Koletzko B, Sauerwald T, et al. Breast feeding and obesity: Cross Sectional study. BMJ. 1999;319(7203):147–50.

34. Harder T, Bergmann R, Kallischnigg G, Plagemann A. Duration of breastfeeding and risk of overweight: a meta-analysis. Am J Epidemiol. 2005;162(5):397–403.

35. Arenz S, Rückerl R, Koletzko B, Von Kries R. Breast-feeding and childhood obesity – a systematic review. Int J Obes. 2004;28(10):1247–56.

36. Butte NF. The role of breastfeeding in obesity. Pediatr Clin North Am. 2001;48(1):189–98.

37. Mayer-Davis EJ, Rifas-Shiman SL, Zhou L, Hu FB, Colditz GA, Gillman MW. Breast-feeding and risk for childhood obesity. Diabetes Care. 2006;29(10):2231.

38. Horta BL, Bahl R, Martines JC, Victora CG. Evidence on the long-term effects of breastfeeding. Geneva: World Health Organization; 2007.

39. Gillman MW, Rifas-Shiman SL, Camargo CA Jr, et al. Risk of overweight among adolescents who were breastfed as infants. J Am Med Assoc. 2001;285(19):2461–67.

40. Bogen DL, Hanusa BH, Whitaker RC. The effect of breast-feeding with and without formula use on the risk of obesity at 4 years of age. Obesity. 2004;12(9):1527–35.

41. Grummer-Strawn LM, Mei Z. Does breastfeeding protect against pediatric overweight? Analysis of longitudinal data from the centers for disease control and prevention pediatric nutrition surveillance system. Pediatrics. 2004;113(2): e81–6.

42. Nelson MC, Gordon-Larsen P, Adair LS. Are adolescents who were breast-fed less likely to be overweight? Analyses of sibling pairs to reduce confounding. Epidemiology. 2005;16(2):247.

43. Kramer MS, Chalmers B, Hodnett ED, et al. Promotion of breastfeeding intervention trial (PROBIT): a randomized trial in the republic of Belarus. J Am Med Assoc. 2001;285(4):413–20.

44. Stettler N, Zemel BS, Kumanyika S, Stallings VA. Infant weight gain and childhood overweight status in a multicenter, cohort study. Pediatrics. 2002;109(2):194–99.

45. Dewey KG. Growth characteristics of breast-fed compared to formula-fed infants. Biol Neonate. 1998;74:94–105.

46. Elobeid MA, Allison DB. Putative environmental-endocrine disruptors and obesity: a review. Curr Opin Endocrinol Diabetes Obes. 2008;15(5):403.

47. Kleinman RE, editor. Pediatric nutrition handbook. 5th ed. Chicago, IL: American Academy of Pediatrics; 2004.

48. Finley D, Lonnerdal B, Dewey K, Grivetti L. Breast milk composition: fat content and fatty acid composition in vegetarians and non-vegetarians. Am J Clin Nutr. 1985;41(4):787–800.

49. Dennison BA, Erb TA, Jenkins PL. Television viewing and television in bedroom associated with overweight risk among low-income preschool children. Pediatrics. 2002;109(6):1028–35.

50. Gordon-Larsen P, McMurray RG, Popkin BM. Determinants of adolescent physical activity and inactivity patterns. Pediatrics. 2000;105(6):E83.

51. Fisher JO, Birch LL. Fat preferences and fat consumption of 3- to 5-year-old children are related to parental adiposity. J Am Diet Assoc. 1995;95(7):759–64.

52. Birch LL. Effects of peer models' food choices and eating behaviors on preschoolers' food preferences. Child Dev. 1980;51:489–96.

53. Birch LL. Development of food preferences. Annu Rev Nutr. 1999;19(1):41–62.

54. Taheri S, Lin L, Austin D, Young T, Mignot E. Short sleep duration is associated with reduced leptin, elevated ghrelin, and increased body mass index. PLoS Med. 2004;1(3):210.

55. Reilly JJ, Armstrong J, Dorosty AR, et al. Early life risk factors for obesity in childhood: Cohort study. BMJ. 2005;330(7504):1357.

56. Cappuccio FP, Taggart FM, Kandala NB, Currie A. Meta-analysis of short sleep duration and obesity in children and adults. Sleep. 2008;31(5):619.

57. Horta BL, Gigante DP, Osmond C, Barros FC, Victora CG. Intergenerational effect of weight gain in childhood on offspring birthweight. Int J Epidemiol. 2009;38(3):724–32.

58. Davis MM, McGonagle K, Schoeni RF, Stafford F. Grandparental and parental obesity influences on childhood overweight: implications for primary care practice. J Am Board Fam Med. 2008;21(6):549.

8 Intrauterine Growth Retardation

Ken K. Ong

CONTENTS

Key Words: Barker, developmental origin, birth weight, SGA, IUGR, thrifty phenotype, thrifty genotype

INTRODUCTION

The secular trends towards increasing prevalence of overweight and obesity are detectable even in very young pre-school age children. For example, analysis of routine health check data in the UK showed a steady rise in mean body weight and BMI between 1989 and 1998 in children aged just 3–4 years old *(1)*. Such findings indicate that our attention to the aetiology, prediction and prevention of obesity should start very early on in life to include even antenatal and early infancy factors.

In contrast to body weight in early childhood, there is little evidence that mean birth weight has changed appreciably over time, at least in western Europe *(2)*; however in countries in rapid developmental transition, the increasing prevalence of maternal obesity and gestational diabetes has led to a rising incidence of neonatal macrosomia (birth weight > 4000 g) *(3)*. Birth weight is positively associated with later BMI in most studies, suggesting that larger babies are more likely to become obese *(4)*. However BMI is an imprecise marker of adiposity, and in studies that use more accurate measures of body composition it is evident that larger babies are more likely to have greater lean body mass but not greater fat mass as children *(5)*, adolescents *(6)* and older adults *(7)*. Rather, it appears that low birth weight babies, born following intrauterine growth restriction, are more likely to become fatter and have higher risks for obesity-related diseases in later life, an observation that was originally reported by David Barker and colleagues and which led to the eponymous "Barker Hypothesis" described below.

From: *Contemporary Endocrinology: Pediatric Obesity: Etiology, Pathogenesis, and Treatment*
Edited by: M. Freemark, DOI 10.1007/978-1-60327-874-4_8,
© Springer Science+Business Media, LLC 2010

THE BARKER HYPOTHESIS

The observation that low birth weight is associated with increased risk of cardiovascular disease was prompted by the strong geographical association between areas in England and Wales with the highest infant mortality rates in 1921–1925 and the highest ischaemic heart disease mortality rates in 1968–1978 (8). Remarkably, Barker and Osmond's initial proposition in 1986, that the transition from poor nutrition in early life to a subsequent affluent diet might increase the susceptibility to obesity-related disease (8), remains the most widely held explanation. Over the following decade, those authors and others established the epidemiological associations between small size at birth and various adulthood disease risks, including cardiovascular disease (9), hypertension (10), type 2 diabetes (11) and stroke (12). Other low birth weight associations include ageing (13), ovarian hyperandrogenism and menstrual irregularities (14). The persistence of such associations after exclusion of preterm infants and adjustment for gestational age meant that reduced or restricted fetal growth was the implicated exposure, although more recent studies show that preterm infants also have increased risks for type 2 diabetes (15). Furthermore, the continuum in disease risks across the whole spectrum of birth weights indicated that these associations reflected the effects of common determinants of fetal growth, rather than maternal disease or severe placental dysfunction.

Large epidemiological studies using available birth records showed that the association between low birth weight and coronary heart disease was independent of selection bias or potential confounding due to social class or smoking (16). However, where more detailed parameters of fetal growth were available there was no clear consistency regarding which measures of fetal weight, length, placental weight or abdominal circumference were primarily associated with later disease. Furthermore, meta-analyses showed that, as with many other associations, the initial reports tended to report far greater effect sizes than subsequent larger studies (17).

Indeed, in many studies, the association between birth weight and later disease was not apparent until after adjustment was made for adult body weight or BMI, leading to the suggestion that adult size is a much stronger and more robust risk factor than birth weight (17). A more compromising proposal was made by Lucas and colleagues who pointed out that "early size adjusted for later size" is a measure of change in size between the earlier and later measurements, or more accurately centile crossing between birth and adult life (18).

THE DEVELOPMENTAL ORIGINS OF HEALTH AND DISEASE HYPOTHESIS

The Developmental Origins of Health and Disease Hypothesis (DoHAD) arose in the early 2000s from the growing realisation of the correct interpretation of adult body size-adjusted associations with birth weight coupled with epidemiological studies that analysed available information on infant and childhood growth, particularly from Scandinavian populations with remarkably detailed historical childhood records. Having started with a focus on birth weight as a marker of fetal growth, the search for the early origins of health and disease now encompasses the full-range of childhood growth and development and has spawned its own sub-discipline named "lifecourse epidemiology". As anticipated, the associations with postnatal growth and weight gain appear to be stronger than those with birth weight alone. For example, in a study of men with birth and school records in Helsinki, Finland the risk of death from coronary heart disease increased by 14% for each unit (kg/m^3) lower ponderal index at birth and by 22% for each unit (kg/m^2) higher childhood BMI (19). Such observations supported the original postulate that adult disease might be a consequence of poor prenatal nutrition followed by improved postnatal nutrition (8).

In addition to the case-control studies of adult disease outcomes, which made use of archival childhood data, supportive evidence for the role of postnatal growth and weight gain on later disease risks has come from more recent prospective birth cohort studies, which rely on measures of adiposity or biochemical markers of future disease risks. Systematic reviews have summarised the consistent association between rapid weight gain during early life and later increased risks for obesity. There is a two- to threefold increase in overweight or obesity risk in those individuals whose weight crossed upwards during infancy by at least one centile band (e.g. 2nd to 9th centile, or 9th to 25th centile), which is equivalent to a gain in weight SD score ≥ 0.67 (20). No interaction is seen with birth weight, and therefore the effects of rapid infancy weight gain are similar in both SGA and normal birth weight populations. Rather, the key factor linking these observations to low birth weight is that infants who were growth restrained in utero are much more likely than other infants to show rapid postnatal growth, often termed "catch-up" growth as it compensates for the earlier growth deficiency (21).

Rapid infant weight gain has also been associated with subsequent increased body fat, and particularly central or abdominal fat distribution, in studies using the gold standard 4-component model for body composition (22) and MRI assessment of visceral fat in adults (23). Furthermore, even after the completion of centile crossing in overall body weight and length, SGA infants who showed early catch-up growth appear to show an ongoing propensity for gains in adiposity during childhood (24) and even in adult life (25). Other associations of rapid infancy weight gain, which may be highly relevant to its links with later disease risks include: insulin resistance (26), higher blood pressure (27) and also markers of more rapid physical and sexual maturation including higher adrenal androgen levels (28), more rapid skeletal maturation (29) and earlier age at menarche in girls (30). The latter outcomes are particularly pertinent as earlier menarche is independently associated with low birth weight (30,31) and predicts long-term increased risks of obesity and type 2 diabetes in later adult life (32).

While the epidemiological disease associations may appear to be stronger with postnatal growth rather than fetal growth in such observational studies it may be difficult to disentangle the effects of each exposure. Alternatively the two factors might lie on the same causal pathway to later disease. However, efforts to identify and even quantify the relative contributions of antenatal and postnatal factors are essential in order to inform future preventative strategies.

ANTENATAL PATHOGENESIS – ANIMAL MODELS

A variety of animal models have demonstrated that fetal growth restriction leads to increased blood pressure, hyperinsulinaemia and impaired glucose tolerance (33). Intrauterine growth restriction may be achieved by a variety of techniques including bilateral uterine arterial ligation, protein restriction, caloric restriction or glucocorticoid exposure. There is some evidence that in the preimplantation period the fetus may exhibit particular sensitivity to nutrient deficiencies. For example, maternal periconceptional B vitamin and methionine status may influence offspring insulin resistance and blood pressure in sheep (34). Simply changing maternal diet does not necessarily result in hypertensive offspring; the rise in blood pressure may depend critically on both the prevailing conditions and the precise gestational timing. It has been suggested that long-term brain and cardiovascular function may be most sensitive to the influences during the embryonic period, renal outcomes during maximal placental growth and development and adipose tissue and muscle outcomes during the fetal growth phase during the late pregnancy (Fig. 1) (35).

The mechanisms linking early life insults to later disease risk may range from structural changes in organ size and function, such as in kidney nephron numbers, to long-term molecular changes in tissue sensitivity and receptor numbers, and levels of metabolite transporter molecules. There is much interest in the potential role of epigenetics as a mechanism that could explain how short-term discrete exposures during early life may have very long-lasting effects on metabolism and disease risks in later life, and even on the transmission of these changes to future generations (36).

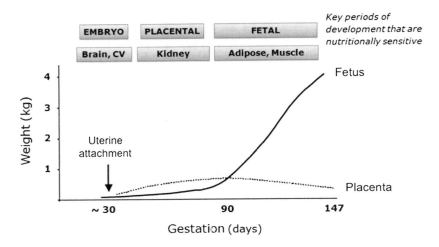

Fig. 1. Summary of the main developmental windows during the reproductive period in sheep during which manipulation of the maternal diet significantly modulates placental and fetal development. *Upper bars* represent windows of developmental plasticity with respect to individual organs. CV, cardiovascular system. Adapted with permission from Symonds et al. *(35)*.

The identification of such long-lasting effects of discrete exposures during critical early developmental periods of life has led to many interesting hypotheses as to why it may be beneficial for an individual organism to make very long-term decisions on metabolism or organ function. Barker and Hales coined the "Thrifty Phenotype" hypothesis to describe how the observed structural and physiological responses to early nutritional insults might enhance fetal survival *(33)*. For example, during settings of overall fetal growth restriction the development in the fetus of peripheral resistance to insulin or insulin-like growth factor-I (IGF-I) could beneficially divert sparse nutrients towards essential head or longitudinal growth. This hypothesis has been further developed in arguments that promote adaptive developmental plasticity as a mechanism that evolved to enhance survival and reproductive success *(37)*.

ANTENATAL PATHOGENESIS – HUMAN STUDIES

The "Thrifty Phenotype" hypothesis was a play of words on the "Thrifty Genotype" hypothesis which was originally proposed by Neel in 1962 to explain the remarkably high prevalence of type 2 diabetes in recently westernised, previously undernourished populations. Essentially, genetic predisposition to type 2 diabetes may have conferred some advantages during earlier times of undernutrition and would now be over-represented in these populations. Specific candidates have included genetic defects in insulin secretion or insulin responsiveness that could link size at birth to later risk for type 2 diabetes. The initial illustration of low birth weight in humans with rare mutations in the glucokinase gene, which cause maturity-onset diabetes in the young (MODY), has been followed up with reports that common type 2 diabetes risk alleles at the *CDKAL1* and *HHEX-IDE* loci are associated with lower birth weight *(38)*. Such genetic variants would not explain why low birth weight babies are more likely to be overweight or fatter in later life, but they might contribute to or modify the risks of disease in those who showed subsequent rapid weight gains.

With regard to antenatal nutritional restriction, the limited studies in humans provide some confirmation of the results of animal models; however the findings are often inconsistent. Ravelli reported that infants exposed to the Dutch famine of 1944–1945 during the first half of pregnancy had higher obesity rates at 19 years of age; in contrast, famine exposure during the last trimester of pregnancy and the first months of life led to lower obesity rates *(39)*. These findings are broadly consistent with a long-term effect of early nutritional deprivation on later regulation of weight gain and adiposity. The precise mechanisms by which this effect is mediated are unclear, but epigenetic events may play a role; for example, periconceptional famine exposure has been related to reduced DNA methylation of the imprinted insulin-like growth factor-II gene (40). However, these findings do not explain why lighter babies at birth are at greater risk of disease, as early gestation famine exposure was associated with slightly larger rather than lower birth weight. Furthermore, studies of other famines, such as the Leningrad Siege, did not confirm these findings, and in rural Gambia, food supplementation increased birth weights only during the wet season when women had negative energy balance due to food shortages and high agricultural workload, but not during the dry season when energy intakes were still only 60% of the recommended dietary allowance (41). This finding suggests that human fetal growth is relatively protected against all except the greatest variations in macronutrient intakes. Maternal micronutrient (such as in Vitamin B12 and folate) deficiencies may play a greater role in the early determination of childhood insulin resistance, but results of early studies will need confirmation in other settings.

Non-nutritional factors could link low birth weight to later risks of obesity-related disease. Fetal growth may be restrained due to maternal smoking, primiparity, maternal disease, such as gestational diabetes or pre-eclampsia, or by less severe increases in blood pressure. Identification of fetal growth restriction by repeated ultrasound measurements is a potential advantage, but is limited by the accuracy of the measurements and limited prediction of low birth weight. Use of individualised birth weight standards that assess birth weight relative to gestational age, gender, maternal height and weight before pregnancy, parity and ethnicity has been shown to provide better identification of "growth-restricted" infants and better prediction of the associated long-term metabolic outcomes (42).

The eventual identification of potentially modifiable determinants of SGA and later obesity-related disease will be informed by more accurate and more objective assessments of specific gestational exposures in the mother, and also by better characterisation of the newborn growth-restricted phenotype. A promising approach is better assessment of body composition and body fat distribution in the newborn. Using whole body magnetic resonance imaging (MRI), Modi and colleagues observed that intra-abdominal adipose tissue depots are remarkably preserved in growth-restricted newborns at birth, and there are wide differences in adipose tissue partitioning between infants of different ethnic backgrounds. Though smaller in weight, length and head circumference, Asian Indian newborns born in India had greater visceral, deep subcutaneous and superficial subcutaneous fat than European newborns born in the UK (43).

EARLY POSTNATAL PATHOGENESIS – ANIMAL MODELS

It is now clear that several of the original animal models of antenatal nutritional growth restriction are accompanied by postnatal over-nutrition. For example, antenatal protein-restricted mice were more susceptible than controls to the excess weight gain induced by postnatal weaning onto a highly palatable "cafeteria" diet. In contrast, postnatal low-protein-restricted mice were resistant to the excess weight gain from a highly palatable diet, indicating that the early environment has long-term consequences for weight gain (44). The combination of antenatal growth restriction and postnatal growth acceleration also leads to a shortened lifespan in mice; this contrasts with the increased longevity in mice with limited growth during the suckling period (45).

The early postnatal period may therefore represent a specific window of opportunity to reset the antenatal "metabolic programme" established in response to fetal growth restriction (37). The clearest evidence for a very specific window comes from studies of the postnatal leptin surge in rodents. Leptin increases fivefold to tenfold during the second postnatal week independent of fat mass, before declining again after weaning. It is thought that this leptin surge may have neurotrophic effects on the maturing neuroendocrine axis. Rats that received injections of leptin between days 3 and 10 showed a transient reduction in weight gain. The effects were more marked in rats that had been severely undernourished in utero (their mothers received 30% of ad libitum intakes); in this group postnatal leptin administration also completely blocked their predisposition to adiposity, insulin resistance and other adverse metabolic parameters (46). However, in male rats of normal pregnancies, the same neonatal leptin treatment increased diet-induced weight gain, hyperinsulinemia and total body adiposity, indicating a complex inter-dependency between the effects of these antenatal and early postnatal signals.

EARLY POSTNATAL PATHOGENESIS – HUMAN STUDIES

Infant growth is highly nutritionally dependent. Energy demands for growth constitute about 35% of total energy requirement during the first 3 months of life, declining rapidly to 17.5% in the next 3 months and to 6% between ages 6 and 12 months, compared to only 1–2% during childhood (47). The observation that earlier versus later timing of catch-up growth within the first 3 months of life is related to more adverse cardiovascular and metabolic risk profiles in early adulthood (48) implicates a role of postnatal nutrition in mediating, or at least moderating, these disease risk associations. The influence of infant nutrition is exemplified by the marked slower weight gain and growth patterns of breast-fed compared to formula-fed infants, at least in western settings (49), and the consistent (albeit modest) protective effects of breast-feeding on later adiposity and obesity risks (50). In contrast, in less developed settings, the protective effects of breast-feeding on gastro-intestinal and respiratory disease advantages usually outweigh its relatively lower nutritional content (51).

With regard to specific infant nutrients, it has been suggested that higher protein intakes during infancy may increase adiposity and subsequent obesity risks (52); however, such associations have not yet been widely confirmed. The role of infant protein intake, and specifically dairy milk protein intake, on infant growth and weight gain has been most robustly tested in a multicentre-randomised clinical trial (53). Infants who were randomised to the lower-protein formula showed slower gains in weight and BMI, but not in length, compared to infants on the high-protein, but isocaloric, formula, and their weight-for-length was similar to a breast-fed reference group (53).

However, simple alterations in formula milk content or composition on their own may not have major long-term effects on the trajectory of postnatal growth. It is unclear how postnatal catch-up weight gain is regulated in infants who were growth restricted in utero, although their lower leptin levels at birth point to an antenatal setting of infant appetite. Inheritance of common genetic variants associated with lower satiety and increased susceptibility to obesity may also have very early postnatal manifestations. Protein is generally agreed to be the most satiating macronutrient; therefore, potential (side-)effects of lower infant intakes of total calories or protein on reduced levels of satiety (54) may limit the reliance on such approaches to reduce rapid infant weight gain and prevent childhood obesity. In addition to the traditional biological determinants of infant weight gain and growth, it is likely that parental attitudes to infant feeding and growth (55) and policy factors may also contribute to the wide variations in infant growth rates (56). In 2006 the WHO published the first international growth charts which placed breast-fed infants as the standard for optimal growth and nutrition. The application of such charts in the UK was estimated to increase the number of infants classified as overweight by 35% and to reduce substantially the number of infants (wrongly) classified as underweight by around 85% (56). These studies indicate the potential major impact of appropriate growth standards and policies to set a lower trajectory of infant weight gain.

FUTURE STRATEGIES – HEALTHY CATCH-UP GROWTH

Significant short- and long-term benefits of postnatal catch-up growth, particularly in developing settings *(57)*, contrast with the increased risks of future obesity-related disease, and this risk-benefit balance for the fetal growth-restrained infant has been termed "the catch-up dilemma". In SGA children who remain short, there is evidence that growth hormone therapy may achieve the beneficial gains in long-term height and even cognitive function, but without the increased adiposity and metabolic disadvantages normally associated with early spontaneous, appetite-driven, catch-up growth *(58)*. While a pharmaceutical approach in all SGA children should not be contemplated, those studies illustrate the potential for different pathways of postnatal catch-up growth leading to differences in future disease risks (Fig. 2).

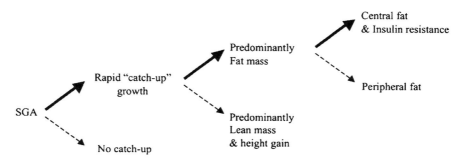

Fig. 2. Schematic diagram of the common SGA pathway of rapid postnatal catch-up weight gain leading to increased total and central adiposity *(bold arrows)*. Alternative putative pathways to healthy catch-up growth are shown by the *dotted arrows*. Reproduced with permission from Ong *(58)*.

In general birth cohort studies, heterogeneity is also detectable between infancy gains in BMI and adiposity versus growth in length and lean mass. These differences may be under endocrine or genetic control *(59)*. IGF-I is a major regulator of bone and skeletal muscle growth and is itself nutritionally regulated during early infancy, with higher levels seen in formula milk-fed infants than in breast-fed infants. In normal infants, higher IGF-I levels were associated with subsequent greater gains in length and lesser gains in BMI and adiposity *(59)*. IGF-I may therefore regulate the more favourable partitioning of infant weight gain into greater statural growth rather than adiposity, or it may at least represent an informative biomarker of those future growth patterns.

Finally, in addition to identifying the optimal nutrient composition and quantity, the promotion of healthy infant growth will require recognition of antenatal and infant drivers of appetite and growth, and also engagement with the prevailing parental attitudes and beliefs.

Editor's Questions and Author's Response

- **Type 2 diabetes reflects the convergence of defects in insulin secretion and insulin action. Do you think that intrauterine growth retardation limits beta cell replication in the perinatal period and thereby predisposes to subsequent development of type 2 diabetes?**

- Yes, this is a distinct possibility. Animal models show that fetal growth restriction leads to a reduction in beta cell numbers, which contributes to the subsequent beta cell failure and hyperglycaemia (Gatford et al., 2008). Similarly, in a birth cohort study we reported that thinness at birth was associated with a lower childhood disposition index, which is a marker of beta cell function corrected for degree of insulin resistance (Ong et al., 2004). It is conjectured that beta cell numbers do not regenerate after the perinatal period and therefore your insulin secretory capacity is fixed in response to the prevailing level of nutrition during fetal and early infant life. This could be one mechanism to explain why low birth weight infants have a limited metabolic capacity to respond to large transitions nutritional status if they become obese in later life.

There is evidence that neonatal administration of exendin-4, a pancreatic beta cell trophic factor and oral anti-diabetic agent, restores the defect in beta cell mass in fetal growth-restricted rats (Stoffers et al., 2003). This raises the intriguing possibility that future interventions in low birth weight babies during early infancy might prevent their later development of type 2 diabetes.

- **Some have argued that caloric deprivation during pregnancy or intrauterine growth retardation can cause premature activation of the hypothalamic-pituitary-adrenal axis, exposing the fetus and newborn infant to excessive glucocorticoid levels. Others find alterations in growth-restricted animals that might enhance glucocorticoid action. How do you interpret the roles of glucocorticoids in the intrauterine programming of metabolic disease?**

- Elegant animal models of glucocorticoid administration, or genetic modification of cortisol metabolism, demonstrate that increased glucocorticoid activity can link low birth weight to later insulin resistance and associated disease risks (Seckl and Holmes, 2007). However, in humans the role of the hypothalamic-pituitary-adrenal axis in explaining the epidemiological associations with low birth weight is not yet clear. While there are some epidemiological studies linking low birth weight to later cortisol levels such reports are inconsistent (Ong, 2005).

   Repeated high-dose maternal corticosteroid therapy is now well established for the prevention of neonatal respiratory distress syndrome following preterm labour and also for in utero prevention of genital abnormalities in female infants with congenital adrenal hyperplasia. These treatments have good safety profiles and appear to have little or no impact on birth weight (Crowther and Harding, 2007), growth or blood pressure in young children (Crowther et al., 2007). However, long-term follow-up of such offspring is clearly needed to finally establish or refute these arguments.

Crowther CA, Doyle LW, Haslam RR, Hiller JE, Harding JE, Robinson JS. Outcomes at 2 years of age after repeat doses of antenatal corticosteroids. N Engl J Med. 2007;357:1179–1189.

Crowther CA, Harding JE. Repeat doses of prenatal corticosteroids for women at risk of preterm birth for preventing neonatal respiratory disease. Cochrane Database Syst Rev. 2007. CD003935.

Gatford KL, Mohammad SN, Harland ML, De Blasio MJ, Fowden AL, Robinson JS, Owens JA. Impaired beta-cell function and inadequate compensatory increases in beta-cell mass after intrauterine growth restriction in sheep. Endocrinology 2008;149:5118–5127.

Ong K. Adrenal function of low-birth weight children. Endocr Dev 2005;8:34–53.

Ong KK, Petry CJ, Emmett PM, Sandhu MS, Kiess W, Hales CN, Ness AR, the-ALSPAC-Study-Team, Dunger DB. Insulin sensitivity and secretion in normal children related to size at birth, postnatal growth, and plasma insulin-like growth factor-I levels. Diabetologia 2004;47:1064–1070.

Seckl JR, Holmes MC. Mechanisms of disease: glucocorticoids, their placental metabolism and fetal 'programming' of adult pathophysiology. Nat Clin Pract Endocrinol Metab. 2007;3:479–488.

Stoffers DA, Desai BM, DeLeon DD, Simmons RA. Neonatal exendin-4 prevents the development of diabetes in the intrauterine growth retarded rat. Diabetes 2003;52:734–740.

REFERENCES

1. Buchan IE, Bundred PE, Kitchiner DJ, Cole TJ. Body mass index has risen more steeply in tall than in short 3-year olds: serial cross-sectional surveys 1988–2003. Int J Obes (Lond) Jan 2007;31(1):23–29.
2. Cole TJ. Secular trends in growth. Proc Nutr Soc May 2000;59(2):317–324.
3. Bergmann RL, Richter R, Bergmann KE, Plagemann A, Brauer M, Dudenhausen JW. Secular trends in neonatal macrosomia in Berlin: influences of potential determinants. Paediatr Perinat Epidemiol Jul 2003;17(3):244–249.
4. Sorensen HT, Sabroe S, Rothman KJ, Gillman M, Fischer P, Sorensen TI. Relation between weight and length at birth and body mass index in young adulthood: cohort study. BMJ 1 Nov 1997;315(7116):1137.

5. Murphy MJ, Metcalf BS, Jeffery AN, Voss LD, Wilkin TJ. Does lean rather than fat mass provide the link between birth weight, BMI, and metabolic risk? EarlyBird 23. Pediatr Diabetes Aug 2006;7(4):211–214.

6. Singhal A, Fewtrell M, Cole TJ, Lucas A. Low nutrient intake and early growth for later insulin resistance in adolescents born preterm. Lancet Mar 29 2003;361(9363):1089–1097.

7. Yliharsila H, Kajantie E, Osmond C, Forsen T, Barker DJ, Eriksson JG. Birth size, adult body composition and muscle strength in later life. Int J Obes (Lond) Sep 2007;31(9):1392–1399.

8. Barker DJ, Osmond C. Infant mortality, childhood nutrition, and ischaemic heart disease in England and Wales. Lancet 10 May 1986;1(8489):1077–1081.

9. Barker DJ, Winter PD, Osmond C, Margetts B, Simmonds SJ. Weight in infancy and death from ischaemic heart disease. Lancet 1989;2(8663):577–580.

10. Barker DJ, Osmond C, Golding J, Kuh D, Wadsworth ME. Growth in utero, blood pressure in childhood and adult life, and mortality from cardiovascular disease. BMJ 4 Mar 1989;298(6673):564–567.

11. Hales CN, Barker DJ, Clark PM, et al. Fetal and infant growth and impaired glucose tolerance at age 64. BMJ 1991;303(6809):1019–1022.

12. Martyn CN, Barker DJ, Osmond C. Mothers' pelvic size, fetal growth, and death from stroke and coronary heart disease in men in the UK. Lancet 1996;348(9037):1264–1268.

13. Aihie Sayer A, Cooper C, Barker DJ. Is lifespan determined in utero? Arch Dis Child 1997;77:F.

14. Ibanez L, Potau N, Francois I, de Zegher F. Precocious pubarche, hyperinsulinism, and ovarian hyperandrogenism in girls: relation to reduced fetal growth. J Clin Endocrinol Metabol 1998;83(10):3558–3562.

15. Hovi P, Andersson S, Eriksson JG, et al. Glucose regulation in young adults with very low birth weight. N Engl J Med 17 May 2007;356(20):2053–2063.

16. Leon DA, Lithell HO, Vagero D, Koupilova I, Mohsen R, Berglund L. Reduced fetal growth rate and increased risk of death from ischaemic heart disease: cohort study of 15 000 Swedish men and women born 1915–29. BMJ 1998;317: 241–244.

17. Huxley R, Neil A, Collins R. Unravelling the fetal origins hypothesis: is there really an inverse association between birthweight and subsequent blood pressure? Lancet 31 Aug 2002;360(9334):659–665.

18. Lucas A, Fewtrell MS, Cole TJ. Fetal origins of adult disease – the hypothesis revisited. BMJ 1999;319:245–249.

19. Eriksson JG, Forsen T, Tuomilehto J, Winter PD, Osmond C, Barker DJ. Catch-up growth in childhood and death from coronary heart disease: longitudinal study. BMJ 1999;318:427–431.

20. Ong KK, Loos RJ. Rapid infancy weight gain and subsequent obesity: systematic reviews and hopeful suggestions. Acta Paediatr Aug 2006;95(8):904–908.

21. Ong KK, Ahmed ML, Emmett PM, Preece MA, Dunger DB, the-ALSPAC-Study-Team. Association between postnatal catch-up growth and obesity in childhood: prospective cohort study. BMJ 2000;320:967–971.

22. Chomtho S, Wells JC, Williams JE, Davies PS, Lucas A, Fewtrell MS. Infant growth and later body composition: evidence from the 4-component model. Am J Clin Nutr Jun 2008;87(6):1776–1784.

23. Demerath EW, Reed D, Choh AC, et al. Rapid postnatal weight gain and visceral adiposity in adulthood: the Fels longitudinal study. Obesity (Silver Spring) 2009;17:2060–2066.

24. Ibanez L, Ong K, Dunger DB, de Zegher F. Early development of adiposity and insulin resistance after catch-up weight gain in small-for-gestational-age children. J Clin Endocrinol Metab Jun 2006;91(6):2153–2158.

25. Meas T, Deghmoun S, Armoogum P, Alberti C, Levy-Marchal C. Consequences of being born small for gestational age on body composition: an 8-year follow-up study. J Clin Endocrinol Metab Oct 2008;93(10):3804–3809.

26. Ong KK, Petry CJ, Emmett PM, et al. Insulin sensitivity and secretion in normal children related to size at birth, postnatal growth, and plasma insulin-like growth factor-I levels. Diabetologia 2004;2004(47):1064–1070.

27. Adair LS, Martorell R, Stein AD, et al. Size at birth, weight gain in infancy and childhood, and adult blood pressure in 5 low- and middle-income-country cohorts: when does weight gain matter? Am J Clin Nutr May 2009;89(5): 1383–1392.

28. Ong KK, Potau N, Petry CJ, et al. Opposing influences of prenatal and postnatal weight gain on adrenarche in normal boys and girls. J Clin Endocrinol Metab Jun 2004;89(6):2647–2651.

29. Demerath EW, Jones LL, Hawley NL, et al. Rapid infant weight gain and advanced skeletal maturation in childhood. J Pediatr 14 May 2009;155(3):355–361.

30. Ong KK, Emmett P, Northstone K, et al. Infancy weight gain predicts childhood body fat and age at menarche in girls. J Clin Endocrinol Metab 24 Feb 2009;94(5):1527–1532.

31. Adair LS. Size at birth predicts age at menarche. Pediatrics 2001;107(4):e59.

32. Lakshman R, Forouhi N, Luben R, et al. Association between age at menarche and risk of diabetes in adults: results from the EPIC-Norfolk cohort study. Diabetologia 5 Mar 2008;51(5):781–786.

33. Hales CN, Desai M, Ozanne SE. The thrifty phenotype hypothesis: how does it look after 5 years? Diabetic Med 1997;14(3):189–195.

34. Sinclair KD, Allegrucci C, Singh R, et al. DNA methylation, insulin resistance, and blood pressure in offspring determined by maternal periconceptional B vitamin and methionine status. Proc Natl Acad Sci U S A 4 Dec 2007;104(49):19351–19356.

35. Symonds ME, Stephenson T, Gardner DS, Budge H. Long-term effects of nutritional programming of the embryo and fetus: mechanisms and critical windows. Reprod Fertil Dev 2007;19(1):53–63.

36. Gluckman PD, Hanson MA, Buklijas T, Low FM, Beedle AS. Epigenetic mechanisms that underpin metabolic and cardiovascular diseases. Nat Rev Endocrinol Jul 2009;5(7):401–408.

37. Gluckman PD, Hanson MA, Bateson P, et al. Towards a new developmental synthesis: adaptive developmental plasticity and human disease. Lancet 9 May 2009;373(9675):1654–1657.

38. Freathy RM, Bennett AJ, Ring SM, et al. Type 2 diabetes risk alleles are associated with reduced size at birth. Diabetes Jun 2009;58(6):1428–1433.

39. Ravelli GP, Stein ZA, Susser MW. Obesity in young men after famine exposure in utero and early infancy. N Engl J Med 1976;295(7):349–353.

40. Heijmans BT, Tobi EW, Stein AD, et al. Persistent epigenetic differences associated with prenatal exposure to famine in humans. Proc Natl Acad Sci U S A 4 Nov 2008;105(44):17046–17049.

41. Prentice AM, Whitehead RG, Watkinson M, Lamb WH, Cole TJ. Prenatal dietary supplementation of African women and birth-weight. Lancet 1983;1(8323):489–492.

42. Verkauskiene R, Figueras F, Deghmoun S, Chevenne D, Gardosi J, Levy-Marchal M. Birth weight and long-term metabolic outcomes: does the definition of smallness matter? Horm Res 2008;70(5):309–315.

43. Modi N, Thomas EL, Uthaya SN, Umranikar S, Bell JD, Yajnik C. Whole body magnetic resonance imaging of healthy newborn infants demonstrates increased central adiposity in Asian Indians. Pediatr Res 28 Jan 2009;65(5):584–587.

44. Ozanne SE, Lewis R, Jennings BJ, Hales CN. Early programming of weight gain in mice prevents the induction of obesity by a highly palatable diet. Clin Sci (Lond) Feb 2004;106(2):141–145.

45. Ozanne SE, Hales CN. Lifespan: catch-up growth and obesity in male mice. Nature 29 Jan 2004;427(6973):411–412.

46. Vickers MH, Gluckman PD, Coveny AH, et al. Neonatal leptin treatment reverses developmental programming. Endocrinology Oct 2005;146(10):4211–4216.

47. FAO. Human energy requirements: report of a Joint FAO/WHO/UNU Expert Consultation. Food and Nutrition Technical Report Series 1. 2004.

48. Leunissen RW, Kerkhof GF, Stijnen T, Hokken-Koelega A. Timing and tempo of first-year rapid growth in relation to cardiovascular and metabolic risk profile in early adulthood. J Am Med Assoc 3 Jun 2009;301(21):2234–2242.

49. Ong KK, Preece MA, Emmett PM, Ahmed ML, Dunger DB. Size at birth and early childhood growth in relation to maternal smoking, parity and infant breast-feeding: longitudinal birth cohort study and analysis. Pediatr Res Dec 2002;52(6):863–867.

50. Arenz S, Ruckerl R, Koletzko B, von Kries R. Breast-feeding and childhood obesity – a systematic review. Int J Obes Relat Metab Disord Oct 2004;28(10):1247–1256.

51. Fawzi WW, Forman MR, Levy A, Graubard BI, Naggan L, Berendes HW. Maternal anthropometry and infant feeding practices in Israel in relation to growth in infancy: the North African infant feeding study. Am J Clin Nutr Jun 1997;65(6):1731–1737.

52. Rolland-Cachera MF, Deheeger M, Akrout M, Bellisle F. Influence of macronutrients on adiposity development: a follow up study of nutrition and growth from 10 months to 8 years of age. Int J Obes Relat Metab Disord Aug 1995;19(8): 573–578.

53. Koletzko B, von Kries R, Closa R, et al. Lower protein in infant formula is associated with lower weight up to age 2 y: a randomized clinical trial. Am J Clin Nutr. 2009;89(6):1836–45.

54. Kalhan SC. Optimal protein intake in healthy infants. Am J Clin Nutr Jun 2009;89(6):1719–1720.

55. Lucas P, Arai L, Baird J, Kleijnen J, Law C, Roberts H. A systematic review of lay views about infant size and growth. Arch Dis Child Feb 2007;92(2):120–127.

56. Wright C, Lakshman R, Emmett P, Ong K. Implications of adopting the WHO 2006 Child Growth Standard in the UK: two prospective cohort studies. Arch Dis Child 1 Oct 2007;93(7):566–569.

57. Victora CG, Adair L, Fall C, et al. Maternal and child undernutrition: consequences for adult health and human capital. Lancet 26 Jan 2008;371(9609):340–357.

58. Ong KK. Catch-up growth in small for gestational age babies: good or bad? Curr Opin Endocrinol Diabetes Obes Feb 2007;14(1):30–34.

59. Ong K, Langkamp M, Ranke M, et al. Insulin like growth factor-I concentrations in infancy predict differential gains in body length and adiposity: the Cambridge baby growth study. Am J Clin Nutr 2009;90(1):156–161.

9 Gestational Diabetes

Dana Dabelea

CONTENTS

Key Words: Intrauterine, macrosomia, fetal growth, type 2 diabetes, maternal, insulin

INTRODUCTION

The prevalence of obesity has been increasing dramatically in the United States over the past decades in each race/ethnic group, in both men and women and in adults as well as children (1–3). From NHANES 2003–2004 data, 18.8% of children aged 6–11 years were overweight, compared to 6.5% of children in 1976–1980 (4). Among youth aged 12–19 years, prevalence of overweight increased from 5% in the late 1970s to 17.4% in 2003–2004 (4). Moreover, the distribution of body mass index (BMI) has shifted in a skewed fashion, such that the heaviest children have become even heavier over time (5). Overweight is now present at increasingly younger ages, indicating that risk factors for this condition start operating early in life (3). As in adults, obesity in childhood and adolescence is associated with adverse short- and long-term chronic outcomes, such as the insulin resistance syndrome, type 2 diabetes, cardiovascular disease, and increased cardiovascular mortality (6–8).

Fetal life is considered one of the critical periods when an exposure may have lifelong effects, through biological programming, on the structure or function of organs, tissues, and body systems. These early effects may be modified by later life exposures (through biological interaction) to determine future chronic disease risk (9). Determining which and how early-life factors operate among youth to promote the development of obesity is the first step toward prevention of both childhood and adult obesity.

From: *Contemporary Endocrinology: Pediatric Obesity: Etiology, Pathogenesis, and Treatment*
Edited by: M. Freemark, DOI 10.1007/978-1-60327-874-4_9,
© Springer Science+Business Media, LLC 2010

FETAL PROGRAMMING: A CONCEPTUAL FRAMEWORK

The notion that inadequate "nutrition" at critical periods of development in fetal life is a key determinant of childhood and adult health has important implications *(10–12)*. The hypothesis of fetal over-nutrition or fuel-mediated teratogenesis *(13)* proposed in the 1950s by Pederson postulates that intrauterine exposure to hyperglycemia causes permanent changes in the fetus of a woman with diabetes in pregnancy, leading to malformations, macrosomia, and an increased risk of developing obesity and type 2 diabetes later in life. In the 1980s this hypothesis was broadened to include the possibility that other fuels, such as free fatty acids, ketone bodies, and amino acids, also increase fetal growth *(13)*. Most studies of "fetal over-nutrition" have focused on maternal diabetes. Recent evidence, however, suggests that exposure to maternal diabetes represents the extreme of a distribution of altered maternal fuels to which the fetus is exposed in pregnancies complicated by obesity.

CONSEQUENCES OF EXPOSURE TO DIABETES DURING PREGNANCY

Exposure to altered glucose–insulin metabolism (or frank diabetes) in utero predisposes to fetal macrosomia and may increase the risks for obesity and metabolic consequences of obesity later in life, including during childhood and adolescence *(14)*.

Fetal Growth. Infants of diabetic mothers display excess fetal growth, often, but not always, resulting in macrosomia *(15)*. This increases the risks for cesarean delivery and traumatic birth injury *(15)*. Excess fetal growth is thought to be caused by increased substrate availability, including but not necessarily limited, to glucose. While maternal glucose freely crosses the placenta to the fetus, maternal insulin does not *(13)*. As a result, the fetus receives excess nutrients, and the fetal pancreas responds by producing increased insulin to meet the excessive glucose load. Insulin acts as an anabolic hormone in the fetus, promoting adiposity and, to a lesser extent, linear growth.

There is evidence that increased adiposity is already present at birth in infants of mothers with gestational diabetes. Catalano et al. *(16)* studied a group of 195 infants of mothers with gestational diabetes and 220 infants of mothers with normal glucose tolerance and found that fat mass, but not birth weight or fat-free mass, was 20% higher in the infants exposed to diabetes in utero. Maternal fasting glucose level measured during the oral glucose tolerance test was the strongest correlate of infant adiposity, further supporting the hypothesis that the degree of hyperglycemia determines the metabolic effects on the neonate. This suggests that, even in the absence of macrosomia, the exposure to the diabetic intrauterine milieu causes alterations in fetal growth patterns, which likely predispose neonatal overweight.

Childhood Growth and Obesity. The role of exposure to diabetes in utero on subsequent infant and childhood growth, obesity, and type 2 diabetes has been prospectively examined in two studies: the Pima Indian Study and the Diabetes in Pregnancy Study at Northwestern University in Chicago. The offspring of Pima Indian women with pre-existent type 2 diabetes and gestational diabetes were larger for gestational age at birth, and, at every age, they were heavier for height than the offspring of prediabetic or non-diabetic women *(14,17,18)*. Even in normal birth weight offspring of diabetic pregnancies, childhood obesity was still more common than among offspring of non-diabetic pregnancies *(19)*.

Researchers at The Diabetes in Pregnancy Center at Northwestern University have reported excessive growth in offspring of women with diabetes during pregnancy *(20)*. By age 8 years the children were, on average, 30% heavier than expected for their heights. In this study, amniotic fluid insulin was collected at 32–38 weeks of gestation. At the age of 6 years there was a significant positive association between amniotic fluid insulin levels and childhood obesity, as estimated by the symmetry index. The amniotic insulin concentrations in children who had a symmetry index of less than 1.0 (86.1 pmol/l,

14.4 µU/ml) or between 1.0 and 1.2 (69.9 pmol/l, 11.7 µU/ml) at 6 years of age were only half of those measured in the more obese children who had a symmetry index greater than 1.2 (140.5 pmol/l, 23.4 µU/ml, $p < 0.05$ for each comparison). Thus, this study demonstrated a direct correlation between one measure of the altered diabetic intrauterine environment and the degree of obesity in children and adolescents.

Not all studies have shown as clear an association between exposure to maternal diabetes in utero and childhood adiposity (21,22). The Growing Up Today Study (21) measured rates of obesity among 9- to 14-year-old offspring of mothers with gestational diabetes. Each 1-kg increase in birth weight was associated with a 40% increased odds of being overweight (>95th percentile) as an adolescent; even when maternal BMI and other potential mediators were taken into account, there remained a 30% increased odds of being overweight per 1-kg increase in birth weight. Exposure to gestational diabetes in utero was also associated with a 40% increased odds of being overweight as an adolescent, although these odds were attenuated when further adjustments were made for birth weight (odds ratio 1.3, 95% confidence interval 0.9–1.9) and maternal BMI (odds ratio 1.2, 95% confidence interval 0.8–1.7). While these results suggest that any increase in childhood obesity associated with exposure to gestational diabetes is not independent of birth weight and maternal obesity, there are important limitations to this study. All data were collected by questionnaire, and self-reported weight may be inaccurate. In addition, only about half of the mothers with children agreed to have the study contact their children, and of the eligible children only 68% of the girls and 58% of the boys completed the questionnaires, for an overall response rate of 34%. Moreover, a retrospective chart review by Whitaker et al. (22) found no difference in overweight (≥85th percentile for weight) for children aged 5–10 years according to maternal gestational diabetes status.

The inconsistencies in these results may be partly explained by differences in exposure prevalence across populations studied. The rates of obesity and diabetes (including diabetes in pregnancy) in Pima Indians exceed those of nearly all other populations. Additional studies are needed to evaluate the effect of intrauterine diabetes exposure on fetal and childhood growth among different ethnic groups and among populations with milder degrees of hyperglycemia.

Abnormal Glucose Tolerance and Risk for Type 2 Diabetes. For more than 30 years, Pima Indian women have had routine oral glucose tolerance tests approximately every 2 years as well as during pregnancy (18). Women who had diabetes before or during pregnancy were termed diabetic mothers; those who developed diabetes only after pregnancy were termed prediabetic mothers. By age 5–9 and 10–14 years, type 2 diabetes was present almost exclusively among the offspring of diabetic women. In all age groups there was significantly more diabetes in the offspring of diabetic women than in those of prediabetic and non-diabetic women, and there were much smaller differences in diabetes prevalence between offspring of prediabetic and non-diabetic women (23). Recently, the SEARCH Case–Control Study (SEARCH CC) provided novel evidence that intrauterine exposure to maternal diabetes and obesity are important determinants of type 2 diabetes in youth of other racial/ethnic groups (non-Hispanic white, Hispanic, and African-American), together contributing to 47% of type 2 diabetes in the offspring (24).

Cardiovascular Abnormalities. Animal studies have shown that exposure to diabetes in utero can induce cardiovascular dysfunction in adult offspring (25). Few human studies have examined cardiovascular risk factors in offspring of diabetic pregnancies. By 10–14 years, offspring of diabetic pregnancies enrolled in the Diabetes in Pregnancy follow-up study at Northwestern University had significantly higher systolic and mean arterial blood pressure than offspring of non-diabetic pregnancies (20). Higher concentrations of markers of endothelial dysfunction (ICAM-1, VCAM-1, E-selectin) as well as increased cholesterol-to-HDL ratio were reported among offspring of mothers with type 1 diabetes compared with offspring of non-diabetic pregnancies, independent of current body mass index (26). Recently, the Pima Indian investigators have shown that, independent of adiposity, 7- to

11-year-old offspring exposed to maternal diabetes during pregnancy have significantly higher systolic blood pressure than offspring of mothers who did not develop type 2 diabetes until after the index pregnancy (27). These data suggest that in utero exposure to diabetes confers risks for the development of cardiovascular disease later in life that are independent of adiposity and may be exerted in concert with genetic predisposition to diabetes or cardiovascular disease.

DOES MATERNAL DIABETES TYPE MATTER?

Several studies have found that the effects of exposure to diabetes in utero on future obesity are similar for pregnancies complicated by pre-existing type 1, type 2, or gestational diabetes (14,20). Weiss et al. (28) compared the offspring of women with type 1 diabetes to offspring of women without diabetes and reported that at age 5–15 years they had significantly higher BMI, greater insulin resistance, and more than a threefold increased odds of type 2 diabetes. Amniotic fluid insulin levels were associated with offspring BMI and insulin resistance, further supporting the influence of the fetal metabolic environment on development of obesity and type 2 diabetes.

In a study of impaired glucose tolerance in the offspring of mothers with type 1, type 2, and gestational diabetes, Silverman et al. found that the risk of impaired glucose tolerance was not different by type of maternal diabetes (29). Rather, impaired glucose tolerance was closely related to the amniotic fluid insulin levels, which are indicative of the degree of fetal hyperinsulinemia. Sobngwi and colleagues also confirmed that impaired glucose tolerance and defective insulin secretory responses in adults are associated with exposure to pre-gestational type 1 diabetes in utero (30). The control population in this study was a group of adult offspring of fathers with type 1 diabetes; in theory, this controls for confounding by genetic susceptibility. These results further support the conclusion that hyperglycemia and other fuel alterations in pregnancies complicated by diabetes, and not the etiology of the mother's diabetes, are the important factors influencing risk of obesity and glucose metabolism abnormalities in the offspring.

In the Pima Indian population, Franks and colleagues found that maternal glucose levels are associated with excess fetal growth and later risk of diabetes even among women with normal glucose tolerance (31). Birth weight was found to increase significantly with each standard deviation increase in maternal blood glucose level, and the risk of type 2 diabetes in the offspring increased 30% with each standard deviation increase in maternal glucose level. The presence of excess risk of metabolic abnormalities in offspring even in glucose tolerant mothers suggests that exposure to hyperglycemia is a continuous risk factor, and prevention of long-term consequences in the offspring may require improvement in glycemia even in pregnancies uncomplicated by diabetes.

PROGRAMMING OF FETAL GROWTH AND ADIPOSITY BY MATERNAL OBESITY

Much less is known about whether and how fetal programming is driven by exposure in utero to maternal obesity in the absence of diabetes. Multiple factors have been associated with fetal growth, in addition to maternal glucose intolerance: age, parity, race/ ethnicity, weight, weight gain, smoking status, and fetal gender (32,33). Black race, female infant gender, and younger maternal age are associated with risk of fetal growth restriction (34–36) while advancing parity and higher maternal body size are associated with larger babies (36). Interestingly, paternal contribution to fetal growth seems less important (32). Maternal height and "frame size," regarded as markers of lifelong nutritional status, are important determinants of fetal growth (37). Birth weight was shown to increase linearly with increasing pre-pregnancy BMI and with increasing weight gain during pregnancy (38,39).

An important question is whether exposure to maternal obesity during pregnancy in the absence of frank diabetes is also associated with increased obesity in the offspring, above and beyond genetic susceptibility. Vohr et al. found that maternal pre-pregnancy weight and weight gain during pregnancy were significant predictors not only of macrosomia but also of neonatal adiposity (based on skinfold assessment) among both infants of GDM mothers and control infants (40). Moreover, these patterns of adiposity at birth persisted at age 1 year (41). Using data from more than 3,000 children available through the National Longitudinal Survey of Youth, Salsberry et al. found that the risk that a child would be overweight at a young age increases with maternal pre-pregnancy BMI (42). Recent findings indicate that children exposed to maternal obesity, in the absence of gestational diabetes, are at increased risk of developing the metabolic syndrome during adolescence (43). This suggests that metabolic factors that affect fetal growth and perinatal outcomes are present in obese mothers who do not fulfill the diagnostic criteria for gestational diabetes. Similarly, in SEARCH CC, exposure to maternal obesity in utero was associated with 2.8-fold increased odds for type 2 diabetes in multi-ethnic youth, independent of exposure to diabetes during pregnancy (24).

GENETIC, FAMILIAL, OR SPECIFIC INTRAUTERINE EFFECTS?

It is clear that the above associations are partly due to increased genetic susceptibility to obesity and diabetes inherited by offspring from their mothers. Shared genes certainly account for some of the similarity in maternal and offspring weight and risk for type 2 diabetes (44). However, there is also strong evidence that excess growth experienced by offspring of diabetic mothers is not due to genetic factors alone. First, obesity is no more common in the offspring of women in whom diabetes developed after delivery than in those of non-diabetic women (14,45). Second, obesity and diabetes in the offspring of diabetic women cannot be accounted for by maternal obesity (14,19,24). Third, the excessive growth seen in the offspring of diabetic mothers is not found in offspring of diabetic fathers in either the Joslin Clinic or the Pima Indian series (46).

While these findings provide evidence that genetic confounding does not explain all of the effects of maternal diabetes during pregnancy on the risks of obesity and type 2 diabetes in the offspring, there are genetic mutations which have been shown to cause obesity and type 2 diabetes and are maternally transmitted (47). Therefore, the ideal way to remove possible confounding by genetic predisposition is to examine sibling pairs in which one sibling is born before and one is born after the onset of their mother's diabetes (48). The Pima Indian studies have examined the effect of intrauterine exposure to diabetes on risk for obesity among discordant siblings (48). The mean body mass index in the 62 Pima Indian non-diabetic siblings born after the onset of the mother's diabetes, i.e., the offspring of the diabetic woman, was significantly higher (mean BMI difference: 2.6 kg/m^2) than among the 121 non-diabetic siblings who were not exposed to diabetes in utero, e.g., born before the onset of the mother's diabetes. In contrast, there was no significant difference between siblings born before or after their father was diagnosed with type 2 DM (mean BMI difference: 0.4 kg/m^2) (48). These data support the hypothesis that exposure to DM in utero has effects on offspring body size that are distinct from, or act in concert with, genetic susceptibility to obesity. They point toward the role of altered maternal fuels, especially hyperglycemia, as mediators of fetal growth and risk of obesity in offspring exposed to maternal diabetes in utero.

The Growing Up Today Study (21), on the other hand, found that the 40% increased odds of being overweight among 9- to 14-year-old offspring of mothers with gestational diabetes was no longer significant when adjustment was made for birth weight and reported maternal BMI; the latter is considered a surrogate for genetic susceptibility for obesity. These findings suggest that either shared adverse lifestyle habits among mothers and daughters or maternal transmission of susceptibility genes account for part of the increased risk of obesity among offspring of mothers with gestational diabetes in addition to the intrauterine exposure to diabetes per se.

Alternatively, since insulin resistance in the mother spares glucose, amino acids, and fatty acids for placental-fetal transport *(37,49)*, it can be hypothesized that obese or diabetic pregnant women, who have severe insulin resistance, transport an excess of nutrients to the fetus. This results in fetal adiposity *(37)*. This hypothesis is entirely compatible with the original "fuel-mediated teratogenesis" hypothesis *(13)*, as long as the metabolic pathways responsible for the abnormal fetal growth and development are also associated with an increased risk of later-life chronic disorders such as obesity, type 2 diabetes, and cardiovascular disease. Data in rats *(50)* show that pre-gestational obesity induced by overfeeding leads to obesity, metabolic alterations, and increased adipose tissue cellularity in the offspring. Importantly, in these models, the process is independent of inherited genetic influences.

POSSIBLE MECHANISMS RESPONSIBLE FOR THE INTRAUTERINE EFFECTS

Despite the evidence from animal and human studies that exposure to maternal diabetes and obesity in utero may have long-term programming consequences on the offspring, the specific mechanisms responsible for these effects are not fully understood.

Dysregulation of the Adipo-insular Axis. One of the proposed mechanisms is a resetting of the adipo-insular axis in exposed newborns. The adipo-insular axis is a bi-directional feedback loop involving leptin released by adipocytes and insulin released by pancreatic β-cells *(51)*. As body fat stores increase, leptin levels increase, which in turn reduce insulin production. Increased levels of insulin stimulate the biosynthesis and secretion of leptin from adipocytes *(51)*. This feedback loop found in animal studies *(52,53)* is now also supported by human data *(51)*.

Several studies suggest that the adipo-insular feedback loop may be programmed in utero *(54–56)*. Elevated cord blood leptin concentrations were found in infants of mothers with type 1 diabetes (24.7 ng/ml) and of mothers with gestational diabetes (29.3 ng/ml), as compared with controls (7.9 ng/ml) *(57)*, even after controlling for differences in birth weight. This suggests a direct influence of maternal hyperglycemia on fetal fat mass and leptin levels. In two other studies, exposure to gestational diabetes was associated with both hyperleptinemia and hyperinsulinemia in the newborn *(54,58)*. This suggests that fetal over-nutrition by exposure to maternal diabetes and obesity in utero may lead to increased insulin secretion and adiposity in the offspring despite an increase in plasma leptin concentrations, which are unable to control the release of insulin and the increase in fetal adiposity *(54)*. Induction of leptin resistance in utero may therefore be hypothesized as a potential mechanism for later development of obesity in offspring exposed to over-nutrition in utero. Inefficient leptin action programmed in utero may lead to hyperphagia, decreased fat oxidation, increased tissue triglyceride levels, insulin resistance, and obesity later in life *(51,59,60)*.

Fetal Malprogramming of Hypothalamic Neurons. "Functional teratogenesis." An interesting hypothesis relating hormonal changes present at birth in offspring exposed to diabetes in utero has been formulated by Plageman et al. *(61)*. When present in increased concentrations during critical ontogenetic periods, hormones (such as insulin and leptin) can act as "endogenous functional teratogens" *(61,62)*. As example, untreated diabetes in pregnant rats leads to "malprogramming" of hypothalamic neuropeptidergic neurons in offspring, leading to increased orexigenic neuropeptide Y and agouti-related peptide, which could contribute to hyperphagia and later development of overweight. Islet transplantation in pregnant rats with gestational diabetes normalizes blood glucose and prevents these acquired alterations *(63)*.

Defective Insulin Secretion in Offspring Exposed to Maternal Diabetes. In Goto-Kakizaki (GK) rats, the diabetic syndrome is produced by streptozotocin injection or glucose infusion. These rats do not have any genetic predisposition for diabetes nor can their diabetes be classified as type 1 or 2.

In these studies, hyperglycemia in the mother during pregnancy leads to impairment of glucose tolerance and decreased insulin action and secretion in adult offspring (64,65).

Impaired insulin secretion (66) has also been observed in human studies. Among 104 normal glucose tolerant Pima Indian adults, the acute insulin response was 40% lower in offspring of diabetic versus prediabetic mothers (67). In a different population, Sobngwi et al. (30) showed that adult offspring of women with type 1 diabetes during pregnancy had a significantly decreased insulin secretory response to glucose when compared with offspring of type 1 diabetic fathers, while there were no differences between groups with respect to insulin action. Based on the observations made in rats and supported by the human findings, it may be hypothesized that exposure to hyperglycemia during critical periods of fetal development "programs" the developing pancreas in a way that leads to a subsequent impairment in insulin secretion. This, coupled with an increased risk for obesity, resulting from over-nutrition in utero, may lead to an early onset of type 2 diabetes, especially in individuals at high genetic risk.

CLINICAL AND PUBLIC HEALTH IMPLICATIONS

The long-term effects of exposure to maternal diabetes during childhood and over the life-course have been described as a vicious cycle (68). Children whose mothers had diabetes during pregnancy are at increased risk of becoming obese and developing diabetes at young ages. Many of these female offspring already have diabetes or abnormal glucose tolerance by the time they reach their childbearing years, thereby perpetuating the cycle. A remaining research need is to derive risk estimates for childhood obesity, impaired glucose tolerance, and type 2 diabetes that are attributable to exposure to maternal diabetes in utero, in various racial/ethnic groups.

If maternal obesity during pregnancy drives fuel-mediated teratogenesis, the public health consequences are enormous, since obesity is widespread and increasing. Studies are needed to disentangle the relative contributions of various fuels to the long-term effects on childhood risks for obesity and impaired glucose metabolism in offspring of obese pregnant women.

Finally, more information is needed to determine the most effective strategies and interventions to address the risk of chronic metabolic diseases in the infant of the diabetic mother. However, it is increasingly clear that public health efforts to prevent obesity and type 2 diabetes should focus not only on adult lifestyle risk factors but also on prenatal exposure to hyperglycemia and obesity in utero. Reduced obesity in women of reproductive age and prevention of excessive weight gain during pregnancy not only may decrease the risk of gestational diabetes in the mother but will likely also reduce the risk of excess fetal growth, future obesity, and type 2 diabetes in the offspring.

REFERENCES

1. Mokdad AH, Serdula MK, Dietz WH, Bowman BA, Marks JS, Koplan JP. The continuing epidemic of obesity in the United States. J Am Med Assoc. 2000;284:1650–1.
2. Mokdad AH, Serdula MK, Dietz WH, Bowman BA, Marks JS, Koplan JP. The spread of the obesity epidemic in the United States. J Am Med Assoc. 1999;282:1519–22.
3. Ogden CL, Flegal KM, Carroll MD, Johnson CL. Prevalence and trends in overweight among US children and adolescents, 1999–2000. J Am Med Assoc. 2002;288 14:1728–32.
4. Wang Y, Beydoun MA. The obesity epidemic in the United States – gender, age, socioeconomic, racial/ethnic, and geographic characteristics: a systematic review and meta-regression analysis. Epidemiol Rev. 2007;29:6–28.
5. Flegal KM, Troiano RP. Changes in the distribution of body mass index of adults and children in the US population. Int J Obes Relat Metab Disord. 2000;24:807–18.
6. Freedman DS, Dietz WH, Srinivasan SR, Berenson GS. The relation of overweight to cardiovascular risk factors among children and adolescents: the Bogalusa Heart Study. Pediatrics. 1999;103:1175–82.

7. Must A, Jacques PF, Dallal GE, Bajema CJ, Dietz WH. Long-term morbidity and mortality of overweight adolescents. A follow-up of the Harvard Growth Study of 1922 to 1935. N Engl J Med. 1992;327:1350–55.

8. Must A, Anderson SE. Effects of obesity on morbidity in children and adolescents. Nutr Clin Care. 2003;6:4–12.

9. Ben Shlomo Y, Kuh D. A life course approach to chronic disease epidemiology: conceptual models, empirical challenges and interdisciplinary perspectives. Int J Epidemiol. 2002;31:285–93.

10. Barker DJ, Fall CH. Fetal and infant origins of cardiovascular disease. Arch Dis Child. 1993;68:797–99.

11. Barker DJ, Gluckman PD, Godfrey KM, Harding JE, Owens JA, Robinson JS. Fetal nutrition and cardiovascular disease in adult life. Lancet. 1993;341:938–41.

12. Barker DJ. In utero programming of chronic disease. Clin Sci (Colch). 1998;95:115–28.

13. Freinkel N. Banting Lecture 1980. Of pregnancy and progeny (review). Diabetes. 1980;29:1023–35.

14. Pettitt DJ, Baird HR, Aleck KA, Bennett PH, Knowler WC. Excessive obesity in offspring of Pima Indian women with diabetes during pregnancy. N Engl J Med. 1983;308:242–45.

15. Jansson T, Cetin I, Powell TL, Desoye G, Radaelli T, Ericsson A, et al. Placental transport and metabolism in fetal overgrowth – a workshop report. Placenta. 2006;27 Suppl A:S109–13.

16. Catalano PM, Thomas A, Huston-Presley L, Amini SB. Increased fetal adiposity: a very sensitive marker of abnormal in utero development. Am J Obstet Gynecol. 2003;189:1698–704.

17. Pettitt DJ, Nelson RG, Saad MF, Bennett PH, Knowler WC. Diabetes and obesity in the offspring of Pima Indian women with diabetes during pregnancy. Diabetes Care. 1993;16:310–14.

18. Pettitt DJ, Bennett PH, Knowler WC, Baird HR, Aleck KA. Gestational diabetes mellitus and impaired glucose tolerance during pregnancy. Long-term effects on obesity and glucose tolerance in the offspring. Diabetes. 1985;34 Suppl 2: 119–22.

19. Pettitt DJ, Knowler WC, Bennett PH, Aleck KA, Baird HR. Obesity in offspring of diabetic Pima Indian women despite normal birth weight. Diabetes Care. 1987;10:76–80.

20. Silverman BL, Rizzo T, Green OC, Cho NH, Winter RJ, Ogata ES, et al. Long-term prospective evaluation of offspring of diabetic mothers. Diabetes. 1991;40 Suppl 2:121–25.

21. Gillman MW, Rifas-Shiman S, Berkey CS, Field AE, Colditz GA. Maternal gestational diabetes, birth weight, and adolescent obesity. Pediatrics. 2003;111:e221–6.

22. Whitaker RC, Pepe MS, Seidel KD, Wright JA, Knopp RH. Gestational diabetes and the risk of offspring obesity. Pediatrics. 1998;101:E91–7.

23. Dabelea D, Pettitt DJ. Intrauterine diabetic environment confers risks for type 2 diabetes mellitus and obesity in the offspring, in addition to genetic susceptibility. J Pediatr Endocrinol Metab. 2001;14:1085–91.

24. Dabelea D, Mayer-Davis EJ, Lamichhane AP, D'Agostino RB Jr, Liese AD, Vehik KS, et al. Association of intrauterine exposure to maternal diabetes and obesity with type 2 diabetes in youth: the SEARCH Case-Control study. Diabetes Care. 2008;31 7:1422–6.

25. Holemans K, Gerber RT, Meurrens K, De Clerck F, Poston L, Van Assche FA. Streptozotocin diabetes in the pregnant rat induces cardiovascular dysfunction in adult offspring. Diabetologia. 1999;42:81–89.

26. Manderson JG, Mullan B, Patterson CC, Hadden DR, Traub AI, McCance DR. Cardiovascular and metabolic abnormalities in the offspring of diabetic pregnancy. Diabetologia. 2002;45:991–96.

27. Bunt JC, Tataranni PA, Salbe AD. Intrauterine exposure to diabetes is a determinant of hemoglobin A(1)c and systolic blood pressure in pima Indian children. J Clin Endocrinol Metab. 2005;90:3225–9.

28. Weiss PA, Scholz HS, Haas J, Tamussino KF, Seissler J, Borkenstein MH. Long-term follow-up of infants of mothers with type 1 diabetes: evidence for hereditary and nonhereditary transmission of diabetes and precursors. Diabetes Care. 2000;23:905–11.

29. Silverman BL, Metzger BE, Cho NH, Loeb CA. Impaired glucose tolerance in adolescent offspring of diabetic mothers: Relationship to fetal hyperinsulinism. Diabetes Care. 1995;18:611–17.

30. Sobngwi E, Boudou P, Mauvais-Jarvis F, Leblanc H, Velho G, Vexiau P, et al. Effect of a diabetic environment in utero on predisposition to type 2 diabetes. Lancet. 2003;361:1861–5.

31. Franks PW, Looker HC, Kobes S, Touger L, Tataranni PA, Hanson RL, et al. Gestational glucose tolerance and risk of type 2 diabetes in young Pima Indian offspring. Diabetes. 2006;55:460–65.

32. Catalano PM, Drago NM, Amini SB. Factors affecting fetal growth and body composition. Am J Obstet Gynecol. 1995;172:1459–63.

33. Sacks DA. Fetal macrosomia and gestational diabetes: what's the problem? Obstet Gynecol. 1993;81:775–81.

34. Wen SW, Goldenberg RL, Cutter GR, Hoffman HJ, Cliver SP, Davis RO, et al. Smoking, maternal age, fetal growth, and gestational age at delivery. Am J Obstet Gynecol. 1990;162:53–58.

35. Meis PJ, Michielutte R, Peters TJ, Wells HB, Sands RE, Coles EC, et al. Factors associated with term low birthweight in Cardiff, Wales. Paediatr Perinat Epidemiol. 1997;11:287–97.

36. Goldenberg RL, Cliver SP. Small for gestational age and intrauterine growth restriction: definitions and standards. Clin Obstet Gynecol. 1997;40:704–14.

37. Perry IJ, Lumey LH. Fetal growth and development: the role of nutrition and other factors. In: Kuh D, Ben-Shlomo Y, editors. A life course approach to chronic disease epidemiology. Oxford: Oxford University Press; 2004. pp. 345–71.

38. Luke B. Nutritional influences on fetal growth. Clin Obstet Gynecol. 1994;37:538–49.

39. Abrams BF, Berman CA. Nutrition during pregnancy and lactation. Prim Care. 1993;20:585–97.

40. Vohr BR, McGarvey ST, Coll CG. Effects of maternal gestational diabetes and adiposity on neonatal adiposity and blood pressure. Diabetes Care. 1995;18:467–75.

41. Vohr BR, McGarvey ST. Growth patterns of large-for-gestational-age and appropriate-for-gestational-age infants of gestational diabetic mothers and control mothers at age 1 year. Diabetes Care. 1997;20:1066–72.

42. Salsberry PJ. Why are some children still uninsured? J Pediatr Health Care. 2003;17:32–38.

43. Boney CM, Verma A, Tucker R, Vohr BR. Metabolic syndrome in childhood: association with birth weight, maternal obesity, and gestational diabetes mellitus. Pediatrics. 2005;115:e290–6.

44. Rankinen T, Zuberi A, Chagnon YC, Weisnagel SJ, Argyropoulos G, Walts B, et al. The human obesity gene map: the 2005 update. Obesity (Silver Spring). 2006;14:529–644.

45. White P. Childhood diabetes: its course, and influence on the second and third generations. Diabetes. 1960;9:345–48.

46. Pettitt DJ, Knowler WC. Long-term effects of the intrauterine environment, birth weight, and breast-feeding in Pima Indians. Diabetes Care. 1998;21 Suppl 2:B138–41.

47. Perucca-Lostanlen D, Narbonne H, Hernandez JB, Staccini P, Saunieres A, Paquis-Flucklinger V, et al. Mitochondrial DNA variations in patients with maternally inherited diabetes and deafness syndrome. Biochem Biophys Res Commun. 2000;277:771–75.

48. Dabelea D, Hanson RL, Lindsay RS, Pettitt DJ, Imperatore G, Gabir MM, et al. Intrauterine exposure to diabetes conveys risks for type 2 diabetes and obesity: a study of discordant sibships. Diabetes. 2000;49:2208–11.

49. Catalano PM, Kirwan JP, Haugel-de Mouzon S, King J. Gestational diabetes and insulin resistance: role in short- and long-term implications for mother and fetus. J Nutr. 2003;133:1674S–83S.

50. Kartik S, Harrell A, Liu X, Gilchrist JM, Ronis MJ, Badger TM. Maternal obesity at conception programs obesity in the offspring. Am J Physiol Regul Integr Comp Physiol. 2008;291:528–38.

51. Kieffer TJ, Habener JF. The adipoinsular axis: effects of leptin on pancreatic beta-cells. Am J Physiol Endocrinol Metabol. 2000;278:E1–14.

52. Seufert J, Kieffer TJ, Habener JF. Leptin inhibits insulin gene transcription and reverses hyperinsulinemia in leptin-deficient ob/ob mice. Proc Natl Acad Sci USA. 1999;96:674–79.

53. Seufert J, Kieffer TJ, Leech CA, Holz GG, Moritz W, Ricordi C, et al. Leptin suppression of insulin secretion and gene expression in human pancreatic islets: implications for the development of adipogenic diabetes mellitus. J Clin Endocrinol Metab. 1999;84:670–76.

54. Simmons D, Breier BH. Fetal overnutrition in polynesian pregnancies and in gestational diabetes may lead to dysregulation of the adipoinsular axis in offspring. Diabetes Care. 2002;25:1539–44.

55. Mantzoros CS, Rifas-Shiman SL, Williams CJ, Fargnoli JL, Kelesidis T, Gillman MW. Cord blood leptin and adiponectin as predictors of adiposity in children at 3 years of age: a prospective cohort study. Pediatrics. 2009;123:682–89.

56. Muhlhausler BS, Adam CL, Findlay PA, Duffield JA, McMillen IC. Increased maternal nutrition alters development of the appetite-regulating network in the brain. FASEB J. 2006;20:1257–59.

57. Persson B, Westgren M, Celsi G, Nord E, Ortqvist E. Leptin concentrations in cord blood in normal newborn infants and offspring of diabetic mothers. Horm Metab Res. 1999;31:467–71.

58. Wolf HJ, Ebenbichler CF, Huter O, Bodner J, Lechleitner M, Foger B, et al. Fetal leptin and insulin levels only correlate inlarge-for-gestational age infants. Eur J Endocrinol. 2000;142:623–29.

59. Kieffer TJ, Heller RS, Habener JF. Leptin receptors expressed on pancreatic beta-cells. Biochem Biophys Res Commun. 1996;224:522–27.

60. Seufert J, Kieffer TJ, Leech CA, Holz GG, Moritz W, Ricordi C, et al. Leptin suppression of insulin secretion and gene expression in human pancreatic islets: implications for the development of adipogenic diabetes mellitus. J Clin Endocrinol Metab. 1999;84:670–76.

61. Plagemann A. 'Fetal programming' and 'functional teratogenesis': on epigenetic mechanisms and prevention of perinatally acquired lasting health risks. J Perinat Med. 2004;32:297–305.

62. McMillen IC, Edwards LJ, Duffield J, Muhlhausler BS. Regulation of leptin synthesis and secretion before birth: implications for the early programming of adult obesity. Reproduction. 2006;131:415–27.

63. Franke K, Harder T, Aerts L, Melchior K, Fahrenkrog S, Rodekamp E, et al. 'Programming' of orexigenic and anorexigenic hypothalamic neurons in offspring of treated and untreated diabetic mother rats. Brain Res. 2005;1031:276–83.

64. Gauguier D, Bihoreau M-T, Ktorza A, Berthault M-F, Picon L. Inheritance of diabetes mellitus as consequence of gestational hyperglycemia in rats. Diabetes. 1990;39:734–9.

65. Aerts L, Sodoyez-Goffaux F, Sodoyez JC, Malaisse WJ, Van Assche FA. The diabetic intrauterine milieu has a long-lasting effect on insulin secretion by B cells and on insulin uptake by target tissues. Am J Obstet Gynecol. 1988;159:1287–92.

66. Hultquist GT, Olding LB. Pancreatic-islet fibrosis in young infants of diabetic mothers. Lancet. 1975;2:1015–6.

67. Gautier JF, Wilson C, Weyer C, Mott D, Knowler WC, Cavaghan M, et al. Low acute insulin secretory responses in adult offspring of people with early onset type 2 diabetes. Diabetes. 2001;50:1828–33.

68. Pettitt DJ, Knowler WC. Diabetes and obesity in the Pima Indians: a crossgenerational vicious cycle. J Obes Weight Regul. 1988;7:61–5.

V THE ROLES OF DIET AND ENERGY EXPENDITURE IN OBESITY PATHOGENESIS

10 The Role of Diet

Laura Johnson and Susan Jebb

CONTENTS

Key Words: Diet, fiber (fibre), fat, sugar, energy density

One of the few things certain about obesity is that weight is gained only when energy intake (EI) exceeds energy needs for a prolonged period of time. However, EI must be considered in the context of an individual's energy requirements. When expressed per kilogram of body weight, energy needs in children are much greater than those in adults owing to the demands of growth and development (*1*). Obesity results not from a high absolute energy intake, which may match energy needs in a growing, physically active child, but from intake which exceeds energy needs on a regular basis. Variation in physical activity can mean that energy needs of children of the same age can differ by as much as 1 MJ (Fig. 1). It is the coupling of intake and expenditure that is key, and the search for specific dietary factors that increase the risk of obesity is therefore a quest for factors that undermine the homeostatic control of food intake.

Innate appetite control mechanisms in children appear to be more robust than in adults. Multiple studies have shown that young children compensate well for excessive EI at one meal by reducing EI at the next meal whereas energy compensation in adults is less effective (*2,3*). However, the efficiency of appetite control mechanisms declines with age even in childhood; by the time of the "adiposity rebound" at age 5–7 years, the effect of poor diets on weight gain becomes increasingly apparent. This may explain why the prevalence of obesity tends to be highest in older children (*4,5*). Unfortunately, by this stage inappropriate eating habits may have become established behaviours.

Moreover, individual variation in the precision of appetite regulation means that some children are at higher risk even at a very young age (*6,7*). During infancy, formula feeding (*8*) and early weaning (*9*) are associated with rapid weight gain, which is a strong risk factor for childhood obesity (*10*).

From: *Contemporary Endocrinology: Pediatric Obesity: Etiology, Pathogenesis, and Treatment*
Edited by: M. Freemark, DOI 10.1007/978-1-60327-874-4_10,
© Springer Science+Business Media, LLC 2010

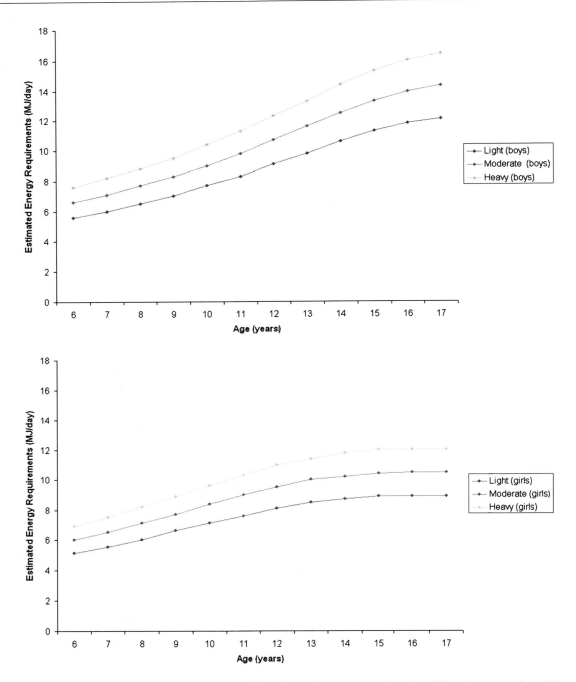

Fig. 1. Variation in energy requirements among girls and boys by age and activity level (based on equations *(1)*).

Considering the marked increase in the prevalence of obesity in children over the last 20 years it is unlikely that innate child appetite traits have altered significantly. In contrast, changes in diet have been profound and likely explain, at least in part, the rapid increase in the prevalence of obesity in recent times.

DIETARY FAT

The role of dietary fat in the aetiology of obesity is a hotly debated topic (11,12). Mechanistically, dietary fat is a obvious contender as a risk factor for obesity because it is the most energy-dense macronutrient (supplying 9 vs. 4 kcal/g for carbohydrate), the most palatable, least satiating macronutrient, and the last in the oxidative hierarchy to be used as fuel (13).

Prospective studies on the impact of fat intake on weight gain in children, however, have produced equivocal results. In a study of US children, each extra 1% of energy from fat was associated with a 0.18 kg/m^2 increase in BMI; in contrast, a study of French children showed no evidence of an association between fat intake and excessive growth (14,15). This is in spite of broadly similar study designs which included children aged 2–8 years, a modest sample size ($n = 70$ or 112), detailed measures of diet (diary or diet history), moderate % fat intakes ($\sim$32% of total energy), and adjustment for confounding factors. In the largest study of fat intake, which included 10,796 US children aged 9–14 years in the 'Growing Up Today' cohort, there was also no evidence of an effect on obesity (16). If fat intake per se does have an effect on the risk of obesity in childhood then the impact appears to be small.

FIBRE INTAKE

Fibre adds bulk to the diet, slows gastric emptying, lengthens transit time through the gastro-intestinal tract, impedes digestion, and increases satiety (17). Prospective cohorts demonstrate that high-fibre intakes attenuate long-term weight gain and reduce the risk of obesity in adults (17). Conventionally, recommendations for a high-fibre intake have been avoided for children as too much fibre may limit EI, retard growth, and reduce the absorption of minerals (18). However, at present fibre intake among children is low, and in light of the growing childhood obesity epidemic a modest increase in fibre intake may be beneficial (19).

Nevertheless, the evidence for a relationship between fibre and weight gain in children is limited. Two prospective studies of US children found no evidence of an association between low-fibre intake and excessive weight gain. In the first study 1,379 low-income preschool children in the WIC (Women, Infants and Children) nutrition program were followed for 9 months; no association was found between fibre intake (g/d) and annual weight gain (20). In the 'Growing Up Today' cohort of more than 10,000 children aged 9–14 years, fibre intake (g/d) was unrelated to annual body weight change after 3 years of follow-up (16). A third study of 328 German children also found no evidence of an effect of fibre intake on BMI or % body fat change from age 2 to 7 years (21). In these studies fibre intake ranged from 10 to 16 g/d, which is well below the recommended 19–38 g/d for 1- to 18-year-olds in the United States (22). If fibre intakes were higher then an effect on weight gain might be observed. Accordingly, while there is paucity of evidence to suggest that fibre intakes have contributed to the rise in obesity in children, studies of the effect of increasing fibre intakes to attenuate excess weight gain are warranted.

DIETARY ENERGY DENSITY

Dietary energy density (DED) refers to the amount of energy consumed per unit weight of food. The effect of DED on energy intake (EI) has been assessed in laboratory-based experimental studies. Meals with high DED lead to greater intakes of energy than meals with low DED because adults and children tend to consume a *constant weight* of food when differences in energy density are unknown. This concept is referred to as passive overconsumption (23,24). It is unclear if passive consumption occurs outside the laboratory; some data suggest that free-living adults make conscious choices to reduce portion sizes of more energy-dense foods when they know the energy content of those foods (25).

Fat is a key determinant of energy density and may explain the relationship between DED and EI. However, adult studies that manipulated fat content while keeping DED constant found that the effect of DED is independent of fat intake (26,27). Water contributes more to the weight of foods than any macronutrient; thus energy-dense foods are not just high in fat but also dry (28). For example, a dry food like biscuits (e.g. cream crackers, which is 13% fat, 10% protein and 4% water) and a high-fat food like cheese (e.g. Cheddar, which is 35% fat, 26% protein, and 35% water) can have similar energy densities (29). Importantly DED encompasses all foods likely to lead to an increase in EI and weight gain and so may be a better measure of an obesogenic diet better than fat or fibre intake alone.

Evidence from observational studies supports the theory that DED has a greater impact on fat mass as children get older (25). One prospective analysis of 2,275 English children aged 10 years enrolled in the Avon Longitudinal Study of Parents and Children (ALSPAC) found a linear association between DED and fat mass measured 3 years later. Each 1 kJ/g DED at age 10 years was associated with 0.16 ± 0.06 kg more fat mass at age 13 years (30). In contrast data from 600 children in a sub-sample of ALSPAC at the age of 5 years showed no evidence of a linear association between DED and fatness at 9 years. However, there was a non-linear association between DED at age 7 years and excessive fatness at age 9 years (defined as the top quintile of fat mass index), so that each 1 kJ/g DED increased the risk of excess adiposity by 36% (31). A similar non-linear association was observed in a small study of Northern Irish children (n = 48), which found that each 1 kJ/g DED at age 7 years was associated with a 90% increase in the risk of excess fat gain between the ages of 7 and 15 years (defined by the top tertile of change in fat mass index) (32). The changing effect of DED on fatness with age suggests that overconsumption in response to energy-dense foods may become more likely as children get older because innate appetite control becomes more susceptible to disruption by external cues such as high palatability.

FOODS

Focusing on single nutrients is potentially flawed as foods are made up of many nutrients that may interact to affect the risk of obesity. For example, high-fat foods, but not high-fat intake, were associated with increased weight gain, and high-fibre foods, but not high-fibre intakes, were associated with decreased weight gain over a 1-year period in 2- to 5-year-old US children (20).

Two food groups that have received particular attention with respect to the risk of obesity are sugar-sweetened beverages and fruits and vegetables. Sugar-sweetened beverages (SSB) increase EI and promote weight gain since liquid calories elicit a poor satiety response relative to solid food (33). Birch and Fisher reviewed studies in children in which ad libitum EI was measured following a high- or low-calorie drink (2). Collectively this research shows that pre-school children consistently reduce their EI in response to a high-energy drink compared to a low-energy drink; thus overall EI is not increased. However, the ability to respond to energy from SSB may not be perfect; one study reported that the reduction in EI at the subsequent meal was only 45% of the extra energy ingested (34). Furthermore, energy compensation declines with age. It is possible that young children are less susceptible to the effects of high-energy drinks compared with adolescents.

A wealth of research, summarised in seven reviews published in the last 3 years, suggests that sugary drinks are associated with a small increase in the risk of obesity in children (35). However, two different meta-analyses (36,37) found no effect of SSB on weight or BMI gain in children. Prospective studies of the association between SSB consumption and direct measures of fat mass in children also support a weak or null effect. A study of 208 Canadian adolescents (33), a study of 190 US girls aged 8–12 years (38), and data from the ALSPAC study when children were 5, 7, and 9 years old (39) all found no evidence of a longitudinal association between SSB consumption and increased body fat. In two of these studies SSB consumption accounted for just 3–4% of energy intake, which is much lower than that observed in US studies that did find evidence of an association with BMI. Overall the case for a specific role of sugar-sweetened drinks in encouraging obesity in children is supported by experimental studies but confirmation of an effect in observational studies of free-living children tends to be limited to specific samples of US adolescents where consumption of SSB may be particularly high. Nonetheless, such drinks add energy to the diet in the absence of other essential nutrients and it is logical to replace SSB with water or low-energy alternatives.

A high consumption of fruits and vegetables may protect against excess weight gain as they are high in fibre and water, both of which lower DED. The most recent data from the Health Survey for England (5) indicate that although fruit and vegetable consumption has increased recently it is still low in children and has declined over the last 40 years (40), suggesting that they may have a role in the emergence of the obesity epidemic.

A recent review of fruit and vegetable intake and obesity in children has highlighted the need for more research in this area (41). The only prospective analyses of the association between fruit and vegetable intake and obesity in young people are from the United States (20,42,43). Data from the 'Growing Up Today' cohort describing food intake, physical activity, height, and weight on a yearly basis over 3 years showed a small inverse relationship between vegetable intake and BMI among boys. Each serving of vegetables was associated with a 0.003 kg/m^2 decrease in annual BMI change, which was attenuated by the inclusion of EI in the model. There was no evidence of a relationship between fruit consumption and BMI in either boys or girls (43). In samples of 2- to 5-year-old children in the Women, Infants and Children (WIC) special supplemental nutrition programs in New York and North Dakota, neither vegetables nor fruits were associated with weight change (20,42).

Fruit and vegetable intake is almost universally lower than recommended levels in both the United States and the United Kingdom and it is prudent to continue to promote increased consumption (5,44). The absence of fruits and vegetables is associated with a lower DED and plays a significant role in a dietary pattern associated with obesity (45). Moreover, intervention studies in adults have shown promising results of increasing fruits and vegetables for weight loss and maintenance (46).

DIETARY PATTERNS

Identifying foods associated with obesity may account for interactions between nutrients but ignores the inherent complexity of diets, which are composed of many foods eaten in varying combinations. Analyses of patterns of food consumption or dietary patterns are a relatively new area of research in relation to obesity in children but they offer a more comprehensive assessment of the role of diet in obesity and may be more easily translated into food-based dietary guidelines.

Dietary patterns can be characterised in two ways: based on the data and based on hypotheses. Data-driven methods, like factor or cluster analysis, produce common patterns of food consumption, which may or may not be related to the disease of interest. In contrast, hypothesis-driven methods, like diet indices or reduced rank regression, use prior knowledge of causal mechanisms to extract dietary patterns that characterise specific features of consumption, e.g. an energy-dense, high-fat, and low-fibre diet. For each child a dietary pattern score is calculated from intakes of all food groups so that high scores represent consumption of a specific combination of foods.

Common patterns of food consumption have been characterised in four samples of UK, Korean, and US children. Infant dietary patterns during weaning were assessed at age 6 months in the Southampton Women's Survey (SWS). An 'infant guidelines' pattern was observed that included high intakes of breast milk, fruits, vegetables, meat, fish, and home-prepared foods. Surprisingly this pattern was associated with both greater skinfold thickness at 12 months and a greater gain in skinfold thickness between 6 and 12 months, which was independent of previous breastfeeding and age at introduction of solids. In a sample of 5-year-old Korean children, a pattern that included many meats and fast foods such as hamburgers and pizza was associated with a 77% (95% CI = 6–294%) higher risk of overweight (defined by BMI 85th Korean reference percentiles) *(47)*. A small cluster (12%) of 9- to 10-year-old girls in the National Heart, Lung, and Blood Institute Growth and Health Study ate a 'healthy' diet characterised by a high intake of fruits, vegetables, dairy, and grains and a low intake of sweetened drinks, sweets, fried foods, burgers, and pizza. At 10 years follow-up white, but not black, girls in this 'healthy eating' cluster had a lower waist circumference *(48)*.

UK data from food frequency questionnaires completed at age 3, 4, 7, and 9 years of age in ALSPAC suggested that a food pattern characterised by high consumption of soft drinks, crisps, chocolates, and biscuits was common at all ages *(49)*. However, there was no association between this dietary pattern at age 3 and risk of overweight at age 7 years *(50)*. Using more detailed data and a hypothesis-based approach, an energy-dense, high-fat, and low-fibre dietary pattern was extracted from food diaries collected in the same cohort at age 5 and 7 years *(45)*. A high pattern score was associated with very low intake of foods like fresh fruits and vegetables and high-fibre bread, alongside a high intake of foods like crisps and snacks, chocolates, and confectioneries (as indicated by pattern loadings, Fig. 2).

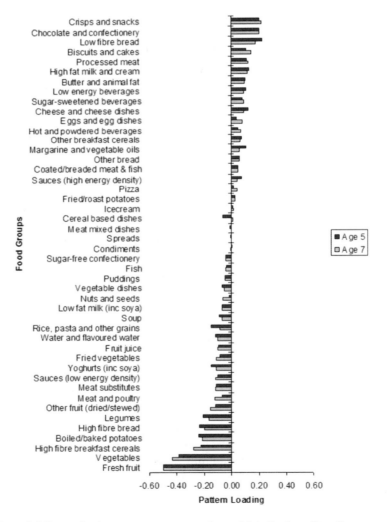

Fig. 2. The contribution of different food groups to an energy-dense, high-fat, low-fibre dietary pattern in the ALSPAC cohort *(57)*.

An increase of 1 SD of pattern score at ages 5 and 7 years, respectively, was associated with an extra 0.15 and 0.28 kg of fat mass at age 9 years.

The analysis of dietary patterns combines many small effects from individual foods and nutrients and has produced the most consistent evidence to date for dietary causes of obesity. Figure 3 illustrates the relative estimated impact of nutrients, beverages, and the whole diet consumed at age 5 or 7 years on excess adiposity at age 9 years and shows that the effect of an energy-dense, high-fat, low-fibre dietary pattern was larger than the effect of DED, fibre, or fat intake alone on the risk of excess adiposity. *These findings suggest that the diet as a whole is a more important determinant of obesity risk than any single food or nutrient.*

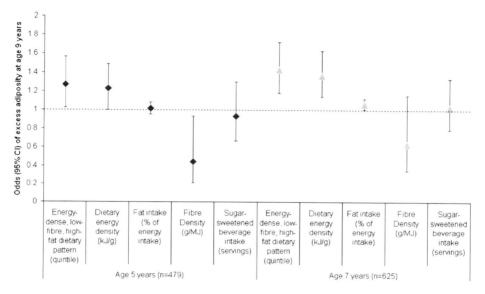

Fig. 3. Data from ALSPAC illustrating the relative impact of fat, fibre, energy density, sugar-sweetened beverages, and dietary pattern score at age 5 or 7 years on the odds of excess adiposity (top quintile of fat mass index) at age 9 years after adjusting for sex, TV watching, maternal education, maternal BMI, child weight status at baseline, and misreporting of EI *(57)*.

EATING BEHAVIOUR

One explanation for the mixed findings in relation to diet and obesity is that the impact of diet on excessive weight gain may be limited to those with an underlying behavioural susceptibility. Behavioural traits proposed to encourage overconsumption such as a fast eating rate, poor sensitivity to satiety, heightened food responsiveness, and a tendency to eat palatable food in the absence of hunger have been characterised in children using experimental methods and psychometric questionnaires *(51)*. Some cross-sectional studies suggest that these eating behaviour traits are related to weight, but few longitudinal studies have been performed to confirm an association with greater weight gain over time *(52)*. The Viva la Familia study measured how much palatable food was eaten in the absence of hunger by 879 overweight Hispanic children and found an association with BMI at follow-up 1 year later; interestingly, it was not independent of baseline BMI *(53)*, suggesting that eating behaviours are entrained at an early age and that the connection between appetite and food intake may be dysregulated in overweight children.

Indeed, there is evidence that genetic variation underlies differences in obesogenic eating behaviour traits *(54)*, which could explain why some children seem to gain more weight than others when exposed to the modern food environment. One study of Swedish parents and their children indicated that consumption of sweets and soft drinks was related to high scores on an external eating scale. If individual eating behaviour increases exposure to an obesogenic-type diet this may create a synergistic effect (55). However, data from ALSPAC exploring the interaction between DED at age 10 years and the FTO gene, which has been associated with eating behaviour in children (56), found independent effects, suggesting that eating behaviour and diet simply combine additively to increase the risk of obesity (30). This is an emerging area of research that deserves more attention in the future.

SUMMARY

Establishing the role of diet in the aetiology of obesity in children is fraught with methodological difficulties associated with self- or parent-reported measures of diet and reliance on indirect indicators of fat mass such as BMI. Many studies of the impact of nutrients like fat and fibre report mixed results; however, DED seems to be emerging as a strong risk factor. Single food groups tend to have a limited impact on weight gain. The most consistent evidence is for sugar-sweetened beverages, though the effect is small. The concept of dietary patterns combines the many small effects of various foods and nutrients and provides a more reliable assessment of long-term obesity risk. Ultimately excess weight gain is a consequence of surplus EI from any source. A balanced diet that combines many fruits, vegetables, high-fibre cereals, wholemeal breads, and low-fat meats and limits energy-dense snacks like chocolates, crisps, confectioneries, white bread, and processed meat is most likely to prevent excessive weight gain in children.

Meanwhile, research to develop new approaches to facilitate dietary change is urgently required. An increasing number of families are seeking to make healthier choices but are thwarted by the availability, accessibility, and marketing of less healthy options, often with economic incentives to encourage bulk purchases or supersizing. Changes in the wider food environment are a necessary component alongside individual decision-making to drive population-wide changes in dietary habits to favour weight control.

Editor's Comment and Question and Authors' Response

- **As noted here and in Chapter 1 by Popkin, the consumption of sugar-sweetened beverages by children has increased dramatically during the past generation. Indeed, simple elimination of sugary drinks can reduce body weight rapidly (though in many cases transiently) in some obese teenagers. Much concern has been raised about the pathogenic role of fructose, a major component of table sugar, high-fructose corn syrup, juice concentrates, and honey. Unlike glucose, fructose is taken up rapidly by the liver after GI absorption and appears to promote hepatic fat deposition and post-prandial hypertriglyceridaemia, particularly in insulin-resistant subjects. LDL cholesterol levels may also increase in normoinsulinaemic subjects (Schaefer et al., 2009). On the other hand, fructose raises insulin levels to a far lesser degree than glucose; moreover, central metabolism of fructose may promote food intake, while central metabolism of glucose suppresses feeding (Land and Cha, 2009).**

As you note, there is considerable controversy over the role of fructose in body fat deposition and weight gain. Some investigators using high levels of fructose feeding (25% of daily energy) show induction of visceral adiposity and insulin resistance (Stanhope et al., 2008). Others are not yet convinced (White, 2008) and argue, as you do, against focusing on single macronutrient in the battle against weight gain (Schaefer et al., 2009).

There is also much discussion about the roles of vitamins and micronutrients (vitamin D, carotenoids, magnesium, selenium, etc.) in obesity pathogenesis. What is your view?

- Some micronutrients may be associated with obesity risk but this is most likely explained by the kind of dietary pattern associated with obesity, which is energy dense, high in fat and low in fibre, and also coincidentally nutrient poor. There is no convincing mechanistic evidence that any associations between obesity and micronutrient intakes are causal.

Land MD, Cha SH. BBRC. 2009;382:1–5.
Schaefer EJ, et al. J Nutr. 2009;139:1257S–62S.
Stanhope KL, et al. Am J Clin Nutr. 2008;87:1194–203.
White JS. Am J Clin Nutr. 2008;88:1716S–21S.

REFERENCES

1. Torun B. Energy requirements of children and adolescents. Public Health Nutr. 2005;8(7A):968–93.
2. Birch LL, Fisher JO. Food intake regulation in children: fat and sugar substitutes and Intake. Ann N Y Acad Sci. 1997;819:194–220.
3. Birch LL, Deysher M. Caloric compensation and sensory specific satiety: evidence for self regulation of food intake by young children. Appetite. 1986;7:323–31.
4. Ogden CL, Carroll MD, Curtin LR, McDowell MA, Tabak CJ, Flegal KM. Prevalence of overweight and obesity in the United States, 1999–2004. J Am Med Assoc. 2006;295(13):1549–55.
5. Health Survey for England. HSE 2007 latest trends: children trend tables 2007. London: The Information Centre for Health and Social Care, IC. National Health Service, NHS; 2008.
6. Cecil JE, Palmer CN, Wrieden W, et al. Energy intakes of children after preloads: adjustment, not compensation. Am J Clin Nutr. 2005;82(2):302–08.
7. Johnson SL. Improving preschoolers' self-regulation of energy intake. Pediatrics. 2000;106(6):1429–35.
8. Griffiths LJ, Smeeth L, Hawkins SS, Cole TJ, Dezateux C. Effects of infant feeding practice on weight gain from birth to 3 years. Arch Dis Child. 2009;94:577–82.
9. Baker JL, Michaelsen KF, Rasmussen KM, Sorensen TIA. Maternal prepregnant body mass index, duration of breast-feeding, and timing of complementary food introduction are associated with infant weight gain. Am J Clin Nutr. 2004;80(6):1579–88.
10. Ong KK, Loos RJF. Rapid infancy weight gain and subsequent obesity: systematic reviews and hopeful suggestions. Acta Paediatr. 2006;95(8):904–08.
11. Bray GA, Popkin BM. Dietary fat intake does affect obesity! Am J Clin Nutr. Dec 1998;68(6):1157–73.
12. Willett WC, Leibel RL. Dietary fat is not a major determinant of body fat. Am J Med. 2002;113(Suppl 9B):47S–59S.
13. Prentice AM. Macronutrients as sources of food energy. Public Health Nutr. 2005;8(7a):932–39.
14. Rolland-Cachera MF, Deheeger M, Akrout M, Bellisle F. Influence of macronutrients on adiposity development: a follow-up study of nutrition and growth from 10 months to 8 years of age. Int J Obes. 1995;19:573–78.
15. Skinner JD, Bounds W, Carruth BR, Morris M, Ziegler P. Predictors of children's body mass index: a longitudinal study of diet and growth in children aged 2–8 y. Int J Obes. 2004;28(4):476–82.
16. Berkey CS, Rockett HRH, Field AE, et al. Activity, dietary intake, and weight changes in a longitudinal study of preadolescent and adolescent boys and girls. Pediatrics. 2000;105(4):E56.
17. Howarth NCMS, Saltzman EMD, Roberts SBPD. Dietary fiber and weight regulation. Nutr Rev. 2001;59(5):129–39.
18. Edwards CA, Parrett AM. Dietary fibre in infancy and childhood. Proc Nutr Soc. 2003;62(1):17–23.
19. Williams CL. Dietary fiber in childhood. J Pediatr. 2006;149(5 Suppl 1):S121–30.
20. Newby PK, Peterson KE, Berkey CS, Leppert J, Willett WC, Colditz GA. Dietary composition and weight change among low-income preschool children. Arch Pediatr Adolesc Med. 2003;157(8):759–64.
21. Buyken AE, Cheng G, Gunther ALB, Liese AD, Remer T, Karaolis-Danckert N. Relation of dietary glycemic index, glycemic load, added sugar intake, or fiber intake to the development of body composition between ages 2 and 7 y. Am J Clin Nutr. 2008;88(3):755–62.
22. Gidding SS, Dennison BA, Birch LL, et al. Dietary recommendations for children and adolescents: a guide for practitioners: consensus statement from the American Heart Association. Endorsed by the American Academy of Pediatrics. Circulation. 2005;112(13):2061–75.

23. Rolls BJ. The relationship between dietary energy density and energy intake. Physiol Behav. 14 Jul 2009;97(5):609–15. See also Fisher JO, Liu Y, Birch LL, Rolls BJ. Effects of portion size and energy density on young children's intake at a meal. Am J Clin Nutr 2007;86(1):174–79.

24. Leahy KE, Birch LL, Rolls BJ. Reducing the energy density of an entree decreases children's energy intake at lunch. J Am Diet Assoc. 2008;108(1):41–48.

25. Johnson L, Wilks DC, Lindroos AK, Jebb SA. Reflections from a systematic review of dietary energy density and weight gain: is the inclusion of drinks valid? Obes Rev. 2009;10:681–92.

26. Bell EA, Rolls BJ. Energy density of foods affects energy intake across multiple levels of fat content in lean and obese women. Am J Clin Nutr. 2001;73(6):1010–18.

27. Stubbs RJ, Ritz P, Coward WA, Prentice AM. Covert manipulation of the ratio of dietary fat to carbohydrate and energy density: effect on food intake and energy balance in free-living men eating ad libitum. Am J Clin Nutr. 1995;62(2): 330–37.

28. Drewnowski A, Almiron-Roig E, Marmonier C, Lluch A. Dietary energy density and body weight: is there a relationship? Nutr Rev. 2004;62(11):403–13.

29. Holland B, Welch AA, Unwin ID. McCance and Widdowson's the composition of foods. 5th ed. London: The Royal Society of Chemistry and MAFF; 1991.

30. Johnson L, van Jaarsveld CHM, Emmett PM, et al. Dietary energy density affects fat mass in early adolescence and is not modified by FTO variants. PLoS ONE. 2009;4(3):e4594.

31. Johnson L, Mander AP, Jones LR, Emmett PM, Jebb SA. A prospective analysis of dietary energy density at age 5 and 7 years and fatness at 9 years among UK children. Int J Obes. 2007;32(4):586–93.

32. McCaffrey TA, Rennie KL, Kerr MA, et al. Energy density of the diet and change in body fatness from childhood to adolescence; is there a relation? Am J Clin Nutr. 2008;87(5):1230–37.

33. DiMeglio DP, Mattes RD. Liquid versus solid carbohydrate: effects on food intake and body weight. Int J Obes. 2000;24(6):794–800.

34. Johnson SL, Birch LL. Parents' and children's adiposity and eating style. Pediatrics. 1994;94(5):653–61.

35. Gibson S. Sugar-sweetened soft drinks and obesity: a systematic review of the evidence from observational studies and interventions. Nutr Res Rev. 2008;21(02):134–47.

36. Vartanian LR, Schwartz MB, Brownell KD. Effects of soft drink consumption on nutrition and health: a systematic review and meta-analysis. Am J Public Health. 2007;97:667–75.

37. Forshee RA, Anderson PA, Storey ML. Sugar-sweetened beverages and body mass index in children and adolescents: a meta-analysis. Am J Clin Nutr. 2008;87(6):1662–71.

38. Phillips SM, Bandini LG, Naumova EN, et al. Energy-dense snack food intake in adolescence: longitudinal relationship to weight and fatness. Obes Res. 2004;12(3):461–72.

39. Johnson L, Mander AP, Jones LR, Emmett PM, Jebb SA. Is sugar-sweetened beverage consumption associated with increased fatness in children? Nutrition. 2007;23(7–8):557–63.

40. Cavadini C, Siega-Riz AM, Popkin BM. US adolescent food intake trends from 1965 to 1996. BMJ. 2000;83(1): 18–24.

41. Newby PK. Plant foods and plant-based diets: protective against childhood obesity? Am J Clin Nutr. May 2009;89(5):1572S–87S.

42. Faith MS, Dennison BA, Edmunds LS, Stratton HH. Fruit juice intake predicts increased adiposity gain in children from low-income families: weight status-by-environment interaction. Pediatrics. 2006;118(5):2066–75.

43. Field AE, Gillman MW, Rosner B, Rockett HR, Colditz GA. Association between fruit and vegetable intake and change in body mass index among a large sample of children and adolescents in the United States. Int J Obes. 2003;27(7): 821–26.

44. US Department of Agriculture USDA, US Department of Health and Human Services USHHS. Dietary Guidelines for Americans (http://www.health.gov/dietaryguidelines/dga2005/document/pdf/DGA2005.pdf): US Department of Agriculture and US Department of Health and Human Services; 2005 (Accessed 24/05/2009).

45. Johnson L, Mander AP, Jones LR, Emmett PM, Jebb SA. Energy-dense, low-fiber, high-fat dietary pattern is associated with increased fatness in childhood. Am J Clin Nutr. 2008;87(4):846–54.

46. Rolls BJ, Ello-Martin JA, Tohill BC. What can intervention studies tell us about the relationship between fruit and vegetable consumption and weight management? Nutr Rev. 2004;62(1):1–17.

47. Shin KO, Oh S-Y, Park HS. Empirically derived major dietary patterns and their associations with overweight in Korean preschool children. Br J Nutr. 2007;98:416–21.

48. Ritchie LD, Spector P, Stevens MJ, et al. Dietary patterns in adolescence are related to adiposity in young adulthood in black and white females. J Nutr. 2007;137(2):399–406.

49. Northstone K, Emmett PM. Are dietary patterns stable throughout early and mid-childhood? A birth cohort study. Br J Nutr. 2008;100:1069–76.

50. Reilly JJ, Armstrong J, Dorosty AR, et al. Early life risk factors for obesity in childhood: cohort study. BMJ. 2005;330:1357.

51. Carnell S, Wardle J. Measuring behavioural susceptibility to obesity: validation of the child eating behaviour questionnaire. Appetite. 2007;48(1):104–13.

52. Llewellyn C, Carnell S, Wardle J. Eating behaviour and weight in children. In: Moreno L, Pigeot I, Ahrens W (eds.). Epidemiology of obesity in children and adolescents – prevalence and aetiology. Vol 1. New York, NY: Springer; 2009.

53. Butte NF, Cai G, Cole SA, et al. Metabolic and behavioral predictors of weight gain in Hispanic children: the Viva la Familia Study. Am J Clin Nutr. 2007;85(6):1478–85.

54. Carnell S, Haworth CMA, Plomin R, Wardle J. Genetic influence on appetite in children. Int J Obes. 2008;32:1468–73.

55. Elfhag K, Tholin S, Rasmussen F. Consumption of fruit, vegetables, sweets and soft drinks are associated with psychological dimensions of eating behaviour in parents and their 12-year-old children. Public Health Nutr. 2008;11:914–23.

56. Wardle J, Carnell S, Haworth CM, Farooqi IS, O'Rahilly S, Plomin R. Obesity associated genetic variation in FTO is associated with diminished satiety. J Clin Endocrinol Metab. 2008;93(9):3640–43.

57. Johnson L. Dietary determinants of fat mass in children. Cambridge: MRC Human Nutrition Research, University of Cambridge; 2008.

11 Energy Expenditure in Children: The Role of *NEAT*

Lorraine Lanningham-Foster and James A. Levine

Contents

Key Words: Energy expenditure, metabolic rate, physical activity, exercise, school, neighborhood

INTRODUCTION: ENERGY EXPENDITURE

By the law of conservation of energy, body fat increases when energy intake is consistently greater than energy expenditure. Excess body fat and obesity are the result of sustained positive energy balance *(1)*. The pandemic of obesity has spread from the United States to Europe and is now emerging in middle- and even low-income countries *(2)*. In the United States, for example, since the 1970s the weight of the average person has increased by ~12 kg; importantly this trend affects all ages, races, and socio-economic groups *(3)*. Because of the health *(3,4)* and economic costs of obesity *(5)* the urgency to understand why humans are gaining weight has intensified.

It is accepted that nutritional quality is often poor *(6)*. However, there is controversy as to whether increased energy intake has accompanied the obesity epidemic. For example, in Britain, obesity rates have doubled since the 1980s yet energy intake appears to have decreased *(7)*. The NHANES surveys in the United States are difficult to interpret because the method used to examine energy intake changed

From: *Contemporary Endocrinology: Pediatric Obesity: Etiology, Pathogenesis, and Treatment*
Edited by: M. Freemark, DOI 10.1007/978-1-60327-874-4_11,
© Springer Science+Business Media, LLC 2010

between surveys *(8,9)*. In the absence of firm data that link increased dietary intake to obesity *(10)*, the role of energy expenditure in human energy balance has come under greater scrutiny.

Classically, there are three components of human daily energy expenditure (Fig. 1a): basal metabolic rate, the thermic effect of food, and activity thermogenesis. Basal metabolic rate is the energy required for core body functions and is measured at complete rest without food *(15,16)*. It accounts for about 60% of daily energy expenditure in a sedentary person. Nearly all of its variability (~80% of the variance) is accounted for by body size – or more precisely lean body mass; the bigger a person, the greater his/her basal metabolic rate *(17)*. The thermic effect of food (TEF) is the energy expended in response to a meal; it is the energy associated with digestion, absorption, and fuel storage *(17,18)*. The thermic effect of food accounts for about 10% of daily energy needs and does not vary greatly between people. The remaining component, activity thermogenesis, can be sub-divided into exercise and non-exercise activity thermogenesis (NEAT).

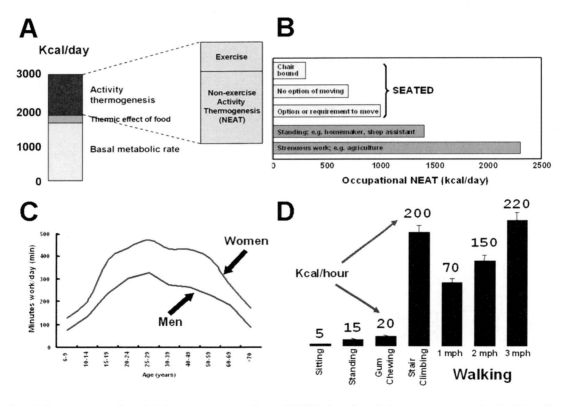

Fig. 1. (**a**) Components of total daily energy expenditure (TDEE) in a free-living sedentary adult. (**b**) The effect of occupational intensity on energy expenditure [data from *(11)*]. (**c**) Work burdens for women and men from the Ivory Coast versus age [from *(12,13)*]. (**d**) Energy expenditure above resting for a variety of activities [data from *(14)*].

Despite more limited information on energy expenditure in children compared to adults, there are some key differences between children and adults. Children have a higher basal metabolic rate compared to adults *(19–21)*. As children mature, there is a gradual decrease in energy expenditure with increasing age. The changes in energy expenditure appear to be related most closely to changes in body composition that occur around the time of puberty. There also appear to be hormonal influences such that there is a larger increase in fat-free mass in boys compared to girls. Energy requirements are thus increased, with the greatest increase for boys, at the start of puberty. Variation in energy expenditure has been explored in relationship to obesity in children. Although obese children spend less time engaged in physical activity, they do not have a reduced resting metabolic rate or thermic effect of food.

MEASUREMENT OF ENERGY EXPENDITURE AND NEAT

The measurement of energy expenditure associated with rest, activity, the utilization of food, and NEAT has been explained in-depth previously *(22,23)*. There are, however, many important considerations for performing these measurements in children compared to adults. General methods for measurement of energy expenditure are described here with emphasis on appropriate procedures used with children.

Basal Metabolic Rate and Resting Energy Expenditure

BMR should be measured in individuals who slept at the site of measurement overnight. For this reason it is generally not practical to routinely perform this measurement in young children. A more common approach would be to measure the energy expenditure associated with rest. Resting energy expenditure (REE) should be performed in the postprandial state, at least 6 h after consumption of any calories or performing any rigorous activity. For children, it is ideal to complete this measurement first thing in the morning after an overnight fast. Children should be fully rested while supine for 60 min prior to the measurement. A common technique is to allow the child to watch an age-appropriate video while resting.

The measurement should be performed with the child supine. A single pillow may support the child's head and/or the head of the bed should be at a 10° vertical tilt. The child should be in thermal comfort and the room should not be brightly lit. Children should be encouraged to lie motionless and should not be allowed to talk. The age of the child may impair their ability to remain motionless for long periods and researchers often develop creative approaches to encouraging appropriate behavior. For example, a simple technique of giving a child a laboratory timer so that they know how much time they have to lie still may be helpful. The measurement period should last for 20 min.

Thermic Effect of Food

Measurement of the thermic effect of food is also challenging in younger children. However, the measurement may be more ideal in school-age children, ideally at the age of 10 and above. Optimally, a measurement of resting energy expenditure should be performed first, then the child is provided a meal. The energy content of the food should be known precisely and should be 400 kcal or greater. Providing the child with food that they prefer to eat is critical. Parent involvement with food choices is preferred over allowing the child to select the foods. Energy expenditure should then be measured for 360 min or until energy expenditure falls to within 5% of the resting energy expenditure. For those using hood-based systems (with response time 2 min), energy expenditure can be measured every 15 min out of 30 min to avoid subject agitation. The thermic effect of food is calculated from the area under curve describing the energy expenditure above resting energy expenditure (EE-REE) versus time. Some would argue that it is of value to also measure the thermic effect of non-caloric meals.

Energy Expenditure of Physical Activities

Points of reference are important. Resting energy expenditure should be measured first, and then the energy expenditure of the posture of reference should be measured while the child is motionless. For example, for measuring the energy expenditure of desk work at school, sitting energy expenditure should be measured as the point of reference. For measuring the energy expenditure of standing in the school play yard, standing energy expenditure should be measured as the point of reference. A creative approach may be required: standing or sitting motionless is not the natural mode of activity.

Distraction is a common technique; children are frequently allowed to watch age-appropriate videos during measurement of activity energy expenditure. Measurement of energy expenditure during the performance of the activity of interest should be performed for 10–15 min if the calorimeter has a response time of 2 min. Where calorimeter response times are longer, the measurement period needs to be prolonged so that steady-state energy expenditure is reached. However, in working with children it is ideal to use equipment with lower response times to minimize the length of the measurement period. The energy expenditure for the activity can be calculated as the steady-state energy expenditure for that activity minus (or divided by) either the energy expenditure of the posture of reference or the resting energy expenditure.

Defining Exercise and NEAT

Exercise is defined as "bodily exertion for the sake of developing and maintaining physical fitness," for example, sport or visiting the gym *(24)*. The vast majority of world-dwellers do not participate in exercise as so defined, and for them, exercise activity thermogenesis is zero. Importantly too, the vast majority of "exercisers" participate in exercise for less than 2 h/week and for them, exercise accounts for an average energy expenditure of less than 100 kcal/day. *Given that most children do not participate in organized sport activity (see below), their energy expenditure from exercise (as defined above) per se is low.*

NEAT is the energy expenditure of all physical activities other than volitional sporting-like exercise. NEAT includes all those activities that render us vibrant, unique, and independent beings such as dancing, going to work or school, shoveling snow, playing the guitar, swimming, or walking in the modern mall. NEAT is expended every day and can most easily be classified as NEAT associated with occupation and NEAT associated with leisure. In children, the concept of NEAT may be slightly different compared to adults as children more commonly engage in NEAT associated with leisurely play. A child's frequent participation in bouts of activity is important for proper development; this is true not only in humans, but across several species. School-age children confined to the limitations of their environments are likely to engage in NEAT associated with leisure and NEAT associated with school. *Indeed, for most children, the total energy expenditure associated with NEAT exceeds greatly the energy expenditure associated with volitional sport-like exercise (see Energy Equivalents of Daily Activity in the Appendix).*

NEAT Energy Expenditure

NEAT is commonly measured by one of two approaches. The first is to measure or estimate total NEAT. Here, total daily energy expenditure is measured using techniques such as the doubly labeled water method *(25–27)* or gas and/or heat exchange (room calorimetry) and from it Resting Energy Expenditure + Thermic Effect of Food + Exercise Activity Thermogenesis (EAT) is subtracted [TOTAL NEAT = TEE − (REE+TEF+EAT)]. The second approach is the factorial approach whereby the components of NEAT are quantified and total NEAT calculated by summing these components. This approach is frequently used for estimating NEAT in free-living children. First, a child's physical activities are recorded over the time period of interest (e.g., 7 days), for example, using accelerometry *(28)*. The energy equivalent of each of these activities is determined. The time spent in each activity is then multiplied by the energy equivalent for that activity. These values are then summed to derive an estimate of NEAT. The advantage of this approach is that the components of NEAT can be defined. This final point is critical because the components of NEAT in children and adults are likely different and customization based on the individual's activity patterns is beneficial in more accurately determining NEAT.

NEAT VARIABILITY

Daily energy expenditure varies substantially *(11)*. In fact highly active adults expend three times more energy per day than inactive adults *(11)* and this marked variability in daily energy expenditure is even greater when data from non-industrialized countries are considered *(29,12)*. Overall, for two adults *of similar size*, daily energy expenditure varies by as much as 2,000 calories per day. As noted above, basal metabolic rate is largely accounted for by body size and the thermic effect of food is small. Thus, activity thermogenesis must vary by as much as 2,000 calories per day. Given that volitional exercise makes only a minor contribution to activity thermogenesis in most people, this wide variation in daily activity thermogenesis must be explained by NEAT.

In adults, occupation is a key determinant of NEAT. For someone of average age, sex, and weight, occupational NEAT varies as shown in Fig. 1b. If an average person were to go and work in agriculture, their NEAT could theoretically increase by 1,500 kcal/day *(12)*.

Understanding the role of occupation on NEAT is far from straightforward, however, because occupation-related NEAT is overlaid simultaneously by societal *and* biological drives. In Fig. 1c the occupational NEAT of more than 5,000 dwellers from agricultural regions of the Ivory Coast is shown. Each individual was followed for 7 days by a trained enumerator and all their daily tasks were recorded using one of 200 numeric codes. First, the societal effect of sex on work burdens can be seen; women work more than men. In these societies, the societal construct is that women conduct all (>95%) of domestic tasks and about a third of agricultural tasks. Men work exclusively in agriculture and have greater leisure time than women *(12)*. Second, these data demonstrate the interaction of ageing on work participation, noting that this population is unfettered by retirement policy. As ageing occurs, occupational NEAT declines (Fig. 1c) *(13)*. Across all species that have been studied, non-exercise activity levels decline with ageing *(30)*. These data thereby depict the interplay of both society and biology. Other studies *(11)* and these suggest that occupation is the major predictor of NEAT in adults; active work can expend 1,500 kcal/day more than a sedentary job *(29,12)*.

Variability in leisure *(31)* also accounts for substantial variability in NEAT. The energy expended in several activities is shown in Fig. 1d *(14)*. Consider that a child returns home from school by parent car at 4 pm. From then until bedtime at 9 pm the primary activity may be to operate the television remote control or video game control in a semi-recumbent position. For these 5 h, the average energy expenditure above resting would approximate 8% and the NEAT will thus approximate 25 kcal for the evening (0.08 × 1,500 BMR × (5/24) h). Now imagine he/she becomes aware of the soccer tryouts after school, the neighborhood park, and the possibility of walking to school. The child then decides to undertake these tasks. The increase in energy expenditure would be equivalent to walking approximately 1–2 mph for the same period of leisure time (4–9 pm). NEAT then increases to 625–935 kcal for the evening (2 or 3 × 1,500 BMR × (5/24) h). Thus, for this hypothetical child, the variance in leisure time NEAT has the potential of impacting energy expenditure by almost 1,000 kcal/day. Thus leisure activities range from almost complete rest to those that are highly energized. Since NEAT can vary dramatically among individuals, could NEAT be important in weight gain?

NEAT IN WEIGHT GAIN AND OBESITY

In humans, the manipulation of energy balance is associated with changes in NEAT. In one study *(32)*, 12 pairs of twins were overfed by 1,000 kcal/day. There was a fourfold variation in weight gain, which by definition must have reflected substantial variance in energy expenditure. Since the changes in energy expenditure were not accounted for by changes in basal metabolic rate or sport-like exercise, changes in NEAT were implicated indirectly. Interestingly, twinness accounted for a substantial minority of the inter-individual variance in weight gain, suggesting that NEAT is under both environmental and biological/genetic influences. When positive energy balance is imposed through overfeeding, NEAT increases *(33,34)*. Moreover, the change in NEAT is predictive of fat gain *(35)*. Those who with overfeeding increase their NEAT the most gain the least fat (Fig. 2a). Those who with overfeeding do not increase their NEAT gain the most fat. Therefore, NEAT is fundamentally important in human fat gain.

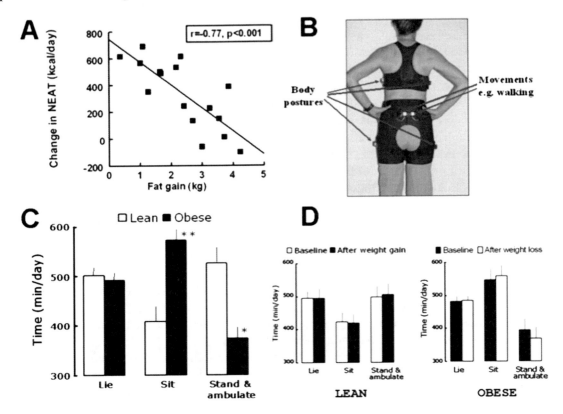

Fig. 2. (**a**) Fat gain versus changes in NEAT with 8 weeks of overfeeding by 1,000 kcal/day in 16 lean, sedentary volunteers *(35)*. (**b**) Posture and activity sensing undergarments *(36)*. (**c**) Time allocation for components of NEAT in 10 sedentary lean and 10 obese individuals during weight maintenance feeding *(36)*. (**d**) Time allocation for components of NEAT in lean subjects before and after weight gain and obese subjects before and after weight loss *(36)*.

If people who fail to increase NEAT with overfeeding gain excess body fat, could there be a NEAT deficit in obesity? To examine this question, we integrated micro-sensors into undergarments (Fig. 2b). These sensors allowed body postures and movements, especially walking, to be quantified every half second for 10 days. The data (Fig. 2c) demonstrated that obese subjects were seated for 2½ h/day more than lean subjects. The lean sedentary volunteers stood and walked more than 2 h/day longer than obese subjects. Importantly the lean subjects lived in a similar environment and had similar jobs compared to the obese subjects. Because all the components of energy expenditure were measured it could be calculated that if the obese subjects were to adopt the same NEAT-o-type as the lean subjects, they might expend an additional 350 calories/day. Thus NEAT and specifically walking are of substantial energetic importance in obesity. Lean individuals exploit opportunities to walk, where the obese find opportunities to sit.

We have also quantified differences in daily standing/walking times between normal weight and overweight children. These initial studies indicate that normal weight children stand for longer periods of time each day compared to overweight children; however, the difference is slightly less (90 min compared to 2 h) than that in adults. The significance of this lower difference in standing/walking time in children compared to adults needs to be explored, despite the complexity of performing such evaluations. Our findings suggest that there are developmental influences on NEAT across the life span and that these influences are different in lean compared to obese individuals.

It might seem obvious that because people with obesity are heavier, they sit more than lean people. However, these differences do not reflect greater body weight alone. When lean adult subjects gained weight through overfeeding, their tendency to stand/ambulate persisted (Fig. 2d). When obese subjects became lighter, their tendency to sit did not change (Fig. 2b).

Thus, obesity is associated with a NEAT defect that predisposes obese people to sit *(37)*. Lean people have an innate tendency to stand and walk. These findings appear to be true in children as well as adults.

NEAT CHILDREN

Obesity prevalence among children is at the highest levels measured; presently 15% of US boys and girls aged 6–11 years are overweight *(38)*. Obesity among children has increased more rapidly in the last 30 years and this is now occurring worldwide. The situation, however, is projected to get far worse because there are now three times more obese children than there were two decades ago *(39–41)*. Childhood obesity is a global epidemic with unheralded health consequences *(42,43)*. These rising obesity rates have been, in part, blamed upon increasing sedentariness *(44–47)*. Sitting in front of a television, video game, or computer screen has been consistently associated with low levels of physical activity *(47)*. Weekly screen time in children is as high as 55 h/week *(48)* and the average home in the United States has a television on for 8 h/day *(49)*. Although many programs have attempted to separate children from the screen, these activities are highly valued and children are resistant to giving them up *(50)*. There is therefore an urgent need to devise approaches that render children active; the school is the obvious place to start.

As to why physical activity became drained from school is uniformly explained by a decrease in the prioritization of physical activity relative to other learning objectives on the school calendar. This occurred concomitantly with decreased fiscal allocation of resources for physical activity. This is equally true in the Unites States, European countries, China, North Korea, and Australia. Interestingly, facilities for physical activity (e.g., gym, playground, or field) are often present and qualified teachers are available (albeit often few in numbers). However, even elementary schools do not have daily programmed activity; middle schools rarely have compulsory daily activity and most children report that they do not get regular physical activity. In high schools the story is even worse, at least in the United States; here many schools offer physical education as a one semester optional course to meet a minimal state requirement for physical education. Most children do not participate in physical activity most days of the week.

Of course, school systems cannot shoulder the blame for childhood obesity, but schools used to compel daily activity and school is where our children spend most of their weekdays. Furthermore children used to walk or ride their bikes to school, whereas now they invariably ride on a bus or in a car. It only takes a moment of thought to realize that educational standards are irrelevant if children grow up entrained to be sedentary and unhealthy.

It is imperative for both health and fiscal reasons that effective childhood obesity prevention and intervention programs be developed immediately. Previous approaches to reverse low levels of physical activity in children have generally focused on impacting the behaviors that children and their parents engage in at school and/or at home. However, these approaches in general vary in success and overall have failed. Rather than trying to impact behavior one wonders whether a redesigned physical infrastructure could impact how children behave.

Despite efforts to promote NEAT and activity within the boundaries of the traditional school system, there is a growing realization that these efforts have failed and are likely to continue to do so. That being understood, focus is intensifying as to whether school infrastructure and operational systems can be altered to promote NEAT and daily activity and reverse obesity. By examining this question under the headings of (a) the student, (b) the classroom, (c) the school, and (d) the environment external to school, the conclusion is drawn that a multifaceted approach can be readily applied to effectively change the nature of school from chair imprisoned to NEAT enhanced.

NEAT SCHOOL

There are four aspects one needs to consider when redesigning the school to promote health. The first is the individual. The second is their immediate space – the classroom. The third is the general space – the school itself. The fourth is the external space – the out-of-school environment. Let us consider these one by one.

THE INDIVIDUAL

The individual space of a pupil can most easily be summarized as a desk–chair space or more pejoratively a "desk sentence." Even from pre-school, students are conditioned to be desk-bound. The focus on educational discipline for centuries has been to maintain children at their desks. This enables a teacher to organize a group of individuals whose natural tendency is to move.

An important question is why we should contemplate changing desk-based learning when this learning approach preceded the obesity epidemic. This argument ignores three issues. The first is that desk-based learning evolved at the time when children would invariably walk to school and be active in their leisure time. For example, many children had documented walk times of more than 4 h/day in their commute to school prior to 1900. The second issue is the assumption that children learn best while seated; the Socratic Peripatetic School in ancient Athens invoked ambulation as the standard form of learning and a multitude of scholars have worked standing or in motion; Einstein was said to solve the riddle of relativity while riding his bicycle. The third issue is that it is an assumption that children learn best while seated; the evidence for this is absent. There is no education compulsion for children to learn while seated at a desk. In fact our studies indicate that if you give a child a chance to move, they will do so and will learn better. If the notion of a 'student sitting at a desk' is dispelled, enormous educational possibilities result.

Examples of NEAT Solutions

1. It is possible for students to use lightweight podium desks that are height adjusted. This enables a student to sit or stand as she wishes and also to define her work space as she chooses; desks can be moved to where the student wishes to learn.
2. A student can use aluminum lightweight portable personalized white boards that she can move to her chosen workspace. This enables a teacher (in motion too) to write personally for a student and for a student to write on a board in response.
3. Mobile technologies can be applied. A student using a wireless Ethernet-connected portable computer can gain and deliver knowledge anywhere in the school system. The weight of a portable laptop computer is often less than standard book bags *(51)*. The technologies allow a student and teacher to communicate privately and at distance. Other mobile technologies (e.g., mobile audio devices) enable a student to receive educational materials while in motion (e.g., audio materials heard while walking or spelling words practiced while playing basketball).
4. Personalized health-sensing technologies can be worn by students. Students already oftentimes wear identity cards. Similarly, students' NEAT and cafeteria food choices can be logged on a portable device

and fed back to students to provide them with information and feedback. For example, a student who meets his activity goal for the week could be rewarded and a student who eats pizza everyday for a week could be sent "an eat cool" advisory.

THE CLASSROOM

Once the chairs and desks have been removed from a traditional classroom, it looks very different (Fig. 3). In fact, the role of the space itself comes under question. The Merriam-Webster definition of a classroom is "a space where a body of students meeting regularly to study the same subject" *(24)*. As soon as the desks and chairs are dispensed with, we can consider changes in classroom setting. For example, Can park land function as a classroom (San Francisco has city-wide wireless Internet and so educational materials could be accessed at any time from anywhere in the city)? Can a walking track be a classroom? Once desk and chairs are no longer needed the answers to these two questions could be "yes."

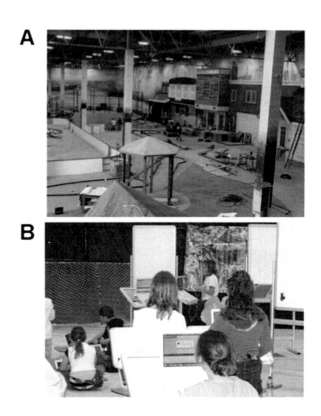

Fig. 3. A sample, NEAT-promoting school of the future.

Examples of NEAT Solutions

1. *Open-format classrooms.* An open-format classroom is a traditional classroom space from which the desks and tables have been removed. An open-format classroom has several advantages over the traditional desk–chair approach. First students can define their own space and their own groupings; some students like to work collaboratively, whereas other students do not. Second, a teacher can direct students within the space so that different educational objectives can be mirrored by different physical layouts. Third, different technologies (such as those described above) can be introduced but only as

needed. For example, in a mathematics lesson, a teacher may want to teach students from a white board (wall mounted) at the front of the classroom and so laptop computers would not be used inside the room. Alternatively, a teacher may want to teach biology using video clips from a local hospital's operating room, and here students would need to have their laptop video-cams linked to the hospital.

2. *Un-roomed classrooms.* The theme of mobility can take students out of the traditional four-walled classroom (noting the definition of a "classroom" above). The "classroom" can become a gymnasium, a park, or a walking track. This approach has several advantages as well as drawbacks. A major advantage is that a four-walled space is not needed, so this frees up traditional school classroom "real estate." A consequence of this could be that fewer classrooms are needed for a given school. Also, the un-roomed classroom creates novel educational paradigms; for example, virtual classrooms can evolve to bring geographically separated students under one educational environment and educators with unique skills to students who would not otherwise benefit. Moving-wall systems can be used to "create" classrooms ad hoc in undefined space as the need arises.

Drawbacks that educators report are the issues of acoustics and behavioral issues. Acoustics in free-living space is difficult for three reasons: (a) noise transition from source to listener. This can be helped using high-quality mobile transmission systems; (b) the effect of extraneous noise such as traffic. Theoretically this is helped (but only to a degree) using noise-cancelling technology; and (c) multi-person communication. Even though traditional teaching is from teacher to students [see (a)], an important part of the educational experience is the vocal interchange between students; this can be challenging even with advanced mobile, acoustic systems. The second drawback of wall-less learning can broadly be defined as "behavioral issues." This does not necessarily refer to issue of disciplinary control but rather to the nature of group-dynamics *(52)*. There is a general belief that education benefits from the process of group-dynamics and this can potentially be stultified by learning either while in motion (e.g., on a walking track) or with virtual learning environments. Although this is intuitively true, evidence is lacking.

THE SCHOOL

When considering how the school itself (Fig. 3) can contribute to NEAT-enhanced active learning, two broad categories need to be considered: the first is organizational infrastructure and the second is physical infrastructure. At an organizational level there are several important areas. For example, Are policies in place that promote NEAT and physical activity throughout the school day? Does lesson organization permit or enhance NEAT? Does recess allocation and organization permit and promote physical activity? Does the school week allocate time to physical activity?

Have safety and legal issues been anticipated?

What is important to appreciate is that organizational issues are often inexpensive or even cost-neutral.

With respect to physical infrastructure, there are also several considerations. For example, Is there adequate space to promote daylong physical activity? Are the resources available to recreate, redesign, and retool classrooms to promote activity? Is the physical infrastructure used wisely to promote daylong physical activity? Are new schools NEAT-compliant?

Possible NEAT Solutions

Let us examine NEAT solutions for an entire school first from an organizational perspective and then with respect to physical infrastructure.

1. *Leadership.* The role of school leadership in promoting daylong physical activity and NEAT cannot be understated. The school principal needs to *drive* the initiative for NEAT-enhanced active schooling. Leadership invariably, however, needs to emanate from beyond the individual school itself; there needs

to be support from regional and even national school authorities (see below). Within the school, there must be support beyond the principal, including teachers, janitors, kitchen staff, mechanics, and grounds staff.

2. *Lesson organization to promote NEAT.* There are obvious examples of how important lesson organization can be. For example, say a biology teacher wishes to teach her biology class at a local nature reserve; those lessons will need to be scheduled to enable the students to arrive on site in a timely fashion. More radical approaches can be contemplated; for example, several sports- and arts-orientated schools schedule all formal education in the morning to enable students to ski or learn ballet in the afternoon; these students generally exceed educational standards. One could therefore envisage a health-promotion school with the same educational organization, where half the day is allocated to healthy pursuits. On a more subtle level, lessons can be organized in such a way as to maximize the distance between the classrooms so that students have to walk the greatest possible distance between lessons. NEAT-based scheduling has tremendous potential power to increase daytime NEAT.

3. *Recess.* In North American schools recess has contracted to the point where oftentimes it serves only to enable children to eat and use bathrooms. Recreational time during the day is diminishing. This also in part reflects the pressures that many educational systems impose with respect to meeting educational goals. Increasing recess-associated physical activity necessitates that recess time is available to students but also that the time is used efficiently.

4. *Allocating time in the school week for physical activity.* The obvious opportunity here is to reverse the astonishing decline in compulsory physical education that has occurred in many high-income countries. What should the goal be? The NEAT deficit in children is about 90 min/day. The notion that all children should be active in school for three 30-min sessions per day seems excessive. However, consider a school in North Dakota that engages all children in 30-min walks at the beginning of the school day, after lunch, and at the end of the school day. The walking segments at the beginning and end of the school day are supervised through a volunteer program and the school bus system is not unduly inconvenienced. In this model, school education time is unaffected. More subtle approaches can also be used; for example, specific school corridors can be pre-allocated for specific classes so that lesson-time walking is encouraged.

5. Recognizing non-traditional activities as being health positive is simply a state of mind. Most children do not engage in formal sports. There is a need to encourage children to pursue activities that they enjoy and that *foster lifelong participation*. Examples include skate-boarding, using rollerblades, dancing, yoga, and talking to friends on the phone while walking. Emphasizing the pleasure of participating over "winning" is often important too.

6. Contrary to expectations, it is not complicated to devise legal waivers for most activities at school; this should not be seen as a barrier to promoting daylong, enjoyable, and healthy activities at school.

NEAT solutions for an entire school also involve infrastructural considerations.

1. *Adequate space.* A common misconception is that a school needs to be completely rebuilt to render it activity promoting. Oftentimes reallocating preexisting resources and space can create a physical infrastructure to promote NEAT and activity. For example, an old disused play area can be converted into an engaging climbing play ground that invites and stimulates activity. Disused concrete areas can be rebuilt into skateboard parks. An unused wall can become a climbing wall. Parts of walkways can be designated for roller-blade use. Cycle paths can be designated and even mountain bike trails designed. Walks between school areas can be made more engaging using culture and art projects. Unused open spaces can be used as an arena to encourage music and outdoors dancing. Careful review of existing spaces can yield remarkable results at little cost. Safety issues, however, must be considered.

2. Resource availability is often cited as the key limiting factor for promoting school-based physical activity. This chapter, however, argues strongly against this. Nonetheless, increasing the resources available to a school can help promote physical activity. Such resources can range from small amounts of

money to purchase equipment such as carts containing recess equipment through major grants to convert schools into health-promoting environments. Fund raising from the student body, school districts, funding agencies, and industry are all potential sources of funding. None should be overlooked.

3. The efficient use of physical infrastructure is important for promoting daylong activity. If a school elects to build a skateboard park in its concrete area, will this wonderful area be used for only 1 h a day? Could recess times be staggered to give more children more opportunities? Could sports facilities (e.g., gymnasiums) that are normally closed on weekends be opened (often using community volunteers) to enable children to play in out-of-school hours and weekends? Conversely, could community facilities such as swimming pools be better shared with schools that do not have such opportunities? The efficient use of existing resources can oftentimes triple their use.

4. Building new schools. New schools are built in every major populous center every year. Without rebuilding existing schools, it is self-evident to build new schools from the "bottom-up" (Wifi to bike track) to be NEAT and activity promoting.

THE OUT-OF-SCHOOL ENVIRONMENT

Understanding the role of the school day in promoting a child's physical activity cannot ignore the role of the external world on the school and vice versa.

Possible NEAT Solutions

The external world affects how a school functions in many ways. Governmental and regional policies, for example, can create mandates to promote physical activity and health. Resource allocations for children engaged in these programs can be diverted from health promotion budgets rather than school ones. Play areas for out-of-school activities can be rendered safe through police allocation; similarly children can be encouraged to walk or cycle to school assuming city planners recognize the need for walkways and safe cycle paths that override busy streets. In the same way that school-based solutions for obesity may exploit environmental re-engineering, so too can compatible programs be derived for adult workplaces.

What is often overlooked is how a school can interface with its external environment. This occurs in two ways. First, a program delivered to children can be complemented by a program delivered to their families. There is widespread potential to use the school premises (and infrastructure) to achieve this goal as well. In so doing, broad-based partnerships between schools and the communities they serve can be strengthened. The second element is even more important. Obese children are likely to become obese adults. What happens in school today affects the nation tomorrow. If children leave the school systems profoundly unhealthy, they are likely to remain this way for life. On the other hand, an education that provides an approach to lifelong activity and fun could be one of the most valuable educational elements a child takes away from the NEAT-enhanced school of tomorrow.

CONCLUSION

It is recognized that the primary goal of school is to educate children. Since the inception of modern schooling, this mandate has been understood to represent the obligation to provide broad-based education that serves a student lifelong. Examples include the commonplace inclusion of sex education in the curriculum plus the presence of broadening experiences such as drama. It has long been understood that the role of school extends beyond trigonometry and Shakespeare. There is also a universal recognition that childhood obesity is rising unabated at catastrophic rates. Since most children in developed countries attend school, our schools are an obvious place to consider obesity intervention and prevention.

Over the last few decades, the emphasis in the sciences was on changes in nutritional quality being the principal driver in the obesity epidemic. However, the emphasis has shifted over the last 5 years toward the belief that energy expenditure, in particular NEAT, is at the crux of the obesity epidemic.

Exercise is associated with considerable health benefit including diminished rates of diabetes, heart disease, and possibly cancer and is associated with prolongation of life span *(53)*; the converse appears to be true for inactivity *(54)*. If so, increasing NEAT might confer health benefit and longer life.

ACKNOWLEDGMENTS

Sources of support: Supported by grants DK56650, DK63226, DK66270, DK50456 (Minnesota Obesity Center), HD52001, and RR-0585 from the US Public Health Service and by the Mayo Foundation and by a grant to the Mayo Foundation.

Editor's Comments and Question and Authors' Response

- **We face an educational crisis in the United States, with high school dropout rates approximating 35–40% in major urban centers. Measures of educational achievement appear to have declined at the population level, and a significant percentage of children are under pharmacotherapy for behavior control. Thus educators MUST seek new approaches to improve school satisfaction and performance.**

  "Open" schools and classrooms have been implemented successfully in some locales when supported strongly by parents, teachers, administrators, and the community. On the other hand, open classrooms have been criticized for their failure to provide "structure" for children from chaotic home situations and for those with attention deficit disorders and other learning disabilities. Some teachers find it difficult or impossible to maintain a stable, tranquil, effective, and safe learning environment in the open classroom setting.

  Would an expanded traditional school day that includes three 30-min periods of vigorous non-competitive play accomplish the NEAT goals that you seek to achieve, if combined with (a) limits on "screen time" at home and (b) government policies and a built environment that promote walking to and from school?

- An alternative to open classrooms, which in many school districts are untenable, is to modulate the school day within the preexisting infrastructure. Examples include (a) "walk-to-school" programs, (b) evening use of school gyms for urban sports activities, (c) changing unused concrete areas to skateboard parks, (d) mandating certain classes to be walking based, or (e) "top-and-tail" programs where the first and last 30 min of the school day are active. It is clear, however, whatever options are selected, that school leadership is critical. Also, such activities need to be integrated across the school workforce (e.g., a school walking program without support from the janitorial staff is likely to fail). Government actions are viewed often as intrusive. However, in October of 2009 the Australian Government recommended the ban of all screen time for under-2's and a 1-h limit for 2–5-year olds; these recommendations are likely to be implemented across all state-supported entities such as day care centers.

REFERENCES

1. Levine JA. Nonexercise activity thermogenesis–liberating the life-force. J Intern Med. 2007;262:273–87.
2. World Health Organization. Obesity: preventing and managing the global epidemic. Geneva: World Health Organization; 1997.
3. Fontaine KR, Redden DT, Wang C, Westfall AO, Allison DB. Years of life lost due to obesity. J Am Med Assoc. 2003;289:187–93.
4. http://www.cdc.gov/nchs/data/ad/ad347.pdf
5. Finkelstein E, Fiebelkorn C, Wang G. The costs of obesity among full-time employees. Am J Health Promot. 2005;20:45–51.
6. Seidell JC. Prevention of obesity: the role of the food industry. Nutr Metab Cardiovasc Dis. 1999;9:45–50.
7. Prentice AM, Jebb SA. Obesity in Britain: gluttony or sloth? BMJ. 1995;311:437–39.
8. Kant AK, Graubard BI. Secular trends in patterns of self-reported food consumption of adult Americans: NHANES 1971–1975 to NHANES 1999–2002. Am J Clin Nutr. 2006;84:1215–23.
9. http://archive.nlm.nih.gov/proj/dxpnet/nhanes/docs/nhanesDocs.php
10. Lanningham-Foster L, Nysse LJ, Levine JA. Labor saved, calories lost: the energetic impact of domestic labor-saving devices. Obes Res. 2003;11:1178–81.
11. Black AE, Coward WA, Cole TJ, Prentice AM. Human energy expenditure in affluent societies: an analysis of 574 doubly-labelled water measurements. Eur J Clin Nutr. 1996;50:72–92.
12. Levine JA, Weisell R, Chevassus S, Martinez CD, Burlingame B, Coward WA. The work burden of women. Science. 2001;294:812.
13. Levine J, Heet J, Burlingame B. Aging on the job. Sci Aging Knowledge Environ. 2006;2006:pe16.
14. Levine JA, Schleusner SJ, Jensen MD. Energy expenditure of nonexercise activity. Am J Clin Nutr. 2000;72: 1451–54.
15. Daan S, Masman D, Strijkstra A, Verhulst S. Intraspecific allometry of basal metabolic rate: relations with body size, temperature, composition, and circadian phase in the kestrel, Falco tinnunculus. J Biol Rhythms. 1989;4:267–83.
16. Ford LE. Some consequences of body size. Am J Physiol. 1984;247:H495–507.
17. Donahoo WT, Levine JA, Melanson EL. Variability in energy expenditure and its components. Curr Opin Clin Nutr Metab Care. 2004;7:599–605.
18. Hill JO, DiGirolamo M, Heymsfield SB. Thermic effect of food after ingested versus tube-delivered meals. Am J Physiol. 1985;248:E370–4.
19. Bitar A, Vermorel M, Fellmann N, Coudert J. Twenty-four-hour energy expenditure and its components in prepubertal children as determined by whole-body indirect calorimetry and compared with young adults. Am J Clin Nutr. 1995;62:308–15.
20. Bitar A, Vernet J, Coudert J, Vermorel M. Longitudinal changes in body composition, physical capacities and energy expenditure in boys and girls during the onset of puberty. Eur J Nutr. 2000;39:157–63.
21. Molnar D, Schutz Y. The effect of obesity, age, puberty and gender on resting metabolic rate in children and adolescents. Eur J Pediatr. 1997;156:376–81.
22. Levine JA. Non-exercise activity thermogenesis (NEAT). Nutr Rev. 2004;62:S82–97.
23. Levine JA. Measurement of energy expenditure. Public Health Nutr. 2005;8:1123–32.
24. Merriam-Webster Collegiate Dictionary. 11th ed. Springfield, MA: Merriam-Webster Inc.; 2003.
25. Coward WA. Stable isotopic methods for measuring energy expenditure. The doubly-labelled-water (2H2(18)O) method: principles and practice. Proc Nutr Soc. 1988;47:209–18.
26. Coward WA, Roberts SB, Cole TJ. Theoretical and practical considerations in the doubly-labelled water (2H2(18)O) method for the measurement of carbon dioxide production rate in man. Eur J Clin Nutr. 1988;42:207–12.
27. Hoos MB, Plasqui G, Gerver WJ, Westerterp KR. Physical activity level measured by doubly labeled water and accelerometry in children. Eur J Appl Physiol. 2003;89:624–26. Epub 2003 Jul 9.
28. Lanningham-Foster LM, Jensen TB, McCrady SK, Nysse LJ, Foster RC, Levine JA. Laboratory measurement of posture allocation and physical activity in children. Med Sci Sports Exerc. 2005;37:1800–5.
29. Coward WA. Contributions of the doubly labeled water method to studies of energy balance in the Third World. Am J Clin Nutr. 1998;68:962S–9S.
30. Westerterp KR. Daily physical activity and ageing. Curr Opin Clin Nutr Metab Care. 2000;3:485–88.
31. Prentice AM, Leavesley K, Murgatroyd PR, et al. Is severe wasting in elderly mental patients caused by an excessive energy requirement? Age Ageing. 1989;18:158–67.
32. Bouchard C, Tremblay A, Despres JP, et al. The response to long-term overfeeding in identical twins. N Engl J Med. 1990;322:1477–82.
33. Klein S, Goran M. Energy metabolism in response to overfeeding in young adult men. Metabolism. 1993;42:1201–5.

34. Diaz EO, Prentice AM, Goldberg GR, Murgatroyd PR, Coward WA. Metabolic response to experimental overfeeding in lean and overweight healthy volunteers. Am J Clin Nutr. 1992;56:641–55.
35. Levine JA, Eberhardt NL, Jensen MD. Role of nonexercise activity thermogenesis in resistance to fat gain in humans. Science. 1999;283:212–14.
36. Levine JA, Lanningham-Foster LM, McCrady SK, et al. Interindividual variation in posture allocation: possible role in human obesity. Science. 2005;307:584–86.
37. Tryon WW, Goldberg JL, Morrison DF. Activity decreases as percentage overweight increases. Int J Obes Relat Metab Disord. 1992;16:591–95.
38. Marsh HW, Hau KT, Sung RY, Yu CW. Childhood obesity, gender, actual-ideal body image discrepancies, and physical self-concept in Hong Kong children: cultural differences in the value of moderation. Dev Psychol. 2007;43:647–62.
39. Ogden CL, Fryar CD, Carroll MD, Flegal KM. Mean body weight, height, and body mass index, United States 1960–2002. Advance data from vital and health statistics. vol 347. Hyattsville, MD: National Center for Health Statistics; 2004.
40. Hedley AA, Ogden CL, Johnson CL, Carroll MD, Curtin LR, Flegal KM. Prevalence of overweight and obesity among US children, adolescents, and adults, 1999–2002. J Am Med Assoc. 2004;291:2847–50.
41. Freedman DS, Ogden CL, Berenson GS, Horlick M. Body mass index and body fatness in childhood. Curr Opin Clin Nutr Metab Care. 2005;8:618–23.
42. James WP. The epidemiology of obesity. Ciba Found Symp. 1996;201:1–11. discussion 11–16, 32–36.
43. James PT, Leach R, Kalamara E, Shayeghi M. The worldwide obesity epidemic. Obes Res. 2001;9(Suppl 4):228S–33S.
44. Dietz WH, Gortmaker SL. Preventing obesity in children and adolescents. Annu Rev Public Health. 2001;22:337–53.
45. Cole TJ, Bellizzi MC, Flegal KM, Dietz WH. Establishing a standard definition for child overweight and obesity worldwide: international survey. BMJ. 2000;320:1240–43.
46. Dietz W. Physical activity and childhood obesity. Nutrition. 1991;7:295–6.
47. Must A, Bandini LG, Tybor DJ, Phillips SM, Naumova EN, Dietz WH. Activity, inactivity, and screen time in relation to weight and fatness over adolescence in girls. Obesity (Silver Spring). 2007;15:1774–81.
48. Vandewater EA, Bickham DS, Lee JH. Time well spent? Relating television use to children's free-time activities. Pediatrics. 2006;117:e181–91.
49. Nielsen ACC. Nielsen report on television. Northbrook, IL: AC Nielsen Co., Media Research Division; 1998.
50. Faith MS, Berman N, Heo M, et al. Effects of contingent television on physical activity and television viewing in obese children. Pediatrics. 2001;107:1043–48.
51. Motmans RR, Tomlow S, Vissers D. Trunk muscle activity in different modes of carrying schoolbags. Ergonomics. 2006;49:127–38.
52. Schaber PL. Incorporating problem-based learning and video technology in teaching group process in an occupational therapy curriculum. J Allied Health. 2005;34:110–16.
53. US Department of Health and Human Services CfDaP, National Center for Chronic Disease Prevention and Health Promotion. Physical activity and health: a report of the surgeon general. Atlanta, GA: US Department of Health and Human Services CfDaP, National Center for Chronic Disease Prevention and Health Promotion; 1996.
54. Blair SN, Brodney S. Effects of physical inactivity and obesity on morbidity and mortality: current evidence and research issues. Med Sci Sports Exerc. 1999;31:S646–62.

VI METABOLIC COMPLICATIONS OF CHILDHOOD OBESITY

12 Childhood Obesity and the Regulation of Growth, Thyroid Function, Sexual Development, and Calcium Homeostasis

Michael Freemark

CONTENTS

Key Words: Growth hormone, insulin-like growth factor (IGF), thyroid hormone, cortisol, prolactin, pseudohypoparathyroidism, adrenarche, puberty, gynecomastia, vitamin D, bone

Certain endocrine and metabolic disorders cause mild to moderate weight gain and fat deposition. Excess fat storage in turn can have profound effects on intermediary metabolism and endocrine function. We begin this section with a brief discussion of endocrine disorders that promote excess weight gain. We then review the effects of obesity on linear growth and bone maturation, thyroid function, sexual development, adrenal function, and calcium homeostasis and bone mineralization. Subsequent chapters in this volume discuss the implications of obesity for insulin production and action and the regulation of glucose tolerance, blood pressure, lipid metabolism and atherogenesis, sleep hygiene, and hepatic function.

METABOLIC AND HORMONAL DISORDERS CAUSING EXCESS FAT DEPOSITION

Hormonal disorders commonly associated with weight gain and increases in the ratio of fat to lean body mass include growth hormone (GH) deficiency, hypothyroidism, glucocorticoid excess, and the polycystic ovarian syndrome (PCOS, Table 1). Fat deposition in GH deficiency results from heightened insulin sensitivity, impaired lipolysis, sarcopenia, and induction of 11β-hydroxysteroid dehydrogenase 1 (11β-HSD1) in visceral or abdominal fat, which favors local overproduction of cortisol *(1)*. Hypothyroidism promotes weight gain by reducing resting energy expenditure, while glucocorticoid excess causes hyperphagia, adipogenesis, and muscle wasting. Ovarian hyperandrogenism/PCOS is

From: *Contemporary Endocrinology: Pediatric Obesity: Etiology, Pathogenesis, and Treatment*
Edited by: M. Freemark, DOI 10.1007/978-1-60327-874-4_12,
© Springer Science+Business Media, LLC 2010

Table 1
Mechanisms of Weight Gain in Hormonal Disorders

GH deficiency
> Increased insulin sensitivity
>
> Increased lipogenesis, decreased lipolysis
>
> Increased 11 beta HSD-1 in abdominal/viceral fat
>
> Sarcopenia and decreased resting energy expenditure

Hypothyroidism
> Reduced resting energy expenditure
>
> Decreased exercise
>
> ? sarcopenia

Glucocorticoid excess
> Hyperphagia
>
> Increased adipogenesis
>
> Sarcopenia

PCOS/Ovarian hyperandrogenism
> ? hyperinsulinemia

Hyperprolactinemia (variable weight gain)
> Hypogonadism
>
> ? increased food intake
>
> ? increased adipogenesis

Hypothalamic obesity
> Central leptin resistance with hyperphagia
>
> Heightened vagal tone with hyperinsulinemia
>
> GH deficiency, hypothyroidism, +/– precocious puberty, hyperprolactinemia
>
> Glucocorticoid excess (surgical and post-op periods)

associated with insulin resistance and hyperinsulinemia; given the ability of insulin to stimulate ovarian androgen production (see below), it may be a consequence as well as a cause of obesity.

Hypothalamic damage or disease can cause insatiable appetite and progressive weight gain. Reductions in basal metabolic rate and physical activity contribute to hypothalamic obesity (see Chapter 2 by Lustig). Deficiencies of GH, thyroid hormone, and glucocorticoids are common in this setting and some patients have precocious puberty, which can promote fat deposition, particularly in girls. The insatiable appetite and obesity probably result from central leptin resistance and heightened vagal tone with hyperinsulinemia. The use of high-dose glucocorticoids around the time of surgery facilitates weight gain; hyperprolactinemia, which has been associated with weight gain in adults and children (2,3), may also contribute.

GH deficiency, hypothyroidism, glucocorticoid excess, and pseudohypoparathyroidism (which can be accompanied by hypothyroidism as well as GH deficiency) are associated with short stature and/or decreased height velocity. In contrast, stature and height velocity are normal or increased in "exogenous" obesity (see below). Laboratory testing in an obese child is unlikely to reveal an underlying hormonal disorder (other than insulin resistance and glucose intolerance) if the height, growth velocity, pubertal development, and menstrual function are appropriate for age and family history. It should be noted, however, that linear growth and bone maturation may not be reduced in children with adrenal tumors that produce androgens as well as cortisol. Moreover, linear growth may appear normal or even increased in GH-deficient or hypothyroid patients who also have precocious puberty.

EFFECTS OF OBESITY ON LINEAR GROWTH AND BONE MATURATION

Final adult height in otherwise normal obese children generally falls within two standard deviations of target height. However, rates of linear growth and bone maturation are often increased in obese pre- and peri-pubertal children despite marked reductions in basal and stimulated plasma growth hormone (GH) concentrations and a reduction in circulating GH half-life (4). The reduction in GH secretion in obese children and adults has been ascribed to negative feedback by free fatty acids, a reduction in plasma ghrelin (a GH secretagogue produced by the stomach), and nutrient-stimulated increases in IGF-1 production. Total IGF-1 and IGF binding protein (BP)-3 concentrations in obese subjects are typically normal or only mildly elevated; this may reflect in part the production of IGF-1 and IGF BP-3 by white adipose tissue (5,6) and/or an increase in hepatic GH sensitivity, resulting from induction of hepatic GH receptors by hyperinsulinemia (Fig. 1). Induction of GH receptor expression in obesity is suggested by an increase in levels of GH binding protein (7), the circulating form of the extracellular GH receptor domain, and by heightened production of IGF-1 following a single dose of GH (8).

Total IGF-2 concentrations were elevated in obese adults in two studies but were normal in a study of obese adolescents (9). Many investigations find reductions in serum IGF binding proteins 1 and 2 (IGFBP-1 and BP-2), which correlate inversely with plasma insulin concentrations and liver fat content (10,11). The reductions in IGFBPs 1 and 2 are postulated to increase the bioavailability of IGF-1,

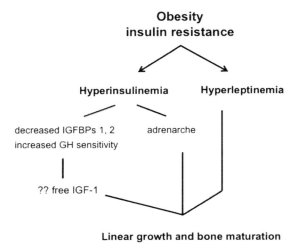

Fig. 1. Mechanisms that may explain the normal or increased rates of growth and bone maturation in pre- and peri-pubertal obese children. IGF, insulin-like growth factor; BP, binding protein. An increase in adrenal androgen production in obese children with precocious adrenarche may also accelerate bone maturation.

which may thereby maintain or increase linear growth in obesity despite diminished GH secretion. "Free" IGF-1 levels have been found to be elevated in some, but not all, studies of obese adults *(12,13)*; however, a recent investigation found that the bioactivity of IGF-1, as assessed by a kinase receptor activation assay, was normal in obese women. The ratio of bioactive IGF-1 to total IGF-1, however, was increased *(14)*.

Reductions in plasma IGF BP-1 or 2 concentrations in insulin-resistant obese subjects may facilitate weight gain because overexpression of IGFBP-1 or 2 in transgenic mice reduces adipogenesis and prevents diet-induced obesity. Interestingly BP-1 excess reduces insulin sensitivity but BP-2 excess improves glucose tolerance *(15,16)*

The effects of IGF-1 on growth and bone maturation may be potentiated by insulin-induced increases in adrenal androgen production (Fig. 1 and below); bone age may be advanced as much as 1 year in children with precocious adrenarche, which is more common in obese children. The hyperleptinemia of obesity also appears to play a role (Fig. 1). Circulating leptin levels rise in proportion to body (particularly subcutaneous) fat stores and are higher in girls than in boys. Leptin stimulates proliferation of isolated mouse and rat osteoblasts and increases the width of the chondroprogenitor zone of the mouse mandible in vivo. Conversely, leptin deficiency in ob/ob mice reduces cortical bone mass but increases trabecular mass *(17)*; leptin treatment increases femoral length, bone area, and bone mineral content *(18)* and may promote the differentiation of osteoblasts from bone marrow stem cells *(17)*. The effects of leptin may be exerted in concert with IGF-1 because leptin increases IGF-1 receptor expression in mouse chondrocytes *(19)*. Nevertheless, linear growth is normal in patients with congenital deficiencies of leptin or the leptin receptor *(20,21)*.

THYROID FUNCTION

Plasma T4 and TSH levels generally fall within the normal range in obese subjects but triiodothyronine concentrations are mildly elevated, a consequence of nutrient-dependent T4 to T3 conversion [*(4)*, Fig. 2]. The elevation of T3 increases resting energy expenditure and may thereby limit further weight gain. Caloric restriction and weight loss, on the other hand, decrease total and free T4 and T3 levels, reducing energy expenditure and thereby facilitating weight regain.

The effects of caloric excess and deprivation on thyroid hormone levels are mediated in part by leptin-dependent effects on hypothalamic TRH production (Fig. 2; see also Chapter 28 by Lechan and Fekete). Thyroid hormone levels are variably low in leptin receptor-deficient humans and are reduced in leptin receptor-deficient db/db mice. Leptin treatment reverses the loss of TSH pulsatility

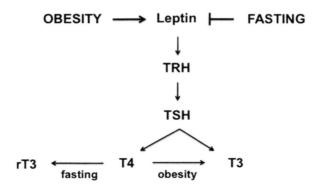

Fig. 2. Hyperleptinemia and nutrient-dependent conversion of T4 to T3 can increase T3 levels in obesity; fasting reduces T4 and T3 production and increases the conversion of T4 to inactive reverse T3 (rT3).

that accompanies short-term fasting and normalizes thyroid hormone levels following longer-term caloric restriction. These actions are mediated by direct effects of leptin/STAT-3 signaling on TRH transcription and indirect effects on TRH production mediated by increases in αMSH and reductions in agouti-related peptide (AgRP) and neuropeptide Y *(22,23)*.

GONADAL FUNCTION AND PUBERTAL DEVELOPMENT

A recent study found that obesity in early childhood (age 36–54 months) and excessive weight gain between 3 and 9 years of age increase the risks of precocious thelarche and may reduce the age of menarche *(24)*. Since leptin promotes gonadotropin secretion and rises transiently before the onset of puberty in normal weight children, it is possible that the hyperleptinemia of obesity promotes early sexual maturation, at least in girls.

More commonly, obese girls and boys develop precocious adrenarche without true puberty, and teenage obese girls are prone to ovarian hyperandrogenism with mild hirsutism, acne, anovulation, and menstrual irregularity. The pathogenesis of precocious adrenarche and ovarian hyperandrogenism remains poorly understood. However, insulin and IGF-1 in excess act in synergy with adrenocorticotrophic hormone (ACTH) and luteinizing hormone (LH) to stimulate the production of androgens from adrenocortical cells and ovarian theca cells, respectively. These effects are mediated through induction of P450c17α hydroxylase activity. The biologic availability of ovarian and adrenal androgens is increased because insulin suppresses hepatic sex hormone binding globulin (SHBG) expression and reduces plasma SHBG concentrations. Free androgens increase the frequency of gonadotropin-releasing hormone (GnRH) pulses and the ratio of LH to follicle-stimulating hormone (FSH), thereby exacerbating thecal androgen production. The increase in free androgens may induce precocious adrenarche in pre-pubertal girls and boys and may cause anovulation and hirsutism in adolescent girls and young women [*(25,26)*, Fig. 3; see also Chapter 24 by Franks and Joharatnam].

Free and total testosterone levels are generally normal in obese boys but may decline with dramatic weight gain in association with a fall in gonadotropin levels. These changes can reverse with weight

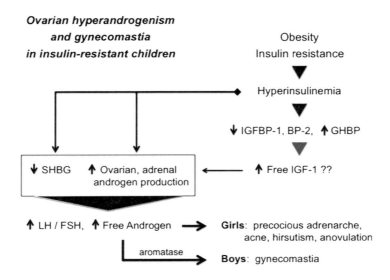

Fig. 3. Development of ovarian hyperandrogenism and gynecomastia in obese adolescents. IGF, insulin-like growth factor; BP, binding protein; GHBP, growth hormone binding protein; SHBG, sex hormone binding globulin; LH, luteinizing hormone; FSH, follicle-stimulating hormone.

loss. Aromatization of androstenedione in adipose tissue increases plasma estrone concentrations, causing gynecomastia in adolescent boys.

In rare cases the gynecomastia and ovarian hyperandrogenism in obese children are caused by hyperprolactinemia. Prolactin levels are typically normal or low in obese children or adults. However, hyperprolactinemia deriving from a pituitary tumor may be associated with weight gain in children as well as adults (2,3).

GLUCOCORTICOID PRODUCTION AND TURNOVER

The abdominal weight gain, striae, hirsutism, and menstrual irregularity that may accompany obesity are often confused with Cushing's syndrome. In contrast to "exogenous" obesity, Cushing's syndrome is typically associated with linear growth failure and delayed bone maturation (unless a primary adrenal tumor produces excess androgens as well as glucocorticoids) as well as hemorrhagic/violaceous, rather than pink, striae. Basal plasma, salivary, and urinary free cortisol concentrations and basal ACTH levels in obese, non-Cushingoid children generally fall within the normal range, and diurnal variation and the response to dexamethasone are maintained (27). However, body fat mass correlates with total excretion of glucocorticoid metabolites, suggesting that obesity is accompanied by increased cortisol secretion and turnover.

Changes in tissue glucocorticoid metabolism may modulate fat distribution and peripheral insulin sensitivity (28). For example, polymorphisms in the glucocorticoid receptor have been associated with obesity, hypertension, and insulin resistance in some studies in adults. Additional investigations suggest that overexpression of 11 beta hydroxysteroid dehydrogenase type 1 ($11\beta HSD_1$) in visceral adipose tissue may exacerbate weight gain by increasing local production of cortisol from inactive cortisone. In contrast, other studies find lower expression of $11\beta HSD_1$ in preadipocytes of obese, non-diabetic adults (29); the expected reduction in tissue cortisol concentrations is postulated to counteract the insulin resistance and weight gain in obese patients. An increase in $11\beta HSD_1$ expression after weight loss may facilitate adipose cortisol production, adipogenesis, and weight rebound.

CALCIUM HOMEOSTASIS, BONE MINERALIZATION, AND FRACTURES

Adolescents and adults with severe obesity, particularly those with dark skin, often have reduced circulating levels of 25-hydroxyvitamin D (25OHD). One study (30) found that 25OHD levels were less than 20 ng/ml in 78.4% of markedly obese (BMI 43.3) African-American teenage girls (mean age 14 years). The prevalence of vitamin D deficiency is lower in obese whites than in black or Hispanic children (31): in a total of 127 obese adolescents (mean age 13 years, BMI 36.4), vitamin D deficiency was noted in 43.6% of Hispanics and 48.7% of African-Americans but only 10.2% of Caucasians; levels of 25OHD correlated inversely with serum parathyroid hormone (PTH). A more recent investigation (32) showed that 17 of 58 obese adolescents (mean 14.9 years, BMI 36, 66% female, 14% black) had 25OHD levels below 20 ng/ml; however, none had elevated (>65 ng/ml) PTH levels, and bone mineral content and density fell within the normal range.

The reductions in 25OH vitamin D levels in obese children may be explained by decreased intake of vitamin D-containing dairy products, decreased cutaneous synthesis of vitamin D3 (in persons of color), and/or reduced bioavailability of vitamin D3 owing to deposition in adipose tissue (33). 25OHD levels in adults are inversely proportional to visceral and subcutaneous fat stores and measures of insulin sensitivity (34). Recent evidence suggests that 1,25 diOH vitamin D inhibits expression of peroxisome-proliferator-activated receptor gamma (PPARγ) and c/EBPα, providing a mechanism by which vitamin D deficiency may promote adipogenesis (35). However, no studies thus far have demonstrated that Vitamin D treatment can prevent or reverse weight gain in obese subjects.

Some studies show variable decreases in bone mineral content in obese subjects; others find that overweight and obese children have normal or increased bone mass compared with lean children. Yet the incidence of extremity fractures appears to be higher in obese than in lean children *(36,37)*; experiments in mice suggests that high-fat feeding increases bone density but reduces bone strength, bending stiffness, and fracture resistance *(38)*. Overall bone quality appears to reflect a number of genetic and environmental factors including milk intake and sun exposure, consumption of carbonated beverages, and physical activity, which promotes bone accrual and strength *(39)*.

REFERENCES

1. Agha A, Monson JP. Modulation of glucocorticoid metabolism by the growth hormone: IGF-1 axis. Clin Endocrinol (Oxford). 2007;66:459–65.
2. Colao A, Sarno AD, Cappabianca P, Briganti F, Pivonello R, Somma CD, Faggiano A, Biondi B, Lombardi G. Gender differences in the prevalence, clinical features and response to cabergoline in hyperprolactinemia. Eur J Endocrinol. 2003;148(3):325–31.
3. Gillam MP, Molitch ME, Lombardi G, Colao A. Advances in the treatment of prolactinomas. Endocr Rev. 2006;27: 485–534.
4. Douyon L, Schteingart DE. Effect of obesity and starvation on thyroid hormone, growth hormone and cortisol secretion. Endocrinol Metab Clin North Am. 2002;31:173–89.
5. Wabitsch M, Heinze E, Debatin KM, Blum WF. IGF-I- and IGFBP-3-expression in cultured human preadipocytes and adipocytes. Horm Met Res. 2000;32:555–9.
6. Peter MA, Winterhalter KH, Boni-Schnetzler M, Froesch ER, Zapf J. Regulation of insulin-like growth factor-I (IGF-I) and IGF-binding proteins by growth hormone in rat white adipose tissue. Endocrinology. 1993;133:2624–31.
7. Kratzsch J, Dehmel B, Pulzer F, et al. Increased serum GHBP levels in obese pubertal children and adolescents: relationship to body composition, leptin and indicators of metabolic disturbances. Int J Obes. 1997;21:1130–6.
8. Gleeson HK, Lissett CA, Shalet SM. Insulin-like growth factor-I response to a single bolus of growth hormone is increased in obesity. J Clin Endocrinol Metab. 2005;90:1061–7.
9. Wabitsch M, Blum WF, Muche R, Heinze E, Haug C, Mayer H, Teller W. Insulin-like growth factors and their binding proteins before and after weight loss and their associations with hormonal and metabolic parameters in obese adolescent girls. Int J Obes Relat Metab Disord. 1996;20(12):1073–80.
10. Wheatcroft SB, Kearney MT. IGF-dependent and IGF-independent actions of IGF-binding protein-1 and -2: implications for metabolic homeostasis. Trends Endocrinol Metab. 2009;20:153–62.
11. Kotronen A, Lewitt M, Hall K, Brismar K, Yki-Jarvinen H. Insulin-like growth factor binding protein 1 as a novel specific marker of hepatic insulin sensitivity. J Clin Endocrinol Metab. 2008;93:4867–72.
12. Frystyk J, Skjaerbaek C, Vestbo E, Fisker S, Orskov H. Circulating levels of free insulin-like growth factors in obese subjects: the impact of type 2 diabetes. Diabetes Metab Res Rev. 1999;15:314–22.
13. Rasmussen MH, Juul A, Kjems LL, Hilsted J. Effects of short-term caloric restriction on circulating free IGF-I, acid-labile subunit, IGF-binding proteins (IGFBPs)-1-4, and IGFBPs-1-3 protease activity in obese subjects. Eur J Endocrinol. 2006;155(4):575–81.
14. Frystyk J, Brick DJ, Gerweck AV, Utz AL, Miller KK. Bioactive insulin-like growth factor-1 in obesity. J Clin Endocrinol Metab. 2009;94:3093–7.
15. Rajkumar K, Modric T, Murphy LJ. Impaired adipogenesis in insulin-like growth factor binding protein-1 transgenic mice. J Endocrinol. 1999;162(3):457–65.
16. Wheatcroft SB, Kearney MT, Shah AM, Ezzat VA, Miell JR, Modo M, Williams SC, Cawthorn WP, Medina-Gomez G, Vidal-Puig A, Sethi JK, Crossey PA. IGF-binding protein-2 protects against the development of obesity and insulin resistance. Diabetes. 2007;56(2):285–94.
17. Cirmanova V, Bayer M, Starka L, Zajickova K. The effect of leptin on bone: an evolving concept of action. Physiol Res. 2008;57(Suppl 1):S143–51.
18. Steppan CM, Crawford DT, Chidsey-Frink KL, Ke H, Swick AG. Leptin is a potent stimulator of bone growth in ob/ob mice. Regul Pept. 2000;92:73–8.
19. Maor G, Rochwerger M, Segev Y, Phillip M. Leptin acts as a growth factor on the chondrocytes of skeletal growth centers. J Bone Miner Res. 2002;17:1034–43.
20. Montague CT, Farooqi IS, Whitehead JP, Soos MA, Rau H, Wareham NJ, Sewter CP, Digby JE, Mohammed SN, Hurst JA, Cheetham CH, Earley AR, Barnett AH, Prins JB, O'Rahilly S. Congenital leptin deficiency is associated with severe early-onset obesity in humans. Nature. 1997;387(6636):903–8.

21. Farooqi IS, Wangensteen T, Collins S, Kimber W, Matarese G, Keogh JM, Lank E, Bottomley B, Lopez-Fernandez J, Ferraz-Amaro I, Dattani MT, Ercan O, Myhre AG, Retterstol L, Stanhope R, Edge JA, McKenzie S, Lessan N, Ghodsi M, De Rosa V, Perna F, Fontana S, Barroso I, Undlien DE, O'Rahilly S. Clinical and molecular genetic spectrum of congenital deficiency of the leptin receptor. N Engl J Med. 2007;356(3):237–47.

22. Feldt-Rasmussen U. Thyroid and leptin. Thyroid. 2007;17:413–9.

23. Hollenberg AN. The role of the thyrotropin-releasing hormone (TRH) neuron as a metabolic sensor. Thyroid. 2008;18:131–8.

24. Lee JM, Appugliese D, Kaciroti N, Corwyn RF, Bradley RH, Lumeng JC. Weight status in young girls and the onset of puberty. Pediatrics. 2007;119:e624–30.

25. Sam S, Dunaif A. Polycystic ovary syndrome: syndrome XX? Trends Endocrinol Metab. 2003;14:365–70.

26. Chang RJ. The reproductive phenotype in polycystic ovary syndrome. Nat Clin Pract Endocrinol Metab. 2007;3(10):688–95.

27. Artz E, Haqq A, Freemark M. Hormonal and metabolic consequences of childhood obesity. Endocrinol Metab Clin North Am. 2005;34(3):643–58.

28. Wake DJ, Rask E, Livingstone DEW, Soderberg S, Olsson T, Walker BR. Local and systemic impact of transcriptional up-regulation of 11β-hydroxysteroid dehydrogenase type 1 in adipose tissue in human obesity. J Clin Endocrinol Metab. 2003;88:3983–8.

29. Tomlinson JW, Moore JS, Clark PM, Holder G, Shakespeare L, Stewart PM. Weight loss increases 11β-hydroxysteroid dehydrogenase type 1 expression in human adipose tissue. J Clin Endocrinol Metab. 2004;89:2711–6.

30. Ashraf A, Alvarez J, Saenz K, Gower B, McCormick K, Franklin F. Threshold for effects of vitamin D deficiency on glucose metabolism in obese female African-American adolescents. J Clin Endocrinol Metab. 2009;94:3200–6.

31. Alemzadeh R, Kichler J, Babar G, Calhoun M. Hypovitaminosis D in obese children and adolescents: relationship with adiposity, insulin sensitivity, ethnicity, and season. Metabolism. 2008;57:183–91.

32. Lenders CM, Feldman HA, Von Scheven E, et al. Relation of body fat indexes to vitamin D status and deficiency among obese adolescents. Am J Clin Nutr. 2009;90:459–67.

33. Wortsman J, Matsuoka LY, Chen TC, Lu Z, Holick MF. Decreased bioavailability of vitamin D in obesity. Am J Clin Nutr. 2000;72(3):690–3.

34. Cheng S, Massaro JM, Fox CS, Larson MG, Keyes MJ, McCabe EL, Robins SJ, O'Donnell CJ, Hoffmann U, Jacques PF, Booth SL, Vasan RS, Wolf M, Wang TJ. Adiposity, cardiometabolic risk, and vitamin D status: the Framingham Heart Study. Diabetes. 2010; 59(1):242–8.

35. Wood RJ. Vitamin D and adipogenesis: new molecular insights. Nutr Rev. 2008;66:40–6.

36. Taylor ED, Theim KR, Mirch MC, Ghorbani S, Tanofsky-Kraff M, Adler-Wailes DC, Brady S, Reynolds JC, Calis KA, Yanovski JA. Orthopedic complications of overweight in children and adolescents. Pediatrics. 2006;117(6):2167–74.

37. Rana AR, Michalsky MP, Teich S, Groner JI, Caniano DA, Schuster DP. Childhood obesity: a risk factor for injuries observed at a level-1 trauma center. J Pediatr Surg. 2009;44:1601–5.

38. Ionova-Martin SS, Do SH, Barth HD, et al. Reduced size-independent mechanical properties of cortical bone in high fat diet-induced obesity. Bone. 2010;46(1):217–25.

39. Manias K, McCabe D, Bishop N. Fractures and recurrent fractures in children: varying effects of environmental factors as well as bone size and mass. Bone. 2006;39:652–7.

13 Pathogenesis of Insulin Resistance and Glucose Intolerance in Childhood Obesity

Ram Weiss, Anna Cali, and Sonia Caprio

CONTENTS

Key Words: Insulin resistance, pre-diabetes, visceral fat, skeletal muscle, liver, type 2 diabetes, metabolic syndrome, brown adipose tissue (BAT)

Obesity in children and adults is associated with resistance to the metabolic effects of insulin. The term "insulin resistance" is commonly used to describe the resistance of skeletal muscle and liver to insulin-dependent glucose metabolism: insulin resistance reduces myocellular glucose uptake and utilization, increases hepatic glucose production, and facilitates adipose tissue lipolysis. Reductions in hepatic insulin clearance and a compensatory up-regulation of beta cell insulin secretion lead to hyperinsulinemia.

It is important to recognize that the process of insulin resistance is tissue and pathway selective. Thus certain actions of insulin in liver (e.g., lipoprotein synthesis and suppression of sex hormone binding globulin and IGF binding protein-1), skin, ovary, and kidney are preserved; this explains in part the clinical manifestations of insulin resistance, which include dyslipidemia, acanthosis nigricans, hyperandrogenism, and hypertension. Together with glucose intolerance, these disorders are postulated to drive the development of atherogenesis and to increase the risk of cardiovascular disease in susceptible individuals (1).

Insulin resistance can be induced by changes in metabolic demand during the lifespan: examples include the transient insulin resistance of puberty (2), pregnancy, and acute illness. Sensitivity to insulin declines progressively with age and may be influenced by the macronutrient composition of the diet (3). The clinical manifestations of insulin resistance depend upon the duration of the underlying disorder and on the susceptibility of the individual; thus the acute and long-term effects of insulin resistance are modulated by familial, genetic, racial, and ethnic factors.

From: *Contemporary Endocrinology: Pediatric Obesity: Etiology, Pathogenesis, and Treatment*
Edited by: M. Freemark, DOI 10.1007/978-1-60327-874-4_13,
© Springer Science+Business Media, LLC 2010

PATHOPHYSIOLOGY OF INSULIN RESISTANCE

The most common cause of insulin resistance in the pediatric age group is obesity. Most obese children and adults are insulin resistant; however even severely obese children can in some cases be highly insulin sensitive, normotensive, normolipidemic, and euglycemic *(4)*. The relationship between obesity and peripheral insulin resistance depends more on the distribution of lipid (or "lipid partitioning") in specific fat depots than on the absolute amount of fat per se. Different lipid depots have distinct metabolic characteristics reflected in their adipocytokine and cytokine secretion profiles *(5)*, sensitivity to hormones such as norepinephrine or insulin, and anatomical blood supply and drainage (portal vs. systemic) *(6)*. Increased visceral fat accumulation in obese children is associated with increased insulin resistance *(7)* and the clustering and heightened expression of cardiovascular risk factors *(8)* (Figs. 1 and 2). Some obese children manifest a unique lipid partitioning pattern characterized by a large visceral fat depot and a relatively smaller subcutaneous fat depot. Children with a predominance of visceral fat have adverse metabolic profiles in comparison with those with larger subcutaneous

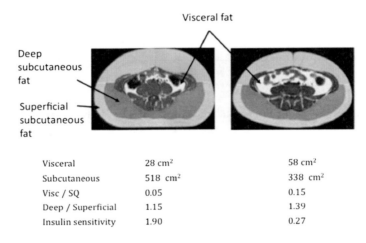

Visceral	28 cm²	58 cm²
Subcutaneous	518 cm²	338 cm²
Visc / SQ	0.05	0.15
Deep / Superficial	1.15	1.39
Insulin sensitivity	1.90	0.27

Fig. 1. Representative MRI images of Caucasian female subjects with low and high levels of visceral fat. Note the inverse relationship between visceral fat and insulin sensitivity (Matsuda index). Adapted from Taksali et al. *(9)*.

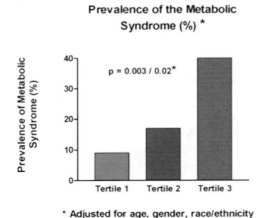

Fig. 2. Relation of tertiles of visceral fat and the prevalence of the metabolic syndrome. Adapted from Taksali et al. *(9)*.

fat depots, even when the latter have greater BMI and percent body fat *(9)*. Thus, the subcutaneous fat depot, localized more in the lower body region than in the upper body region *(10)*, serves as a "metabolic sink" that accumulates fat in states of excess energy intake/low energy output. Individuals with the ability to store excess fat in lower body subcutaneous depots appear to be able to gain excess weight without developing significant insulin resistance. In contrast, those with low capacity to store excess lipid in subcutaneous depots tend to accumulate fat in visceral depots and in insulin responsive tissues such as muscle and liver and develop insulin resistance.

The skeletal muscle is the primary site for post-prandial glucose uptake and utilization. Intramyocellular lipid deposition is higher in obese than in lean subjects (Fig. 3) and correlates inversely with peripheral insulin sensitivity *(11)* (Fig. 4) and is increased in offspring of patients with T2DM and in obese children with impaired glucose tolerance *(12)*. The effect of lipid within the myocyte on insulin signal transduction is indirect and probably mediated by several fatty acid derivatives such as ceramide, diacylglycerol, and fatty acyl CoA as well as reactive oxygen species that inhibit insulin signaling *(13)*. Similarly, hepatic fat accumulation is strongly associated with obesity and with hepatic resistance to the effects of insulin on glucose metabolism; it is also associated with an adverse cardiovascular risk profile in children (see Chapter 15 by Alisi et al., this volume).

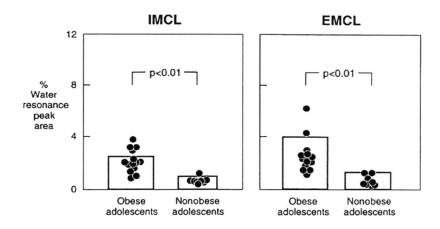

Fig. 3. Intramyocellular lipid (IMCL) and extramyocellular lipid (EMCL) content in lean and obese adolescents. From Sinha et al. *(11)* with permission.

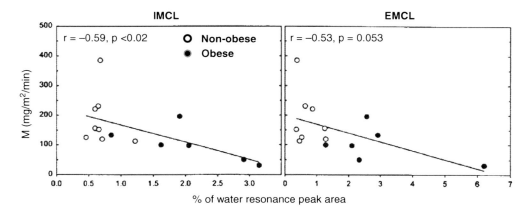

Fig. 4. Relation of intramyocellular lipid (IMCL) and extramyocellular lipid (EMCL) content to whole-body insulin sensitivity in lean and obese adolescents. Redrawn from Sinha et al. *(11)* with permission.

As the liver governs glucose metabolism in the fasting state and the muscle affects glucose metabolism mainly in the post-absorptive state, significant hepatic insulin resistance may have a stronger impact on fasting glucose levels and on the early post-absorptive suppression of hepatic gluconeogenesis following a meal. In contrast, muscle lipid deposition has a greater impact on post-prandial glucose levels. Combined resistance in skeletal muscle and liver induces a rise in blood glucose, which is noted first in the post-prandial state. This triggers an adaptive increase in beta cell insulin secretion and a reduction in hepatic insulin clearance. The net result is an increase in circulating insulin levels (hyperinsulinemia). In early stages, hyperinsulinemia maintains euglycemia; however, persistent insulin resistance imposes a continuous burden on beta cell insulin secretion. In the long run, this may contribute to beta cell failure *(14,15)*. The induction of adipose tissue lipolysis in insulin resistance raises circulating free fatty acids, which stimulate insulin secretion initially but ultimately reduce beta cell function in the presence of hyperglycemia. The high levels of insulin increase renal sodium retention, reduce uric acid clearance *(16)*, and promote ovarian androgen production *(17)*. Hyperinsulinemia may also activate the sympathetic nervous system *(18)* and impact the metabolism and secretion of pro-inflammatory cytokines as well as coagulation mediators *(19)*.

Some suggest that hepatic deposition of lipid is not a primary process but a "normal" response to elevated circulating insulin levels induced by muscle insulin resistance; they argue that hepatic steatosis is a consequence, not a culprit, of the adverse metabolic phenotype characteristic of insulin-resistant individuals. Exposure of the liver to hyperinsulinemia, along with increased free fatty acid flux, likely contributes to the dyslipidemia observed in individuals with insulin resistance. This dyslipidemia consists of elevated triglycerides, reduced HDL-cholesterol, and an increased concentration of small LDL particles, which are integral to the pathogenesis of atherosclerotic heart disease *(20,21)* (see also Chapter 14 by McCrindle, this volume).

In summary, peripheral tissue resistance to the action of insulin, specifically in metabolic pathways related to glucose metabolism in the muscle and liver, results in a compensatory hyperinsulinemia. Selective preservation of insulin signaling pathways yields a clinical picture characterized by dyslipidemia (specifically elevated triglycerides, low HDL-cholesterol, and the presence of small LDL particles), hypertension, and ovarian hyperandrogenism. Altered glucose metabolism, manifested as impaired fasting glucose, impaired glucose tolerance, or overt diabetes, reflects the inability of beta cells to secrete insulin in amounts sufficient to overcome insulin resistance. Insulin resistance and hyperinsulinemia enhance the expression of pro-inflammatory cytokines and factors related to hyper-coagulability. The clustering of these factors accelerates the process of atherogenesis and cardiovascular disease.

EPIDEMIOLOGY OF ALTERED GLUCOSE METABOLISM IN CHILDHOOD

The epidemic of childhood obesity has been accompanied by a sharp increase in the incidence of type 2 diabetes (T2DM) in the pediatric age group. T2DM represents the end of a spectrum of altered glucose metabolism that includes at least two pre-diabetic conditions: impaired glucose tolerance (IGT) and impaired fasting glucose (IFG). As not all those with a pre-diabetic condition progress to develop T2DM, the prevalence of these pre-diabetic conditions is much greater than that of overt diabetes. Recent data from the SEARCH for Diabetes study in the United States showed that the prevalence of T2DM in Caucasians (at ages 10–19 years) was 0.18/1,000, with higher rates in female than in male subjects (0.22 vs. 0.15 per 1,000, $p = 0.01$). The incidence of type 2 diabetes was 3.7/100,000, with similar rates for female and male subjects (3.9 vs. 3.4 per 1,000, respectively, $p = 0.3$) *(22)*. Among African-American youth aged 10–19 years, the prevalence (per 1,000) of T2DM was 1.06 (0.93–1.22) and the annual incidence (per 100,000) was 19.0 (16.9–21.3). For T2DM, the rates were $6.9/10^5$ (5.7–8.4) and $4.8/10^5$ (3.8–6.0) for female and male subjects, respectively *(23)*. It should be noted that the SEARCH study excluded all subjects in seropositivity to islet antigens, even if they had a phenotype and family history characteristics of patients with type 2 diabetes. Nevertheless, among Hispanic female subjects aged 15–19 years, the incidence of type 2 diabetes exceeded that of type 1 diabetes ($p < 0.05$). The incidence of type 1 and type 2 diabetes for Hispanic male subjects aged 15–19 years was not significantly different (24). In the most conservative estimate, more than 20,000 obese children in the European Union have T2DM, while more than 400,000 have impaired glucose tolerance (25). Among US adolescents, the unadjusted prevalences of IFG, IGT, or either one were 13.1, 3.4, and 16.1%, respectively, with overweight adolescents having a 2.6-fold higher rate than those with normal weight (1.3–5.1) (26). These data indicate that alterations in glucose metabolism, specifically of pre-diabetic conditions, are common among obese children and adolescents. Moreover, T2DM, previously considered rare in childhood, must now figure prominently in the differential diagnosis of any overweight or obese adolescent with hyperglycemia.

PATHOPHYSIOLOGY OF ALTERED GLUCOSE METABOLISM IN CHILDHOOD

The development of T2DM involves at least two mechanisms relevant to glucose metabolism pathways: increased peripheral insulin resistance and a failure of beta cell function to compensate adequately for such resistance. The most common cause of insulin resistance in childhood is obesity, which reduces insulin action in otherwise healthy individuals and exacerbates pre-existing insulin resistance in those with a predisposing condition. Predisposing factors include ethnic background (African-American, Hispanic, Native American, Asian, and Pacific Islander), a family history of T2DM in first-degree relatives, prematurity and intrauterine growth retardation, a history of exposure to gestational diabetes, sedentary behavior, and, possibly, specific macro and micronutrients in the diet (27).

Obese children and adolescents with pre-diabetic conditions have marked peripheral insulin resistance in comparison to normal glucose tolerant peers (28). While glucose tolerant subjects have varying degrees of insulin sensitivity (29), pre-diabetic subjects uniformly have very low insulin sensitivity. Development of insulin resistance triggers a compensatory increase in circulating insulin levels that is achieved by two independent mechanisms: increased secretion of insulin from pancreatic beta cells and reduced clearance of insulin by the liver (30). The relation of insulin secretion to insulin resistance is hyperbolic (best described as sensitivity × secretion = constant) and is called the disposition index (DI) (31). As an individual's DI is largely genetically determined, one can have various degrees of insulin sensitivity for a given DI during the lifespan; yet as the degree of insulin sensitivity declines in a given individual, the demand for beta cell insulin secretion must increase (32) (Fig. 5). Failure to maintain adequate insulin secretion will translate to a new and lower DI that manifests as a relative hyperglycemia in comparison to the previous steady state.

Early defects in beta cell function have been demonstrated in obese children and adolescents with IGT and with T2DM. In the face of comparable degrees of insulin resistance, individuals with IGT display a pattern of first-phase insulin secretion that is reduced in comparison to those with normal glucose tolerance yet greater than those with T2DM. Second-phase insulin secretion is initially preserved in those with IGT but is reduced in those with early T2DM (33). Thus, T2DM in obese adolescents manifests a dual defect in both phases of insulin secretion following glucose challenge and thus represents overt beta cell failure.

Mathematical modeling of beta cell function indices derived from oral glucose tolerance tests (OGTTs) demonstrates subtle yet significant defects in beta cell function in the various pre-diabetic conditions in obese youth. First-phase insulin secretion is progressively lower in IFG, IGT, and IFG/IGT, respectively, compared with NGT. Second-phase insulin secretion is significantly reduced only in the IFG/IGT group. Thus, IFG in obese adolescents is linked primarily to alterations in glucose

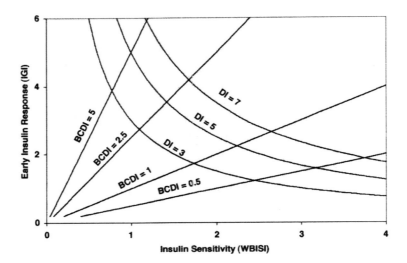

Fig. 5. Relation of OGTT-derived indexes of insulin secretion and sensitivity and their interactions. As shown, for a given DI, as insulin sensitivity is lower, early insulin response is higher. This translates to a greater BCDI (beta cell demand index), reflecting the metabolic burden placed on the β-cell in order to maintain a constant DI and normal glucose homeostasis. From Weiss et al. *(15)* with permission.

sensitivity of first-phase insulin secretion and liver insulin sensitivity. The IGT group has a more severe degree of peripheral insulin resistance and reduction in first-phase secretion. IFG/IGT is hallmarked by profound insulin resistance and by a new additional defect in second-phase insulin secretion. Thus, although we tend to categorize degrees of glucose intolerance based on thresholds for clinical purposes, the deterioration from normal glucose tolerance to T2DM represents a continuum that culminates as a significant defect of beta cell function. Milder defects in beta cell function can be detected even in subjects with glucose levels in the "high normal" range. However, beta cell function deteriorates further as glucose tolerance worsens *(34)*: isolated IGT, manifested as elevated 2-h glucose levels during an OGTT, represents an early first-phase beta cell defect, while the combination of impaired fasting glucose and IGT is associated with more profound beta cell dysfunction.

Reductions in peripheral insulin resistance, whether achieved by diet-induced weight loss, exercise, or pharmacologic interventions, allow the affected individual to shift along the DI curve to a new steady state in which beta cell capacity is sufficient to maintain euglycemia. It is currently unclear if increases in insulin sensitivity can fully restore beta cell function once an individual has developed overt glucose intolerance.

DYNAMICS OF PRE-DIABETIC CONDITIONS

Not all obese children and adolescents with a pre-diabetic status progress to develop overt diabetes. For example, some adolescents with pre-diabetes at mid-puberty revert to normal glucose tolerance upon completion of pubertal development. The progression from IGT to T2DM is associated with a continuous reduction in insulin sensitivity, tightly linked to significant weight gain *(35)*. Indeed, changes in insulin sensitivity, mostly associated with weight dynamics, are the main predictors of changes in the 2-h glucose level during an OGTT. However, the progression from normal glucose metabolism to IGT or T2DM also reflects a defect in beta cell function manifest as impaired responsiveness to a rapid dynamic change in glucose *(36)*. The defect in beta cell function can be demonstrated using the DI, which deteriorates progressively from normal to impaired glucose

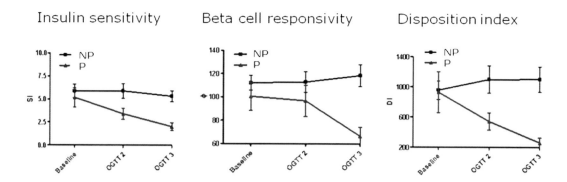

Fig. 6. Progression of glucose intolerance in insulin-resistant adolescents. NP, non-progressors, i.e., insulin-resistant patients who did not develop impaired glucose tolerance (IGT); P, progressors, i.e., those who progressed to IGT. Adapted from Cali et al. *(36)*.

metabolism to overt diabetes *(37)*. In combination with an increase in insulin resistance over time, a fall in beta cell insulin secretion leads to deteriorating glucose tolerance and eventually to impaired glucose tolerance (Fig. 6).

Persistent or progressive insulin resistance imposes a beta cell burden that is likely to translate to beta cell failure in predisposed individuals. Long-term exposure to inflammatory factors and free fatty acidemia play important contributory roles. On the other hand, those with good beta cell function may compensate adequately for marked insulin resistance for prolonged periods of time. Importantly, fasting levels of insulin or C-peptide are poor predictors of future deterioration in glucose tolerance; it takes a glucose challenge (oral or intravenous) to uncover subtle defects in beta cell function that reveal an individual's vulnerability.

An OGTT is a useful tool for assessing glucose tolerance in obese youth. Adults with IGT have residual beta cell function less than 50% of baseline; this may also be true in children. The reproducibility of the OGTT has been questioned; however, documentation of IGT on even a single study demonstrates the vulnerability of the patient to beta cell dysfunction in the advent of further weight gain, pregnancy, or treatment with glucocorticoids. IGT is a dynamic condition and represents a narrow window of opportunity; children and adolescents with IGT should therefore be a primary focus of preventive and therapeutic efforts.

INSULIN RESISTANCE ("METABOLIC") SYNDROME IN CHILDHOOD

The metabolic syndrome, also known as "the insulin resistance" syndrome, describes a cluster of cardiovascular risk factors that have been shown to predict the development of cardiovascular disease (CVD) *(38,39)* and type 2 diabetes (T2DM) *(40)*. The syndrome is characterized by abdominal adiposity, dyslipidemia, hypertension, and glucose intolerance *(41)*. Some have questioned the clinical utility of the term in adults *(42)* and in children *(43)* and advocate addressing individual risk factors in their clinical context. This debate has important clinical implications with regard to treatment decisions; yet it must be understood that the pathophysiological changes that lead to the metabolic syndrome have common features in people of all ages and are postulated to drive the development of atherogenesis and cardiovascular disease.

One must also appreciate that cardiovascular risk factors such as elevated fasting glucose or the degree of obesity represent continuous variables. For example, increasing BMI during childhood represents a continuous risk factor for the development of coronary heart disease in adulthood *(44)*;

nevertheless, severely obese children have a significantly worse metabolic phenotype in comparison with moderately obese children and are at higher risk for cardiovascular disease (45). Likewise, a seemingly "upper normal" fasting glucose level in the context of obesity during late adolescence may signify future risk of type 2 diabetes (46), and a rise in triglyceride levels within the "normal range" in late adolescence can predict the development of diabetes (47) and of coronary heart disease (48).

Another issue that adds complexity to any definition of the metabolic syndrome is its generalizability for populations of different ethnic backgrounds. IGT and type 2 diabetes are more common in ethnic minorities in the United States (49) and in some European countries (50). A potential explanation is that ethnic minority youth are more obese and more insulin resistant than their Caucasian peers (51) and have different lipid partitioning profiles when matched for BMI. Moreover, non-obese Hispanic and African-American children have increased insulin secretion and reduced hepatic insulin clearance relative to Caucasian children matched for degree of insulin sensitivity (52). Thus, assessments of insulin sensitivity based on fasting or post-prandial insulin levels may in the future have to be ethnicity-specific. Moreover, anthropometric measures such as visceral and subcutaneous fat content should be ethnicity-sensitive and derived from outcome data of the relevant populations (53).

SUMMARY

Insulin resistance, which is common among obese children and adolescents, manifests as a cluster of cardiovascular risk factors that include dyslipidemia, hypertension, and altered glucose metabolism. While cardiovascular disease is rarely observed in childhood, altered glucose metabolism manifests early and is commonly seen in obese youth. Obese individuals who exhibit an increase in the ratio of intra-abdominal to subcutaneous fat and deposition of lipid in insulin responsive tissues are mostly insulin resistant. Glucose intolerance reflects the confluence of severe insulin resistance and beta cell dysfunction, emerging most commonly in those with a family history of T2DM, intrauterine exposure to diabetes, or intrauterine growth retardation.

Editor's Questions and Authors' Response

- **Visceral adipose tissue is said to be more "metabolically active" than subcutaneous tissue with higher rates of lipolysis; this is said to explain the increases in free fatty acids and heightened liver fat deposition in people with visceral adiposity. Given the overall mass of the visceral fat depot, however, some investigators argue that circulating FFA are derived primarily from non-visceral stores. In your opinion, why does visceral fat play such an important role in the pathogenesis of insulin resistance?**

- As previously shown by Jensen et al, visceral fat contributes free fatty acids to the circulation in proportion to its overall size in comparison to total fat. The difference is that these free fatty acids reach the liver via the portal and not via the systemic circulation. It is postulated that free fatty acids reach the liver in high concentrations and have a local effect in various signal transduction pathways. Moreover, visceral fat seems to have a different secretion profile of adipocytokines and of inflammatory cytokines in comparison to subcutaneous fat. The pro-inflammatory molecules secreted from visceral fat act locally in the liver and likely affect muscle glucose uptake and the secretion of insulin from pancreatic beta cells.

- **The relative amount of visceral fat in obese African-American teenagers is significantly less than that in BMI-matched Caucasians. Yet the rates of type 2 diabetes in African-American adolescents are at least twofold to fourfold higher than those in Caucasians. How do you explain this apparent paradox?**

- Indeed, African-American children tend to have less visceral fat in comparison to their Caucasian peers, yet have a greater prevalence of diabetes. This paradox can be explained by the fact that the relation of insulin secretion and insulin sensitivity (i.e., the disposition index) is different between these groups. This translates to a greater insulin response in the face of the same degree of insulin sensitivity in African-American lean and obese children in comparison to Caucasians. That means in the face of marked insulin resistance characteristic of severe obesity, African-Americans must produce more insulin to maintain glucose tolerance. This greater beta cell demand predisposes them to earlier beta cell failure. In addition, higher rates of type 2 diabetes in African-Americans might be explained in part by dietary factors.

Editor's Comments

- The discussion in this chapter focuses largely on the distribution and metabolic activity of white adipose tissue, which is designed for energy storage. But newborn infants also contain large masses of *brown adipose tissue (BAT)*, which is essential for thermogenesis. The major depot of BAT (interscapular) regresses after birth. Until recently, it was thought that stores of BAT in older children and adults were too limited to exert a significant impact on energy balance. However, recent investigations show that BAT can be detected in the supraclavicular and paraspinal regions in a significant percentage of women and men (Saito et al., 2009; Au-Yong et al., 2009; van Marken Lichtenbelt et al., 2009; Cypess et al., 2009). The BAT is a mixture of brown and white adipocytes and stains positively for uncoupling protein-1 (UCP-1). The mass of BAT appears to correlate inversely with age, ambient temperature, light exposure, BMI, and visceral fat mass. The role of BAT in energy homeostasis in children and adolescents is currently unknown; but since BAT appears to protect against obesity and diabetes in mice (Almind et al., 2007), it is possible that the ratio of BAT/visceral fat may prove to be a determinant of childhood weight gain and metabolic function.

- The authors demonstrate convincingly that type 2 diabetes is the end result of a process of metabolic decompensation in which beta cell dysfunction is superimposed upon pre-existing insulin resistance. Formal glucose tolerance testing is useful for assessing states of pre-diabetes [impaired fasting glucose (100–125 mg%) and/or impaired glucose tolerance (2 h glucose 140–199 mg%)] and for identification of overt type 2 diabetes. However, the validity and clinical utility of the OGTT have been questioned: it may be difficult to bring certain adolescents to the clinic in early morning for a 2–4 h test and the results may vary over time. An American Diabetes Association expert panel (Nathan et al., 2009) recently suggested that measurement of HbA1c provides a clinically useful assessment of glucose intolerance in adults; values equal to or exceeding 6.5% were considered diagnostic of diabetes. Others have argued that a combination of fasting blood glucose and HbA1c may reduce the need for a formal GTT to diagnose impaired glucose tolerance (Manley et al., 2009). HbA1c can be measured under random conditions and provides an assessment of glucose exposure for the past 3 months. Values can be misleading in patients with hemoglobinopathies or in other states of increased red blood cell turnover. Nevertheless, the test can provide valuable information in children as well as adults; in our experience, HbA1c values equal to or exceeding 6.5% are commonly associated with impaired glucose tolerance or overt type 2 diabetes, and impaired fasting glucose is common in patients with A1c values ranging from 6 to 6.4%. Still, the precise relationship between HbA1c and the OGTT should be assessed in pediatric patients.

Almind K, Manieri M, Sivitz WI, Cinti S, Kahn CR. Ectopic brown adipose tissue in muscle provides a mechanism for differences in risk of metabolic syndrome in mice. Proc Natl Acad Sci USA. 2007 Feb 13;104(7):2366–71.

Au-Yong IT, Thorn N, Ganatra R, Perkins AC, Symonds ME. Brown adipose tissue and seasonal variation in humans. Diabetes. 2009 Nov;58(11):2583–7.

Cypess AM, Lehman S, Williams G, Tal I, Rodman D, Goldfine AB, Kuo FC, Palmer EL, Tseng YH, Doria A, Kolodny GM, Kahn CR. Identification and importance of brown adipose tissue in adult humans. N Engl J Med. 2009 Apr 9;360(15):1509–17.

Manley SE, Sikaris KA, Lu ZX, Nightingale PG, Stratton IM, Round RA, Baskar V, Gough SC, Smith JM. Validation of an algorithm combining haemoglobin A(1c) and fasting plasma glucose for diagnosis of diabetes mellitus in UK and Australian populations. Diabet Med. 2009 Feb;26(2):115–21.

Nathan DH et al.; International Expert Committee. International Expert Committee report on the role of the A1C assay in the diagnosis of diabetes. Diabetes Care. 2009 Jul;32(7):1327–34.

Saito M, Okamatsu-Ogura Y, Matsushita M, Watanabe K, Yoneshiro T, Nio-Kobayashi J, Iwanaga T, Miyagawa M, Kameya T, Nakada K, Kawai Y, Tsujisaki M. High incidence of metabolically active brown adipose tissue in healthy adult humans: effects of cold exposure and adiposity. Diabetes. 2009 Jul;58(7):1526–31.

van Marken Lichtenbelt WD, Vanhommerig JW, Smulders NM, Drossaerts JM, Kemerink GJ, Bouvy ND, Schrauwen P, Teule GJ. Cold-activated brown adipose tissue in healthy men. N Engl J Med. 2009 Apr 9;360(15):1500–8.

REFERENCES

1. Reaven GM. Role of insulin resistance in human disease. Diabetes. 1988;37:1595–607.

2. Goran MI, Gower BA. Longitudinal study on pubertal insulin resistance. Diabetes. 2001;50(11):2444–50.

3. Lutsey PL, Steffen LM, Stevens J. Dietary intake and the development of the metabolic syndrome: the Atherosclerosis Risk in Communities study. Circulation. 2008;117(6):754–61.

4. Weiss R, Taksali SE, Dufour S, Yeckel CW, Papademetris X, Cline G, Tamborlane WV, Dziura J, Shulman GI, Caprio S. The "obese insulin-sensitive" adolescent: importance of adiponectin and lipid partitioning. J Clin Endocrinol Metab. 2005;90(6):3731–37.

5. Matsuzawa Y, Funahashi T, Nakamura T. Molecular mechanism of metabolic syndromeX: contribution of adipocy-tokines adipocyte-derived bioactive substances. Ann N Y Acad Sci. 1999;892:146–54.

6. Wajchenberg BL. Subcutaneous and visceral adipose tissue: their relation to the metabolic syndrome. Endocr Rev. 2000;21(6):697–738.

7. Cruz ML, Bergman RN, Goran MI. Unique effect of visceral fat on insulin sensitivity in obese Hispanic children with a family history of type 2 diabetes. Diabetes Care. 2002;25(9):1631–36.

8. Bacha F, Saad R, Gungor N, Janosky J, Arslanian SA. Obesity, regional fat distribution, and syndrome X in obese black versus white adolescents: race differential in diabetogenic and atherogenic risk factors. J Clin Endocrinol Metab. 2003;88(6):2534–40.

9. Taksali SE, Caprio S, Dziura J, Dufour S, Calí AM, Goodman TR, Papademetris X, Burgert TS, Pierpont BM, Savoye M, Shaw M, Seyal AA, Weiss R. High visceral and low abdominal subcutaneous fat stores in the obese adolescent: a determinant of an adverse metabolic phenotype. Diabetes. 2008;57(2):367–71.

10. Jensen MD. Role of body fat distribution and the metabolic complications of obesity. J Clin Endocrinol Metab. 2008;93(11 Suppl 1):S57–63.

11. Sinha R, Dufour S, Petersen KF, LeBon V, Enoksson S, Ma YZ, Savoye M, Rothman DL, Shulman GI, Caprio S. Assessment of skeletal muscle triglyceride content by (1)H nuclear magnetic resonance spectroscopy in lean and obese adolescents: relationships to insulin sensitivity, total body fat, and central adiposity. Diabetes. 2002;51(4):1022–27.

12. Weiss R, Dufour S, Taksali SE, Tamborlane WV, Petersen KF, Bonadonna RC, Boselli L, Barbetta G, Allen K, Rife F, Savoye M, Dziura J, Sherwin R, Shulman GI, Caprio S. Prediabetes in obese youth: a syndrome of impaired glucose tolerance, severe insulin resistance, and altered myocellular and abdominal fat partitioning. Lancet. 2003;362(9388):951–57.

13. Shulman GI. Cellular mechanisms of insulin resistance. J Clin Invest. 2000;106(2):171–76.

14. Stumvoll M, Tataranni PA, Stefan N, Vozarova B, Bogardus C. Glucose allostasis. Diabetes. 2003;52(4):903–9.

15. Weiss R, Cali AM, Dziura J, Burgert TS, Tamborlane WV, Caprio S. Degree of obesity and glucose allostasis are major effectors of glucose tolerance dynamics in obese youth. Diabetes Care. 2007;30(7):1845–50.

16. Facchini F, Chen YD, Hollenbeck CB, Reaven GM. Relationship between resistance to insulin-mediated glucose uptake, urinary uric acid clearance, and plasma uric acid concentration. J Am Med Assoc. 1991;266(21):3008–11.

17. Dunaif A. Insulin resistance and the polycystic ovary syndrome: mechanism and implications for pathogenesis. Endocr Rev. 1997;18(6):774–800.

18. Anderson EA, Hoffman RP, Balon TW, Sinkey CA, Mark AL. Hyperinsulinemia produces both sympathetic neural activation and vasodilation in normal humans. J Clin Invest. 1991;87(6):2246–52.

19. Van Gaal LF, Mertens IL, De Block CE. Mechanisms linking obesity with cardiovascular disease. Nature. 2006;444(7121):875–80.

20. Grundy SM. Hypertriglyceridemia, atherogenic dyslipidemia, and the metabolic syndrome. Am J Cardiol. 1998;81: 18–25B.

21. Festa A, Williams K, Hanley AJ, Otvos JD, Goff DC, Wagenknecht LE, Haffner SM. Nuclear magnetic resonance lipoprotein abnormalities in prediabetic subjects in the Insulin Resistance Atherosclerosis Study. Circulation. 2005;111:3465–72.

22. Bell RA, Mayer-Davis EJ, Beyer JW, D'Agostino RB Jr, Lawrence JM, Linder B, Liu LL, Marcovina SM, Rodriguez BL, Williams D, Dabelea D, SEARCH for Diabetes in Youth Study Group. Diabetes in non-Hispanic white youth: prevalence, incidence, and clinical characteristics: the SEARCH for Diabetes in Youth Study. Diabetes Care. 2009;32(Suppl 2):S102–11.

23. Mayer-Davis EJ, Beyer J, Bell RA, Dabelea D, D'Agostino R Jr, Imperatore G, Lawrence JM, Liese AD, Liu L, Marcovina S, Rodriguez B, SEARCH for Diabetes in Youth Study Group. Diabetes in African American youth: prevalence, incidence, and clinical characteristics: the SEARCH for Diabetes in Youth Study. Diabetes Care. 2009;32(Suppl 2):S112–22.

24. Lawrence JM, Mayer-Davis EJ, Reynolds K, Beyer J, Pettitt DJ, D'Agostino RB Jr, Marcovina SM, Imperatore G, Hamman RF. SEARCH for Diabetes in Youth Study Group. Diabetes in Hispanic American youth: prevalence, incidence, demographics, and clinical characteristics: the SEARCH for Diabetes in Youth Study. Diabetes Care. 2009;32(Suppl 2):S123–32.

25. Lobstein T, Jackson-Leach R. Estimated burden of paediatric obesity and co-morbidities in Europe. Part 2. Numbers of children with indicators of obesity-related disease. Int J Pediatr Obes. 2006;1(1):33–41.

26. Li C, Ford ES, Zhao G, Mokdad AH. Prevalence of pre-diabetes and its association with clustering of cardiometabolic risk factors and hyperinsulinemia among U.S. adolescents: National Health and Nutrition Examination Survey 2005–2006. Diabetes Care. 2009;32(2):342–47.

27. Weiss R, Kaufman FR. Metabolic complications of childhood obesity: identifying and mitigating the risk. Diabetes Care. 2008;31(Suppl 2):S310–6.

28. Weiss R, Dufour S, Taksali SE, Tamborlane WV, Petersen KF, Bonadonna RC, Boselli L, Barbetta G, Allen K, Rife F, Savoye M, Dziura J, Sherwin R, Shulman GI, Caprio S. Prediabetes in obese youth: a syndrome of impaired glucose tolerance, severe insulin resistance, and altered myocellular and abdominal fat partitioning. Lancet. 2003;362(9388):951–57.

29. Weiss R, Taksali SE, Dufour S, Yeckel CW, Papademetris X, Cline G, Tamborlane WV, Dziura J, Shulman GI, Caprio S. The "obese insulin-sensitive" adolescent: importance of adiponectin and lipid partitioning. J Clin Endocrinol Metab. 2005;90(6):3731–37.

30. Weiss R, Dziura JD, Burgert TS, Taksali SE, Tamborlane WV, Caprio S. Ethnic differences in beta cell adaptation to insulin resistance in obese children and adolescents. Diabetologia. 2006;49(3):571–79.

31. Kahn SE, Prigeon RL, McCulloch DK, Boyko EJ, Bergman RN, Schwartz MW, Neifing JL, Ward WK, Beard JC, Palmer JP, Porte D. Quantification of the relationship between insulin sensitivity and beta-cell function in human subjects. Evidence for a hyperbolic function. Diabetes. 1993;42(11):1663–72.

32. Weiss R, Cali AM, Dziura J, Burgert TS, Tamborlane WV. Caprio S Degree of obesity and glucose allostasis are major effectors of glucose tolerance dynamics in obese youth. Diabetes Care. 2007;30(7):1845–50.

33. Weiss R, Caprio S, Trombetta M, Taksali SE, Tamborlane WV, Bonadonna R. Beta-cell function across the spectrum of glucose tolerance in obese youth. Diabetes. 2005;54(6):1735–43.

34. Yeckel CW, Taksali SE, Dziura J, Weiss R, Burgert TS, Sherwin RS, Tamborlane WV, Caprio S. The normal glucose tolerance continuum in obese youth: evidence for impairment in beta-cell function independent of insulin resistance. J Clin Endocrinol Metab. 2005;90(2):747–54.

35. Weiss R, Taksali SE, Tamborlane WV, Burgert TS, Savoye M, Caprio S. Predictors of changes in glucose tolerance status in obese youth. Diabetes Care. 2005;28(4):902–9.

36. Cali AM, Man CD, Cobelli C, Dziura J, Seyal A, Shaw M, Allen K, Chen S, Caprio S. Primary defects in beta-cell function further exacerbated by worsening of insulin resistance mark the development of impaired glucose tolerance in obese adolescents. Diabetes Care. 2009;32(3):456–61.

37. Bacha F, Gungor N, Lee S, Arslanian SA. In vivo insulin sensitivity and secretion in obese youth: what are the differences between normal glucose tolerance, impaired glucose tolerance, and type 2 diabetes? Diabetes Care. 2009; 32(1):100–5.

38. Gami AS, Witt BJ, Howard DE, Erwin PJ, Gami LA, Somers VK, Montori VM. Metabolic syndrome and risk of incident cardiovascular events and death: a systematic review and meta-analysis of longitudinal studies. J Am Coll Cardiol. 2007;49(4):403–14.

39. Pyorala M, Miettinen H, Halonen P, Laakso M, Pyorala K. Insulin resistance syndrome predicts the risk of coronary heart disease and stroke in healthy middle-aged men: the 22-year follow-up results of the Helsinki Policemen Study. Arterioscler Thromb Vasc Biol. 2000;20:538–44.

40. Cornier MA, Dabelea D, Hernandez TL, Lindstrom RC, Steig AJ, Stob NR, Van Pelt RE, Wang H, Eckel RH. The metabolic syndrome. Endocr Rev. 2008;29(7):777–822.

41. Reaven GM. Role of insulin resistance in human disease. Diabetes. 1988;37:1595–607.

42. Kahn R, Buse J, Ferrannini E, Stern M, American Diabetes Association. European Association for the Study of Diabetes. The metabolic syndrome: time for a critical appraisal: joint statement from the American Diabetes Association and the European Association for the Study of Diabetes. Diabetes Care. 2005;28(9):2289–304.

43. Brambilla P, Lissau I, Flodmark CE, Moreno LA, Widhalm K, Wabitsch M, Pietrobelli A. Metabolic risk-factor clustering estimation in children: to draw a line across pediatric metabolic syndrome. Int J Obes (Lond). 2007;31(4):591–600.

44. Baker JL, Olsen LW, Sørensen TI. Childhood body-mass index and the risk of coronary heart disease in adulthood. N Engl J Med. 2007;357(23):2329–37.

45. Freedman DS, Mei Z, Srinivasan SR, Berenson GS, Dietz WH. Cardiovascular risk factors and excess adiposity among overweight children and adolescents: the Bogalusa Heart Study. J Pediatr. 2007;150(1):12–17.

46. Tirosh A, Shai I, Tekes-Manova D, Israeli E, Pereg D, Shochat T, Kochba I, Rudich A, Israeli Diabetes Research Group. Normal fasting plasma glucose levels and type 2 diabetes in young men. N Engl J Med. 2005;353(14):1454–62.

47. Tirosh A, Shai I, Bitzur R, Kochba I, Tekes-Manova D, Israeli E, Shochat T, Rudich A. Changes in triglyceride levels over time and risk of type 2 diabetes in young men. Diabetes Care. 2008;31(10):2032–37.

48. Tirosh A, Rudich A, Shochat T, Tekes-Manova D, Israeli E, Henkin Y, Kochba I, Shai I. Changes in triglyceride levels and risk for coronary heart disease in young men. Ann Intern Med. 2007;147(6):377–85.

49. Dabelea D, Pettitt DJ, Jones KL, Arslanian SA. T2DM mellitus in minority children and adolescents: an emerging problem. Endocrinol Metab Clin North Am. 1999;28:709–29.

50. Haines L, Wan KC, Lynn R, Barrett TG, Shield JP. Rising incidence of type 2 diabetes in children in the U.K. Diabetes Care. 2007;30(5):1097–101.

51. Arslanian SA. Metabolic differences between Caucasian and African-American children and the relationship to T2DM mellitus. J Pediatr Endocrinol Metab. 2002;15(Suppl 1):509–17.

52. Arslanian SA, Saad R, Lewy V, Danadian K, Janosky J. Hyperinsulinemia in African-American children: decreased insulin clearance and increased insulin secretion and its relationship to insulin sensitivity. Diabetes. 2002;51:3014–19.

53. Misra A, Wasir JS, Vikram NK. Waist circumference criteria for the diagnosis of abdominal obesity are not applicable uniformly to all populations and ethnic groups. Nutrition. 2005;21(9):969–76.

14 Pathogenesis and Management of Dyslipidemia in Obese Children

Brian W. McCrindle

CONTENTS

Key Words: Cholesterol, triglycerides, lipoprotein, free fatty acids, cardiovascular disease, metabolic syndrome, diet, statin, bile acid, fibrate, nicotinic acid

INTRODUCTION AND SUMMARY

Lipid abnormalities are common in overweight and obese children and adolescents. The underlying pathogenesis is complex, most closely related to visceral adiposity, and driven by insulin resistance and high levels of circulating free fatty acids. Clinically, dyslipidemia is characterized by a triad of abnormalities including elevated triglycerides, decreased high-density lipoprotein (HDL) levels, and qualitative changes in low-density lipoprotein (LDL) particles, which become smaller, denser, and more atherogenic. These lipid abnormalities cluster with other metabolic risk factors and contribute to the definition of metabolic syndrome in adults and emerging definitions of metabolic syndrome in children. The evaluation of overweight and obese children and adolescents should include a fasting lipid profile and a detailed family history for risk factors and cardiovascular disease. Healthy lifestyle and weight management counseling are essential. Exercise and activity interventions associated with decreases in visceral adiposity and increases in muscle mass can improve lipid abnormalities even before significant weight loss is achieved. Dietary strategies aimed at reducing refined carbohydrates and fat intake, while increasing intake of fiber and fish oil, can have an important impact on triglyceride levels. Few patients will meet criteria for starting lipid-lowering drug therapy unless there are important concomitant morbidities such as diabetes or hypertension or an underlying familial dyslipidemia. Identification and effective management of lipid abnormalities in this setting are important in order to prevent and reverse accelerated atherosclerosis.

From: *Contemporary Endocrinology: Pediatric Obesity: Etiology, Pathogenesis, and Treatment*
Edited by: M. Freemark, DOI 10.1007/978-1-60327-874-4_14,
© Springer Science+Business Media, LLC 2010

PATHOPHYSIOLOGIC ASPECTS

Basic Lipid Metabolism

Lipoprotein particles. In order for lipids to be transported in the hydrophilic environment of the circulation they must be packaged within particles that give them a hydrophilic surface. Lipoprotein particles consist of a hydrophobic core of triglycerides and cholesterol esters surrounded by a hydrophilic bilayer of phospholipids facing outward and free cholesterol facing inward. Embedded in the surface are various regulatory proteins responsible for receptor recognition and metabolic functions. These particles are characterized by their internal density, which is lower if there is a greater proportion of triglycerides and higher if there is a greater proportion of cholesterol esters. They are also characterized by their size and by the types of proteins on their surface.

Transport and metabolism of exogenous lipids. Dietary triglycerides (broken down to monoglycerides and free fatty acids [FFA]) and cholesterol (broken down to unesterified cholesterol and FFA) are absorbed from the intestinal lumen into the intestinal villae where they are reassembled as triglycerides and cholesterol esters. These are then packaged as very large buoyant particles called chylomicrons, which enter the circulation via the lymphatic system. Chylomicrons are characterized primarily by the presence of apolipoproteins B48, C-II, and E. As they circulate, the triglycerides are metabolized by peripheral lipoprotein lipase residing on endothelial cells. Triglycerides are removed and hydrolyzed to FFA and monoglycerol, with the FFA being taken up by muscle cells as an energy source and by adipocytes for storage. The particle shrinks in size and increases in density to become a chylomicron-remnant particle, which is cleared by the liver through interaction with particle surface apolipoprotein E and hepatocyte low-density lipoprotein (LDL)-like receptors.

Transport and metabolism of endogenous lipids. FFA taken up by the liver serve as substrates for triglyceride synthesis and stimulate production of apolipoprotein B. Endogenesis synthesis of free cholesterol within hepatocytes from acetyl CoA is mediated by a rate-limiting enzyme, 3-hydroxy-3-methyl-glutaryl coenzyme A (HMG-CoA) reductase. The triglycerides are incorporated with esterified cholesterol into lipoprotein particles called very-low-density lipoproteins (VLDL), which have surface apolipoproteins B100 and E. The triglycerides within circulating VLDL particles are metabolized by lipoprotein lipase and apolipoproteins C-II and C-III, causing the particle to become smaller and denser (higher proportion of cholesterol ester content). This forms an intermediate density lipoprotein (IDL). IDL can be cleared by the liver via hepatocyte LDL receptors by recognition of apolipoprotein E. Additionally, the triglyceride within IDL is further metabolized by lipoprotein lipase and hepatic lipase, causing the particle to become even smaller and more denser, forming a low-density lipoprotein (LDL). LDL particles may deliver their cholesterol esters to macrophages and other tissues through a non-receptor-mediated uptake, often after oxidation. LDL particles are cleared from the circulation by the liver through recognition of surface apolipoprotein B100 by the hepatocyte LDL receptor.

The pathway by which cholesterol is transported away from peripheral cells and tissues, such as macrophages and arterial wall foam cells, to the liver for uptake and excretion into bile is referred to as reverse cholesterol transport. Free cholesterol is removed from peripheral cells by the interaction of apolipoprotein A-I on the nascent HDL particle (a flattened disc-like structure) with the ATP-binding membrane cassette (ABC) transporter, ABCA1. The cholesterol in the nascent HDL is esterified by lecithin cholesterol acyl transferase (LCAT), with apolipoprotein A-I as a co-factor, producing a more mature, larger, and more spherical HDL particle with cholesterol ester in its core. Less than half the time, this HDL particle can deliver its cholesterol ester to the liver through the interaction of apolipoprotein A-I with the HDL receptor (also called scavenger receptor type I). The cholesterol delivered to the liver may be excreted into bile either as cholesterol or by conversion of cholesterol into bile acids. Alternatively, HDL can transfer cholesterol esters to the apolipoprotein B-containing lipoproteins (VLDL, IDL, and LDL) in exchange for their triglyceride by the cholesterol ester transfer protein (CETP).

Pathogenesis of obesity-related lipid abnormalities. The pathogenesis of the lipid abnormalities associated with obesity has been well described, although the relative contributions of various driving forces continue to be debated *(1–4)*. The manifest lipid abnormalities, characterized by low levels of HDL-C, high triglycerides, and the presence of qualitative changes in LDL, rendering it a smaller, denser and more atherogenic particle, are referred to as the lipid triad. The triad is accompanied by a host of other associated lipid abnormalities, which are listed in Table 1.

Table 1
Lipid Abnormalities Associated with the Metabolic Syndrome and Obesity

Increased plasma VLDL-C
Increased plasma remnant particles
Elevated non-HDL-C
Elevated serum triglycerides
Preponderance of small, dense LDL particles
Elevated apolipoprotein B
Reduced concentration of HDL-C
Presence of small, dense HDL particles
Decreased apolipoprotein A-1
Increased apolipoprotein C-III
Increased plasma free fatty acid levels
Postprandial lipemia

VLDL-C, very-low-density lipoprotein cholesterol; HDL-C, high-density lipoprotein cholesterol; LDL, low-density lipoprotein; apo, apolipoprotein.
The basic pathophysiology underlying the lipid triad is shown in Fig. 1.

Overproduction of VLDL. The features of the lipid triad are primarily explained by an increase in the number of VLDL particles which have higher relative content of triglycerides. Overproduction of VLDL is driven by increased delivery of FFA to the liver, with subsequent increased synthesis of triglycerides as well as apolipoprotein B100. The excess FFA are derived from adipose tissue and from hydrolysis of triglycerides from VLDL which, under normal circumstances, are taken up by muscle as an energy source and by adipose tissue for storage. The insulin resistance associated with visceral adiposity appears to be a key factor. Increased release of FFA from adipocytes occurs when visceral adipose triglyceride stores are increased and insulin resistance results in lack of inhibition of hormone-sensitive lipase. In extra-adipose tissues, the resistance to insulin impairs the activation of lipoprotein lipase, which favors the accumulation of VLDL particles.

The lipid triad. The increased plasma triglyceride level is a direct reflection of overproduction and inadequate uptake and utilization of VLDL particles. The fall in HDL results from chemical transformation of the particle. Cholesterol ester transfer protein mediates an exchange of triglyceride in VLDL for cholesterol esters in HDL, resulting in a relative increase in triglyceride in HDL. The triglyceride in HDL is then metabolized by the action of hepatic lipase, creating a smaller, denser particle, as well as free apolipoprotein A-I. This altered HDL particle is more readily cleared from plasma or excreted via the kidney, resulting in lower circulating HDL-C levels.

A similar process results in the production of small, dense LDL particles. Cholesterol ester transfer protein-mediated exchange of triglyceride from VLDL with cholesterol ester from LDL results in a triglyceride-enriched LDL particle, which becomes smaller and denser as triglycerides are metabolized

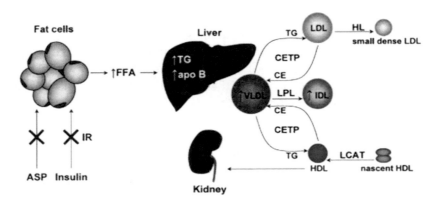

Fig. 1. Pathophysiology of the obesity-related lipid triad. Lack of sensitivity of the metabolically active adipocyte to the regulatory effects of insulin and acylation stimulating protein result in the increased release of circulating free fatty acids. These contribute excessive substrate for triglyceride production, stimulate production of apolipoprotein B in the liver, which are then incorporated into an increased production of triglyceride-enriched VLDL particles. Triglyceride from VLDL is exchanged with cholesterol esters from both LDL and HDL particles, a process mediated by cholesterol ester transfer protein. Hepatic lipase metabolizes the triglyceride content of both HDL and LDL, resulting in smaller, denser particles. For LDL, this results in a more atherogenic particle, and for HDL, this results in increased catabolism and clearance. Reproduced with permission from Mudd et al. *(13).* apo, apolipoprotein; ASP, acylation stimulating protein; CE, cholesterol ester; CETP, cholesterol ester transfer protein; FFA, free fatty acids; HDL, high-density lipoprotein; HL, hepatic lipase; IDL, intermediate-density lipoprotein; IR, insulin resistance; LCAT, lecithin cholesterol acyl transferase; LDL, low-density lipoprotein; TG, triglyceride; VLDL, very-low-density lipoprotein.

by hepatic lipase. These particles are more atherogenic, in that they more easily enter and are retained with the arterial wall, with subsequent oxidation and glycation, inducing foam cell formation and endothelial dysfunction.

FFA and hyperglycemia. Incomplete oxidation of FFA can generate metabolites like kiacyglycerol, ceramide, and reactive oxygen species which can increase hepatic gluconeogenesis, reduce insulin-dependent glucose uptake in skeletal muscle, and impair glucose-stimulated insulin secretion in pancreatic beta cells. In the aggregate, these effects contribute to hyperglycemia. Many of the effects of increased FFA are similar to the effects of decreased adiponectin, another feature of increased visceral adiposity. The effects of FFA and hypoadiponectinemia are potentiated by inflammatory cytokines produced in response to chronic inflammation in visceral adipose tissue (see Chapter 13 by Weiss et al., this volume).

CLINICAL ASPECTS

Assessment and Interpretation

When to assess. Recommendations for the assessment of lipid abnormalities for children and adolescents differ depending on the context. For the *general population*, initial guidelines from an NIH Expert Panel published in 1992 advocated both a population-based and a high-risk individual-based strategies *(5).* The population-based strategy did not recommend universal lipid assessment, but rather dietary goals to be applied to the general population. These aimed at shifting lipid levels for all children and adolescents. The *high-risk individual*-based strategy was a selective screening and tiered intervention algorithm aimed at identifying those children most at risk of having a clinically significant elevation of LDL. Decisions to screen were based on a family history of hypercholesterolemia and/or the presence of premature atherosclerotic cardiovascular disease events or morbidity in first-degree relatives. Children without available family history data could be screened if other risk factors were present, including obesity. Initial screening consisted of a fasting total cholesterol assessment or a full lipoprotein profile. Stratification of abnormalities directing the intensity of further assessment and intervention were based on the average of two fasting LDL results. Primary criticisms of these guidelines included (a) the lack of reliability of family history as an entry criterion for screening; (b) the limited focus on LDL; (c) the single cutpoint applied across age, sex, and ethnicity; and, eventually (d) the failure to address the emerging epidemic of childhood obesity.

Some of these concerns have led to recent modifications, including the addition of overweight and obesity as entry criteria for screening, the confirmation of the safety but limited efficacy of fat and cholesterol dietary restrictions, and a clarification of the role of lipid-lowering drug therapy (6). These modifications were adopted into the recent guidelines from the American Academy of Pediatrics, with minor differences (7). Most recently, the National Heart, Lung and Blood Institute has again convened an Expert Panel to develop best evidence-based risk factor guidelines for children and adolescents that can incorporate recommendations for each of the individual risk factors and behaviors in an integrated approach. In this way, guidelines for management of lipid abnormalities (including abnormalities of triglycerides and non-HDL) are more explicitly defined in relation to the presence and management of other risk factors and risk conditions (http://www.nhlbi.nih.gov/guidelines/cvd_ped/).

Recommendations for the evaluation of overweight or obese children and adolescents (defined by BMI percentile ≥85th percentile) now include assessment of a lipid profile obtained after at least a 12-h overnight fast (8,9). Canadian guidelines recommend that a fasting lipid profile be performed for overweight and obese children aged 10 years and older, although earlier screening is recommended at younger ages if the family history is positive for hyperlipidemia or premature atherosclerotic cardiovascular disease (9). US guidelines have no age restriction (8). The inclusion of waist circumference as an additional indicator of risk of lipid abnormalities in the setting of childhood obesity has been advocated (10).

What to assess. A fasting lipid profile includes assessment in plasma of total cholesterol, triglycerides, and HDL-C, with calculation of LDL-C using the Friedewald formula (LDL-C = total cholesterol – HDL-C – [triglycerides/5]; measurements in mg/dl) (11). For children with triglyceride levels ≥400 mg/dl, the Friedewald calculation of LDL-C is invalid. While direct methods of LDL-C measurement are more accurate than the Friedewald calculation, they remain primarily a specialized tool (12).

These laboratory assessments measure the cholesterol content attributable to a class of lipoprotein particles, but do not assess the number or characteristics of these particles. The addition of measurement of apolipoprotein B has been advocated as measure of the number of atherogenic particles and a more accurate assessment of LDL-C, as well as an indirect indicator of the presence of small, dense LDL particles (13,14). Likewise, assessment of apolipoprotein A-I levels may be an indirect indicator of the number and size of HDL particles. A number of specialized methods have been developed to more directly determine lipoprotein particle size and concentration, but they are not widely available or utilized at present (15–17). Distributions of values, demographic correlates, and relationship to measures of adiposity have been shown in children in the Bogalusa Heart Study, with a suggestion that they may provide a better understanding of the relationship between early lipid abnormalities and cardiovascular risk (18,19). They have been shown in adults to provide a more accurate assessment of risk of cardiovascular disease and may identify patients with "normal" levels of LDL-C who may benefit from LDL-lowering therapy (20). This may be of particular relevance for patients with overweight and obesity. In children, variations in subclasses of VLDL have been noted in relation to measures of adiposity, with significant racial differences (21).

In summary, a standard fasting lipid profile may give an accurate evaluation of abnormalities of triglyceride and HDL-C levels and a less accurate assessment of abnormalities of LDL-C levels, but does not provide specific information regarding VLDL-C levels or qualitative abnormalities in HDL and LDL particle characteristics and subclasses prevalent in the setting of the metabolic syndrome. Nonetheless, it does provide sufficient information for screening and clinical decision-making.

Definition of abnormal. Normal lipid values are based on representative population-based standardized assessments of fasting lipid profiles. Definitions of abnormality for children and adolescents are based on the magnitude of deviation from the central value of the distribution, usually based on percentile cutpoints. Table 2 gives a classification scheme based roughly on LDL-C, non-HDL-C, and triglyceride values above the 75th percentile (borderline) and 95th percentile (abnormal), or HDL-C levels below the 10th percentile. The normal values derived from the Lipid Research Clinics (LRC) Program Prevalence Study, which included a cross-sectional assessment of predominately white children and adolescents and are the cutpoints used in the original NIH Expert Panel recommendations *(22,24–26)*. This study determined age and gender-related maturational associations with lipid values. These cutpoints have been used as the basis for classifying dyslipidemia in both NIH Expert Panel and AAP lipid guidelines for children and adolescents. They do not, however, take into account maturational changes with age and differences with respect to sex and race.

Table 2
Classification of Plasma Lipid Concentrations (mg/dl) for Children and Adolescents[a]

Laboratory parameter	Acceptable	Borderline	Abnormal
Total cholesterol	<170	170–199	≥200
LDL-C	<110	110–129	≥130
HDL-C	>45	40–45	<40
Triglycerides			
<10 years of age	<75	75–99	≥100
10–19 years of age	<90	90–129	≥130
Non-HDL-C[b]	<120	120–144	≥145

[a]Based on a standard fasting lipid profile *(22)*.
[b]From the Bogalusa Heart Study *(23)*.

The National Health and Nutrition Examination Survey (NHANES) is a contemporary series of cross-sectional assessments based on a sampling strategy within the general population and, thus, has greater validity than the Lipid Research Clinics Program Prevalence Study. NHANES data have been used to determine the distribution of lipid values and associations with age, sex and race, and trends over time. Age and sex-specific normal values are linked to the cutpoints for young adults used for the Adult Treatment Panel (ATP) III recommendations, which are calibrated to risk of cardiovascular disease in adults *(27,28)*. For males' ages 12–20 years, high borderline and high cutpoints correspond to the 86th and 97th percentiles respectively for total cholesterol, the 86th and 98th percentiles for LDL-C, and the 89th and 95th percentiles for triglycerides, with low HDL-C defined as below the 26th percentile. For females' ages 12–20 years, high borderline and high cutpoints correspond to the 78th and 94th percentiles respectively for total cholesterol, the 83th and 95th percentiles for LDL-C, and the 89th and 95th percentiles for triglycerides, with low HDL-C defined as below the 26th percentile. Growth curves are provided with these cutpoints modeled over the age spectrum. Comparison of the lipid classification schemes from the LRC and NHANES as applied to several population-based cohort study datasets has shown that the age and sex-specific cutpoints from NHANES are more predictive of low HDL-C levels in adults but less predictive of high total cholesterol, LDL-C and triglyceride levels *(29)*. It might be argued that for clinical purposes, the simpler cutpoints from the LRC be preferred over the more complex cutpoints from NHANES, especially given that exact specification of future risk of atherosclerotic cardiovascular disease remains unclear.

The role of race and sex in relation to lipid values has been addressed in several studies. After puberty, young white males have been shown to have significant adverse changes in total cholesterol, LDL-C, VLDL-C, and HDL-C levels, with less significant changes for white and black females and black males *(30)*. Race differences in triglycerides and VLDL-C between blacks and whites have been noted, with higher VLDL-C and triglyceride levels in whites and slightly higher HDL-C in blacks *(21,31)*. White males have lower HDL-C levels than black males and white females. Although differences in lipid values are evident relevant to race and sex, the magnitude of these differences is felt to be sufficiently small such that their specification regarding cutpoints would add complexity without significantly enhancing relevance.

Lipid abnormalities and subsequent development of cardiovascular disease. The relationship of lipid abnormalities identified in youth with the subsequent development of atherosclerotic cardiovascular disease in adulthood is an important issue, which would provide the necessary imperative to identify and treat lipid abnormalities in youth. Only indirect evidence is available. The Bogalusa Heart Study performed serial cross-sectional assessments in a biracial community and has reported normal lipid values and important correlates, including associations with the degree of atherosclerotic arterial involvement both in pathologic studies and studies using non-invasive vascular markers *(32–35)*. This study and other similar studies were also instrumental in confirming tracking of lipid abnormalities from childhood and adolescence into adulthood, particularly when measures of adiposity are taken into account *(36–38)*. An autopsy analysis of 34 subjects (mean age 18 years) who had participated in the Bogalusa Heart Study *(39)* showed that percent surface involvement of the aorta with fatty streaks correlated with total cholesterol ($r = 0.67$) and LDL-C ($r = 0.67$). The relationship with LDL-C was linear, suggesting the absence of a clear cutpoint for increased risk. Associations with VLDL-C, HDL-C, and triglycerides were weaker and non-significant. Percent surface involvement of the coronary arteries with fatty streaks correlated only with VLDL-C ($r = 0.41$). A later Bogalusa Heart Study analysis of autopsies of 204 participants ages 2–39 (death from various causes) showed similar correlations between vascular involvement and total cholesterol and LDL-C *(35)*.

Importantly, the number of risk factors had an exponential and non-linear relationship with percent surface involvement of the coronary arteries with fibrous plaques *(35)*. This finding would suggest that the clustering of lipid abnormalities and other obesity-related risk factors (as in the metabolic syndrome) greatly accelerates the atherosclerotic process. This hypothesis is supported by studies of carotid atherogenesis in living subjects. Carotid intima-media thickness (CIMT) was assessed in 486 adults ages 25–37 years who were serially assessed in the Bogalusa Heart Study *(40)*. Increased CIMT was independently related to childhood measures of higher LDL-C and BMI, adulthood measures of higher LDL-C and systolic blood pressure and lower HDL-C, and long-term cumulative burden of LDL-C and HDL-C. The relationships with LDL-C and CIMT appeared to slightly non-linear, with some acceleration in the upper quartile of LDL-C values. In a study pooling data from several cohorts, the presence of dyslipidemia in association with overweight and obesity in adolescents has been shown to be associated with increased CIMT in young adulthood, more so than in the presence of dyslipidemia alone *(41)*. These observations provide an important imperative for prevention, detection, and treatment of lipid abnormalities and associated metabolic co-morbidities in overweight and obese youth.

Lipid abnormalities as components of definitions of the metabolic syndrome. The metabolic syndrome remains a controversial concept when applied to children and adolescents, and it is unclear what additional information is derived from its application to a population experiencing changes in growth and development (42). The dichotomous categorization of what, in reality, is a continuous marker of risk may oversimplify a complex pathophysiologic process that remains incompletely understood. Some have argued that there is currently insufficient evidence to define the metabolic syndrome in children and adolescents (43,44). The relationship of the metabolic syndrome to measures of adiposity appears to be non-linear, with the risk of metabolic syndrome increasing dramatically when measures of adiposity exceed the 85th–95th percentile. A study using NHANES data showed prevalence of metabolic syndrome in 12–19-year-old adolescents to be 0.1% for those with BMI <85th percentile, 6.8% for those with BMI at the 85th to <95th percentiles, and 28.7% for those with BMI >95th percentile (45).

Yet, in terms of lipid abnormalities, the use of the concept of metabolic syndrome may raise the imperative to evaluate and treat high-risk patients more aggressively. Therapies can be aimed at altering the underlying pathophysiologic milieu generating the metabolic syndrome, which is the main goal of lifestyle interventions aimed at reducing adiposity. Alternatively, therapies can be aimed at the individual risk factor components, including lipid abnormalities, but in an integrated manner.

Despite controversy regarding the conceptualization of the metabolic syndrome in youth, many definitions have been proposed, leading to differing estimates of prevalence (46). Most of the definitions are based on extrapolations of definitions developed for adults and differ in the components included and their cutpoints for defining abnormalities (Table 3) (50). Definitions include values from a fasting lipid profile, predominately HDL-C and triglyceride levels; patients taking lipid-lowering drugs are considered to have met the lipid abnormality criteria. The definition proposed by the International Diabetes Federation seems to be gaining popularity, mainly because it represents a compromise between single cutpoints across age and gender groups and strict use of percentile cutpoints.

Table 3
Fasting Lipid Abnormalities Contributing to Definitions of Metabolic Syndrome in Children

	HDL-C	Triglycerides
Cook (45)	≤40 mg/dl	≥110 mg/dl
De Ferranti (47)	<50 mg/dl in girls	
	<45 mg/dl in boys	≥100 mg/dl
Weiss (48)	<5th percentile	>95th percentile
IDF (49)		
6 to <10 years	No cutpoint	No cutpoint
10–16 years[a]	≤40 mg/dl	≥150 mg/dl
≥17 years[a]	≤50 mg/dl in girls	≥150 mg/dl
	≤40 mg/dl in boys	≥150 mg/dl

[a]Children and adolescents aged 10 years and older who are taking lipid-lowering drugs are to be considered as having met the lipid abnormality criteria.
dl, deciliter; HDL-C, high-density lipoprotein cholesterol; IDF, International Diabetes Federation; mg, milligrams.

Lipid abnormalities remain one of the most prevalent components in the setting of metabolic syndrome. From NHANES data, triglyceride levels >110 mg/dl were noted in 23.4% of the general population of 12–19-year-old adolescents, with a prevalence of 17.6% for those with BMI <85th percentile, 33.5% for those at the 85th to <95th percentile, and 51.8% for those with BMI >95th percentile

(45). Likewise, HDL-C levels ≤40 mg/dl were noted in 23.3%, with a prevalence of 17.7% for those with BMI <85th percentile, 32.3% for those at the 85th to <95th percentile, and 50.0% for those with BMI >95th percentile. In a case-control study of children and adolescents, fasting triglyceride levels were strongly associated with higher degrees of adiposity, but no differences were noted between moderately versus severely obese subjects (Fig. 2) *(48)*. A gradient of lower HDL-C was also noted, with a less marked gradient for higher LDL-C. There was a non-linear association between lipid values and insulin resistance. Of note, the 95th percentile of the LDL-C distribution for each adiposity category did not exceed 110 mg/dl; thus, it would be unlikely for even a severely obese child or adolescent to meet criteria for starting a lipid-lowering drug.

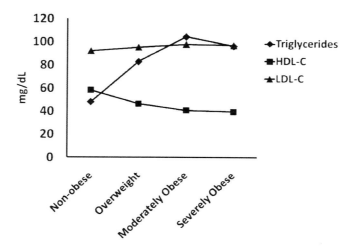

Fig. 2. Mean fasting lipid value related to level of adiposity. Non-obese = BMI <85th percentile; overweight = BMI 85th–97th percentile; moderately obese – BMI Z-score 2.0–2.5; severely obese = BMI Z-score >2.5. dl, deciliter; HDL-C, high-density lipoprotein cholesterol; LDL-C, low-density lipoprotein cholesterol; mg, milligrams.

Consideration has been given as to the inclusion of other lipid abnormalities in the definition of metabolic syndrome. Non-HDL-C is a readily available parameter from a standard fasting lipid profile and has some validity for measurement in non-fasting samples as well *(51)*. It is felt to represent the level of all classes of atherogenic lipoprotein particles. It has been shown to be a marker for diabetes risk in adolescents, a relationship that is strengthened in the presence of obesity *(52)*. Further study using NHANES data suggests that non-HDL-C is significantly related to the number of components of the metabolic syndrome present in adolescents *(53)*. Non-HDL-C assessed during childhood has been shown to be as predictive as other lipid parameters in relation to CIMT in young adults *(51)*. Population-based values from the Bogalusa Heart Study are available *(23)*.

Contribution of obesity-related lipid abnormalities to other dyslipidemias and risk conditions. The dyslipidemia associated with obesity may in some cases be superimposed upon the metabolic abnormalities in other primary lipid disorders. For example, obese patients with *primary hypercholesterolemia* secondary to LDL-receptor mutations may have concomitant reductions in HDL-C and elevations in plasma triglycerides *(54,55)*. In other conditions, obesity may exacerbate or unmask an underlying primary predisposition for lipid abnormalities, particularly those associated with overproduction of VLDL and *primary hypertriglyceridemias* (Table 4) *(56)*.

Familial combined hyperlipidemia is a genetically heterogenous condition; the inheritance pattern is usually autosomal dominant *(57–59)*. There is considerable variation of phenotypic expression both within and between affected family members *(60)*. Lipid features include elevations in total cholesterol (more specifically associated with increased LDL-C or non-HDL-C), triglycerides (concomitantly

Table 4
Etiology of Hypertriglyceridemia

Genetic disorders
Lipoprotein lipase deficiency
Apolipoprotein C-II deficiency
Familial hypertriglyceridemia (hyperprebetalipoproteinemia)
Familial dysbetalipoproteinemia
Familial combined hyperlipidemia
Metabolic disorders
Diabetes mellitus
Obesity and insulin resistance
Fatty liver disease
Hypothyroidism[a]
Nephrotic syndrome[a]
Drugs and medications (also see Appendix)
Alcohol
Estrogens
Androgens
Corticosteroids
β-blockers, thiazides
Isotretinoin
Valproic acid
Antiretroviral protease inhibitors
Atypical antipsychotics

[a]Less common; hypercholesterolemia dominant abnormality.

associated with decreased HDL-C), or both. It is also associated with an increased risk of premature cardiovascular disease, recently been shown to be manifest as increased carotid intima-media thickness in children, and vulnerability to the metabolic syndrome *(61)*. The phenotype has many similarities to the lipid triad of abnormalities associated with the metabolic syndrome. Differentiating familial combined hyperlipidemia from the classic dyslipidemia of obesity can be challenging, particularly as they often coexist in the same patient *(59)*. This is particularly true for children and adolescents, where the metabolic abnormalities associated with obesity may be necessary for the clinical condition to manifest *(62)*. Indeed, the primary underlying pathophysiology is an overproduction of VLDL, a feature that shares with obesity-related dyslipidemia. Clinical features that may distinguish familial combined hyperlipidemia from obesity-related dyslipidemia are the presence of higher fasting levels of LDL-C, apolipoprotein B, and non-HDL than would be seen in the metabolic syndrome, together with a positive family history of variable lipid abnormalities and premature cardiovascular disease.

Familial dysbetalipoproteinemia is an autosomal recessive condition manifest as elevated total cholesterol, non-HDL-C and triglycerides, with decreased HDL-C *(63)*. Apolipoprotein E can exist as three isoforms, designated ApoE2, ApoE3, and ApoE4. Homozygosity for ApoE2 occurs in about

1 in 170 people and results in decreased hepatic clearance of VLDL and intermediate lipoprotein particles, as well as an overproduction of VLDL. It is associated with an increased risk of premature cardiovascular disease. The lipid abnormalities are usually not manifest during childhood, but can be unmasked in the presence of obesity and metabolic syndrome.

Lipid abnormalities associated with overweight and obesity can contribute important cardiovascular risk in the setting of high-risk clinical conditions other than primary lipid disorders (64). *High-risk conditions* are those that may be associated with coronary artery disease before 30 years of age; these include type-1 diabetes (mixed dyslipidemia), chronic renal disease (mixed dyslipidemia), heart transplantation recipients (lipid abnormalities associated with chronic inflammation and immunosuppressive medications), and patients who have had Kawasaki disease with persistence of coronary artery aneurysms (low HDL-C associated with subclinical inflammation). *Moderate-risk conditions* are those associated with accelerated atherosclerosis and cardiovascular disease; these include type-2 diabetes (mixed dyslipidemia), chronic inflammatory diseases such as systemic lupus erythematosus and juvenile rheumatoid arthritis (lipid abnormalities associated with chronic inflammation and medications), and patients who have had Kawasaki disease with regression of coronary artery aneurysms (low HDL-C). *At-risk conditions* are those associated with accelerated atherosclerosis as assessed by epidemiologic evidence; these include post-cancer treatment survivors, patients with congenital heart disease, and patients who have had Kawasaki disease without detected coronary artery involvement. Evaluation of children and adolescents with any of these conditions requires a fasting lipid profile and attention to the level of adiposity. The magnitude of the risk may influence decisions regarding aggressiveness of treatment for the lipid abnormalities and the target lipid levels to be achieved.

Intervention

Lifestyle management. Healthy behavior change remains the cornerstone of therapy for obesity-related lipid abnormalities. Therapy is aimed at reducing adiposity and improving the metabolic milieu, but therapy may also be targeted directly toward the lipid abnormalities.

Dietary management. Dietary management is aimed at restricting intake of saturated fat, cholesterol, and simple carbohydrates, with consideration of increasing dietary fiber and omega-3 fatty acids. Consultation and counseling with a registered dietician are recommended. Specific recommendations are noted in Table 5.

The safety of the fat- and cholesterol-restricted diet in the general pediatric population has been demonstrated in some large-scale clinical trials. The Dietary Intervention Study in Children (DISC) was a randomized trial of an intensive fat- and cholesterol-restricted dietary intervention in prepubertal children with increased LDL-C who were below the thresholds at which drug therapy would be considered (65). After 3 years, there was no impact of the dietary intervention on growth, development, and nutritional indices. However, the degree of LDL-C reduction was modest (mean –3.2 mg/dl). The effect was maintained for up to 7 years of follow-up (66). The Special Turku Coronary Risk Factor Intervention Project (STRIP) randomized 7-month-old infants to an intervention aimed at restricting dietary fat and cholesterol and increasing the proportion of mono- and polyunsaturated fat. At the age of 5 years, boys had a 9% lower LDL-C level, with no significant difference noted in girls (67). There was no impact on growth, development, or nutritional indices. A follow-up study at age 7 years confirmed persistence of the relative reductions in total cholesterol and LDL-C levels in boys, together with larger LDL particle size, effects that were not observed in girls (68).

Small studies of dietary alterations in hyperlipidemic children have shown that substitution with soy-based protein may increase HDL-C and lower VLDL-C levels and triglycerides and may lower LDL-C levels (69,70). Dietary enrichment with rapeseed or canola oil has been shown to lower triglyceride and VLDL-C levels (71). Higher fructose consumption has been linked to small, dense LDL particles, and lower intakes of antioxidant vitamins may promote subclinical inflammation.

Table 5
Dietary Recommendations for Targeting Lipid Abnormalities

Reducing LDL-C, non-HDL-C levels
- Restrict proportion of total calories to:
    25–30% from fat
    $\leq$7% from saturated fat
- Restrict cholesterol intake to <200 mg/day
- Preferred use of monounsaturated fat
- Avoidance of trans fats
- Consideration of use of fat sources enriched with plant
    sterol/stanol esters
- Increased consumption of dietary fiber

Reducing triglyceride levels
- Restrict proportion of total calories to:
    25–30% from fat
    $\leq$7% from saturated fat
- Restrict cholesterol intake to <200 mg/day
- Preferred use of monounsaturated fat
- Avoidance of trans fats
- Increased consumption of dietary fiber
- Decrease sugar intake, particularly sugar sweetened drinks
- Increase dietary fish intake as a source of omega-3 fatty acids

HDL-C, high-density lipoprotein cholesterol; LDL-C, low-density
lipoprotein cholesterol; mg, milligram.

Inflammation has increasingly emerged as an important factor in atherogenesis *(72)*. Intake of antioxidant vitamins has not been shown to be of benefit in adults, but in children and adolescents with familial hyperlipidemia, it has been associated with improvements in endothelial function and lipoprotein subclasses *(73,74)*. A clinical trial of docosohexanoic acid in children and adolescents with familial hyperlipidemia found increases in total cholesterol, LDL-C and HDL-C, and an improvement in endothelial function *(75)*. There is some clinical trial evidence to support the use of plant sterol-/stanol-enriched fat sources and dietary fiber enrichment. Plant sterols/stanols have been shown to result in modest reductions in LDL-C but no improvement in endothelial function *(76–80)*, while dietary fiber supplementation has been shown to have a variable effect in lowering triglyceride levels *(81,82)*. Increased fish consumption and fish oil (omega-3 fatty acids) supplementation has been recommended for lowering triglyceride levels, although clinical trial evidence in children is lacking *(83)*. The use of other nutritional supplements has not been well studied or, in the case of garlic extract supplements, has been shown to be of no benefit *(84)*.

Physical activity and sedentary pursuits. Increasing daily physical activity levels is an essential goal in healthy lifestyle behavior change. Several studies have reported favorable changes in lipid abnormalities in response to physical activity in children. A randomized trial in obese adolescents showed that high-intensity training was more effective than no training in reducing plasma triacylglycerol levels, total cholesterol to HDL-C ratio, and diastolic blood pressure *(85)*. Subjects with the most severe lipid abnormalities experienced the most marked effects of high-intensity training, including a beneficial effect on LDL particle size. However, the high-intensity program did not improve adiposity compared to a moderate-intensity program. Another clinical study demonstrated that higher intensity physical activity is more strongly associated with reductions in LDL-C in children than is the total energy spent on physical activity (86). Exercise training in prepubertal children has been shown to reduce LDL-C and increase HDL-C independent of changes in exercise capacity or adiposity (87). In an evaluation of the use of a resistance exercise program in male adolescents, reductions in LDL-C and increases in HDL-C were noted in the absence of changes in body composition (88).

Some clinical trials, particularly those with a predominant exercise training component, have shown improvements in non-invasive vascular markers despite the lack of significant changes in indices of adiposity other than improvements in visceral adiposity and increases in muscle mass (89,90). A recent review suggests that aerobic physical activity, particularly higher intensity exercise, reduces visceral adiposity, with attendant improvements in metabolic indices (91). Evidence was less compelling for an independent effect of resistance training. Therefore, an ideal exercise prescription as part of the management of lipid abnormalities in obese youth may be one that includes 30–60 min/day of higher intensity physical activity combined with resistance exercise.

In concert with the promotion of physical activity there should be a reduction in the amount of time spent in sedentary pursuits. Limitations on the amount of time spent on watching television, playing video and computer games, and text messaging should be established. Media-based sedentary pursuits should be limited to ≤1–2 h/day (92).

Drug therapy. Drug therapy for lipid abnormalities in the setting of childhood obesity should be reserved for: (a) those with severe abnormalities that persist after attempts at reduction in adiposity and adoption of healthy lifestyle behavior change or (b) those with additional risk factors and high-risk conditions. Recommendations for decision-making regarding drug therapy independent of obesity are available, including how to use these medications in children and adolescents (6). The goal of drug therapy is to reduce lipid abnormalities ideally into the normal range, but minimally into the borderline high range (Table 2).

Short-term clinical trials provide support for the use of several classes of medications in children and adolescents with primary lipid disorders (Table 6). There have, however, been no clinical trials of lipid-lowering therapy in obese children and adolescents.

Bile acid sequestrants bind bile acids in the intestinal lumen and prevent their enterohepatic reuptake, thus removing them from the cholesterol pool. Synthesis of replacement bile salts leads to depletion of intracellular cholesterol in hepatocytes; this in turn leads to upregulation of LDL receptors in order to increase cellular uptake of cholesterol, which increases the clearance of circulating LDL. These agents cause a modest decrease in LDL-C but increase in triglyceride levels. In addition, they are associated with gastrointestinal symptoms and poor palatability, leading to poor compliance. They are now used in patients with mild lipid abnormalities or in combination with a statin for those with severe lipid abnormalities.

Cholesterol absorption inhibitors inhibit intestinal absorption of cholesterol and plant sterols, which leads to upregulation of hepatic LDL receptors and increased LDL clearance. These agents cause a modest decrease in LDL-C but have limited or no effect on triglycerides and HDL-C levels. They are predominately used in combination with a statin, although recent studies of their use as monotherapy are encouraging.

The primary therapy of obesity-related lipid abnormalities includes the use of the *3-hydroxyl-3-methyl-glutaryl coenzyme A (HMG-CoA) reductase inhibitors*, or *statins*. Statins inhibit HMG-CoA reductase, a rate-limiting enzyme in pathway of endogenous cholesterol synthesis. This leads to intracellular cholesterol depletion, resulting in upregulation of LDL receptors and increased LDL-C clearance. These agents are very effective in lowering LDL-C, with some increase in HDL-C levels. In addition, the statins have important beneficial pleotropic effects. Adverse effects are uncommon; they include myopathy, rhabdomyolysis, and increases in serum hepatic transaminases. They have been

Table 6
Clinical Trials of Drug Therapy of Lipid Abnormalities in Children and Adolescents

Study	Medication	Subjects/gender condition	Daily dose	Effect on lipid profile			
				TChol (%)	LDL-C (%)	HDL-C (%)	TG (%)
Bile acid sequestrants							
Tonstad (93) RCT 1 year	Cholestyramine	96/both HFH	8 g	−12	−17	+8	NA
McCrindle (94) RCT cross-over 2 × 8 weeks	Cholestyramine	40/both HFH	8 g	−7 to −11	−10 to −15	+2 to +4	+6 to +9
Tonstad (95) RCT 8 weeks Open label 44–52 weeks	Colestipol	27/both HFH	2–12 g	−17	−20	−7	−13
McCrindle (96) RCT cross-over 2 × 18 weeks	Colestipol	36/ both HFH FCH	10 g	−7	−10	+2	+12
Stein (97) RCT 8 weeks Open label 18 weeks	Colesevelam	191/both HFH	1.875 g 3.75 g	−3 −7	−6 −13	+5 +8	+6 +5
Cholesterol absorption inhibitors							
Yeste (98) Open label 12 months	Ezetimibe	6/both PH 11/both HFH	10 mg 10 mg	−31 −26	−42 −30	NC −16	NC NC
Clauss (99) Open label 3.5 months	Ezetimibe	26/both HFH 10/both FCH	10 mg 10 mg	−22 −13	−26 −19	NC NC	NC NC

HMG-CoA reductase inhibitors (statins)

Vander Graf (100) Open label 2 years	Fluvastatin	85/both HFH	80 mg	−27	−34	+5	−5
Lambert (101) RCT 8 weeks	Lovastatin	69 males HFH	10 mg 20 mg 30 mg 40 mg	−17 −19 −21 −29	−21 −24 −27 −36	+9 +2 +11 +3	−18 +9 +3 −9
Stein (102) RCT 48 weeks	Lovastatin	132 males HFH	10 mg 20 mg 40 mg	−13 −19 −21	−17 −24 −27	+4 +4 +5	+4 +8 +6
Clauss (103) RCT 24 weeks	Lovastatin	54 females HFH	40 mg	−22	−27	+3	−23
Knipscheer (104) RCT 12 weeks	Pravastatin	72/both HFH	5 mg 10 mg 20 mg	−18 −17 −25	−23 −24 −33	+4 +6 +11	+2 +7 +3
Wiegman (105) RCT 2 years	Pravastatin	214/both HFH	20–40 mg	−19	−24	+6	−17
Rodenburg (106) Open label 2.1–7.4 years	Pravastatin	186 both HFH	20 or 40 mg	−23	−29	+3	−2
de Jongh (107) RCT 48 weeks	Simvastatin	173/both HFH	10–40 mg	−31	−41	+3	−9
de Jongh (108) RCT 28 weeks	Simvastatin	50/both HFH	40 mg	−30	−40	+5	−17
McCrindle (109) RCT	Atorvastatin	187/both HFH/Severe	10–20 mg	−30	−40	+6	−13
Other agents							
Colletti (110) Open label 1–19 months	Niacin	21 both Severe	500–2,200 mg	−13	−17	+4	+13

(Continued)

Table 6
(continued)

Study	Medication	Subjects/gender condition	Daily dose	Effect on lipid profile			
				TChol (%)	LDL-C (%)	HDL-C (%)	TG (%)
Wheeler (111) RCT 8 weeks	Bezafibrate	14 both HFH	10–20 mg/kg	–22	NC	+15	–23
McCrindle (96) RCT cross-over 2 × 18 weeks	Pravastatin and Colestipol	36/both HFH FCH	Pravastatin, 10 mg (with Colestipol, 5 g)	–13	–17	+4	+8
Van der Graaf (112) RCT 6 and 27 weeks; Open label to 53 weeks	Simvastatin and Ezetimide	248/both HFH	Simvastatin 10–40 mg with Ezetimide 10 mg	–38	–49	+7	–17

NA, not available; NC, not calculated; TC, total cholesterol; HFH, heterozygous familial hypercholesterolemia; FCH, familial combined hyperlipidemia; FH, familial hyperlipidemia; RCT, randomized clinical trial; Severe, severe hyperlipidemia.

shown to have no effect on growth and development but should not be used in prepubertal children who do not have primary familial hyperlipidemia or severe hyperlipidemia.

Fibric acid derivatives, or fibrates, seem ideally suited for management of obesity-related lipid abnormalities. As agonists for nuclear peroxisome proliferator-activated receptor (PPAR)-alpha, they upregulate lipoprotein lipase and downregulate apolipoprotein C-III, which increase the degradation of VLDL-C and triglycerides. They may also decrease hepatic synthesis of VLDL-C by stimulating oxidation of free fatty acids and reducing their contribution to triglyceride synthesis. Fibrates increase expression of the genes encoding for apolipoproteins A-I and A-II, impacting HDL metabolism. As a result, they lower non-HDL-C and triglyceride levels, with increases in HDL-C levels and particle size and increases in LDL particle size. Adverse effects are rare; they include myositis (particularly when administered in combination with a statin), anemia, and gastrointestinal complaints. Despite their theoretic potential, there are almost no pediatric data regarding their use.

Nicotinic acid formulations also seem ideally suited for treatment of obesity-related lipid abnormalities, as they inhibit release of free fatty acids from adipose tissue and reduce VLDL-C and LDL-C production and HDL-C degradation. They effectively lower non-HDL-C, LDL-C, and triglycerides and raise HDL-C levels. Their main limitation is prevalent and symptomatic adverse effects,

Table 7
Risk Factors and Risk Conditions Influencing Decision-Making Regarding Management of Lipid Abnormalities

---

Positive family history – The presence of premature (<55 years in males, <65 years in females) cardiovascular disease in a parent or grandparent manifest as:

    Events: sudden cardiac death, onset of angina, myocardial infarction, stroke

    Objectively diagnosed disease

    Related procedures: angioplasty or arterial stent placement, coronary artery bypass grafting

High-level risk factors

- Hypertension requiring drug therapy (blood pressure ≥99th percentile + 5 mm Hg)
- Current cigarette smoker

High-risk conditions

- Kawasaki disease with current coronary artery aneurysms
- Post-orthotopic heart transplantation
- Chronic renal disease
- Diabetes mellitus

Moderate level risk factors

- Hypertension not requiring drug therapy
- HDL-C < 40 mg/dl

Moderate-risk conditions

- Kawasaki disease with regressed coronary artery aneurysms
- Nephrotic syndrome
- HIV infection
- Chronic inflammatory disease (SLE, JRA)

BMI, body mass index; dl, deciliter; Hg, mercury; HIV, human immunodeficiency virus; JRA, juvenile rheumatoid arthritis; l, liter; mg, milligrams; mm, millimeters; mmol, millimoles; SLE, systemic lupus erythematosus.

primarily flushing; there are also concerns about hepatic toxicity and poor glycemic control. They are reserved for combination with a statin, and there are almost no pediatric data regarding their use.

Decision-making regarding drug therapy is complex and depends not only on the severity of lipid abnormalities, but the presence and severity of associated risk factors and risk conditions (Table 7). Drug therapy is not usually considered for obese children and adolescents with dyslipidemia until an adequate attempt has been made at healthy lifestyle behavior change; nevertheless, lipid-lowering drugs may be used in patients with severe lipid abnormalities while lifestyle interventions are being pursued. In general, drug therapy is not considered in children younger than 10 years of age, although children aged 8–9 years may be selectively treated if lipid abnormalities are very severe and there is a strong family history of premature cardiovascular disease. Recommendations for patient selection in the setting of obesity are given in Table 8, and guidelines for management of statin therapy for pediatric patients exist (6).

Table 8

Recommendations Regarding Drug Therapy for Obese Children and Adolescents

1. Measure and average values from two fasting lipid profiles
2. Statin therapy may be initiated under the following circumstances (if triglycerides >200 mg/dl may use non-HDL-C cutpoints):

BMI ≥97th percentile

– LDL-C ≥190 mg/dl (non-HDL-C≥205 mg/dl)

– LDL-C 160–189 mg/dl (non-HDL-C 175–204 mg/dl)

– LDL-C 130–159 mg/dl (non-HDL-C 145–174 mg/dl)

+ 1 high-level RF/RC or ≥2 moderate-level RF/RC or clinical CVD

BMI >95th and <97th percentile

– LDL-C ≥190 mg/dl (non-HDL-C≥205 mg/dl)

– LDL-C 160–189 mg/dl (non-HDL-C 175–204 mg/dl)

+ positive family history or 1 high- or moderate-level RF/RC

– LDL-C 130–159 mg/dl (non-HDL-C 145–174 mg/dl)

+ 2 high-level or 1 high- +1 moderate-level RF/RC or clinical CVD

3. The choice of statin is a matter of preference. Start with the lowest dose, monitor for adverse effects, and titrate the dose upward if therapeutic targets are not achieved. Therapeutic target:

   Minimal: LDL-C <130 mg/dl (non-HDL-C <145 mg/dl)

   Ideal: LDL-C <110 mg/dl (non-HDL-C <125 mg/dl)

4. If LDL-C remains ≥130 mg/dl after a sufficient trial of a statin, and TG <200 mg/dl, consideration may be given to adding a bile acid sequestrant or cholesterol absorption inhibitor

5. In high-LDL-C patients, if non-HDL-C remains ≥145 mg/dl after effective LDL-C treatment then target therapy toward reducing triglycerides, by adding a fibrate or nicotinic acid. This should be done in consultation with a lipid specialist

CVD, cardiovascular disease; dl, deciliter; HDL-C, high-density lipoprotein cholesterol; LDL-C, low-density lipoprotein cholesterol; mg, milligram; RF/RC, risk factor/risk condition.

There are concerns that recommendations for drug therapy of lipid abnormalities in the setting of childhood obesity could lead to an epidemic of medication (particularly statin) use. However, a population-based study using NHANES data estimated that under current AAP guidelines, only 0.8% of adolescents would be potentially eligible for treatment of increased LDL-C *(7,113)*. Further analysis has shown that the prevalence of lipid abnormalities is greater in overweight than healthy weight youth and that overweight is associated with lower self-reported health status but not increased health-care expenditures *(114)*. This suggests that lipid abnormalities in overweight youth are not being addressed effectively within the context of the health-care system. Further information from administrative data from 2004 for pediatric patients suggests that the prevalence of statin use currently is extremely low *(115)*. The predominate statin in use was atorvastatin, with a prevalence of use for those aged 12–19 years equal to 0.03%, or 3 per 10,000. With the prevalence of heterozygous familial hypercholesterolemia at 1 in 500, it would appear that only a small proportion of eligible children are currently being treated with drug therapy, despite a clear recommendation. It would seem unlikely that recommendations for drug therapy in the setting of obesity would lead to an epidemic of medication use.

Finally, the use of *pharmacologic agents to improve insulin sensitivity* as a means to manage lipid abnormalities has not been well evaluated in the pediatric population. Metformin has been tested in clinical trials and has shown equivocal results in terms of correction of lipid abnormalities *(116–118)*.

SUMMARY

Lipid abnormalities are a major component of the metabolic syndrome related to childhood overweight and obesity and are characterized by high triglyceride levels, low HDL-C levels, and qualitative changes in LDL particles that make them smaller, denser, and more atherogenic. These abnormalities are primarily driven by elevation in plasma free fatty acids derived from metabolically active visceral adipose tissue, resulting in increased hepatic triglyceride synthesis and overproduction of VLDL particles. Assessment of lipid abnormalities relies on a fasting lipid profile. Reduction in adiposity through healthy lifestyle behavior change is the cornerstone of therapy of lipid abnormalities, although dietary and physical activity interventions may have direct benefits. Rarely, drug therapy may be required, particularly for those with severe lipid abnormalities and associated risk factors and risk conditions. Evidence-based research in many areas is lacking; the intersection of clinical care recommendations with the health-care system has assumed increasing importance *(119–121)*.

Editor's Comments

- Triglyceride levels exceeding 1,000 mg/dl can cause *pancreatitis*; chylomicrons in excess are postulated to impair blood flow in pancreatic capillary beds, leading to ischemic changes, and hydrolysis of TG by pancreatic lipase results in necrosis and inflammation. Concentrated preparations of omega-3 fatty acids ethyl esters, which contain primarily eicosapentaenoic (EPA) and docosahexaenoic (DHA), are approved by the FDA for treatment of severe hypertriglyceridemia (>500 mg/dl) in adults. At a dose of 3–4 g/day they reduce TG levels by 26–47%; this effect is mediated by reductions in hepatic lipogenesis, increases in fatty acid oxidation, and degradation of apoB-100 (Bays et al., 2008). High doses of omega-3 fatty acids can also cause variable increases in LDL-C (10–46%) and HDL-C. Increases in LDL-C levels are most common in patients with the highest TG levels; concomitant use of a statin may be required to reduce cholesterol levels. Other possible adverse effects of pharmacologic doses of omega-3 fatty acids include dyspepsia, decreased platelet aggregation, increases in serum ALT levels, and a transient rise in blood glucose.

- Fish oil, flax seed, and tree nuts contain omega-3 fatty acids, and fish consumption (1–2 servings of oily fish per week, ~250–500 mg EPA and DHA) is associated with reductions in cardiovascular mortality in adults (Lee et al., 2008). However, certain predator fish (tuna, swordfish, shark, mackerel) contain higher levels of methylmercury; consumption should be avoided in pregnant women and young children. Non-predator fish (salmon, shrimp, sardines) contain lower levels of methylmercury, and the levels of mercury in fish oil supplements are negligible.

- New markers of cardiovascular risk will no doubt emerge in the near future. For example, high levels of Lp(a) lipoprotein are associated with coronary artery disease in adults (Clarke et al., 2009); application of new markers in children awaits further study.

Bays HE, Tighe AP, Sadovsky R, Davidson MH. Prescription omega-3 fatty acids and their lipid effects: physiologic mechanisms of action and clinical implications. Expert Rev Cardiovasc Ther. 2008 Mar;6(3):391–409.

Clarke R, Peden JF, Hopewell JC, Kyriakou T, Goel A, Heath SC, Parish S, Barlera S, Franzosi MG, Rust S, Bennett D, Silveira A, Malarstig A, Green FR, Lathrop M, Gigante B, Leander K, de Faire U, Seedorf U, Hamsten A, Collins R, Watkins H, Farrall M; PROCARDIS Consortium. Genetic variants associated with Lp(a) lipoprotein level and coronary disease. N Engl J Med. 2009 Dec 24;361(26):2518–28.

Lee JH, O'Keefe JH, Lavie CJ, Marchioli R, Harris WS. Omega-3 fatty acids for cardioprotection. Mayo Clin Proc. 2008 Mar;83(3):324–32.

REFERENCES

1. Raal FJ. Pathogenesis and management of the dyslipidemia of the metabolic syndrome. Metab Syndr Relat Disord. 2009;7(2):83–88.
2. Therond P. Catabolism of lipoproteins and metabolic syndrome. Curr Opin Clin Nutr Metab Care. 2009;12(4): 366–71.
3. Meshkani R, Adeli K. Hepatic insulin resistance, metabolic syndrome and cardiovascular disease. Clin Biochem. 2009;42(13–14):1331–46.
4. Aguilera CM, Gil-Campos M, Canete R, Gil A. Alterations in plasma and tissue lipids associated with obesity and metabolic syndrome. Clin Sci (Lond). 2008;114(3):183–93.
5. American Academy of Pediatrics. National Cholesterol Education Program: report of the expert panel on blood cholesterol levels in children and adolescents. Pediatrics. 1992;89:525–84.
6. McCrindle BW, Urbina EM, Dennison BA, Jacobson MS, Steinberger J, Rocchini AP, Hayman LL, Daniels SR. Drug therapy of high-risk lipid abnormalities in children and adolescents: a scientific statement from the American Heart Association Atherosclerosis, Hypertension, and Obesity in Youth Committee, Council of Cardiovascular Disease in the Young, with the Council on Cardiovascular Nursing. Circulation. 2007;115(14):1948–67.
7. Daniels SR, Greer FR. Lipid screening and cardiovascular health in childhood. Pediatrics. 2008;122(1):198–208.
8. Barlow SE. Expert committee recommendations regarding the prevention, assessment, and treatment of child and adolescent overweight and obesity: summary report. Pediatrics. 2007;120(Suppl 4):S164–92.
9. Lau DC, Douketis JD, Morrison KM, Hramiak IM, Sharma AM, Ur E. 2006 Canadian clinical practice guidelines on the management and prevention of obesity in adults and children [summary]. CMAJ. 2007;176(8):S1–13.
10. Katzmarzyk PT, Srinivasan SR, Chen W, Malina RM, Bouchard C, Berenson GS. Body mass index, waist circumference, and clustering of cardiovascular disease risk factors in a biracial sample of children and adolescents. Pediatrics. 2004;114(2):e198–205.
11. Friedewald WT, Levy RI, Fredrickson DS. Estimation of the concentration of low-density lipoprotein cholesterol in plasma, without use of the preparative ultracentrifuge. Clin Chem. 1972;18(6):499–502.
12. Tighe DA, Ockene IS, Reed G, Nicolosi R. Calculated low density lipoprotein cholesterol levels frequently underestimate directly measured low density lipoprotein cholesterol determinations in patients with serum triglyceride levels < or =4.52 mmol/l: an analysis comparing the LipiDirect magnetic LDL assay with the Friedewald calculation. Clin Chim Acta. 2006;365(1–2):236–42.
13. Mudd JO, Borlaug BA, Johnston PV, Kral BG, Rouf R, Blumenthal RS, Kwiterovich PO Jr. Beyond low-density lipoprotein cholesterol: defining the role of low-density lipoprotein heterogeneity in coronary artery disease. J Am Coll Cardiol. 2007;50(18):1735–41.

14. Bairaktari ET, Seferiadis KI, Elisaf MS. Evaluation of methods for the measurement of low-density lipoprotein cholesterol. J Cardiovasc Pharmacol Ther. 2005;10(1):45–54.

15. Caulfield MP, Li S, Lee G, Blanche PJ, Salameh WA, Benner WH, Reitz RE, Krauss RM. Direct determination of lipoprotein particle sizes and concentrations by ion mobility analysis. Clin Chem. 2008;54(8):1307–16.

16. Petersen M, Dyrby M, Toubro S, Engelsen SB, Norgaard L, Pedersen HT, Dyerberg J. Quantification of lipoprotein subclasses by proton nuclear magnetic resonance-based partial least-squares regression models. Clin Chem. 2005;51(8):1457–61.

17. Okazaki M, Usui S, Fukui A, Kubota I, Tomoike H. Component analysis of HPLC profiles of unique lipoprotein subclass cholesterols for detection of coronary artery disease. Clin Chem. 2006;52(11):2049–53.

18. Freedman DS, Bowman BA, Otvos JD, Srinivasan SR, Berenson GS. Levels and correlates of LDL and VLDL particle sizes among children: the Bogalusa heart study. Atherosclerosis. 2000;152(2):441–49.

19. Srinivasan SR, Segrest JP, Elkasabany AM, Berenson GS. Distribution and correlates of lipoproteins and their subclasses in black and white young adults. The Bogalusa Heart Study. Atherosclerosis. 2001;159(2):391–97.

20. Otvos JD, Jeyarajah EJ, Cromwell WC. Measurement issues related to lipoprotein heterogeneity. Am J Cardiol. 2002;90(8A):22i–9i.

21. Freedman DS, Bowman BA, Otvos JD, Srinivasan SR, Berenson GS. Differences in the relation of obesity to serum triacylglycerol and VLDL subclass concentrations between black and white children: the Bogalusa Heart Study. Am J Clin Nutr. 2002;75(5):827–33.

22. National Cholesterol Education Program (NCEP). Highlights of the report of the expert panel on blood cholesterol levels in children and adolescents. Pediatrics. 1992;89(3):495–501.

23. Srinivasan SR, Myers L, Berenson GS. Distribution and correlates of non-high-density lipoprotein cholesterol in children: the Bogalusa Heart Study. Pediatrics. 2002;110(3):e29.

24. Christensen B, Glueck C, Kwiterovich P, Degroot I, Chase G, Heiss G, Mowery R, Tamir I, Rifkind B. Plasma cholesterol and triglyceride distributions in 13,665 children and adolescents: the Prevalence Study of the Lipid Research Clinics Program. Pediatr Res. 1980;14(3):194–202.

25. Beaglehole R, Trost DC, Tamir I, Kwiterovich P, Glueck CJ, Insull W, Christensen B. Plasma high-density lipoprotein cholesterol in children and young adults. The Lipid Research Clinics Program Prevalence Study. Circulation. 1980;62(4 Pt 2):IV83–92.

26. Tamir I, Heiss G, Glueck CJ, Christensen B, Kwiterovich P, Rifkind BM. Lipid and lipoprotein distributions in white children ages 6–19 yr. The Lipid Research Clinics Program Prevalence Study. J Chronic Dis. 1981;34(1):27–39.

27. Jolliffe CJ, Janssen I. Distribution of lipoproteins by age and gender in adolescents. Circulation. 2006;114(10):1056–62.

28. Third Report of the National Cholesterol Education Program (NCEP). Expert panel on detection, evaluation, and treatment of high blood cholesterol in adults (adult treatment panel III) final report. Circulation. 2002;106(25):3143–421.

29. Magnussen CG, Raitakari OT, Thomson R, Juonala M, Patel DA, Viikari JS, Marniemi J, Srinivasan SR, Berenson GS, Dwyer T, Venn A. Utility of currently recommended pediatric dyslipidemia classifications in predicting dyslipidemia in adulthood: evidence from the Childhood Determinants of Adult Health (CDAH) Study, Cardiovascular Risk in Young Finns Study, and Bogalusa Heart Study. Circulation. 2008;117(1):32–42.

30. Srinivasan SR, Wattigney W, Webber LS, Berenson GS. Race and gender differences in serum lipoproteins of children, adolescents, and young adults–emergence of an adverse lipoprotein pattern in white males: the Bogalusa Heart Study. Prev Med. 1991;20(6):671–84.

31. Chen W, Srinivasan SR, Bao W, Wattigney WA, Berenson GS. Sibling aggregation of low- and high-density lipoprotein cholesterol and apolipoproteins B and A-I levels in black and white children: the Bogalusa Heart Study. Ethn Dis. 1997;7(3):241–49.

32. Freedman DS, Cresanta JL, Srinivasan SR, Webber LS, Berenson GS. Longitudinal serum lipoprotein changes in white males during adolescence: the Bogalusa Heart Study. Metabolism. 1985;34(4):396–403.

33. Berenson GS. Bogalusa Heart Study: a long-term community study of a rural biracial (Black/White) population. Am J Med Sci. 2001;322(5):293–300.

34. Li S, Chen W, Srinivasan SR, Bond MG, Tang R, Urbina EM, Berenson GS. Childhood cardiovascular risk factors and carotid vascular changes in adulthood: the Bogalusa Heart Study. J Am Med Assoc. 2003;290(17):2271–76.

35. Berenson GS, Srinivasan SR, Bao W, Newman WP III, Tracy RE, Wattigney WA. Association between multiple cardiovascular risk factors and atherosclerosis in children and young adults. The Bogalusa Heart Study. N Engl J Med. 1998;338(23):1650–56.

36. Clarke WR, Schrott HG, Leaverton PE, Connor WE, Lauer RM. Tracking of blood lipids and blood pressures in school age children: the Muscatine study. Circulation. 1978;58(4):626–34.

37. Freedman DS, Shear CL, Srinivasan SR, Webber LS, Berenson GS. Tracking of serum lipids and lipoproteins in children over an 8-year period: the Bogalusa Heart Study. Prev Med. 1985;14(2):203–16.

38. Porkka KV, Viikari JS, Taimela S, Dahl M, Akerblom HK. Tracking and predictiveness of serum lipid and lipoprotein measurements in childhood: a 12-year follow-up. The Cardiovascular Risk in Young Finns study. Am J Epidemiol. 1994;140(12):1096–110.

39. Newman WP III, Freedman DS, Voors AW, Gard PD, Srinivasan SR, Cresanta JL, Williamson GD, Webber LS, Berenson GS. Relation of serum lipoprotein levels and systolic blood pressure to early atherosclerosis. The Bogalusa Heart Study. N Engl J Med. 1986;314(3):138–44.

40. Li S, Chen W, Srinivasan SR, Bond MG, Tang R, Urbina EM, Berenson GS. Childhood cardiovascular risk factors and carotid vascular changes in adulthood: the Bogalusa Heart Study. J Am Med Assoc. 2003;290(17):2271–76.

41. Magnussen CG, Venn A, Thomson R, Juonala M, Srinivasan SR, Viikari JS, Berenson GS, Dwyer T, Raitakari OT. The association of pediatric low- and high-density lipoprotein cholesterol dyslipidemia classifications and change in dyslipidemia status with carotid intima-media thickness in adulthood evidence from the cardiovascular risk in Young Finns Study, the Bogalusa Heart Study, and the CDAH (Childhood Determinants of Adult Health) Study. J Am Coll Cardiol. 2009;53(10):860–69.

42. Battista M, Murray RD, Daniels SR. Use of the metabolic syndrome in pediatrics: a blessing and a curse. Semin Pediatr Surg. 2009;18(3):136–43.

43. Steinberger J, Daniels SR, Eckel RH, Hayman L, Lustig RH, McCrindle B, Mietus-Snyder ML. Progress and challenges in metabolic syndrome in children and adolescents: a scientific statement from the American Heart Association Atherosclerosis, Hypertension, and Obesity in the Young Committee of the Council on Cardiovascular Disease in the Young; Council on Cardiovascular Nursing; and Council on Nutrition, Physical Activity, and Metabolism. Circulation. 2009;119(4):628–47.

44. Morrison JA, Ford ES, Steinberger J. The pediatric metabolic syndrome. Minerva Med. 2008;99(3):269–87.

45. Cook S, Weitzman M, Auinger P, Nguyen M, Dietz WH. Prevalence of a metabolic syndrome phenotype in adolescents. Findings from the Third National Health and Nutrition Examination Survey, 1988–1994. Arch Pediatr Adolesc Med. 2003;157:821–27.

46. Cook S, Auinger P, Li C, Ford ES. Metabolic syndrome rates in United States adolescents, from the National Health and Nutrition Examination Survey, 1999–2002. J Pediatr. 2008;152(2):165–70.

47. de Ferranti SD, Gauvreau K, Ludwig DS, Neufeld EJ, Newburger JW, Rifai N. Prevalence of the metabolic syndrome in American adolescents: findings from the Third National Health and Nutrition Examination Survey. Circulation. 2004;110(16):2494–97.

48. Weiss R, Dziura J, Burgert TS, Tamborlane WV, Taksali SE, Yeckel CW, Allen K, Lopes M, Savoye M, Morrison J, Sherwin RS, Caprio S. Obesity and the metabolic syndrome in children and adolescents. N Engl J Med. 2004;350(23):2362–74.

49. Zimmet P, Alberti G, Kaufman F, Tajima N, Silink M, Arslanian S, Wong G, Bennett P, Shaw J, Caprio S. The metabolic syndrome in children and adolescents. Lancet. 2007;369(9579):2059–61.

50. Mancini MC. Metabolic syndrome in children and adolescents – criteria for diagnosis. Diabetol Metab Syndr. 2009;1(1):20.

51. Frontini MG, Srinivasan SR, Xu JH, Tang R, Bond MG, Berenson G. Utility of non-high-density lipoprotein cholesterol versus other lipoprotein measures in detecting subclinical atherosclerosis in young adults (The Bogalusa Heart Study). Am J Cardiol. 2007;100(1):64–68.

52. Liu J, Joshi D, Sempos CT. Non-high-density-lipoprotein cholesterol and cardiovascular risk factors among adolescents with and without impaired fasting glucose. Appl Physiol Nutr Metab. 2009;34(2):136–42.

53. Liu J, Wade TJ, Tan H. Cardiovascular risk factors and anthropometric measurements of adolescent body composition: a cross-sectional analysis of the Third National Health and Nutrition Examination Survey. Int J Obes (Lond). 2007;31(1):59–64.

54. Miller S, Manlhiot C, Chahal N, Cullen-Dean G, Bannister L, McCrindle BW. Impact of increasing adiposity in hyperlipidemic children. Clin Pediatr (Phila). 2008;47(7):679–84.

55. Thavendiranathan P, Jones E, Han RK, Cullen-Dean G, Helden E, Conner WT, McCrindle BW. Association between physical activity, adiposity, and lipid abnormalities in children with familial hyperlipidemia. Eur J Cardiovasc Prev Rehabil. 2007;14(1):59–64.

56. Manlhiot C, Larsson P, Gurofsky RC, Smith RW, Fillingham C, Clarizia NA, Chahal N, Clarke JT, McCrindle BW. Spectrum and management of hypertriglyceridemia among children in clinical practice. Pediatrics. 2009;123(2):458–65.

57. Naukkarinen J, Ehnholm C, Peltonen L. Genetics of familial combined hyperlipidemia. Curr Opin Lipidol. 2006;17(3):285–90.

58. Suviolahti E, Lilja HE, Pajukanta P. Unraveling the complex genetics of familial combined hyperlipidemia. Ann Med. 2006;38(5):337–51.

59. Wierzbicki AS, Graham CA, Young IS, Nicholls DP. Familial combined hyperlipidaemia: under-defined and under-diagnosed? Curr Vasc Pharmacol. 2008;6(1):13–22.

60. Gaddi A, Cicero AF, Odoo FO, Poli AA, Paoletti R. Practical guidelines for familial combined hyperlipidemia diagnosis: an up-date. Vasc Health Risk Manag. 2007;3(6):877–86.

61. Juonala M, Viikari JS, Ronnemaa T, Marniemi J, Jula A, Loo BM, Raitakari OT. Associations of dyslipidemias from childhood to adulthood with carotid intima-media thickness, elasticity, and brachial flow-mediated dilatation in adulthood: the Cardiovascular Risk in Young Finns Study. Arterioscler Thromb Vasc Biol. 2008;28(5):1012–17.

62. ter Avest E, Sniderman AD, Bredie SJ, Wiegman A, Stalenhoef AF, de Graaf J. Effect of aging and obesity on the expression of dyslipidaemia in children from families with familial combined hyperlipidaemia. Clin Sci (Lond). 2007;112(2):131–39.

63. Smelt AH, de Beer F. Apolipoprotein E and familial dysbetalipoproteinemia: clinical, biochemical, and genetic aspects. Semin Vasc Med. 2004;4(3):249–57.

64. Kavey RE, Allada V, Daniels SR, Hayman LL, McCrindle BW, Newburger JW, Parekh RS, Steinberger J. Cardiovascular risk reduction in high-risk pediatric patients: a scientific statement from the American Heart Association Expert Panel on Population and Prevention Science; the Councils on Cardiovascular Disease in the Young, Epidemiology and Prevention, Nutrition, Physical Activity and Metabolism, High Blood Pressure Research, Cardiovascular Nursing, and the Kidney in Heart Disease; and the Interdisciplinary Working Group on Quality of Care and Outcomes Research: endorsed by the American Academy of Pediatrics. Circulation. 2006;114(24):2710–38.

65. Efficacy and safety of lowering dietary intake of fat and cholesterol in children with elevated low-density lipoprotein cholesterol. The Dietary Intervention Study in Children (DISC). The Writing Group for the DISC Collaborative Research Group. J Am Med Assoc. 1995;273(18):1429–35.

66. Obarzanek E, Kimm SY, Barton BA, Van Horn LL, Kwiterovich PO Jr, Simons-Morton DG, Hunsberger SA, Lasser NL, Robson AM, Franklin FA Jr, Lauer RM, Stevens VJ, Friedman LA, Dorgan JF, Greenlick MR. Long-term safety and efficacy of a cholesterol-lowering diet in children with elevated low-density lipoprotein cholesterol: seven-year results of the Dietary Intervention Study in Children (DISC). Pediatrics. 2001;107(2):256–64.

67. Rask-Nissila L, Jokinen E, Ronnemaa T, Viikari J, Tammi A, Niinikoski H, Seppanen R, Tuominen J, Simell O. Prospective, randomized, infancy-onset trial of the effects of a low-saturated-fat, low-cholesterol diet on serum lipids and lipoproteins before school age: The Special Turku Coronary Risk Factor Intervention Project (STRIP). Circulation. 2000;102(13):1477–83.

68. Kaitosaari T, Ronnemaa T, Raitakari O, Talvia S, Kallio K, Volanen I, Leino A, Jokinen E, Valimaki I, Viikari J, Simell O. Effect of 7-year infancy-onset dietary intervention on serum lipoproteins and lipoprotein subclasses in healthy children in the prospective, randomized Special Turku Coronary Risk Factor Intervention Project for Children (STRIP) Study. Circulation. 2003;108(6):672–77.

69. Widhalm K, Brazda G, Schneider B, Kohl S. Effect of soy protein diet versus standard low fat, low cholesterol diet on lipid and lipoprotein levels in children with familial or polygenic hypercholesterolemia. J Pediatr. 1993;123(1):30–34.

70. Laurin D, Jacques H, Moorjani S, Steinke FH, Gagne C, Brun D, Lupien PJ. Effects of a soy-protein beverage on plasma lipoproteins in children with familial hypercholesterolemia. Am J Clin Nutr. 1991;54(1):98–103.

71. Gulesserian T, Widhalm K. Effect of a rapeseed oil substituting diet on serum lipids and lipoproteins in children and adolescents with familial hypercholesterolemia. J Am Coll Nutr. 2002;21(2):103–8.

72. Libby P, Ridker PM, Hansson GK. Inflammation in atherosclerosis: from pathophysiology to practice. J Am Coll Cardiol. 2009;54(23):2129–38.

73. Engler MM, Engler MB, Malloy MJ, Chiu EY, Schloetter MC, Paul SM, Stuehlinger M, Lin KY, Cooke JP, Morrow JD, Ridker PM, Rifai N, Miller E, Witztum JL, Mietus-Snyder M. Antioxidant vitamins C and E improve endothelial function in children with hyperlipidemia: Endothelial Assessment of Risk from Lipids in Youth (EARLY) Trial. Circulation. 2003;108(9):1059–63.

74. Mietus-Snyder M, Malloy MJ. Endothelial dysfunction occurs in children with two genetic hyperlipidemias: improvement with antioxidant vitamin therapy. J Pediatr. 1998;133(1):35–40.

75. Engler MM, Engler MB, Malloy M, Chiu E, Besio D, Paul S, Stuehlinger M, Morrow J, Ridker P, Rifai N, Mietus-Snyder M. Docosahexaenoic acid restores endothelial function in children with hyperlipidemia: results from the EARLY Study. Int J Clin Pharmacol Ther. 2004;42(12):672–79.

76. Ketomaki AM, Gylling H, Antikainen M, Siimes MA, Miettinen TA. Red cell and plasma plant sterols are related during consumption of plant stanol and sterol ester spreads in children with hypercholesterolemia. J Pediatr. 2003;142(5):524–31.

77. Amundsen AL, Ose L, Nenseter MS, Ntanios FY. Plant sterol ester-enriched spread lowers plasma total and LDL cholesterol in children with familial hypercholesterolemia. Am J Clin Nutr. 2002;76(2):338–44.

78. Gylling H, Siimes MA, Miettinen TA. Sitostanol ester margarine in dietary treatment of children with familial hypercholesterolemia. J Lipid Res. 1995;36(8):1807–12.

79. de Jongh S, Vissers MN, Rol P, Bakker HD, Kastelein JJ, Stroes ES. Plant sterols lower LDL cholesterol without improving endothelial function in prepubertal children with familial hypercholesterolaemia. J Inherit Metab Dis. 2003;26(4):343–51.

80. Jakulj L, Vissers MN, Rodenburg J, Wiegman A, Trip MD, Kastelein JJ. Plant stanols do not restore endothelial function in pre-pubertal children with familial hypercholesterolemia despite reduction of low-density lipoprotein cholesterol levels. J Pediatr. 2006;148(4):495–500.

81. Dennison BA, Levine DM. Randomized, double-blind, placebo-controlled, two-period crossover clinical trial of psyllium fiber in children with hypercholesterolemia. J Pediatr. 1993;123(1):24–29.

82. Davidson MH, Dugan LD, Burns JH, Sugimoto D, Story K, Drennan K. A psyllium-enriched cereal for the treatment of hypercholesterolemia in children: a controlled, double-blind, crossover study. Am J Clin Nutr. 1996;63(1): 96–102.

83. Goldberg RB, Sabharwal AK. Fish oil in the treatment of dyslipidemia. Curr Opin Endocrinol Diabetes Obes. 2008;15(2):167–74.

84. McCrindle BW, Helden E, Conner WT. Garlic extract therapy in children with hypercholesterolemia. Arch Pediatr Adolesc Med. 1998;152(11):1089–94.

85. Kang HS, Gutin B, Barbeau P, Owens S, Lemmon CR, Allison J, Litaker MS, Le NA. Physical training improves insulin resistance syndrome markers in obese adolescents. Med Sci Sports Exerc. 2002;34(12):1920–27.

86. Craig SB, Bandini LG, Lichtenstein AH, Schaefer EJ, Dietz WH. The impact of physical activity on lipids, lipoproteins, and blood pressure in preadolescent girls. Pediatrics. 1996;98(3 Pt 1):389–95.

87. Tolfrey K, Campbell IG, Batterham AM. Exercise training induced alterations in prepubertal children's lipid-lipoprotein profile. Med Sci Sports Exerc. 1998;30(12):1684–92.

88. Fripp RR, Hodgson JL. Effect of resistive training on plasma lipid and lipoprotein levels in male adolescents. J Pediatr. 1987;111(6 Pt 1):926–31.

89. Woo KS, Chook P, Yu CW, Sung RY, Qiao M, Leung SS, Lam CW, Metreweli C, Celermajer DS. Effects of diet and exercise on obesity-related vascular dysfunction in children. Circulation. 2004;109(16):1981–86.

90. Watts K, Beye P, Siafarikas A, O'Driscoll G, Jones TW, Davis EA, Green DJ. Effects of exercise training on vascular function in obese children. J Pediatr. 2004;144(5):620–25.

91. Kim Y, Lee S. Physical activity and abdominal obesity in youth. Appl Physiol Nutr Metab. 2009;34(4):571–81.

92. Gutin B, Barbeau P, Owens S, Lemmon CR, Bauman M, Allison J, Kang HS, Litaker MS. Effects of exercise intensity on cardiovascular fitness, total body composition, and visceral adiposity of obese adolescents. Am J Clin Nutr. 2002;75(5):818–26.

93. Tonstad S, Knudtzon J, Sivertsen M, Refsum H, Ose L. Efficacy and safety of cholestyramine therapy in peripubertal and prepubertal children with familial hypercholesterolemia. J Pediatr. 1996;129(1):42–49.

94. McCrindle BW, O'Neill MB, Cullen-Dean G, Helden E. Acceptability and compliance with two forms of cholestyramine in the treatment of hypercholesterolemia in children: a randomized, crossover trial. J Pediatr. 1997;130(2): 266–73.

95. Tonstad S, Sivertsen M, Aksnes L, Ose L. Low dose colestipol in adolescents with familial hypercholesterolaemia. Arch Dis Child. 1996;74(2):157–60.

96. McCrindle BW, Helden E, Cullen-Dean G, Conner WT. A randomized crossover trial of combination pharmacologic therapy in children with familial hyperlipidemia. Pediatr Res. 2002;51(6):715–21.

97. Stein EA, Marais AD, Szamosi T, Raal FJ, Schurr D, Urbina EM, Hopkins PN, Karki S, Xu J, Misir S, Melino M. Colesevelam Hydrochloride: Efficacy and Safety in Pediatric Subjects with Heterozygous Familial Hypercholesterolemia. J Pediatr. 2010;156(2):231–36. Epub 2009 Oct 31.

98. Yeste D, Chacon P, Clemente M, Albisu MA, Gussinye M, Carrascosa A. Ezetimibe as monotherapy in the treatment of hypercholesterolemia in children and adolescents. J Pediatr Endocrinol Metab. 2009;22(6):487–92.

99. Clauss S, Wai KM, Kavey RE, Kuehl K. Ezetimibe treatment of pediatric patients with hypercholesterolemia. J Pediatr. 2009;154(6):869–72.

100. van der Graaf A, Nierman MC, Firth JC, Wolmarans KH, Marais AD. de GE. Efficacy and safety of fluvastatin in children and adolescents with heterozygous familial hypercholesterolaemia. Acta Paediatr. 2006;95(11):1461–66.

101. Lambert M, Lupien PJ, Gagne C, Levy E, Blaichman S, Langlois S, Hayden M, Rose V, Clarke JT, Wolfe BM, Clarson C, Parsons H, Stephure DK, Potvin D, Lambert J. Treatment of familial hypercholesterolemia in children and adolescents: effect of lovastatin. Canadian Lovastatin in Children Study Group. Pediatrics. 1996;97(5):619–28.

102. Stein EA, Illingworth DR, Kwiterovich PO Jr, Liacouras CA, Siimes MA, Jacobson MS, Brewster TG, Hopkins P, Davidson M, Graham K, Arensman F, Knopp RH, DuJovne C, Williams CL, Isaacsohn JL, Jacobsen CA, Laskarzewski PM, Ames S, Gormley GJ. Efficacy and safety of lovastatin in adolescent males with heterozygous familial hypercholesterolemia: a randomized controlled trial. J Am Med Assoc. 1999;281(2):137–44.

103. Clauss SB, Holmes KW, Hopkins P, Stein E, Cho M, Tate A, Johnson-Levonas AO, Kwiterovich PO. Efficacy and safety of lovastatin therapy in adolescent girls with heterozygous familial hypercholesterolemia. Pediatrics. 2005;116(3):682–88.

104. Knipscheer HC, Boelen CC, Kastelein JJ, van Diermen DE, Groenemeijer BE, van den Ende A, Buller HR, Bakker HD. Short-term efficacy and safety of pravastatin in 72 children with familial hypercholesterolemia. Pediatr Res. 1996;39(5):867–71.

105. Wiegman A, Hutten BA, de Groot E, Rodenburg J, Bakker HD, Buller HR, Sijbrands EJ, Kastelein JJ. Efficacy and safety of statin therapy in children with familial hypercholesterolemia: a randomized controlled trial. J Am Med Assoc. 2004;292(3):331–37.

106. Rodenburg J, Vissers MN, Wiegman A, van Trotsenburg AS, van der Graaf A, de Groot E, Wijburg FA, Kastelein JJ, Hutten BA. Statin treatment in children with familial hypercholesterolemia: the younger, the better. Circulation. 2007;116(6):664–68.

107. de Jongh S, Ose L, Szamosi T, Gagne C, Lambert M, Scott R, Perron P, Dobbelaere D, Saborio M, Tuohy MB, Stepanavage M, Sapre A, Gumbiner B, Mercuri M, van Trotsenburg AS, Bakker HD, Kastelein JJ. Efficacy and safety of statin therapy in children with familial hypercholesterolemia: a randomized, double-blind, placebo-controlled trial with simvastatin. Circulation. 2002;106(17):2231–37.

108. de Jongh S, Lilien MR, op't Roodt J, Stroes ES, Bakker HD, Kastelein JJ. Early statin therapy restores endothelial function in children with familial hypercholesterolemia. J Am Coll Cardiol. 2002;40(12):2117–21.

109. McCrindle BW, Ose L, Marais AD. Efficacy and safety of atorvastatin in children and adolescents with familial hypercholesterolemia or severe hyperlipidemia: a multicenter, randomized, placebo-controlled trial. J Pediatr. 2003;143(1):74–80.

110. Colletti RB, Neufeld EJ, Roff NK, McAuliffe TL, Baker AL, Newburger JW. Niacin treatment of hypercholesterolemia in children. Pediatrics. 1993;92(1):78–82.

111. Wheeler KA, West RJ, Lloyd JK, Barley J. Double blind trial of bezafibrate in familial hypercholesterolaemia. Arch Dis Child. 1985;60(1):34–37.

112. van der Graaf A, Cuffie-Jackson C, Vissers MN, Trip MD, Gagne C, Shi G, Veltri E, Avis HJ, Kastelein JJ. Efficacy and safety of coadministration of ezetimibe and simvastatin in adolescents with heterozygous familial hypercholesterolemia. J Am Coll Cardiol. 2008;52(17):1421–29.

113. Ford ES, Li C, Zhao G, Mokdad AH. Concentrations of low-density lipoprotein cholesterol and total cholesterol among children and adolescents in the United States. Circulation. 2009;119(8):1108–15.

114. Skinner AC, Mayer ML, Flower K, Weinberger M. Health status and health care expenditures in a nationally representative sample: how do overweight and healthy-weight children compare? Pediatrics. 2008;121(2):e269–77.

115. Lasky T. Statin use in children in the United States. Pediatrics. 2008;122(6):1406–8. author reply 1408.

116. Jones KL, Arslanian S, Peterokova VA, Park JS, Tomlinson MJ. Effect of metformin in pediatric patients with type 2 diabetes: a randomized controlled trial. Diabetes Care. 2002;25(1):89–94.

117. Freemark M, Bursey D. The effects of metformin on body mass index and glucose tolerance in obese adolescents with fasting hyperinsulinemia and a family history of type 2 diabetes. Pediatrics. 2001;107(4):E55.

118. Clarson CL, Mahmud FH, Baker JE, Clark HE, McKay WM, Schauteet VD, Hill DJ. Metformin in combination with structured lifestyle intervention improved body mass index in obese adolescents, but did not improve insulin resistance. Endocrine. 2009;36(1):141–46.

119. Daniels SR, Jacobson MS, McCrindle BW, Eckel RH, Sanner BM. American Heart Association Childhood Obesity Research Summit: executive summary. Circulation. 2009;119(15):2114–23.

120. Daniels SR, Jacobson MS, McCrindle BW, Eckel RH, Sanner BM. American Heart Association Childhood Obesity Research Summit Report. Circulation. 2009;119(15):e489–517.

121. Pratt CA, Stevens J, Daniels S. Childhood obesity prevention and treatment: recommendations for future research. Am J Prev Med. 2008;35(3):249–52.

15 Fatty Liver Disease

Anna Alisi, Melania Manco, Rita Devito, and Valerio Nobili

CONTENTS

Key Words: NAFLD, steatosis, NAHS, aminotranserase, cirrhosis, fructose, insulin resistance, antioxidant, thiazolidinedione

INTRODUCTION

Fatty liver disease, also named hepatic steatosis, is characterized by the accumulation of fat in liver cells. There are several causes of fatty liver in children, including chronic alcohol consumption, B and C viral hepatitis, type-2 diabetes, obesity, and some metabolic aberrations (see Table 1) *(1)*. The most prevalent form of fatty liver is non-alcoholic fatty liver disease (NAFLD), which associates with obesity and the metabolic syndrome *(2,3)*.

NAFLD is a metabolic condition that ranges from liver fat deposition (simple steatosis) to non-alcoholic steatohepatitis (NASH), which may progress to severe fibrosis, cirrhosis, and ultimately hepatocarcinoma both in adults and in children *(4,5)*. Thus, NAFLD broadly describes several diseases which differ widely in prevalence, presentation, and aetiology. This necessitates a personalized approach to diagnosis and treatment.

NAFLD is an increasingly recognized worldwide cause of liver disease *(6,7)*. Even more important may be the fact that NAFLD occurs in children and adolescents, with a prevalence estimated at 3–10% in some populations *(8,9)*. This percentage increases up to 53% in obese children *(10)*. Thus, NAFLD is expected to become the most common cause of paediatric chronic liver disease in the near future.

From: *Contemporary Endocrinology: Pediatric Obesity: Etiology, Pathogenesis, and Treatment*
Edited by: M. Freemark, DOI 10.1007/978-1-60327-874-4_15,
© Springer Science+Business Media, LLC 2010

Table 1
Possible Causes of Fatty Liver in Children and Adolescents

Nutrition	Obesity Severe weight loss due to starvation, and jejunoileal or gastric bypass Total parenteral nutrition Malnutrition
Drugs	Amiodarone; glucocorticoids; tamoxifen; methotrexate; valproid acid; aspirin; antiretroviral therapy
Dysmetabolism	Dyslipidemia, lipoatrophy; Insulin resistance; metabolic syndrome; Type 2 diabetes, polycystic ovary syndrome
Genetic	Lipodystrophy syndromes; cystic fibrosis; hereditary fructose intolerance; galactosemia; α_1-antitrypsin deficiency; Wilson disease, etc.
Others	Inflammatory bowel disease; hepatitis C and B infection; human immunodeficiency virus infection; celiac disease Alcohol Other hepatotoxins

There is therefore an urgent need for early diagnostic measures to evaluate grade and stage of disease, as well as effective and safe therapeutic approaches for the more advanced state of NASH (i.e., the presence of mild and severe fibrosis) (11,12). Most therapeutic modalities, already available or under investigation, target the major pathways thought essential in the pathogenesis of NASH (13). Unfortunately, pathogenic mechanism(s) leading to fatty liver, necro-inflammation, and fibrosis in children, as in adults, are incompletely understood (14).

In this chapter we summarize our understanding of the natural history, epidemiology, pathogenesis, and treatment of paediatric NAFLD/NASH and reflect on future diagnostic and therapeutic approaches.

NATURAL HISTORY

The natural history of NAFLD is still a mystery, because of its complex nature and the scarcity of prospective studies. Fatty liver may progress to NASH slowly over many years or decades, but the prognosis may depend upon the histological subtype at the time of presentation. Adult patients with simple fatty liver (with or without non-specific inflammation) have a generally benign prognosis, whereas those whose having NASH may progress to fibrosis, cirrhosis, and in a few cases to hepatocarcinoma (15,16). However, the precise percentage of patients with the advanced form of disease and the possible predictors of progression are still undefined. Moreover, data on prognosis of NAFLD and its progression in children are even more limited. Nevertheless, it is well documented that fatty liver and steatohepatitis may occur in very young children (17,18). As in adults, paediatric NAFLD presents a small but definite risk of cirrhosis (19,20).

EPIDEMIOLOGY

NAFLD is an increasingly recognized cause of liver disease throughout the world. However, the precise incidence and prevalence of NAFLD, NASH, and hepatic fibrosis remain unknown due to lack of prospective studies. Furthermore, estimates of prevalence vary widely across populations. Finally, screening approaches used to detect fatty liver, including measurements of serum aminotransferases [ALT (alanine aminotransferase), AST (aspartate aminotransferase), and GGT (gamma glutamyl transferase)] and hepatic imaging (ultrasound and magnetic resonance), are insufficient for the estimation of disease prevalence because definitive diagnosis of NAFLD and NASH requires liver biopsy (see diagnostic approach paragraph for references and more details).

Table 2
Epidemiological Data on Paediatric NAFLD/NASH

References	Number of children	NAFLD/NASH prevalence (%)	Diagnostic method
(22)	72	25	ALT
		53	Ultrasound
(19)	742	9.6	Liver biopsy
(23)	332	10	ALT
(24)	3,280	2.2	Liver biopsy, ultrasound, ALT
(25)	48	48	ALT
(21)	127	23	ALT
(26)	84	24	ALT
		77	Ultrasound

Fatty liver and NASH have been reported in all age groups in North and South America, Europe, Australia and Asia, but the disease is most common in obese children and adults (19,21). Studies of obese adolescents conducted in Europe and America found that the prevalence of NAFLD ranged from 2 to 77% (Table 2); this variability reflects differences in diagnostic approach as well as variation in the age, sex, race/ethnicity, and metabolic risk factors of the populations sampled (21–27). Data from NHANES III indicated that 6% of overweight and 10% of obese adolescents had elevated ALT; the CATCH study (Child and Adolescent Trial for Cardiovascular Health) demonstrated that a multivariate model using the combination of sex, race, ethnicity, and BMI predicted serum ALT and accounted for 36% of the individual variance (21,23). The only population-based study using ultrasound documented a prevalence of 2.6% in Japanese children aged 4–12 years; this value increased to 22% in obese subjects (26). SCALE (Study of Child and Adolescent Liver Epidemiology), a 10-year retrospective review of liver histology at autopsy of children aged 2–19 years, estimated that fatty liver occurs in 9% of subjects (19). In all these reports, the ratio of boys to girls with paediatric NAFLD approximates 2:1. The prevalence of paediatric NAFLD peaks at puberty, in association with increases in sex hormones and insulin resistance (28,29).

NAFLD is more common in Hispanic and Asian children than in white and black children (21). Racial/ethnic differences may be related to genetic, environmental, or sociocultural factors as well as differences in body composition, insulin sensitivity, and adipocytokine profile (30–32). Visceral adiposity and insulin resistance and type 2 diabetes are major risk factors.

HISTOLOGICAL FINDINGS

Histological assessments play an important role in the diagnosis and management of NAFLD. Thus it is important to carefully evaluate and discriminate among the different histological features which characterize NAFLD/NASH.

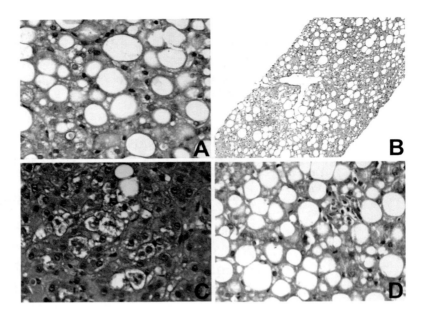

Fig. 1. Major histological features of paediatric NAFLD/NASH. Steatosis is evident in (**a**) (40× magnification) and (**b**) (10× magnification); ballooning and lipogranulomas are present in (**c**) and (**d**), respectively (40× magnification).

The main histological findings in NAFLD/NASH are steatosis, ballooning, inflammation, and fibrosis, but other liver lesions may also be presented (see Fig. 1). However, diagnosis of paediatric NASH can be difficult because all histological features commonly seen in adults are less common in children with definite NASH. The National Institutes of Health NASH Clinical Research Network (NASH CRN) established the heterogeneity of paediatric NASH sub-phenotypes *(11,33)*. Three distinct histological types were identified: type-1 NASH, characterized by steatosis with ballooning degeneration and/or perisinusoidal fibrosis, without portal involvement; type-2 NASH, characterized by steatosis with portal inflammation and/or fibrosis, in the absence of ballooning degeneration or perisinusoidal involvement; and a NASH overlap type, in which characteristics from both types were present *(11,34)*. Most paediatric subjects have type-2 NASH, which is more likely to be associated with advanced fibrosis *(33)*.

Steatosis

Hepatocellular steatosis, the hallmark of NAFLD, is the accumulation of lipids within the cytoplasm of hepatocytes. Two distinct patters of steatosis are recognized morphologically: macrovesicular and microvesicular steatoses (Fig. 1a, b) *(35)*. In macrovesicular steatosis, the hepatocytes are distended by single large fat droplets that displace eccentrically the nucleus. In microvesicular steatosis, the hepatocytes contain multiple small lipid droplets and the nuclei remain centrally placed within the cytoplasm.

Very mild degrees of steatosis can be found in normal liver; lipid vacuoles involving ~5% of hepatocytes are common *(36)*. Pathologic steatosis is most often macrovesicular, but a mixed macro/microvesicular pattern is common. The accumulation of fat in NAFLD is typically concentrated in zone 3 of the acinus with relative sparing of zone 1, but in more severe cases may occupy the whole acinus (Fig. 1a, b) *(37)*.

The severity of steatosis is determined by the extent of parenchymal involvement. Semiquantitative methods based on the percent of surface area involved are useful for grading the steatosis *(38)*.

Ballooning

Ballooning is the descriptive term used to indicate degenerative changes in hepatocytes. Morphologically the ballooned cells show loss of their normal polygonal shape; the cells are swollen and round but may sometimes be spindle shaped (Fig. 1c). Cellular borders are distinct. The cytoplasm is clear, rarefied, and vacuolated and can contain Mallory–Denk bodies, clumps of amorphous eosinophilic or amphophilic intra-cytoplasmic material randomly scattered within the cytoplasm or surrounding the nucleus as a slight irregular ring. Loss or marked diminution of immunohistochemical cytoplasmic staining of Keratin 8/18 may be utilized as a marker of ballooning degeneration (39,40). Light microscopy may not reveal fat vacuoles, but ultrastructurally the ballooned cells contain varying numbers of lipid droplets. Like steatosis, ballooning degeneration in NASH is typically noted in zone 3 of the acinus (41).

Ballooning degeneration is considered to result from intracellular fluid accumulation, a consequence of microtubule dysfunction and impaired protein secretion, and is not unique to steatohepatitis (40,42).

Inflammation

Lobular inflammation is the third major component of NASH and is integral to the diagnosis, even though it is usually mild. The presence of a marked mononuclear cell infiltrate should raise suspicion of a superimposed chronic liver disease (43).

Mononuclear cell infiltration may be observed in lobules or in portal tracts in the active or resolving phase of steatohepatitis. The composition of lobular infiltrates is a mix of lymphocytes and histiocytes, frequently associated with small numbers of polymorphonuclear leukocytes. Lymphocytes are mainly T cells of CD4 and CD8 phenotypes (44). Polymorphonuclear leukocytes may localize in the sinusoids or may cluster around ballooned hepatocytes containing Mallory–Denk bodies (satellitosis) (39).

Histiocytic reactions include activation of Kupffer cells and lipogranulomas. A lipogranuloma is a granulomatous reaction surrounding hepatocytes laden with broken lipids (Fig. 1d). Lipogranulomas contain macrophages, occasional lymphocytes, eosinophils, and giant cells. They may be localized near terminal hepatic venules, scattered throughout the acinus, or confined to the portal tracts. They may be associated with fibrosis, which should not be confused with perisinusoidal fibrosis (39).

Macrophages containing phagocytosed cellular debris and fat vacuoles may be seen in the sinusoids and within the portal tract. As they may persist even after resolution of steatosis in the parenchyma they are useful as hallmarks of past damage (45). Portal chronic inflammation is not required for the diagnosis of NASH even if may be presented in liver biopsies in varying degrees (46).

Fibrosis

Most pathologists do not consider fibrosis obligatory for the diagnosis of NASH; others disagree (39). Classically the fibrosis of NASH manifests in a pericellular "chicken wire" pattern, by which it is distinguished from other causes of steatohepatitis. This pattern results from the deposition of collagen fibers in the perivenular, perisinusoidal spaces of Disse in acinar zone 3, usually in association with the other lesions of steatohepatitis (39) (Fig. 2a). Special histochemical stains for collagen, such as trichrome stain (Masson, Van Gieson) or picrosirius red stain, are required for the detection of fibrosis in the initial stage (Fig. 2b). Hepatic stellate cells, the principal collagen-producing cells in the liver, are considered responsible for the development of fibrosis in NASH, even though the exact pathogenetic mechanism is not still clear.

Portal/periportal and bridging fibrosis can eventually progress to cirrhosis. During progression to cirrhosis the steatosis disappears, while perivenular fibrosis is incorporated in the more extensive bridging fibrosis. Thus the classical characteristics of steatohepatitis are no longer recognizable in more advanced stages of cirrhosis.

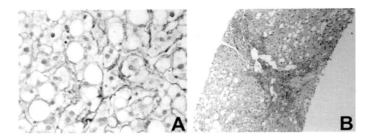

Fig. 2. Appearance of fibrosis in a paediatric patient with NAFLD/NASH. Van Gieson staining is shown in (**a**) (40×
magnification) and (**b**) (10× magnification).

Other histologic findings in NASH may include: acidophilic bodies, which result from hepatocyte apoptosis; megamitochondria; and vacuolated, glycogen-filled nuclei, which may also be seen in
Wilson's disease or in diabetic liver disease.

ETIOPATHOGENESIS

The etiopathogenesis of NAFLD has been long disputed. Several authors have suggested a model
consisting of two or more hits. Liver fat accumulation, which is the suggested "first hit," is thought
to increase vulnerability to possible "second hits," which are responsible for progression to NASH
(47,48). All models of pathogenesis include fat accumulation, insulin resistance, adipocytokines,
oxidative stress, and the innate immune response *(49,50,51,52)*.

In Fig. 3 we summarize some of the key pathogenic mechanisms involved in NAFLD/NASH.

Accumulation of Fat in the Liver

Liver fat accumulation is a consequence of at least three different phenomena: excessive triglyceride
accumulation caused by dietary free fatty acids (FFA), synthesis of hepatic lipids (de novo lipogenesis),
and imbalance influx (mainly dependent on insulin resistance) *(49,53,54)*.

It is widely accepted that dietary habits influence intrahepatic fat accumulation and inflammatory
activity *(55,56)*. Human and animal studies demonstrate that a diet enriched in saturated fat and cholesterol and/or an excess intake of carbohydrates (especially fructose) may be important causes of fatty
liver *(55,56,57,58,59)*. The pivotal role of diet in paediatric NAFLD pathogenesis has been further
validated in some recent studies *(60,61)*.

The control of liver fat synthesis involves a complex network of molecules and nuclear receptors
that regulate enzymes involved in various steps of hepatic lipid metabolism, including FFA uptake
and oxidation, de novo lipogenesis, and triglyceride secretion. The association between hepatic fat
accumulation and insulin resistance does not establish the direction of causality *(62)*. On one hand,
an imbalance between triglyceride synthesis/oxidation/export can increase cellular FFA derivatives
such as diacylglycerol and ceramide. These in turn activate protein kinases that phosphorylate serine
residues in insulin receptor substrate (IRS) proteins and can thereby impair hepatic insulin action.
On the other hand, hepatic insulin resistance caused by inflammatory cytokines and circulating lipids
might induce de novo lipogenesis and increase triglyceride exported as VLDL, thereby causing fatty
liver *(62,63)*. Indeed, FFA derived from diet, adipose lipolysis, and/or de novo hepatic lipogenesis have
an important direct role in the pathogenesis of NAFLD. FFA interact with the receptors involved in
the control of the innate immune response, such as Toll-like receptors (TLR), which activate cellular
apoptosis, induce oxidative stress, and increase cytokine production *(64,65,66)*.

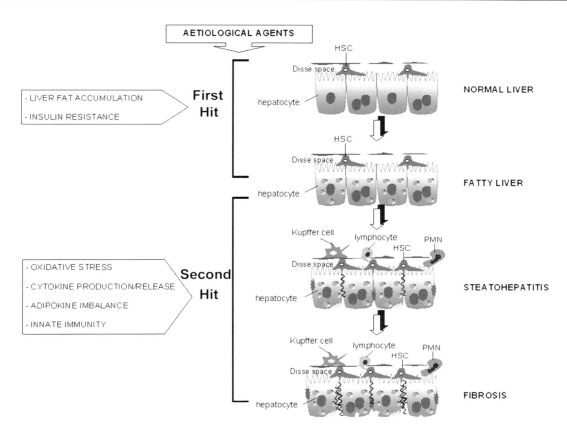

Fig. 3. Pathogenesis of fatty liver and its progression to steatohepatitis and fibrosis. A summary of pathogenetic mechanisms and liver cell modifications during NAFLD/NASH development is shown in this scheme. HSC, hepatic stellate cell; PMN, polymorphonuclear cell.

Role of Insulin Resistance

Insulin resistance is a major risk factor for the development of NAFLD and NASH. Serum ALT levels and liver fat content correlate positively with HOMA-IR, a measure of insulin resistance, and inversely with measures of insulin sensitivity, such as plasma adiponectin and sex hormone binding globulin *(67)*. Moreover, elevated intrahepatic triglyceride content in overweight adolescents is associated with dyslipidemia and with insulin-resistant glucose metabolism in both liver and skeletal muscle *(68)*. Adipose tissue lipolytic activity and serum FFA, markers of insulin resistance, are increased in obese adolescents with NAFLD *(69)*.

As noted previously, *hepatic* insulin resistance may be a consequence or cause of fatty liver disease. In addition, however, the overproduction of FFA and inflammatory cytokines (tumor necrosis factor-alpha, interleukin-6, nuclear factor kappa B, etc) and the fall in adiponectin levels in *systemic* insulin resistance may predispose to hepatic insulin resistance and fatty liver disease; conversely, fatty liver disease and hepatic insulin resistance may precede and contribute to insulin resistance in skeletal muscle and other insulin target tissues, thereby creating a vicious cycle of metabolic dysfunction *(50)*.

Impact of Oxidative Stress

Oxidative stress leads to chemical modification of biological molecules such as DNA, lipids, and proteins *(70)*. Under normal conditions the proper metabolism of liver cells creates a dynamic equilibrium between pro-oxidant molecules (reactive oxygen species, ROS) and antioxidant molecules. Disruption of this balance in favor of pro-oxidant molecules is a phenomenon of cellular oxidative stress that can impair cell function (70).

It is well known that oxidative stress plays a role in the development and progression of NAFLD (71,72). Mitochondrial beta-oxidation is required to prevent fat accumulation in the liver, but excessive and/or incomplete fatty acid oxidation alters physiological cell responses to oxidative stress. This causes an imbalance between intrahepatic antioxidants and reactive oxygen species (73). Accordingly, microvesicular steatosis in children is associated with changes in mitochondrial structure and function; mitochondrial hypertrophy was detected in hepatocytes of an asymptomatic paediatric patient with NAFLD (74,75), and there is a strong interaction between mitochondrial dysfunction and insulin resistance, cytokine production/release, and fibrogenesis (73,76,77). It has been proposed that steatosis makes the liver more susceptible to oxidative/nitrosative/nitrative stress, which is thought to be a stimulus for the progression from simple fatty liver to NASH (77).

The redox state of the cell is conditioned by the ratio of reduced glutathione to oxidized glutathione (GSH/GSSG). In liver cells, the maintenance of GSH levels and the redox state of the cell is a dynamic process insuring the balance between synthesis and utilization of GSH and transport of extracellular GSH and GSSG (78). There are several lines of evidence linking intracellular GSH/GSSG ratio to the pathogenesis of NAFLD/NASH: (i) the level of hepatic GSH is abnormally low in patients with NASH; (ii) GSH levels affect the activation of hepatic stellate cells (HSCs); (iii) paediatric patients with NASH have a decrease in the ratio of blood GSH/GSSG; (iv) depletion of GSH renders the hepatocyte more susceptible to the action of TNF-alpha (pro-apoptotic) and other cytokines, predisposing to the development of NASH; and (v) paediatric patients with NASH exhibit increased hepatic glutathionylated proteins that seem to be related to the state of fibrosis (79,80,81,82).

Function of Inflammatory Cytokines and Adipokines

Inflammatory cytokines implicated as pathogenetic factors in the development of NASH include TNF-alpha and IL-6 (49,83,84). TNF-alpha is expressed and secreted by adipose tissue, stromovascular cells, and endotoxin-activated macrophages (84). A rise in TNF-alpha can induce hepatic insulin resistance, interfering with hepatic glucose uptake and insulin signaling through serine phosphorylation of IRS (85,86). Conversely, a knockout of TNF-α in mice prevents the induction of insulin resistance by a high fat diet. Through induction of cellular apoptosis and production of other inflammatory cytokines (such as TGF beta), TNF-alpha may also play a fundamental role in the pathogenesis of hepatic fibrosis (87). Interestingly, studies in paediatric patients with NASH have revealed a strong correlation between histological liver injury scores and serum TNF-alpha (88).

IL-6 is a cytokine with multiple biological effects ranging from inflammation to tissue injury (84). Type 2 -diabetes and metabolic syndrome are associated with increased circulating levels of IL-6; it is therefore not surprising that plasma IL-6 levels are also high in adult and paediatric patients with NAFLD/NASH (89,90). Produced by adipose tissue, IL-6 can enter the liver portal vein and exert its effects on hepatocytes by activation of IL-6 receptor-dependent pathways, such as suppressor of cytokines-3 (SOCS-3) signaling. The activation of SOCS-3, in turn, inhibits tyrosine phosphorylation of IRS and leads to insulin resistance (48,91). Like TNF-alpha, IL-6 also has pro-inflammatory and pro-fibrogenic properties (85).

Dysregulation of adipocytokines may also play a role in the pathogenesis of fatty liver and steatohepatitis by interfering with insulin signaling and the inflammatory response (84,85,92). In this regard, reductions in adiponectin are among the most important factors. Adiponectin is secreted by adipocytes; it binds to hepatic receptors, increasing hepatic insulin sensitivity and exerting anti-inflammatory effects (84,93,94). Serum adiponectin was decreased in patients with fatty liver disease and NASH, independent of BMI and glycaemia, and in mice with fatty livers *(84,86)*. Serum levels of adiponectin were inversely related to necro-inflammatory activity and grade of fibrosis, even if not clearly associated with the severity of the histological damage *(95)*. Thus adiponectin may normally defend against the development of steatohepatitis; conversely, a fall in adiponectin in obesity and other insulin-resistant states may contribute to progression of fatty liver disease *(96,97)*.

Leptin, produced by white adipose tissue, regulates body weight and energy homeostasis *(98)*. Serum leptin levels are high in obese subjects. Leptin may prevent lipid accumulation in non-adipose tissues such as skeletal muscle, pancreas, and liver through induction of FFA oxidation *(99)*. In addition, leptin may exert beneficial effects on liver function and glucose homeostasis through increases in hepatic insulin sensitivity and reductions in TNF-alpha production and macrophage activation *(99)*. Thus the hyperleptinemia of obesity may be an adaptive response that reduces hepatic inflammation and limits the severity or progression of insulin resistance *(100)*. This may explain why some studies found increased serum levels of leptin in adults and children with NAFLD and steatohepatitis *(101,102)*. No correlation with fibrosis was found in NASH patients, even though leptin is a critical fibrogenic factor in animal models *(101,103)*. Other studies have found no changes in serum leptin levels or associations with the histopathologic profile of NAFLD *(49,104)*.

Resistin in humans circulates as monomeric peptides that may generate oligomeric structures *(105)*. Circulating levels of resistin are increased in mouse models of obesity and in obese humans, at least in some studies *(105,106)*. Resistin is also associated with insulin resistance, diabetes, and inflammation in mice, although in humans its role is not well established *(100,107)*. Recent studies demonstrated that serum resistin levels are increased in patients with NAFLD and associated with histological severity of liver damage (i.e., fibrosis) *(108,109)*. These results have not been confirmed in obese children with NAFLD *(110)*.

Other adipokines associated with NAFLD/NASH in adults include retinol-binding protein-4 (RBP4), plasminogen activator inhibitor (PAI)-1, and visfatin *(111,112)*. Decreased serum levels of RBP4 and increased circulating PAI-1 might be novel markers of severity of paediatric NAFLD *(113)*.

DIAGNOSTIC APPROACHES

Mild enlargement and tenderness of the liver are occasionally noted in NAFLD, but most children are asymptomatic. Detection of NAFLD and assessment of disease severity therefore necessitate laboratory investigation.

Serum Markers

Serum levels of ALT, AST, and GGT are usually (but not always) increased in NAFLD, but values may range from slightly above the normal range to a tenfold increase *(9,114)*. Other forms of liver disease associated with elevated ALT levels and/or steatosis (e.g., viral and autoimmune hepatitis, drug or toxic liver injury including alcohol abuse, Wilson's disease, and alpha1-anti-trypsin deficiency) must be excluded.

Other circulating factors associated with NAFLD/NASH include TNF-alpha, IL-6 and 8, hyaluronic acid (HA), and type-VI collagen *(115,116,117)*. Markers of liver fibrosis include apolipoprotein A1, haptoglobin, alpha$_2$-macroglobulin, HA, and procollagen peptides. Various biochemical markers of fibrosis have been grouped into laboratory panels that have been used for increasing their predictive power. These include: the BARD score, the NAFLD score, the FibroMeter, the Fibrotest/FibroSure, and ELF (enhanced liver fibrosis) markers *(118,119,120)*. Our group has recently demonstrated that ELF markers (HA, procollagen III amino terminal peptide, and tissue inhibitor of metalloproteinase 1) predict liver fibrosis in children with NAFLD *(121)*.

Imaging Techniques

In adults, ultrasound has a sensitivity of 60–94% and a specificity of 73–93% for the diagnosis of liver fat *(122)*. However, ultrasound is unable to detect fat infiltration below 33% or to assess disease severity or the presence or absence of NASH.

Hepatic MRI has a number of advantages including operator independence and reproducibility and includes the possibility of acquiring in-phase (water) and opposed-phase (fat) images in one breath hold. Like ultrasound, MRI cannot distinguish NASH from simple steatosis or detect the presence of fibrosis.

An interesting technique under development is transient elastography (TE) by FibroScan. The detection accuracy of the method increases with worsening grades of fibrosis *(123)*. FibroScan has recently been shown to be an accurate and reproducible technique for identifying significant degrees of fibrosis in children and adults *(124)* (Table 3).

Table 3
Current Non-invasive Techniques for Diagnosis of Paediatric NAFLD/NASH

Serum biomarkers	ALT, AST, and GGT predict the presence of NAFLD but may be normal in some cases
Abdominal ultrasound	Unable to detect fat infiltration below 33% or to differentiate among degrees of the disease and the presence of NASH
Computerized tomography	More sensitive and specific than ultrasound but limited by radiation exposure and the masking effect of iron overload Does not differentiate steatosis from NASH or fibrosis
Magnetic resonance imaging	The most sensitive and specific imaging technique but cannot distinguish simple steatosis from steatohepatitis and/or fibrosis High cost
New approaches	– Markers of extracellular matrix that are related to fibrosis and the development of liver cirrhosis, such as "ELF MARKERS" – Transient elastography (FibroScan) assessment of disease progression

Liver Biopsy

Liver biopsy remains the only reliable way to precisely diagnose NASH and establish the severity of liver injury and presence of fibrosis. Histologic criteria required for the diagnosis of NASH are summarized in Table 4.

Grading and Staging of NAFLD

In an attempt to define and standardize the histopathological diagnosis of NAFLD, a number of systems have been elaborated. Matteoni *et al.* proposed four specific histological patterns of NAFLD: type 1, fatty liver alone; type 2, fatty liver plus lobular inflammation; type 3, steatosis and ballooning degeneration; and type 4, steatosis plus ballooning degeneration plus Mallory body or fibrosis

Table 4
Diagnostic Criteria for NASH

Major criteria	Minor criteria
Steatosis (>5% of hepatocytes)	Mallory–Denk bodies
Ballooning	Apoptosis and necrosis
Lobular inflammation	Megamitochondria
(Fibrosis)	Glycogenated nuclei
	Iron deposition

(125). The grading and staging scheme for NASH proposed by Brunt *et al.* in the same year is based on semiquantitative evaluation of multiple histologic features using the concepts and terminology employed in chronic hepatitis *(126)*. In this scheme 10 histological variables were evaluated for necro-inflammatory activity: macrovesicular steatosis, hepatocellular ballooning and disarray, lobular inflammation, portal inflammation, Mallory's hyaline, acidophil bodies, PAS-D Kupffer cells, glycogenated nuclei, lipogranulomas, and hepatocellular iron. Fibrosis was characterized as perisinusoidal fibrosis, portal fibrosis, and bridging fibrosis.

Table 5
Grading System for NASH

Mild (*grade 1*)	Steatosis (predominantly macrovesicular) involving up to 66% of biopsy; occasional ballooning in zone 3 hepatocytes; scattered intra-acinar inflammation (PMNs or lymphocytes); no portal inflammation
Moderate (*grade 2*)	Steatosis of any degree; obvious ballooning in zone 3; lobular (PMNs or lymphocytes); and portal inflammation mild to moderate; pericellular fibrosis
Severe (*grade 3*)	Panacinar steatosis; obvious ballooning and disarray predominantly in zone 3; mild to moderate intra-acinar inflammation and portal inflammation

A three-tier grading system for pathological diagnosis of NASH was proposed (see Table 5) *(126)*. A limitation of this system is its designation for NASH and not for the full spectrum of NAFLD. To achieve consensus among hepatopathologists and to provide a simplified scoring system for NAFLD, the Pathology Committee of the NASH CRN designed and validated a scoring system applicable to the entire spectrum of NAFLD. Moreover, an NAFLD activity score (NAS) for use in clinical trials was proposed *(127)*.

In developing this scoring system, the semiquantitative system proposed by Brunt was refined and the three features of active injury (steatosis, lobular inflammation, and ballooning) were used to derive a scoring system. The activity score (NAS) was defined as the un-weighted sum of scores of steatosis (graded from 0 to 3), lobular inflammation (graded from 0 to 3), and ballooning (graded from 0 to 2).

Thus the NAS ranges from 0 to 8. An NAS<3 excludes NASH (simple steatosis alone); 3≥NAS<5 is considered borderline; and NAS≥5 is considered diagnostic of NASH *(127)*.

TREATMENT OF FATTY LIVER DISEASE

Therapeutic interventions seek to limit the progression from fatty liver to steatohepatitis and to reverse histological features of necro-inflammation and fibrosis. Limitations of previous therapeutic studies include small numbers of patients and significant differences in diagnostic methods, definitions of fatty liver or steatohepatitis, study design, and outcome measures. An additional limit of existing therapeutic strategies comes from poor understanding of the pathophysiology of fatty liver and steatohepatitis, which confines therapeutic approaches to the treatment of morbidities associated with NAFLD (i.e., obesity, dyslipidemia, insulin resistance, and disordered carbohydrate metabolism) and reduction of oxidative damage *(13,128)*. No treatments target the disease per sè.

Lifestyle Changes

Initial management of an obese child with raised levels of aminotransferases and imaging evidence of fatty liver should focus on gradual weight loss, using a combination of diet and exercise. Indeed, the few available studies demonstrate reductions in aminotransferases and indices of insulin resistance following diet-induced weight loss and changes in lifestyle, which combine calorie-restricted nutritional programs and regular physical exercise *(129)*.

Nevertheless, the particular type of dietary modification that may be beneficial in treating young patients with fatty liver is yet unclear. A pragmatic approach may be to recommend a reduced calorie, balanced diet. Saturated fats and high glycemic foods, including simple sugars, refined grains, rice, and potatoes, should be limited or avoided in favor of whole grains, legumes, and low-glycemic index fruits and vegetables.

Consumption of low-glycemic meals reduces glucose-stimulated insulin secretion, thereby promoting nutrient oxidation and reducing hepatic lipid synthesis and storage. Conversely, simple sugars boost insulin secretion. High consumption of fructose (especially in sweetened beverages) leads to increased de novo lipogenesis and post-prandial hypertriglyceridemia. Fructose consumption induces significant changes in the plasma lipid profile and reduces insulin sensitivity as compared with a glucose-enriched diet. Of note, fructose consumption causes fat to accumulate viscerally, and visceral fat is a strong predictor of intrahepatic fat deposition *(130)*. As compared with other sugars, fructose directly enters the glycolytic/gluconeogenic pathway, resulting in the production of lipogenic substrates such as glucose, glycogen, lactate, and pyruvate. Fructose also promotes lipogenesis via enhanced expression of the sterol regulatory element binding protein 1-c (SREB 1-c). Finally, high consumption of fructose can alter gut microbiota, thus affecting intestinal permeability and promoting metabolic endotoxemia, which can play a pivotal role in the progression from NAFLD to NASH *(56)*.

Consumption of a low-carbohydrate diet (less than 60 g/day) associates with early amelioration of hepatic insulin resistance, as estimated by rate of hepatic glucose production, and with a 30% reduction in the intrahepatic content of triglycerides *(131)*. However, low-carbohydrate regimens may promote excessive consumption of fats, which may be detrimental for intermediate metabolism. Saturated fatty acids stimulate glucose-dependent insulin secretion and promote chronic hyperinsulinemia *(132)*. Conversely, consumption of polyunsaturated fats from fish and flax seed oils has beneficial effects on insulin sensitivity and promotes anti-inflammatory prostaglandin metabolism *(132)*. Essential polyunsaturated fatty acids can reduce fat depots by through activation of peroxisome-proliferator-activated receptors *(133)*, which promotes fatty acid catabolism, and down-regulation of de novo lipogenesis through SREBP pathways *(134)*. On the other hand, arachidonic acid activates Kupffer cells and modulates the fibrogenic response of hepatic stellate cells *(135)*. Moreover, it should be borne in mind that both saturated and unsaturated fats may promote lipid peroxidation, thus exacerbating hepatocyte damage.

Therefore, it seems reasonable to reduce fat intake to less than 20% of total energy intake in obese subjects with NAFLD. Low-glycemic index foods and fibers can help in achieving this goal while avoiding chronic hyperinsulinemia and reducing post-prandial insulin excursions. Intake of antioxidants and vitamins might be beneficial for reversing oxidative damage, though this remains to be established (see below).

It is unknown what percentage of starting weight must be lost or what rate of weight loss must occur to induce significant improvement in hepatic disease in children with NAFLD, but there is consensus that weight loss should be gradual. Preliminary results suggest that the BMI must change by at least 0.5 units *(136)*. Patients should refrain from alcohol or reduce intake to levels less than 20 g/day.

A strategy combining diet and physical exercise seems to be more successful than traditional approaches of fat energy restriction *(42)*. Physical exercise reduces hyperinsulinemia and increases insulin sensitivity and substrate oxidation even without affecting body weight *(137)*. A multidisciplinary approach, which includes the expertise of an endocrinologist, hepatologist, cardiologist, psychologist, and dietician, can ensure weight loss and long-term weight maintenance through permanent change of lifestyle *(138)*.

Bariatric Surgery

The Roux-en-Y-gastric (RYGB) bypass is the only bariatric technique whose use is approved for treatment of morbidly obese adolescents (BMI>40 kg/m^2 or BMI>35 kg/m^2 plus two co-morbidities) by the Food and Drug Administration. RYGB can reverse disordered carbohydrate metabolism and type-2 diabetes and ameliorate features of the metabolic syndrome such as dyslipidemia and hypertension *(139)*. Because of the associations among obesity, insulin resistance, and NASH, bariatric surgery has been proposed as potential treatment in obese adolescents also with NASH *(140)*. However, studies of NASH outcome after bariatric surgery in adolescents are currently lacking. A multicenter study for the follow-up of adolescent bariatric surgery (FABS) is on-going and will conclude in April 2010 (NCT00776776). Experience in adults undergoing bypass surgery demonstrates that fatty liver improves or resolves in most cases, but data on the effects of surgery on necro-inflammation or fibrosis are inconsistent *(141,142,143)*. A transient worsening of liver function may occur early after surgery, probably because rapid weight loss causes a massive flux of fatty acids to the liver *(144,145)*.

Cytoprotective and Antioxidants Agents

Cytoprotective agents and antioxidants have been studied in children with fatty liver as means of addressing the second hit thought to be caused by increased oxidative stress.

Large population surveys found that obese children had lower circulating levels of vitamin E than normal weight subjects *(146)*. Thus, the effectiveness of vitamin E supplementation in the treatment of fatty liver was first investigated in a pilot study, and, then, in follow-up controlled trials *(147,148,149)*.

The first pilot study was uncontrolled and open label. Eleven children who had NASH were prescribed a dose of vitamin E varying from 400 to 1,200 IU/day. Treatment led to improvements in serum aminotransferase levels with no change in BMI or in hepatic fat accumulation on sonogram *(149)*. A subsequent randomized, double-blind placebo-controlled trial comparing vitamin E plus vitamin C versus placebo found treatment with antioxidants to be no better than diet alone in improving levels of liver enzymes and indices of insulin sensitivity after 1 year of treatment *(148)*. The study was prolonged in an open-label fashion for an additional 12 months. At the end of the 2-year follow-up, changes in histological features were assessed in 25 patients treated with vitamin E (600 IU/day) plus vitamin C (500 mg/day) and in 28 patients treated with placebo. All patients were prescribed a diet and regular physical activity. The degree of steatosis, inflammation, and NAS score improved in all patients independent of pharmacological treatment *(147)*.

Other antioxidant agents of potential interest include *S*-adenosyl-methionine, betaine, *N*-acetylcysteine, and lazaroids. Betaine acts as a methyl donor in an alternative pathway for re-methylation of homocysteine to methionine. We are not aware of any controlled studies using these agents in adults or children with fatty liver.

Insulin Sensitizers

Most children with fatty liver disease have hepatic and systemic insulin resistance; this provides a rationale for using insulin sensitizers such as metformin and thiazolidinediones in treatment of NAFLD.

Metformin reduces hepatic glucose production and, to a lesser extent, glycogenolysis and thereby reduces fasting glucose and insulin levels. Metformin alone was administered in a pilot study enrolling 10 children with NAFLD. Use of metformin (500 mg twice/day) was well tolerated and caused reductions in liver fat stores as assessed by MRI after 24 weeks of treatment *(150)*.

However, a follow-up study found no added benefit of metformin on levels of serum aminotransferases, insulin sensitivity, or liver histology in children controlled on diet. The study was double blind in the first 12 months and open in the last 12 months. Controls were the 30 patients who served as controls in the clinical trial for the use of vitamin E *(148,150)*. Twenty-seven patients with biopsy-proven fatty liver and/or steatohepatitis were treated with metformin 1.5 g/day. Twelve patients treated with metformin and 15 controls underwent liver biopsy at the end of the 2-year period. No significant differences were observed between the two arms in terms of laboratory and histological parameters. However, several factors flawed the study, including experimental design, recruitment of controls, and the limited number of patients undergoing liver biopsy.

Hence, there is a strong need for controlled studies to assess the effectiveness of metformin in paediatric NAFLD. Of note, a large, multicenter trial of vitamin E and metformin is underway as part of the NASH clinical research network to evaluate outcomes of treatment in paediatric fatty liver *(143)*.

The PPAR-gamma agonists thiazolidinediones (TZD) are under investigation as treatment for NASH in adults, but have not been studied yet in childhood *(151)*. Apart from their capacity for lowering plasma glucose, TZD have important anti-inflammatory and anti-atherogenic properties *(110)*. Indeed, 55 patients with impaired glucose tolerance or type-2 diabetes and liver biopsy-confirmed non-alcoholic steatohepatitis underwent 6 months of treatment with a hypocaloric diet (a reduction of 500 kcal/day in relation to the calculated daily intake required to maintain body weight) plus pioglitazone (45 mg daily) or a hypocaloric diet plus placebo. Hepatic histologic features, hepatic fat content (assessed by magnetic resonance spectroscopy), and glucose turnover during an oral glucose tolerance test were evaluated prior to and following treatment. Diet plus pioglitazone, as compared with diet plus placebo, improved glycemic control and glucose tolerance, normalized liver aminotransferase levels, decreased hepatic fat content, and increased hepatic insulin sensitivity. Treatment with pioglitazone, as compared with placebo, was associated with improvement in histologic findings with regard to steatosis, ballooning necrosis, and inflammation. Nevertheless, the reduction in fibrosis did not differ significantly from that in the placebo group *(152)*. Thus, TZDs might be useful in the treatment of fatty liver. However, TZDs can cause weight gain, edema, anemia, and bone loss, making them less suitable for use in growing children.

LIPID-LOWERING DRUGS

Lipid-lowering drugs of potential interest for the treatment of fatty liver include fibrates, statins, and resin-binding agents. Fibrates alter lipoprotein metabolism through binding to PPAR alpha, while statins reduce cholesterol synthesis by inhibiting HMG CoA reductase. The effects of fibrates and statins have been investigated in various conditions associated with steatohepatitis in adult patients, but with uncertain results *(153,154)*. A pilot study assessed the effect of simvastatin in a small cohort of adults with NASH followed for 12 months *(155)*. The study was double blind, randomized, and placebo controlled, but included a small number of subjects (*N*=16). Liver biopsy was assessed before and after treatment in 10 patients. Although the treated arm showed a 26% reduction in low-density lipoprotein, there were no statistically significant improvements in serum aminotransferases, hepatic steatosis, necro-inflammatory activity, or stage of fibrosis within or between groups.

Caution must be exercised when prescribing statins to patients with liver disease. Their potential hepatotoxicity requires frequent monitoring of biochemical parameters of hepatic cytolysis and cholestasis. Administration of statins may be contraindicated in patients with advanced or end-stage parenchymal liver disease or with acute liver disease *(156)*.

New Perspectives

The association between small intestinal bacterial overgrowth and steatohepatitis may support the use of prebiotics and probiotics as means for the prevention of steatohepatitis. Modulators of toll-like receptors (TLR) are of potential interest as well *(157)*. Pentoxyfilline, a methylxanthine compound that attenuates TNF-alpha production in peripheral blood and mononuclear cells, represents a potentially interesting approach, as preliminary results in adult patients are encouraging *(158,159)*. The rationale for the use of modulators of TLR or pentoxyfilline comes from evidence supporting a role for the innate immune system in the pathogenesis of NASH, and, particularly, for TNF-alpha in the progression from simple fatty liver to NASH *(157,160)*.

Editor's Questions and Authors' Response

- **What are your indications for liver biopsy in an obese child with elevations in serum ALT, AST, and/or GGT?**

- Assuming that there is nothing to suggest another explanation for hepatic dysfunction, liver biopsy is indicated only in case of persistently elevated liver enzymes following several months of lifestyle intervention. However, the length of this observation period is controversial. In our centre, biopsy is performed after 6 months of unsuccessful lifestyle intervention before starting any pharmacological treatment. In any case, to date, the vast majority of pediatricians do not perform a liver biopsy in this population, thus making a precise estimate of NASH rather difficult.

- **How might the findings of liver biopsy alter your approach to treatment?**

- To date, there is no consensus for pharmacologic treatment of NAFLD. However, there is general agreement on the need for counseling all subjects with NAFLD regarding diet and exercise in order to reduce the underlying insulin resistance. If liver biopsy shows a picture of inflammation or fibrosis, it could be suggested to start a treatment using an antioxidant agent (vitamin E) or metformin (if there is associated IR). Obviously, children showing fibrosis must be monitored carefully during the follow-up period for early signs of liver failure.

REFERENCES

1. Roberts EA. Pediatric nonalcoholic fatty liver disease (NAFLD): a "growing" problem? J Hepatol. 2007;46:1133–42.
2. Kim CH, Younossi ZM. Nonalcoholic fatty liver disease: a manifestation of the metabolic syndrome. Cleve Clin J Med. 2008;75:721–28.

3. Khashab MA, Liangpunsakul S, Chalasani N. Nonalcoholic fatty liver disease as a component of the metabolic syndrome. Curr Gastroenterol Rep. 2008;10:73–80.

4. Caldwell S, Park SH. The epidemiology of hepatocellular cancer: from the perspectives of public health problem to tumor biology. J Gastroenterol. 2009;44(Suppl 19):96–101.

5. Lim YS, Kim WR. The global impact of hepatic fibrosis and end-stage liver disease. Clin Liver Dis. 2008;12: 733–46.

6. Lazo M, Clark JM. The epidemiology of nonalcoholic fatty liver disease: a global perspective. Semin Liver Dis. 2008;28:339–50.

7. Angulo P. Obesity and nonalcoholic fatty liver disease. Nutr Rev. 2007;65(6 Pt 2):S57–63.

8. Papandreou D, Rousso I, Mavromichalis I. Update on non-alcoholic fatty liver disease in children. Clin Nutr. 2007;26:409–15.

9. Mager DR, Roberts EA. Nonalcoholic fatty liver disease in children. Clin Liver Dis. 2006;10:109–31.

10. Dunn W, Schwimmer JB. The obesity epidemic and nonalcoholic fatty liver disease in children. Curr Gastroenterol Rep. 2008;10:67–72.

11. Pardee PE, Lavine JE, Schwimmer JB. Diagnosis and treatment of pediatric nonalcoholic steatohepatitis and the implications for bariatric surgery. Semin Pediatr Surg. 2009;18:144–51.

12. Wieckowska A, Feldstein AE. Diagnosis of nonalcoholic fatty liver disease: invasive versus noninvasive. Semin Liver Dis. 2008;28:386–95.

13. Alisi A, Manco M, Vania A, Nobili V. Pediatric nonalcoholic fatty liver disease in 2009. J Pediatr. 2009;155:469–74.

14. Preiss D, Sattar N. Non-alcoholic fatty liver disease: an overview of prevalence, diagnosis, pathogenesis and treatment considerations. Clin Sci (Lond). 2008;115:141–50.

15. Hashimoto E, Yatsuji S, Tobari M, Taniai M, Torii N, Tokushige K, Shiratori K. Hepatocellular carcinoma in patients with nonalcoholic steatohepatitis. J Gastroenterol. 2009;44(Suppl 19):89–95.

16. Serfaty L, Lemoine M. Definition and natural history of metabolic steatosis: clinical aspects of NAFLD, NASH and cirrhosis. Diabetes Metab. 2008;34(6 Pt 2):634–37.

17. Nobili V, Marcellini M, Devito R, Ciampalini P, Piemonte F, Comparcola D, Sartorelli MR, Angulo P. NAFLD in children: a prospective clinical-pathological study and effect of lifestyle advice. Hepatology. 2006;44:458–65.

18. Fishbein M, Cox S. Non-alcoholic fatty liver disease in a toddler. Clin Pediatr (Phila). 2004;43:483–85.

19. Schwimmer JB, Deutsch R, Kahen T, Lavine JE, Stanley C, Behling C. Prevalence of fatty liver in children and adolescents. Pediatrics. 2006;118:1388–93.

20. Suzuki D, Hashimoto E, Kaneda K, Tokushige K, Shiratori K. Liver failure caused by non-alcoholic steatohepatitis in an obese young male. J Gastroenterol Hepatol. 2005;20:327–29.

21. Schwimmer JB, McGreal N, Deutsch R, Finegold MJ, Lavine JE. Influence of gender, race, and ethnicity on suspected fatty liver in obese adolescents. Pediatrics. 2005;115:e561–5.

22. Franzese A, Vajro P, Argenziano A, Puzziello A, Iannucci MP, Saviano MC, Brunetti F, Rubino A. Liver involvement in obese children. Ultrasonography and liver enzyme levels at diagnosis and during follow-up in an Italian population. Dig Dis Sci. 1997;42:1428–32.

23. Strauss RS, Barlow SE, Dietz WH. Prevalence of abnormal serum aminotransferase values in overweight and obese adolescents. J Pediatr. 2000;136:727–33.

24. Nobili V, Reale A, Alisi A, Morino G, Trenta I, Pisani M, Marcellini M, Raucci U. Elevated serum ALT in children presenting to the emergency unit: relationship with NAFLD. Dig Liver Dis. 2009;41:749–52.

25. Nadeau KJ, Klingensmith G, Zeitler P. Type 2 diabetes in children is frequently associated with elevated alanine aminotransferase. J Pediatr Gastroenterol Nutr. 2005;41:94–98.

26. Chan DF, Li AM, Chu WC, Chan MH, Wong EM, Liu EK, Chan IH, Yin J, Lam CW, Fok TF, Nelson EA. Hepatic steatosis in obese Chinese children. Int J Obes Relat Metab Disord. 2004;28:1257–63.

27. Alisi A, Manco M, Panera N, Nobili V. Association between type two diabetes and non-alcoholic fatty liver disease in youth. Ann Hepatol. 2009;8(Suppl 1):S44–50.

28. Kimata H. Increased incidence of fatty liver in non-obese Japanese children under 1 year of age with or without atopic dermatitis. Publ Health. 2006;120:176–78.

29. Schwimmer JB. Definitive diagnosis and assessment of risk for nonalcoholic fatty liver disease in children and adolescents. Semin Liver Dis. Aug 2007;27(3):312–18.

30. Ogden CL, Flegal KM, Carroll MD, Johnson CL. Prevalence and trends in overweight among US children and adolescents, 1999–2000. J Am Med Assoc. 2002;288:1728–32.

31. Williams DE, Cadwell BL, Cheng YJ, Cowie CC, Gregg EW, Geiss LS, Engelgau MM, Narayan KM, Imperatore G. Prevalence of impaired fasting glucose and its relationship with cardiovascular disease risk factors in US adolescents, 1999–2000. Pediatrics. 2005;116:1122–26.

32. Comuzzie AG, Funahashi T, Sonnenberg G, Martin LJ, Jacob HJ, Black AE, Maas D, Takahashi M, Kihara S, Tanaka S, Matsuzawa Y, Blangero J, Cohen D, Kissebah A. The genetic basis of plasma variation in adiponectin, a global endophenotype for obesity and the metabolic syndrome. J Clin Endocrinol Metab. 2001;86:4321–25.

33. Kleiner DE, Behling CB, Brunt EM, Lavine JE, et al; for the NASH CRN Research Group. Comparison of adult and pediatric NAFLD – confirmation of a second pattern of progressive fatty liver disease in children. J Hepatol. 2006;44:259–60A.

34. Manco M, Marcellini M, Devito R, Comparcola D, Sartorelli MR, Nobili V. Metabolic syndrome and liver histology in paediatric non-alcoholic steatohepatitis. Int J Obes (Lond). 2008;32:381–87.

35. Burt AD, Mutton A, Day CP. Diagnosis and interpretation of steatosis and steatohepatitis. Semin Diagn Pathol. 1998;15:246–58.

36. Paradis V, Bedossa P. Definition and natural history of metabolic steatosis: histology and cellular aspects. Diabetes Metab. 2008;34:638–42.

37. Chalasani N, Wilson L, Kleiner DE, Cummings OW, Brunt EM. Unalp A; NASH Clinical Research Network. Relationship of steatosis grade and zonal location to histological features of steatohepatitis in adult patients with non-alcoholic fatty liver disease. J Hepatol. 2008;48:829–34.

38. Schwenzer NF, Springer F, Schraml C, Stefan N, Machann J, Schick F. Non-invasive assessment and quantification of liver steatosis by ultrasound, computed tomography and magnetic resonance. J Hepatol. 2009;51:433–45.

39. Brunt EM. Nonalcoholic steatohepatitis. Semin Liver Dis. 2004;24:3–20.

40. Lackner C, Gogg-Kamerer M, Zatloukal K, Stumptner C, Brunt EM, Denk H. Ballooned hepatocytes in steatohepatitis: the value of keratin immunohistochemistry for diagnosis. J Hepatol. 2008;48:821–28.

41. Brunt EM, Tiniakos DG. Pathology of steatohepatitis. Best Pract Res Clin Gastroenterol. 2002;16:691–707.

42. Brunt EM, Neuschwander-Tetri BA, Oliver D, Wehmeier KR, Bacon BR. Nonalcoholic steatohepatitis: histologic features and clinical correlations with 30 blinded biopsy specimens. Hum Pathol. 2004;35:1070–82.

43. Brunt EM. Non-alcoholic fatty liver disease in Mac Sween's pathology of the liver. 5th ed. Edinburgh: Churchill Livingstone; 2007. pp. 367–97.

44. Lefkowitch JH, Haythe JH, Regent N. Kupffer cell aggregation and perivenular distribution in steatohepatitis. Mod Pathol. 2002;15:699–704.

45. Ikura Y, Ohsawa M, Suekane T, Fukushima H, Itabe H, Jomura H, Nishiguchi S, Inoue T, Naruko T, Ehara S, Kawada N, Arakawa T, Ueda M. Localization of oxidized phosphatidylcholine in nonalcoholic fatty liver disease: impact on disease progression. Hepatology. 2006;43:506–14.

46. Brunt EM, Kleiner DE, Wilson LA, Unalp A, Behling CE, Lavine JE, Neuschwander-Tetri BA; NASH Clinical Research Network. Portal chronic inflammation in nonalcoholic fatty liver disease (NAFLD): a histologic marker of advanced NAFLD-clinicopathologic correlations from the nonalcoholic steatohepatitis clinical research network. Hepatology. 2009;49:809–20.

47. de Alwis NM, Day CP. Non-alcoholic fatty liver disease: the mist gradually clears. J Hepatol. 2008;48(Suppl 1): S104–12.

48. Day CP. NASH-related liver failure: one hit too many? Am J Gastroenterol. 2002;97:1872–74.

49. Petta S, Muratore C, Craxì A. Non-alcoholic fatty liver disease pathogenesis: the present and the future. Dig Liver Dis. 2009;41:615–25.

50. Tilg H, Moschen AR. Insulin resistance, inflammation, and non-alcoholic fatty liver disease. Trends Endocrinol Metab. 2008;19:371–79.

51. Pessayre D. Role of mitochondria in non-alcoholic fatty liver disease. J Gastroenterol Hepatol. 2007;22(Suppl 1): S20–7.

52. Albano E, Mottaran E, Occhino G, Reale E, Vidali M. Review article: role of oxidative stress in the progression of non-alcoholic steatosis. Aliment Pharmacol Ther. 2005;22(Suppl 2):71–3.

53. Tessari P, Coracina A, Cosma A, Tiengo A. Hepatic lipid metabolism and non-alcoholic fatty liver disease. Nutr Metab Cardiovasc Dis. 2009;19:291–302.

54. Cheung O, Sanyal AJ. Abnormalities of lipid metabolism in nonalcoholic fatty liver disease. Semin Liver Dis. 2008;28:351–9.

55. Musso G, Gambino R, Cassader M. Recent insights into hepatic lipid metabolism in non-alcoholic fatty liver disease (NAFLD). Prog Lipid Res. 2009;48:1–26.

56. Spruss A, Bergheim I. Dietary fructose and intestinal barrier: potential risk factor in the pathogenesis of nonalcoholic fatty liver disease. J Nutr Biochem. 2009;20:657–62.

57. Basciano H, Miller AE, Naples M, Baker C, Kohen R, Xu E, Su Q, Allister EM, Wheeler MB, Adeli K. Metabolic effects of dietary cholesterol in an animal model of insulin resistance and hepatic steatosis. Am J Physiol Endocrinol Metabol. 2009;297:E462–73.

58. Morgan K, Uyuni A, Nandgiri G, Mao L, Castaneda L, Kathirvel E, French SW, Morgan TR. Altered expression of transcription factors and genes regulating lipogenesis in liver and adipose tissue of mice with high fat diet-induced obesity and nonalcoholic fatty liver disease. Eur J Gastroenterol Hepatol. 2008;20:843–54.

59. Omagari K, Kato S, Tsuneyama K, Inohara C, Kuroda Y, Tsukuda H, Fukazawa E, Shiraishi K, Mune M. Effects of a long-term high-fat diet and switching from a high-fat to low-fat, standard diet on hepatic fat accumulation in Sprague-Dawley rats. Dig Dis Sci. 2008;53:3206–4212.

60. Vos MB, Weber MB, Welsh J, Khatoon F, Jones DP, Whitington PF, McClain CJ. Fructose and oxidized low-density lipoprotein in pediatric nonalcoholic fatty liver disease: a pilot study. Arch Pediatr Adolesc Med. 2009;163:674–5.

61. Papandreou D, Rousso I, Malindretos P, Makedou A, Moudiou T, Pidonia I, Pantoleon A, Economou I, Mavromichalis I. Are saturated fatty acids and insulin resistance associated with fatty liver in obese children? Clin Nutr. 2008;27:233–40.

62. Lavoie JM, Gauthier MS. Regulation of fat metabolism in the liver: link to non-alcoholic hepatic steatosis and impact of physical exercise. Cell Mol Life Sci. 2006;63:1393–409.

63. Tsochatzis EA, Manolakopoulos S, Papatheodoridis GV, Archimandritis AJ. Insulin resistance and metabolic syndrome in chronic liver diseases: old entities with new implications. Scand J Gastroenterol. 2009;44:6–14.

64. Baffy G. Kupffer cells in non-alcoholic fatty liver disease: the emerging view. J Hepatol. 2009;51:212–23.

65. Budick-Harmelin N, Dudas J, Demuth J, Madar Z, Ramadori G, Tirosh O. Triglycerides potentiate the inflammatory response in rat Kupffer cells. Antioxid Redox Signal. 2008;10:2009–22.

66. Ginsberg HN. Is the slippery slope from steatosis to steatohepatitis paved with triglyceride or cholesterol? Cell Metab. 2006;4:179–81.

67. Bugianesi E, Gastaldelli A, Vanni E, Gambino R, Cassader M, Baldi S, Ponti V, Pagano G, Ferrannini E, Pizzetto M. Insulin resistance in non-diabetic patients with non-alcoholic fatty liver disease: sites and mechanisms. Diabetologia. 2005;48:634–42.

68. Deivanayagam S, Mohammed BS, Vitola BE, Naguib GH, Keshen TH, Kirk EP, Klein S. Nonalcoholic fatty liver disease is associated with hepatic and skeletal muscle insulin resistance in overweight adolescents. Am J Clin Nutr. 2008;88:257–62.

69. Fabbrini E, deHaseth D, Deivanayagam S, Mohammed BS, Vitola BE, Klein S. Alterations in fatty acid kinetics in obese adolescents with increased intrahepatic triglyceride content. Alterations in fatty acid kinetics in obese adolescents with increased intrahepatic triglyceride content. Obesity (Silver Spring). 2009;17:25–29.

70. Djordjević VB. Free radicals in cell biology. Int Rev Cytol. 2004;237:57–89.

71. Duvnjak M, Lerotić I, Barsić N, Tomasić V, Virović Jukić L, Velagić V. Pathogenesis and management issues for non-alcoholic fatty liver disease. World J Gastroenterol. 2007;13:4539–50.

72. Albano E. New concepts in the pathogenesis of alcoholic liver disease. Expert Rev Gastroenterol Hepatol. 2008;2: 749–59.

73. Marra F, Gastaldelli A, Svegliati Baroni G, Tell G, Tiribelli C. Molecular basis and mechanisms of progression of non-alcoholic steatohepatitis. Trends Mol Med. 2008;14:72–81.

74. Da Silva GH, Coelho KI, Coelho CA, Escanhoela CA. Mitochondrial alterations in nonalcoholic fatty liver disease. Pediatric case description of three submitted sequential biopsies. J Gastrointestin Liver Dis. 2009;18:215–19.

75. Mandel H, Hartman C, Berkowitz D, Elpeleg ON, Manov I, Iancu TC. The hepatic mitochondrial DNA depletion syndrome: ultrastructural changes in liver biopsies. Hepatology. 2001;34:776–84.

76. Begriche K, Igoudjil A, Pessayre D, Fromenty B. Mitochondrial dysfunction in NASH: causes, consequences and possible means to prevent it. Mitochondrion. 2006;6:1–28.

77. Mantena SK, King AL, Andringa KK, Eccleston HB, Bailey SM. Mitochondrial dysfunction and oxidative stress in the pathogenesis of alcohol- and obesity-induced fatty liver diseases. Free Radic Biol Med. 2008;44:1259–72.

78. Han D, Hanawa N, Saberi B, Kaplowitz N. Mechanisms of liver injury. III. Role of glutathione redox status in liver injury. Am J Physiol Gastrointest Liver Physiol. 2006;291:G.

79. Altomare E, Vendemiale G, Albano O. Hepatic glutathione content in patients with alcoholic and non alcoholic liver diseases. Life Sci. 1988;43:991–98.

80. Nobili V, Pastore A, Gaeta LM, Tozzi G, Comparcola D, Sartorelli MR, Marcellini M, Bertini E, Piemonte F. Glutathione metabolism and antioxidant enzymes in patients affected by nonalcoholic steatohepatitis. Clin Chim Acta. 2005;355:105–11.

81. Garcia-Ruiz C, Fernandez-Checa JC. Mitochondrial glutathione: hepatocellular survival-death switch. J Gastroenterol Hepatol. 2006;21:S.

82. Piemonte F, Petrini S, Gaeta LM, Tozzi G, Bertini E, Devito R, Boldrini R, Marcellini M, Ciacco E, Nobili V. Protein glutathionylation increases in the liver of patients with non-alcoholic fatty liver disease. J Gastroenterol Hepatol. 2008;23(8 Pt 2):e457–64.

83. Kotronen A, Yki-Järvinen H. Fatty liver: a novel component of the metabolic syndrome. Arterioscler Thromb Vasc Biol. 2008;28:27–38.

84. Qureshi K, Abrams GA. Metabolic liver disease of obesity and role of adipose tissue in the pathogenesis of nonalcoholic fatty liver disease. World J Gastroenterol. 2007;13:3540–53.

85. Jarrar MH, Baranova A, Collantes R, Ranard B, Stepanova M, Bennett C, Fang Y, Elariny H, Goodman Z, Chandhoke V, Younossi ZM. Adipokines and cytokines in non-alcoholic fatty liver disease. Aliment Pharmacol Ther. 2008;27:412–21.

86. Wang Z, Lv J, Zhang R, Zhu Y, Zhu D, Sun Y, Zhu J, Han X. Co-culture with fat cells induces cellular insulin resistance in primary hepatocytes. Biochem Biophys Res Commun. 2006;345:976–83.

87. Saile B, Matthes N, El Armouche H, Neubauer K, Ramadori G. The bcl, NFkappaB and p53/p21WAF1 systems are involved in spontaneous apoptosis and in the anti-apoptotic effect of TGF-beta or TNF-alpha on activated hepatic stellate cells. Eur J Cell Biol. 2001;80:554–61.

88. Manco M, Marcellini M, Piemonte F, Nobili V. Correlation of serum TNF-α levels and histologic liver injury scores in pediatric NAFLD. Am J Clin Pathol. 2007;127:954–60.

89. Wieckowska A, Papouchado BG, Li Z, Lopez R, Zein NN, Feldstein AE. Increased hepatic and circulating interleukin-6 levels in human nonalcoholic steatohepatitis. Am J Gastroenterol. 2008;103:1372–79.

90. Nobili V, Marcellini M, Giovannelli L, Girolami E, Muratori F, Giannone G, Devito R, De Benedetti F. Association of serum interleukin-8 levels with the degree of fibrosis in infants with chronic liver disease. J Pediatr Gastroenterol Nutr. 2004;39:540–44.

91. Senn JJ, Klover PJ, Nowak IA, Mooney RA. Interleukin-6 induces cellular insulin resistance in hepatocytes. Diabetes. 2002;51:3391–99.

92. Polyzos SA, Kountouras J, Zavos C. Nonalcoholic fatty liver disease: the pathogenetic roles of insulin resistance and adipocytokines. Curr Mol Med. 2009;9:299–314.

93. Kamada Y, Takehara T, Hayashi N. Adipocytokines and liver disease. J Gastroenterol. 2008;43:811–22.

94. Kaser S, Moschen A, Cayon A, Kaser A, Crespo J, Pons-Romero F, Ebenbichler CF, Patsch JR, Tilg H. Adiponectin and its receptors in non-alcoholic steatohepatitis. Gut. 2005;54:117–21.

95. Musso G, Gambino R, Biroli G, Carello M, Fagà E, Pacini G, De Michieli F, Cassader M, Durazzo M, Rizzetto M, Pagano G. Hypoadiponectinemia predicts the severity of hepatic fibrosis and pancreatic B-cell dysfunction in nondiabetic nonobese patients with nonalcoholic steatohepatitis. Am J Gastroenterol. 2005;100:2438–46.

96. Louthan MV, Barve S, McClain CJ, Joshi-Barve S. Decreased serum adiponectin: an early event in pediatric nonalcoholic fatty liver disease. J Pediatr. 2005;147:835–38.

97. Zou CC, Liang L, Hong F, Fu JF, Zhao ZY. Serum adiponectin, resistin levels and non-alcoholic fatty liver disease in obese children. Endocr J. 2005;52:519–24.

98. Friedman JM, Halaas JL. Leptin and the regulation of body weight in mammals. Nature. 1998;395:763–70.

99. Polyzos SA, Kountouras J, Zavos C. Nonalcoholic fatty liver disease: the pathogenetic roles of insulin resistance and adipocytokines. Curr Mol Med. 2009;9:299–314.

100. Bastard JP, Maachi M, Lagathu C, Kim MJ, Caron M, Vidal H, Capeau J, Feve B. Recent advances in the relationship between obesity, inflammation, and insulin resistance. Eur Cytokine Netw. 2006;17:4–12.

101. Marra F, Bertolani C. Adipokines in liver diseases. Hepatology. 2009;50:957–69.

102. Wong VW, Hui AY, Tsang SW, Chan JL, Tse AM, Chan KF, So WY, Cheng AY, Ng WF, Wong GL, Sung JJ, Chan HL. Metabolic and adipokine profile of Chinese patients with nonalcoholic fatty liver disease. Clin Gastroenterol Hepatol. 2006;4:1154–61.

103. Honda H, Ikejima K, Hirose M, Yoshikawa M, Lang T, Enomoto N, Kitamura T, Takei Y, Sato N. Leptin is required for fibrogenic responses induced by thioacetamide in the murine liver. Hepatology. 2002;36:12–21.

104. Pagano C, Soardo G, Esposito W, Fallo F, Basan L, Donnini D, Federspil G, Sechi LA, Vettor R. Plasma adiponectin is decreased in nonalcoholic fatty liver disease. Eur J Endocrinol. 2005;152:113–18.

105. Steppan CM, Bailey ST, Bhat S, Brown EJ, Banerjee RR, Wright CM, Patel HR, Ahima RS, Lazar MA. The hormone resistin links obesity to diabetes. Nature. 2001;409:307–12.

106. Perseghin G, Lattuada G, De Cobelli F, Natali G, Esposito A, Burska A, Belloni E, Canu T, Ragogna F, Scifo P, Del Maschio A, Luzi L. Serum resistin and hepatic fat content in nondiabetic individuals. J Clin Endocrinol Metab. 2006;91:5122–25.

107. Kushiyama A, Shojima N, Ogihara T, Inukai K, Sakoda H, Fujishiro M, Fukushima Y, Anai M, Ono H, Horike N, Viana AY, Uchijima Y, Nishiyama K, Shimosawa T, Fujita T, Katagiri H, Oka Y, Kurihara H, Asano T. Resistin-like molecule beta activates MAPKs, suppresses insulin signaling in hepatocytes, and induces diabetes, hyperlipidemia, and fatty liver in transgenic mice on a high fat diet. J Biol Chem. 2005;280:42016–25.

108. Jiang LL, Li L, Hong XF, Li YM, Zhang BL. Patients with nonalcoholic fatty liver disease display increased serum resistin levels and decreased adiponectin levels. Eur J Gastroenterol Hepatol. 2009;21:662–66.

109. Tsochatzis E, Papatheodoridis GV, Hadziyannis E, Georgiou A, Kafiri G, Tiniakos DG, Manesis EK, Archimandritis AJ. Serum adipokine levels in chronic liver diseases: association of resistin levels with fibrosis severity. Scand J Gastroenterol. 2008;43:1128–36.

110. Chiquette E, Ramirez G, Defronzo R. A meta-analysis comparing the effect of thiazolidinediones on cardiovascular risk factors. Arch Intern Med. 2004;164:2097–104.

111. Thuy S, Ladurner R, Volynets V, Wagner S, Strahl S, Königsrainer A, Maier KP, Bischoff SC, Bergheim I. Nonalcoholic fatty liver disease in humans is associated with increased plasma endotoxin and plasminogen activator inhibitor 1 concentrations and with fructose intake. J Nutr. 2008;138:1452–55.

112. Alkhouri N, Lopez R, Berk M, Feldstein AE. Serum retinol-binding protein 4 (RBP4) levels in patients with nonalcoholic fatty liver disease. J Clin Gastroenterol. 11 Jun 2009;43(10):985–89.

113. Nobili V, Alkhouri N, Alisi A, Ottino S, Lopez R, Manco M, Feldstein AE. Retinol-binding protein 4: a promising circulating marker of liver damage in pediatric nonalcoholic fatty liver disease. Clin Gastroenterol Hepatol. 2009;7:575–79.

114. Nanda K. Non-alcoholic steatohepatitis in children. Pediatr Transplant. 2004;8:613–18.

115. Guha IN, Parkes J, Roderick PR, Harris S, Rosenberg WM. Non-invasive markers associated with liver fibrosis in non-alcoholic fatty liver disease. Gut. 2006;55:1650–60.

116. Ong JP, Elariny H, Collantes R, Younoszai A, Chandhoke V, Reines HD, Goodman Z, Younossi ZM. Predictors of nonalcoholic steatohepatitis and advanced fibrosis in morbidly obese patients. Obes Surg. 2005;15:310–15.

117. Bahcecioglu IH, Yalniz M, Ataseven H, Ilhan N, Ozercan IH, Seckin D, Sahin K. Levels of serum hyaluronic acid, TNF-alpha and IL-8 in patients with nonalcoholic steatohepatitis. Hepatogastroenterology. 2005;52:1549–53.

118. Yilmaz Y, Ulukaya E, Dolar E. The quest for liver fibrosis biomarkers: promises from the enhanced liver fibrosis panel and beyond. Hepatology. 2009;49:1056–1057.

119. Ratziu V, Massard J, Charlotte F, Messous D, Imbert-Bismut F, Bonyhay L, et al. Diagnostic value of biochemical markers (FibroTest-FibroSURE) for the prediction of liver fibrosis in patients with non-alcoholic fatty liver disease. BMC Gastroenterol. 2006;6:6.

120. Guha IN, Parkes J, Roderick P, Chattopadhyay D, Cross R, Harris S, et al. Noninvasive markers of fibrosis in non-alcoholic fatty liver disease: validating the European liver fibrosis panel and exploring simple markers. Hepatology. 2008;47:455–60.

121. Nobili V, Parkes J, Bottazzo G, Marcellini M, Cross R, Newman D, Vizzutti F, Pinzani M, Rosenberg WM. Performance of ELF serum markers in predicting fibrosis stage in pediatric non-alcoholic fatty liver disease. Gastroenterology. 2009;136:160–67.

122. Wieckowska A, McCullough AJ, Feldstein AE. Noninvasive diagnosis and monitoring of nonalcoholic steatohepatitis: present and future. Hepatology. 2007;46:582–89.

123. Friedrich-Rust M, Ong MF, Martens S, Sarrazin C, Bojunga J, Zeuzem S, Herrmann E. Performance of transient elastography for the staging of liver fibrosis: a meta-analysis. Gastroenterology. 2008;134:960–74.

124. Nobili V, Vizzutti F, Arena U, Abraldes JG, Marra F, Pietrobattista A, Fruhwirth R, Marcellini M, Pinzani M. Accuracy and reproducibility of transient elastography for the diagnosis of fibrosis in pediatric nonalcoholic steatohepatitis. Hepatology. 2008;48:442–48.

125. Matteoni CA, Younossi ZM, Gramlich T, Boparai N, Liu YC, McCullough AJ. Nonalcoholic fatty liver disease: a spectrum of clinical and pathological severity. Gastroenterology. 1999;116:1413–19.

126. Brunt EM, Janney CG, Di Bisceglie AM, Neuschwander-Tetri BA, Bacon BR. Nonalcoholic steatohepatitis: a proposal for grading and staging the histological lesions. Am J Gastroenterol. Sept 1999;94:2467–74.

127. Kleiner DE, Brunt EM, Van Natta M, Behling C, Contos MJ, Cummings OW, Ferrell LD, Liu YC, Torbenson MS, Unalp-Arida A, Yeh M, McCullough AJ, Sanyal AJ; Nonalcoholic Steatohepatitis Clinical Research Network. Design and validation of a histological scoring system for nonalcoholic fatty liver disease. Hepatology. 2005;41:1313–21.

128. Balsano C, Alisi A, Nobili V. Liver fibrosis and therapeutic strategies: the goal for improving metabolism. Curr Drug Targets. 2009;10:505–12.

129. Vajro P, Fontanella A, Perna C, Orso G, Tedesco M, De Vincenzo A. Persistent hyperaminotransferasemia resolving after weight reduction in obese children. J Pediatr. 1994;125:239–41.

130. Stanhope KL, Schwarz JM, Keim NL, Griffen SC, Bremer AA, Graham JL, et al. Consuming fructose-sweetened, not glucose-sweetened, beverages increases visceral adiposity and lipids and decreases insulin sensitivity in overweight/obese humans. J Clin Invest. 2009;119:1322–34.

131. Kirk E, Reeds DN, Finck BN, Mayurranjan SM, Patterson BW, Klein S. Dietary fat and carbohydrates differentially alter insulin sensitivity during caloric restriction. Gastroenterology. 2009;136:1552–60.

132. Manco M, Calvani M, Mingrone G. Effects of dietary fatty acids on insulin sensitivity and secretion. Diabetes Obes Metab. 2004;6:402–13.

133. Clarke SD, Jump DB. Polyunsaturated fatty acid regulation of hepatic gene transcription. Lipids. 1996;31(Suppl): S7–11.

134. Kim HJ, Takahashi M, Ezaki O. Fish oil feeding decreases mature sterol regulatory element-binding protein 1 (SREBP-1) by down-regulation of SREBP-1c mRNA in mouse liver. A possible mechanism for down-regulation of lipogenic enzyme mRNAs. A possible mechanism for down-regulation of lipogenic enzyme mRNAs. J Biol Chem. 1999;274:25892–98.

135. Cubero FJ, Nieto N. Ethanol and arachidonic acid synergize to activate Kupffer cells and modulate the fibrogenic response via tumor necrosis factor alpha, reduced glutathione, and transforming growth factor beta-dependent mechanisms. Hepatology. 2008;48:2027–39.

136. Reinehr T, Kiess W, Kapellen T, Andler W. Insulin sensitivity among obese children and adolescents, according to degree of weight loss. Pediatrics. 2004;114:1569–73.

137. Ueno T, Sugawara H, Sujaku K, Hashimoto O, Tsuji R, Tamaki S, Torimura T, Inuzuka S, Sata M, Tanikawa K. Therapeutic effects of restricted diet and exercise in obese patients with fatty liver. J Hepatol. 1997;27:103–7.

138. Brage S, Wedderkopp N, Ekelund U, Franks PW, Wareham NJ, Andersen LB, Froberg K. Objectively measured physical activity correlates with indices of insulin resistance in Danish children. The European Youth Heart Study (EYHS). Int J Obes Relat Metab Disord. 2004;28:1503–8.

139. Inge TH, Miyano G, Bean J, Helmrath M, Courcoulas A, Harmon CM, Chen MK, Wilson K, Daniels SR, Garcia VF, Brandt ML, Dolan LM. Reversal of type 2 diabetes mellitus and improvements in cardiovascular risk factors after surgical weight loss in adolescents. Pediatrics. 2009;123:214–22.

140. Pratt JS, Lenders CM, Dionne EA, Hoppin AG, Hsu GL, Inge TH, Lawlor DF, Marino MF, Meyers AF, Rosenblum JL, Sanchez VM. Best practice updates for pediatric/adolescent weight loss surgery. Obesity (Silver Spring). 2009;17: 901–10.

141. Klein S, Mittendorfer B, Eagon JC, Patterson B, Grant L, Feirt N, Seki E, Brenner D, Korenblat K, McCrea J. Gastric bypass surgery improves metabolic and hepatic abnormalities associated with nonalcoholic fatty liver disease. Gastroenterology. 2006;130:1564–72.

142. Mathurin P, Gonzalez F, Kerdraon O, Leteurtre E, Arnalsteen L, Hollebecque A, Louvet A, Dharancy S, Cocq P, Jany T, Boitard J, Deltenre P, Romon M. Pattou F. The evolution of severe steatosis after bariatric surgery is related to insulin resistance. Gastroenterology. 2006;130:1617–24.

143. Patton HM, Sirlin C, Behling C, Middleton M, Schwimmer JB, Lavine JE. Pediatric nonalcoholic fatty liver disease: a critical appraisal of current data and implications for future research. J Pediatr Gastroenterol Nutr. 2006;43:413–27.

144. Dixon JB, Bhathal PS, Hughes NR, O'Brien PE. Nonalcoholic fatty liver disease: improvement in liver histological analysis with weight loss. Hepatology. 2004;39:1647–54.

145. Luyckx FH, Desaive C, Thiry A, Dewé W, Scheen AJ, Gielen JE, Lefèbvre PJ. Liver abnormalities in severely obese subjects: effect of drastic weight loss after gastroplasty. Int J Obes Relat Metab Disord. 1998;22:222–26.

146. Strauss RS. Comparison of serum concentrations of alpha-tocopherol and beta-carotene in a cross-sectional sample of obese and nonobese children (NHANES III). National Health and Nutrition Examination Survey. J Pediatr. 1999;134:160–65.

147. Nobili V, Manco M, Devito R, Di Ciommo V, Comparcola D, Sartorelli MR, Piemonte F, Marcellini M, Angulo P. Lifestyle intervention and antioxidant therapy in children with nonalcoholic fatty liver disease: a randomized, controlled trial. Hepatology. 2008;48:119–28.

148. Nobili V, Manco M, Devito R, Ciampalini P, Piemonte F, Marcellini M. Effect of vitamin E on aminotransferase levels and insulin resistance in children with non-alcoholic fatty liver disease. Aliment Pharmacol Ther. 2006;24:1553–61.

149. Lavine JE. Vitamin E treatment of nonalcoholic steatohepatitis in children: a pilot study. J Pediatr. 2000;136:734–38.

150. Nobili V, Manco M, Ciampalini P, Alisi A, Devito R, Bugianesi E, Marcellini M, Marchesini G. Metformin use in children with nonalcoholic fatty liver disease: an open-label, 24-month, observational pilot study. Clin Ther. 2008;30:1168–76.

151. Dwivedi S, Havranek R, Fincke C, DeFronzo R, Bannayan GA, Schenker S, Cusi K. A placebo-controlled trial of pioglitazone in subjects with nonalcoholic steatohepatitis. N Engl J Med. 2006;355:2297–307.

152. Belfort R, Harrison SA, Brown K, Darland C, Finch J, Hardies J, et al. A placebo-controlled trial of pioglitazone in subjects with nonalcoholic steatohepatitis. N Engl J Med. 2006;355:2297–307.

153. Laurin J, Lindor KD, Crippin JS, Gossard A, Gores GJ, Ludwig J, Rakela J, McGill DB. Ursodeoxycholic acid or clofibrate in the treatment of non-alcohol-induced steatohepatitis: a pilot study. Hepatology. 1996;23:1464–67.

154. Basaranoglu M, Acbay O, Sonsuz A. A controlled trial of gemfibrozil in the treatment of patients with nonalcoholic steatohepatitis. J Hepatol. 1999;31:384.

155. Nelson A, Torres DM, Morgan AE, Fincke C, Harrison SA. A pilot study using simvastatin in the treatment of nonalcoholic steatohepatitis: a randomized placebo-controlled trial. J Clin Gastroenterol. 2009;43(10):990–94.

156. Anfossi G, Massucco P, Bonomo K, Trovati M. Prescription of statins to dyslipidemic patients affected by liver diseases: a subtle balance between risks and benefits. Nutr Metab Cardiovasc Dis. 2004;14:215–24.

157. Mencin A, Kluwe J, Schwabe RF. Toll-like receptors as targets in chronic liver diseases. Gut. 2009;58:704–20.

158. Adams LA, Zein CO, Angulo P, Lindor KD. A pilot trial of pentoxifylline in nonalcoholic steatohepatitis. Am J Gastroenterol. 2004;99:2365–68.

159. Satapathy SK, Garg S, Chauhan R, Sakhuja P, Malhotra V, Sharma BC, Sarin SK. Beneficial effects of tumor necrosis factor-alpha inhibition by pentoxifylline on clinical, biochemical, and metabolic parameters of patients with nonalcoholic steatohepatitis. Am J Gastroenterol. 2004;99:1946–52.

160. Wullaert A, van Loo G, Heyninck K, Beyaert R. Hepatic tumor necrosis factor signaling and nuclear factor-kappaB: effects on liver homeostasis and beyond. Endocr Rev. 2007;28:365–86.

16 Pathogenesis of Hypertension and Renal Disease in Obesity

Tracy E. Hunley and Valentina Kon

Key Words: Blood pressure, insulin, sympathetic nervous system, renin–angiotensin–aldosterone system, insulin resistance, obesity-related, glomerulopathy, proteinuria

INTRODUCTION

Obesity, hypertension, and renal injury are linked by complex inter-relationships. Obesity-associated metabolic abnormalities promote both systemic hypertension and renal injury; hypertension in turn results from, and contributes to, progressive renal damage, regardless of primary cause. It is now well established that obesity dramatically increases the risks of type-II diabetes and diabetic nephropathy; yet even in the absence of diabetes, obesity predisposes to chronic kidney disease and accelerates its progression. In this chapter we discuss the pathogenesis of hypertension and renal disease in obese adults and children and reflect on their implications for therapy.

HYPERTENSION

Epidemiology

Elevated systemic blood pressure (BP) is a leading contributor to the global disease burden, promoting the development and progression of heart disease, stroke, and kidney damage. The life-threatening complications of chronic hypertension rarely manifest during childhood, but elevated BP among children and adolescents predicts the development of hypertension in adulthood (1), and several intermediate endpoints of hypertensive end-organ damage, including left ventricular hypertrophy, carotid artery intima-media thickness, endothelial dysfunction, proteinuria, and renal scarring are now seen

From: *Contemporary Endocrinology: Pediatric Obesity: Etiology, Pathogenesis, and Treatment*
Edited by: M. Freemark, DOI 10.1007/978-1-60327-874-4_16,
© Springer Science+Business Media, LLC 2010

with increasing frequency in obese children *(2)*. Recent projections indicate that childhood hypertension will contribute significantly to the overall future burden of cardiovascular and renal diseases in adulthood and hasten development of these complications in the pediatric population.

Childhood obesity is now recognized as one of the strongest predictors of hypertension in young adulthood *(2–4)*. Compared with the 25% prevalence of hypertension in adults, only about 3–5% of children are affected. However, establishing pediatric norms and defining hypertension have been complicated by difficulties in obtaining pressure readings in children, a lack of standardization of the measurements, and changes in pressure levels that occur during normal maturational development. The most recent normative BP tables used data acquired from the 1999–2000 National Health and Nutrition Examination Survey (NHANES). BP recordings in 8–17-year olds, collected between 1963 and 1988, documented a decreasing trend for hypertension *(3)*. By contrast, data collected after 1988 revealed a reversal in the downward trend, with both hypertension and pre-hypertension levels increasing in the childhood population. This reversal in the hypertension trend is widely believed to reflect the increasing prevalence of childhood adiposity.

The association between adiposity and hypertension is well established in adults. The prevalence of hypertension is 3 times higher and the incidence 5 times higher in obese adults than in normal weight individuals. It is estimated that at least 50% of the rise in the prevalence of hypertension is attributable to escalating BMI. The obesity–hypertension relationship has now also been convincingly demonstrated in children and adolescents *(2–5)*. Obese children are at threefold higher risk for developing hypertension than non-obese children. As in adults, the risk occurs across the range of BMIs. Thus, some 20–30% of 5–11-year olds with weight >120th percentile of ideal have elevated systolic or diastolic pressure. Overweight adolescents (BMI >75th percentile) have an eightfold increased risk of developing hypertension as adults. The strong association between childhood obesity and hypertension has been confirmed in many parts of the world. As in adults, the prevalence of overweight and elevated blood pressure is higher in Native Americans, African-Americans, Hispanics, and Asians than in white children *(2,3,5–7)*. Citing potential differences and inadequacy in blood pressure measurement techniques and differences in definition of hypertension, some reservations had been raised as to whether obesity-related hypertension in children has affected the overall prevalence of hypertension in the pediatric population. However, using the newest blood pressure criteria for hypertension and pre-hypertension in children, Din-Dzietham et al. demonstrated that development of hypertension lagged behind the uptrend in obesity by 10 years *(6)*. The report concluded that obesity is indeed the most important driving force in childhood hypertension, especially in African-American and Hispanic children. Figure 1 illustrates the recent trends in the impact of obesity on childhood hypertension.

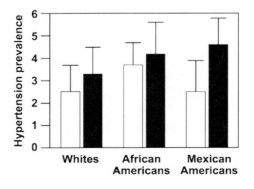

Fig. 1. Impact of obesity rise on hypertension in children. High blood pressure prevalence and 95% confidence interval obtained in 8–17 year olds in the National Health and Nutritional Examination Survey 1963–1988 (NHANES III) *(open columns)* and 1988–1999 (NHANESIV) *(black columns)*. Adapted from Din-Dzietham et al. *(6)*.

Blood Pressure Homeostasis

Blood pressure is the force exerted by the blood against a unit area of vessel wall and is defined as

$$BP = CO \times TPR = (HR \times SV) \times TPR$$

where BP is blood pressure, CO is cardiac output, HR is heart rate, SV is stroke volume, and TPR is the total peripheral resistance. CO and TPR are intimately dependent on the extracellular fluid volume, which is determined primarily by the renal excretion of sodium and water.

Adiposity affects all of these parameters (8). Obese and overweight individuals have increased resting CO by virtue of increased heart rate, which reflects heightened sympathetic tone and reduced vagal tone. Perturbed autonomic regulation has been implicated in obesity-related blunting in heart rate variability that is linked to cardiovascular disease, including hypertension. Obesity also increases stroke volume; this results from expansion in the circulatory volume necessary to perfuse the increased adipose tissue mass and fat-free mass that accompany weight gain. The increased stroke volume also reflects increased ventricular filling pressure and blood volume that follows an increase in tubular sodium reabsorption. As in all hypertensive states, obesity-associated hypertension is associated with impaired pressure natriuresis, a mechanism that normally allows the kidney to regulate systemic BP. Thus, obese individuals have an inappropriately limited natriuretic response to a saline load; this necessitates that obese individuals require a higher blood pressure than those of normal weight to excrete a given sodium load. The mechanisms for impaired renal pressure natriuresis in this setting include augmented sympathetic nervous system activity, activation of the renin–angiotensin–aldosterone system, and increased intrarenal pressure.

The homeostatic mechanisms that maintain the balance between cardiac output and peripheral vascular resistance are disrupted in obesity. Compared with normal weight or obese individuals who are normotensive, peripheral vascular resistance is increased in hypertensive obese individuals despite the increase in CO. This abnormal vascular response is especially apparent in obese/overweight individuals whose fat is centrally distributed. Indeed, even in the absence of overt obesity, there is an independent association between central adiposity and increased CO and/or increased (or insufficiently reduced) vascular resistance. This suggests that the metabolically active visceral fat contributes directly or indirectly to body requirements for blood flow supply.

The underlying mechanisms include enhanced vasoconstriction, endothelial dysfunction with impaired vasodilation, and vascular wall remodeling associated with deposition of lipids, advanced glycation end-products, and extracellular matrix components that impair normal adjustments in vasomotor tone. Early stages of overweight and obesity are characterized by an exaggerated vasoconstrictive response. However, as obesity becomes severe, there ensues a progressive impairment in the vascular response. Such findings suggest that the initially heightened vasomotor response is followed by vascular remodeling that limits the hemodynamic response. Markers of endothelial dysfunction and vessel remodeling, including impaired brachial artery flow-mediated dilation and increased carotid artery intima-media thickness, previously established in adults, have now been well documented in obese children.

Pathophysiologic Mechanisms

SYMPATHETIC NERVOUS SYSTEM ACTIVITY

Direct and indirect evidence supports an important pathophysiological role for an overactive sympathetic nervous system in obesity-associated hypertension (9). Experimental studies show that a high-calorie diet that leads to obesity also causes hypertension. This effect is not observed in obese animals with pharmacologic blockade of α- and β-receptors or animals with bilateral renal denervation that achieve similar weight gain *(10)*. Obese humans have elevated plasma and urinary catecholamine levels as well as heightened sympathetic neural activity *(11)*. A cross-sectional study found that BMI and plasma norepinephrine levels independently predict vasoconstriction and blood pressure elevation in obese hypertensive individuals. This association is especially apparent in children and adults with central obesity *(12)*.

Obesity-related changes in sympathetic tone not only promote vasoconstriction but also impair vasodilation, as assessed by the response to cold stress, mental stress, or handgrip. All vascular beds (e.g., skeletal, mesenteric, renal) may be impacted though their responses to adrenergic stimulation are heterogeneous, modulated by local as well as systemic factors. The physiological mechanisms by which activated sympathetic tone can increase BP include direct vasoconstriction, increases in heart rate and stroke volume that increase cardiac output, and expansion of the extracellular volume by increases in renal tubule sodium reabsorption. These effects are mediated by reductions in insulin sensitivity and concomitant changes in plasma leptin, insulin, adiponectin and free fatty acids, which in combination with activation of the renin–angiotensin system *(9)* heighten sympathetic tone (Fig. 2).

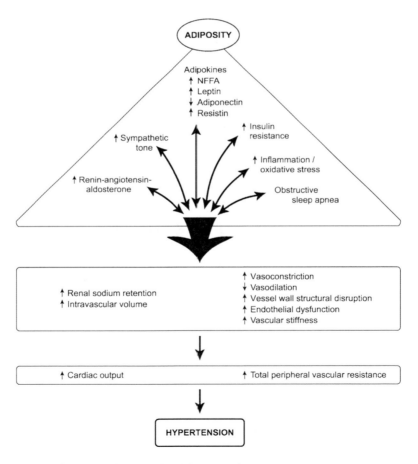

Fig. 2. Mechanisms contributing to obesity-associated hypertension.

Pharmacologic blockade of sympathetic activity with a combined α- and β-adrenergic receptor blocker causes greater reduction in BP in obese than in lean individuals. It is interesting that Pima Indians, who have increased propensity for obesity, do not have heightened sympathetic tone and do not develop hypertension to the same degree as other racial groups. These observations suggest that BP is modulated by ethnic/genetic factors that may counteract the effects of adiposity on sympathetic drive. These factors may promote the differential reactivity of vascular beds. Thus, normotensive obese individuals have elevated sympathetic nerve activity in skeletal muscle but a normal vasodilatative response to α-adrenergic receptor blockade *(13)*. Similar counterbalancing effects may be provided by other vasodilators including nitric oxide and natriuretic peptides or local regulators of sympathetic nerve activity, such as insulin or leptin. Thus, while obesity is regularly accompanied by enhanced sympathetic outflow, the heightened sympathetic tone may be modulated by compensatory mechanisms and/or local factors to achieve the final/sustained vascular tone.

RENIN–ANGIOTENSIN–ALDOSTERONE SYSTEM (RAAS)

The renin–angiotensin–aldosterone system (RAAS) has a causal role in obesity-related hypertension (Fig. 2). Even in the setting of the volume-expanded state that characterizes obesity, all the components of the RAAS are inappropriately normal or elevated *(14)*. Conversely, weight reduction is followed by decrease in RAAS activity. For example, dietary restriction that produced a 5% reduction in weight led to a 7-mmHg reduction in ambulatory systolic blood pressure that was accompanied by a 27% decline in angiotensinogen, 43% decline in renin, 12% reduction in adipose tissue ACE activity, and 20% reduction in the angiotensinogen expression in adipose tissue *(15)*. Mice deficient in components of the RAAS are leaner and gain less weight when fed a high-fat diet than mice with an intact RAAS. White adipose tissue itself (particularly visceral as opposed to subcutaneous adipose) has all the molecular machinery for local angiotensin II (Ang II) generation and Ang II-stimulated signal transduction. Indeed, adipose tissue overexpression of angiotensinogen increases blood pressure in mice *(16)*. Furthermore, an autocrine positive feedback loop for the RAAS appears to amplify generation of its components. Activated RAAS may potentiate obesity by stimulating appetite and by acting as a trophic factor for adipocytes; this increases adipocyte mass and preadipocyte differentiation and fuels a vicious cycle.

Ang II is a powerful stimulus for aldosterone synthesis; yet elevated plasma levels of aldosterone in obesity cannot be explained solely by renin or by elevated potassium levels *(17)*. Moreover, other aldosterone-activating factors originating from adipocytes, including leptin, adiponectin, interleukin-6 (IL-6), or tumor necrosis factor-α (TNF-α), are not involved. Instead, fat cell activation of Wnt-signaling molecules stimulates frizzled receptors in the adrenals to increase secretion of aldosterone as well as cortisol *(18)*. These observations suggest a direct link between adiposity, aldosterone, and hypertension.

HYPERINSULINEMIA/INSULIN RESISTANCE

Hypertension is regularly associated with increased plasma levels of insulin, and experimental and clinical studies find that increased adiposity promotes hyperinsulinemia. Such observations led to the idea that insulin is a key factor underlying obesity-related hypertension. It is true that insulin increases sodium reabsorption and expands extracellular fluid volume but this is not sufficient to produce sustained hypertension. Rather, obesity-associated insulin resistance contributes to hypertension (Fig. 2). The effects of insulin resistance are exerted in combination with other metabolic, hormonal, and hemodynamic disturbances of obesity, such as activated sympathetic tone and increased activity of the RAAS, and increased levels of fatty acids, leptin, resistin, and glucocorticoids.

OBSTRUCTIVE SLEEP APNEA (OSA)

In adults, OSA is an independent risk factor for the presence as well as future development of hypertension. As many as 30% of hypertensive adults have obesity-linked OSA, the severity of which parallels the elevation in blood pressure *(19)*. Even in the absence of obesity, OSA predicts hypertension; conversely, its treatment can in some cases reduce blood pressure. Experimentally, cyclical intermittent upper airway obstruction in non-obese rats and dogs led to hypertension during the waking periods.

OSA in childhood has long been linked to neurocognitive and behavioral problems, but recent studies reveal an association with metabolic and hemodynamic abnormalities, especially in the setting of obesity. Children with OSA have elevated diurnal and nocturnal systolic and diastolic pressure *(20)*. Interestingly, even individuals with primary snoring, which is considered a mild form of OSA, have increased daytime blood pressure with reduced arterial distensibility. It is therefore possible that the link between OSA and hypertension demonstrated in adults begins early in childhood, especially in obese children.

The pathogenesis of increased blood pressure and hypertension with OSA includes recurrent episodes of apnea and intermittent hypoxia/carbon dioxide retention and negative intrathoracic pressures, which depress myocardial contractility, elevate heart rate, and activate the sympathetic nervous system and RAAS. In addition, OSA has been linked to enhanced inflammation and oxidative stress, which likely disrupt nitric oxide bioactivity and lead to endothelial dysfunction and elevated blood pressure.

ADIPOSE TISSUE-RELATED METABOLIC FACTORS

Adiposity. Although increased weight is regularly accompanied by increased blood pressure, there is considerable inter-individual variability and not all obese individuals become hypertensive. As noted above, the divergence between obesity and hypertension has been taken to reflect ethnic and genetic factors as well as the differential impact of varying components of adiposity. There is now strong evidence that fat distribution, specifically visceral adiposity, is a key determinant of hypertension *(21)*. Even normal weight individuals who demonstrate insulin resistance and hypertension have increased intra-abdominal fat mass. Waist circumference and waist-to-height ratios are also good predictors of hypertension in children, especially obese children, suggesting a pathophysiologic role of visceral fat per se *(22)*. Fat mass assessed by bioimpedence correlated not only with established hypertension but also with blood pressure within the entire normal range in healthy children *(23)*.

Visceral fat, as opposed to subcutaneous or intramuscular fat, has strong associations with many pathophysiologic features. Accumulation of large poorly differentiated preadipocytes in visceral fat augments production of bioactive molecules including angiotensinogen, plasminogen activator inhibitor (PAI-1), endothelin, and reactive oxygen species that can vasoconstrict and remodel blood vessels. Moreover, visceral fat is often infiltrated by macrophages that constitute an important source of pro-inflammatory mediators including TNF-α, IL-6, monocyte chemoattractant protein 1 (MCP-1), and inducible nitric oxide synthase (iNOS). Fatty acids released by adipocytes stimulate TNF-α released by macrophages which, in turn, can enhance production of IL-6 by fat cells, further amplifying the inflammatory response. Notably, mice deficient in IL-6 have a blunted hypertensive response to stress *(24)*. Many of the bioactive substances produced by macrophages also inhibit preadipocyte differentiation, further expanding a population of large, dysfunctional, insulin-resistant adipocytes that may fuel the vicious cycle between obesity and hypertension.

Free fatty acids. Non-esterified free fatty acids (NEFFA) derived from lipolysis of triglycerides are major secretory products of adipose tissue. Acute elevation in plasma NEFFA increases blood pressure in experimental animals and humans *(25,26)*. Chronic elevation of NEFFA observed in those with central obesity correlates with elevated blood pressure. Baseline elevation of NEFFA is a highly significant independent risk factor for developing hypertension in non-diabetic, non-hypertensive men. The pathophysiological mechanisms involve stimulation of α-adrenergic tone which causes vasoconstriction, reduces baroreflex sensitivity, and enhances tubular sodium reabsorption. NEFFA also stimulate expression of angiotensinogen in preadipocytes and aldosterone in adrenal cells that can increase blood pressure through vasoconstriction, vascular remodeling, and sodium reabsorption. NEFFA reduce endothelial nitric oxide synthase and thus nitric oxide(NO)-mediated vasodilatation as well as insulin-induced vasodilatation, which is NO-dependent. Finally, NEFFA increase oxidative stress in vivo and in vitro, another mechanism postulated for development of hypertension.

Leptin. Leptin is an adipocyte gene product that regulates food intake, energy expenditure, and intracellular lipid homeostasis. Circulating levels of leptin parallel fat stores, increasing with overfeeding and decreasing with fasting or caloric deprivation. Absence of leptin or a mutation in the leptin receptor causes massive hyperphagia in animals and humans. Yet these mutations are not accompanied by hypertension; this underscores the complexity of leptin modulation of blood pressure.

Increased leptin levels in obesity are associated with increased blood pressure. However, the relationship is modulated by the duration of hyperleptinemia and its site(s) of action (centrally or systemic) *(27)*. Leptin's pressure effect also depends upon the relative contributions of sympathetic tone, endothelin-1, reactive oxygen species, activation of endothelial nitric oxide synthase, and renal regulation of sodium-volume balance. For example, while both intracerebral and systemic infusion of leptin increased sympathetic nerve activity to a similar degree, the lack of pressure elevation following systemic administration indicates a counter-regulatory systemic vasodilation that likely reflects NO production *(28–30)*.

Leptin also modulates renal handling of sodium and water *(29)*. The normal leptin-induced increase in urinary sodium and water excretion is blunted in obesity. The perturbation appears independent of systemic or even renal hemodynamics and may reflect a direct tubular effect. The increase in sodium and water reabsorption appears to reflect enhanced renal sympathetic tone and decreased local NO.

Adiponectin. In contrast to other adipocytokines which are elevated in obesity, adiponectin levels are depressed. Plasma levels are inversely related to obesity and suggest that adiponectin may have protective or adaptive functions. Indeed, adiponectin has insulin-sensitizing, anti-diabetic, anti-inflammatory, and anti-atherogenic effects. Hypoadiponectinemia was shown to be an independent risk factor for hypertension in cross-sectional and prospective studies in lean and obese hypertensive adults and adolescents, even after adjustments for BMI, age, glucose, and cholesterol levels *(31,32)*. It is notable that antihypertensive treatment (ACE inhibition with ramipril or angiotensin receptor antagonism with valsartan) elevates circulating adiponectin level and insulin sensitivity in parallel with their effects on blood pressure. It is of further interest that a subset of obese individuals with adiponectin concentrations similar to those of normal weight subjects did not have metabolic abnormalities including hypertension *(33)*. Experimentally, adiponectin replenishment ameliorated obesity-related hypertension in the KKAy mouse model, while hypertension in salt-fed adiponectin-deficient mice was reversed by adiponectin treatment *(34)*. Hypoadiponectinemia likely contributes to hypertension by way of endothelial dysfunction that is independent of insulin resistance, BMI, or lipid status; adiponectin upregulates endothelial NO synthase expression and reduces ROS production, resulting in heightened NO production and bioavailability in endothelial cells. Experimental and clinical hypoadiponectinemias are associated with endothelial cell dysfunction and impaired endothelium-dependent vasodilation as well as disinhibition of leukocyte–endothelium adhesion and activation of the RAAS.

RENAL DISEASE

Clinical Spectrum of Obesity-Related Glomerulopathy (ORG)

High-grade proteinuria in obese adults that remitted with weight loss and returned with weight gain was first described in 1974 *(35)*. The renal histology was comparable to idiopathic focal segmental glomerulosclerosis (FSGS). The term obesity-related glomerulopathy (ORG) is now used to describe this secondary form of FSGS. From the 1980s to the 1990s, a 10-fold increase in biopsy-proven ORG was noted in adults *(36)*. Underscoring the gravity of ORG in obese adults, the progression to end-stage renal disease occurs in 3% of patients at 2-years follow-up and in 33% at 10 years *(36,37)*.

ORG is increasingly recognized in the pediatric population. One report documented ORG in an 8-year-old child with BMI 58.1 kg/m^2, but in most series ORG is detected in the second decade of life *(36,38–40)*. The clinical characteristics of ORG in pediatric patients are similar to those in adults. The condition is milder than idiopathic FSGS; daily protein excretion is lower (1.8–4.5 g/day), serum albumin is normal or only minimally depressed, and edema is absent or mild. About half of pediatric patients with ORG are hypertensive or hyperlipidemic. Some also have obstructive sleep apnea. Many have been shown to respond to inhibition of the renin–angiotensin system with marked reduction in proteinuria, though as in adults, this may not prevent progressive glomerulosclerosis *(37–39)*. While this chapter focuses primarily on ORG, there is accumulating evidence that obesity potentiates progression of other renal diseases including IgA nephropathy, transplant nephropathy, and renal damage associated with congenitally reduced endowment of nephron number *(41,42)*.

In clinical practice, proteinuria is a well-accepted indicator of renal injury and comprises a spectrum from microalbuminuria (30–300 mg/g creatinine; not detectable by routine urinalysis) to overt proteinuria (>300 mg/g creatinine, detectable by dipstick). As in other glomerulopathies, obesity-associated microalbuminuria appears to be an early indicator of renal damage *(43)*. The prevalence of microalbuminuria in obesity is increased and parallels the BMI. Further, even among normoglycemic first-degree relatives of type-II diabetics, central obesity has been found to be an independent risk factor for microalbuminuria *(44)*. Likewise, in 10,000 young adults, BMI>35 showed significant increases in albuminuria compared to lower BMI groups *(45)*. Albuminuria correlates with substantial renal structural alteration even with normal renal function (see below) *(43)*. As with any renal injury, the presence of hypertension accelerates glomerular injury.

Thus, it is reasonable to assess urine albumin excretion in obese pediatric patients. Children and adolescents with BMI>95th percentile should be assessed for microalbuminuria and glomerular filtration rate by serum creatinine. Thereafter, urine microalbumin should be followed yearly. Currently there are limited data to guide therapeutic interventions, although reports of efficacy by inhibition of the renin–angiotensin system in advanced obesity-related glomerulopathy suggest a potential benefit. Control of hypertension is essential to limit progression of renal disease.

Renal Hemodynamics

There are significant changes in renal hemodynamics even at the early stages of obesity. One study showed that adults with mean BMI 43.8 kg/m^2 had glomerular filtration rate (GFR) 51% higher than that of normal weight controls. The renal plasma flow (RPF) is also elevated, though not to the same degree *(46)*. As a result, the filtration fraction (defined as GFR/RPF) is increased, a hemodynamic adjustment that parallels the degree of BMI and adipose mass *(47,48)*.

Glomerular filtration is determined by the pre- and post-glomerular arteriolar tone, both of which are altered by obesity. Molecular sieving experiments in obese individuals suggest that afferent arteriolar vasodilatation together with efferent arteriolar vasoconstriction contribute to the increase in filtration fraction *(46)*. Experimentally, obese rats have been found to have heightened renal vascular resistance in response to infusions of Ang II. As the Ang II type-I receptor density is highest in the efferent arteriole, these data suggest that obesity promotes renal efferent arteriolar vasoconstriction *(49)*. Furthermore, inhibition of Ang II action in obese subjects increases renal plasma flow, again pointing to efferent arteriolar vasoconstriction as a prominent renal response to obesity *(50)*. Increased filtration fraction has been linked to glomerular injury and scarring through mechanisms that include elevated glomerular pressure and stimulation of local growth factors. In this connection, obesity-induced GFR increase is not fixed. Several studies report that hyperfiltration may normalize following gastroplasty *(51,52)*.

Tubuloglomerular Feedback

Tubuloglomerular feedback (TGF) describes the coupling of each nephron's distal tubule flow to glomerular filtration. Nephron anatomy dictates that the distal tubule signals to its originating glomerulus and contributes to the formation of the macula densa, which encompasses specialized tubular cells abutting the afferent and efferent arterioles. The stimulus to adjust GFR includes the rate of distal tubular flow and the composition of tubular fluid. The signal is perceived in the macula densa and transmitted to the vascular structures of the nephron, particularly the afferent arteriole, which adjusts the rate of filtration. An inverse relationship between tubular flow and filtration is thus established, such that an increase in tubular flow decreases glomerular filtration and vice versa. In simplest terms, increased luminal NaCl leads to a decrease in glomerular filtration through afferent arteriolar vasoconstriction *(53)*.

In obesity, volume expansion is due, at least in part, to increased salt reabsorption in the proximal tubule; this is mediated by increased sympathetic tone, Ang II, adipokines, and increased oncotic pressure of the tubular blood supply caused by glomerular hyperfiltration. By lowering tubular NaCl relative to GFR, these obesity-dependent change mechanisms disrupt the TGF response, preventing suppression of GFR *(54)*. Given the high rate of hypertension in obese individuals, the inadequacy of TGF feedback and failure to constrict the afferent arteriole may allow transmission of systemic BP to the glomerulus, contributing not only to increased GFR but eventually to renal damage *(55)*.

Proteinuria

A hallmark of renal manifestations of obesity/ORG is proteinuria, the magnitude of which is relatively modest and not usually associated with nephrotic syndrome. Thus, presentation with hypoalbuminemia and edema is rare *(36–38)*. The lack of edema may delay detection of proteinuria and increase the chance for progressive glomerulosclerosis and loss of renal function. Indeed, in one study of ORG, those who progressed to end-stage renal failure (ESRD) had elevated serum creatinine at presentation *(37)*. In a Chinese cohort of patients with ORG, protein excretion rose with increasing BMI *(56)*. Yet, the severity of glomerulosclerosis on biopsy was similar across the range of BMI, suggesting that additional intrarenal hemodynamic derangements contributed to excess proteinuria with increasing adiposity.

It should be emphasized, however, that a third of the cohort with biopsy-proven ORG had only mild proteinuria (400 mg/24 h). These findings suggest that the renal pathophysiologic processes that culminate in ORG are already present at a time when proteinuria is only modestly elevated or even before overt proteinuria is detected.

Proteinuria in ORG can in some cases be dramatically lessened with weight loss *(35,57)*. Bariatric surgery has in some studies normalized protein excretion in adult and pediatric patients with ORG *(39,58)*. However, enthusiasm for surgery is tempered by its association with oxalate nephropathy and renal failure post-op *(59)*. As noted previously, pharmacologic agents that reduce blood pressure may (in some but not all cases) reverse microalbuminuria and limit the progression of renal disease in obese subjects.

Renal Morphology

The primary light microscopic feature of ORG that differentiates it from primary FSGS is glomeru-lomegaly *(36,37,60)* (Fig. 3). Increased glomerular filtration due to increased transcapillary hydraulic pressure likely contributes to glomerulomegaly *(60)*. Glomerulomegaly has been linked to the patho-genesis of glomerulosclerosis, with a correlation between glomerular size and degree of sclerosis in a given glomerulus during the early stages of injury *(61)*. Increased glomerular size may not directly cause sclerosis, but may be an early manifestation of processes that promote cell growth and extracel-lular matrix synthesis. Additionally, the link of glomerulomegaly and sclerosis may reflect the limited capacity of mature podocytes to divide. Thus, with increasing glomerular size, the resulting reduc-tion in relative podocyte density may become a stimulus for further injury. In this regard, a study of patients with ORG found that glomerulomegaly was accompanied by a 45% reduction in podocyte density *(60)*. Experimentally, loss of podocytes (through immune targeting) has been shown to induce glomerulosclerosis *(62)*.

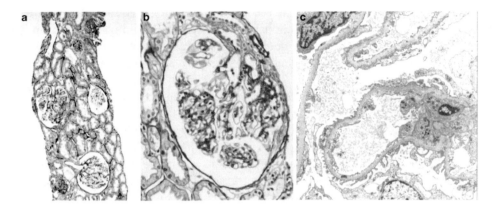

Fig. 3. Morphologic changes of obesity-related glomerulopathy. (**a**) Glomerulomegaly and focal small segmental adhesion with early sclerosis (Jones silver stain, ×100). (**b**) Glomerulomegaly and hilar segmental sclerosis at the vascular pole (periodic acid–Schiff, ×400). (**c**) Transmission electron microscopy showing subtotal foot process effacement (×4,000) *(39)*.

It is important to underscore that progressive glomerular destruction, regardless of cause, will cul-minate in tubulointerstitial fibrosis. It is therefore of interest that compared with idiopathic FSGS, obesity-associated FSGS has less interstitial alpha smooth muscle actin and TGF beta and lower inter-stitial volume, suggesting relative preservation of the tubulointerstitium *(63)*. Such observations may explain the lower rates of progression to ESRD of ORG compared to idiopathic FSGS.

It is interesting that glomerular pathology is also observed in obese patients without clinically appar-ent renal disease. Thus, autopsies of two boys with Prader–Willi syndrome without renal dysfunction or proteinuria revealed marked glomerulomegaly *(64)*. Similarly, examination of renal morphology in extremely obese adults (mean BMI 52 kg/m^2) revealed that 5% of patients had segmental glomeru-losclerosis in 6% of glomeruli. Mean glomerular planar area was 50% higher compared to normal weight controls *(43)*. As noted in other studies, only 4% of these individuals had significant protein-uria (none >500 mg/day). Even obese individuals, considered well enough to serve as renal transplant donors, had 15% larger glomeruli compared to non-obese donors. No data exists as to persistence of glomerulomegaly in these donor kidneys in non-obese recipients, though the possibility of correction in a non-obese milieu seems plausible *(65)*.

Pathophysiologic Mechanisms

Renin–Angiotensin–Aldosterone System (RAAS)

The RAAS is a major regulator of systemic and renal vasomotor tone that affects renal blood flow and glomerular filtration and promotes the growth of renal cells. As noted previously, the adipocytes and infiltrating macrophages of adipose tissue constitute important sources of RAAS components. For example, per weight of tissue, visceral fat expression of angiotensinogen (Aog) is comparable to that of the liver. Circulating levels of Aog correlate with increasing BMI both at normal and elevated weight. Conversely, fasting dramatically reduces adipocyte expression of Aog in experimental animals. Weight loss also reduces the serum levels of angiotensin-converting enzyme (ACE), the predominant enzyme necessary for production of the effector ligand angiotensin II (66). The Ang II type-1 receptor (AT1), primarily responsible for post-glomerular (efferent) anteriolar vasoconstriction, is dramatically elevated in the renal cortex of obese Zucker rats compared to lean Zucker controls (67). Renal AT1 is also upregulated in transgenic mice overexpressing angiotensinogen exclusively in adipocytes (68). These studies suggest that an adipose-derived increase in circulating RAAS ligands and an adipose-driven increase in renal AT1 receptor provide a powerful combination for increasing efferent arteriolar vasoconstriction, glomerular pressure, and cellular proliferation that promote structural damage.

As with other chronic proteinuric glomerulopathies, inhibition of the renin–angiotensin system has been employed successfully to treat obesity-related glomerulopathy. Likewise, aldosterone blockade lessens renal injury in the vascular, glomerular, and tubulointerstitial compartments. These benefits are independent of its antihypertensive effects; presumably, the drugs block the effects of aldosterone on plasminogen activator inhibitor-1 and TGF-β, reactive oxygen intermediates, inflammatory mediators, and podocyte function (69). Aldosterone antagonism attenuates obesity-induced glomerular hyperfiltration in high fat-fed dogs (70). While the role of aldosterone in renal damage in obese humans has not yet been explicitly demonstrated, the compelling nature of animal data has prompted suggestions to use aldosterone antagonism for obesity-related kidney injury (71). The antiproteinuric benefits of angiotensin-converting enzyme inhibition or aldosterone blockade may be reversed by progression of obesity or weight re-gain (37–39).

Metabolic/Adipocyte Factors

Receptors for leptin have been demonstrated in the renal inner medulla and in vascular structures of the renal corticomedullary region. Rapid diuresis follows a single intraperitoneal injection of leptin; this may serve to counterbalance its effect on adrenergic activity. Leptin also affects renal cellular growth. Cultured glomerular endothelial cells proliferate when stimulated by leptin and increase TGF-β production (72). In mesangial cells, leptin increases collagen type I production, cellular hypertrophy (but not proliferation), and the expression of TGF-β receptors, thereby sensitizing them to the increased TGF-β produced by adjacent glomerular endothelial cells (73). Chronic leptin infusion resulted in increased glomerular type-IV collagen as well as an increase in proteinuria in rats. Conversely, in a mouse model of renal tubulointerstitial injury, leptin deficiency was protective. Thus, after unilateral ureteral obstruction, the leptin-deficient mice had less cellular infiltrate, less TGF-β expression, less alpha smooth muscle actin and fibronectin staining, and less interstitial fibrosis than wild-type controls (74).

As noted previously, hypoadiponectinemia is associated with insulin resistance, inflammation, atherosclerosis, and hypertension (32,75). In the kidney, adiponectin supports normal function of the podocyte (76). Thus, adiponectin-null mutant mice have podocyte foot process effacement and albuminuria, both of which normalize with adiponectin treatment. Even wild-type podocytes in culture become more impermeable to albumin when treated with adiponectin. Not surprisingly, adiponectin-null mutant mice have poorer outcomes following renal injury, including increased inflammatory mediators, increased TGF-β, increased glomerular collagen deposition, glomerulomegaly, and albuminuria *(77)*. Taken together, these findings suggest that hypoadiponectinemia may contribute to obesity-related renal injury. Indeed, among obese African-Americans, there is a strong negative correlation between plasma adiponectin levels and albuminuria, pointing to potential podocyte injury *(76)*. Adiponectin deficiency leads to an increase in NADPH oxidase; renal injury augments this deleterious response with increases in urinary reactive oxygen species *(76,77)*. Conversely, adiponectin stimulates phosphorylation of glomerular AMP-activated protein kinase, which inhibits oxidative stress and maintains normal podocyte architecture *(76,78)* (Fig. 4). Pharmacologic maneuvers to raise adiponectin levels (such as PPAR-γ agonists) have been proposed as a potential treatment for ORG *(76)*.

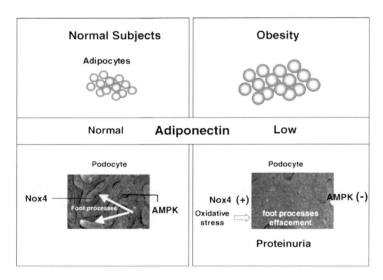

Fig. 4. Adiponectin is essential to normal podocyte function. Low adiponectin in obesity triggers glomerular podocyte effacement and albuminuria. Potential mechanisms include increased oxidative stress through NADPH oxidase 4 (Nox4) enhancement and reduction of 5AMP-activated protein kinase (AMPK) activation. Adapted from Zoccali et al. *(78)*.

Other adipocytokines have relevance for renal damage. For example, TNF-α levels rise with increasing adiposity *(79)* and reduce adiponectin levels. Glomeruli from ORG patients have increased expression of TNF-α and a doubling of TNF receptor 1 *(80)*. These observations suggest that TNF-α may directly contribute to obesity-induced renal damage, possibly through stimulation of TGF-β, macrophage infiltration, and apoptosis.

Circulating levels of interleukin-6 (IL-6) increase with obesity, with as much as 30% derived from adipose tissue *(81)*. IL-6 is the most important regulator of the hepatic acute phase response, which includes C-reactive protein (CRP). Strong epidemiologic data connect CRP with poor cardiovascular outcomes, and CRP may participate directly in vascular wall pathology *(82)*. Visceral adipose volumes were highly correlated with circulating IL-6 and CRP levels in Framingham subjects, and even obese children show dramatic elevation of CRP compared to normal weight controls *(83,84)*. Evidence for IL-6 involvement in vascular and renal disease beyond CRP is found in IL-6 induction of AT1 receptor in vitro and in vivo and subsequent increase in angiotensin-mediated oxidative stress *(79)*. Glomeruli from patients with ORG show a twofold increase in expression of IL-6 signal transducer, pointing to the possibility of direct IL-6 pathogenicity in glomeruli *(80)*. However, whether increased IL-6 plays a pathogenic role in ORG or is only an epiphenomenon is currently not known.

Obesity causes other metabolic disturbances that may contribute to renal damage. Excess intracellular free fatty acids are thought to be shunted toward the production of reactive intermediates such as fatty acyl CoA, diacylglycerol, and ceramide which are cytotoxic. LDL has numerous glomerular effects, promoting mesangial cell proliferation and mesangial cell production of extracellular matrix, plasminogen activator inhibitor (PAI-1), and TGF-β. Sterol regulatory element binding transcription factor-1 (SREBP-1) is upregulated in high-fat-fed, obese C57BL/6 J mice that develop glomerulosclerosis and proteinuria *(85)*. Transgenic overexpression of SREBP-1a resulted in increased lipid accumulation in glomeruli and tubular cells as well as glomerulosclerosis. Conversely, mutant mice with inactivated SREBP-1c were protected from glomerulosclerosis when fed a high-fat diet. Glomerular expression of these lipid-related transporters was upregulated in glomeruli from patients with ORG: fatty acid-binding protein was upregulated fourfold, LDL-receptor twofold, and SREBP-1 twofold *(80)*. Thus, lipid disturbances often associated with obesity provide additional mechanisms for glomerular injury.

SUMMARY

While hypertension and renal damage have long been recognized to be interrelated, obesity dramatically amplifies each of these abnormalities. The obesity epidemic, now well entrenched in the pediatric population, is expected to increase these complications. Current therapies aimed at lessening elevated blood pressure and slowing progressive renal damage will likely be supplemented by interventions aimed at obesity-specific targets.

Editor's Questions and Authors' Response

- **What are the indications for renal biopsy in an obese child with microalbuminuria?**

- Renal biopsy is commonly performed in children with urine albumin excretion exceeding 1 g/day. However, significant renal damage may occur in obese subjects with lower levels of proteinuria and normal renal function; the mean level of proteinuria in a recent series of adults with biopsy-proven ORG was only 400 mg/day. It seems reasonable therefore to consider renal biopsy in obese children and teens with urine albumin excretion >400 mg/g creatinine.

- **Do we have long-term data on the benefits of pharmacologic treatment of microalbuminuria in children?**

- While data on the long-term benefits of treatment with inhibitors/antagonists of the renin–angiotensin system do not exist, biopsy findings of significant structural changes in obese patients with only microalbuminuria suggest a benefit for such intervention. Thus, even in the absence of hypertension or increased creatinine, persistent or increasing microalbuminuria (albumin to creatinine ratio of >30 μg/mg creatinine in a first morning void documented at least 3 times in a 6-month period) warrants treatment with an angiotensin-converting enzyme inhibitor or receptor antagonist. There is currently little data on the use of aldosterone inhibitors in this setting.

REFERENCES

1. Lauer RM, Clarke WR. Childhood risk factors for high adult blood pressure: the Muscatine Study. Pediatrics. Oct 1989;84(4):633–41.

2. Flynn JT. Pediatric hypertension: recent trends and accomplishments, future challenges. Am J Hypertens. Jun 2008;21(6):605–12.

3. National High Blood Pressure Education Program Working Group on High Blood Pressure in Children and Adolescents. The fourth report on the diagnosis, evaluation, and treatment of high blood pressure in children and adolescents. Pediatrics. Aug 2004;114(2 Suppl 4th Report):555–76.

4. Muntner P, He J, Cutler JA, Wildman RP, Whelton PK. Trends in blood pressure among children and adolescents. J Am Med Assoc. 5 May 2004;291(17):2107–13.

5. Sorof JM, Lai D, Turner J, Poffenbarger T, Portman RJ. Overweight, ethnicity, and the prevalence of hypertension in school-aged children. Pediatrics. Mar 2004;113(3 Pt 1):475–82.

6. Din-Dzietham R, Liu Y, Bielo MV, Shamsa F. High blood pressure trends in children and adolescents in national surveys, 1963 to 2002. Circulation. 25 Sept 2007;116(13):1488–96.

7. Ke L, Brock KE, Cant RV, Li Y, Morrell SL. The relationship between obesity and blood pressure differs by ethnicity in Sydney school children. Am J Hypertens. Jan 2009;22(1):52–58.

8. Morse SA, Bravo PE, Morse MC, Reisin E. The heart in obesity-hypertension. Expert Rev Cardiovasc Ther. Jul 2005;3(4):647–58.

9. da Silva AA, do Carmo J, Dubinion J, Hall JE. The role of the sympathetic nervous system in obesity-related hypertension. Curr Hypertens Rep. Jun 2009;11(3):206–11.

10. Kassab S, Kato T, Wilkins FC, Chen R, Hall JE, Granger JP. Renal denervation attenuates the sodium retention and hypertension associated with obesity. Hypertension. Apr 1995;25(4 Pt 2):893–97.

11. Wofford MR, Anderson DC Jr, Brown CA, Jones DW, Miller ME, Hall JE. Antihypertensive effect of alpha- and beta-adrenergic blockade in obese and lean hypertensive subjects. Am J Hypertens. Jul 2001;14(7 Pt 1):694–98.

12. Gilardini L, Parati G, Sartorio A, Mazzilli G, Pontiggia B, Invitti C. Sympathoadrenergic and metabolic factors are involved in ambulatory blood pressure rise in childhood obesity. J Hum Hypertens. Feb 2008;22(2):75–82.

13. Agapitov AV, Correia ML, Sinkey CA, Haynes WG. Dissociation between sympathetic nerve traffic and sympathetically mediated vascular tone in normotensive human obesity. Hypertension. Oct 2008;52(4):687–95.

14. Boustany CM, Bharadwaj K, Daugherty A, Brown DR, Randall DC, Cassis LA. Activation of the systemic and adipose renin-angiotensin system in rats with diet-induced obesity and hypertension. Am J Physiol Regul Integr Comp Physiol. Oct 2004;287(4):R943–9.

15. Engeli S, Bohnke J, Gorzelniak K, et al. Weight loss and the renin–angiotensin–aldosterone system. Hypertension. Mar 2005;45(3):356–62.

16. Massiera F, Bloch-Faure M, Ceiler D, et al. Adipose angiotensinogen is involved in adipose tissue growth and blood pressure regulation. FASEB J. Dec 2001;15(14):2727–29.

17. Lamounier-Zepter V, Ehrhart-Bornstein M, Bornstein SR. Mineralocorticoid-stimulating activity of adipose tissue. Best Pract Res Clin Endocrinol Metab. Dec 2005;19(4):567–75.

18. Schinner S, Willenberg HS, Krause D, et al. Adipocyte-derived products induce the transcription of the StAR promoter and stimulate aldosterone and cortisol secretion from adrenocortical cells through the Wnt-signaling pathway. Int J Obes (Lond). May 2007;31(5):864–70.

19. Pack AI, Gislason T. Obstructive sleep apnea and cardiovascular disease: a perspective and future directions. Prog Cardiovasc Dis. Mar–Apr 2009;51(5):434–51.

20. Li AM, Au CT, Sung RY, et al. Ambulatory blood pressure in children with obstructive sleep apnoea: a community based study. Thorax. Sept 2008;63(9):803–9.

21. Mathieu P, Poirier P, Pibarot P, Lemieux I, Despres JP. Visceral obesity: the link among inflammation, hypertension, and cardiovascular disease. Hypertension. Apr 2009;53(4):577–84.

22. Genovesi S, Antolini L, Giussani M, et al. Usefulness of waist circumference for the identification of childhood hypertension. J Hypertens. Aug 2008;26(8):1563–70.

23. Drozdz D, Kwinta P, Korohoda P, Pietrzyk JA, Drozdz M, Sancewicz-Pach K. Correlation between fat mass and blood pressure in healthy children. Pediatr Nephrol. Sept 2009;24(9):1735–40. Epub 2009 May 28.

24. Lee DL, Leite R, Fleming C, Pollock JS, Webb RC, Brands MW. Hypertensive response to acute stress is attenuated in interleukin-6 knockout mice. Hypertension. Sept 2004;44(3):259–63.

25. de Jongh RT, Serne EH, Ijzerman RG, de Vries G, Stehouwer CD. Free fatty acid levels modulate microvascular function: relevance for obesity-associated insulin resistance, hypertension, and microangiopathy. Diabetes. Nov 2004;53(11):2873–82.

26. Sarafidis PA, Bakris GL. Non-esterified fatty acids and blood pressure elevation: a mechanism for hypertension in subjects with obesity/insulin resistance? J Hum Hypertens. Jan 2007;21(1):12–19.

27. Farooqi IS, Wangensteen T, Collins S, et al. Clinical and molecular genetic spectrum of congenital deficiency of the leptin receptor. N Engl J Med. 18 Jan 2007;356(3):237–47.

28. Dunbar JC, Hu Y, Lu H. Intracerebroventricular leptin increases lumbar and renal sympathetic nerve activity and blood pressure in normal rats. Diabetes. Dec 1997;46(12):2040–43.

29. Villarreal D, Reams G, Freeman RH, Taraben A. Renal effects of leptin in normotensive, hypertensive, and obese rats. Am J Physiol. Dec 1998;275(6 Pt 2):R2056–60.

30. Fruhbeck G. Pivotal role of nitric oxide in the control of blood pressure after leptin administration. Diabetes. Apr 1999;48(4):903–8.

31. Chow WS, Cheung BM, Tso AW, et al. Hypoadiponectinemia as a predictor for the development of hypertension: a 5-year prospective study. Hypertension. Jun 2007;49(6):1455–61.

32. Shatat IF, Freeman KD, Vuguin PM, Dimartino-Nardi JR, Flynn JT. Relationship between adiponectin and ambulatory blood pressure in obese adolescents. Pediatr Res. Jun 2009;65(6):691–95.

33. Aguilar-Salinas CA, Garcia EG, Robles L, et al. High adiponectin concentrations are associated with the metabolically healthy obese phenotype. J Clin Endocrinol Metab. Oct 2008;93(10):4075–79.

34. Ohashi K, Kihara S, Ouchi N, et al. Adiponectin replenishment ameliorates obesity-related hypertension. Hypertension. Jun 2006;47(6):1108–16.

35. Weisinger JR, Kempson RL, Eldridge FL, Swenson RS. The nephrotic syndrome: a complication of massive obesity. Ann Intern Med. Oct 1974;81(4):440–47.

36. Kambham N, Markowitz GS, Valeri AM, Lin J, D'Agati VD. Obesity-related glomerulopathy: an emerging epidemic. Kidney Int. Apr 2001;59(4):1498–509.

37. Praga M, Hernandez E, Morales E, et al. Clinical features and long-term outcome of obesity-associated focal segmental glomerulosclerosis. Nephrol Dial Transplant. Sept 2001;16(9):1790–98.

38. Adelman RD, Restaino IG, Alon US, Blowey DL. Proteinuria and focal segmental glomerulosclerosis in severely obese adolescents. J Pediatr. Apr 2001;138(4):481–85.

39. Fowler SM, Kon V, Ma L, Richards WO, Fogo AB, Hunley TE. Obesity-related focal and segmental glomerulosclerosis: normalization of proteinuria in an adolescent after bariatric surgery. Pediatr Nephrol. Apr 2009;24(4):851–55.

40. Quinlan C, Dorman T, Gill D. A big boy with proteinuria. Focal and segmental glomerulosclerosis. Pediatr Nephrol. Dec 2008;23(12):2175–78.

41. Abitbol CL, Chandar J, Rodriguez MM, et al. Obesity and preterm birth: additive risks in the progression of kidney disease in children. Pediatr Nephrol. Jul 2009;24(7):1363–70.

42. Bonnet F, Deprele C, Sassolas A, et al. Excessive body weight as a new independent risk factor for clinical and pathological progression in primary IgA nephritis. Am J Kidney Dis. Apr 2001;37(4):720–27.

43. Serra A, Romero R, Lopez D, et al. Renal injury in the extremely obese patients with normal renal function. Kidney Int. Apr 2008;73(8):947–55.

44. Chandie Shaw PK, Berger SP, Mallat M, Frolich M, Dekker FW, Rabelink TJ. Central obesity is an independent risk factor for albuminuria in nondiabetic South Asian subjects. Diabetes Care. Jul 2007;30(7):1840–44.

45. Ferris M, Hogan SL, Chin H, et al. Obesity, albuminuria, and urinalysis findings in US young adults from the Add Health Wave III study. Clin J Am Soc Nephrol. Nov 2007;2(6):1207–14.

46. Chagnac A, Weinstein T, Korzets A, Ramadan E, Hirsch J, Gafter U. Glomerular hemodynamics in severe obesity. Am J Physiol Renal Physiol. May 2000;278(5):F817–22.

47. Bosma RJ, Kwakernaak AJ, van der Heide JJ, de Jong PE, Navis GJ. Body mass index and glomerular hyperfiltration in renal transplant recipients: cross-sectional analysis and long-term impact. Am J Transplant. Mar 2007;7(3):645–52.

48. Bosma RJ, van der Heide JJ, Oosterop EJ, de Jong PE, Navis G. Body mass index is associated with altered renal hemodynamics in non-obese healthy subjects. Kidney Int. Jan 2004;65(1):259–65.

49. Stepp DW, Boesen EI, Sullivan JC, Mintz JD, Hair CD, Pollock DM. Obesity augments vasoconstrictor reactivity to angiotensin II in the renal circulation of the Zucker rat. Am J Physiol Heart Circ Physiol. Oct 2007;293(4):H2537–42.

50. Ahmed SB, Fisher ND, Stevanovic R, Hollenberg NK. Body mass index and angiotensin-dependent control of the renal circulation in healthy humans. Hypertension. Dec 2005;46(6):1316–20.

51. Chagnac A, Weinstein T, Herman M, Hirsh J, Gafter U, Ori Y. The effects of weight loss on renal function in patients with severe obesity. J Am Soc Nephrol. Jun 2003;14(6):1480–6.

52. Navarro-Diaz M, Serra A, Romero R, et al. Effect of drastic weight loss after bariatric surgery on renal parameters in extremely obese patients: long-term follow-up. J Am Soc Nephrol. Dec 2006;17(12 Suppl 3):S213–7.

53. Schnermann J, Homer W. Smith Award Lecture. The juxtaglomerular apparatus: from anatomical peculiarity to physiological relevance. J Am Soc Nephrol. Jun 2003;14(6):1681–94.

54. Hashimoto S, Yamada K, Kawata T, Mochizuki T, Schnermann J, Koike T. Abnormal autoregulation and tubuloglomerular feedback in prediabetic and diabetic OLETF rats. Am J Physiol Renal Physiol. Mar 2009;296(3):F598–604.

55. Griffin KA, Kramer H, Bidani AK. Adverse renal consequences of obesity. Am J Physiol Renal Physiol. Apr 2008;294(4):F685–96.

56. Chen HM, Li SJ, Chen HP, Wang QW, Li LS, Liu ZH. Obesity-related glomerulopathy in China: a case series of 90 patients. Am J Kidney Dis. Jul 2008;52(1):58–65.

57. Tran HA. Reversible obesity-related glomerulopathy following weight reduction. Med J Aust. 3 Apr 2006; 184(7):367.

58. Huan Y, Tomaszewski JE, Cohen DL. Resolution of nephrotic syndrome after successful bariatric surgery in patient with biopsy-proven FSGS. Clin Nephrol. Jan 2009;71(1):69–73.

59. Nasr SH, D'Agati VD, Said SM, et al. Oxalate nephropathy complicating Roux-en-Y Gastric Bypass: an underrecognized cause of irreversible renal failure. Clin J Am Soc Nephrol. Nov 2008;3(6):1676–83.

60. Chen HM, Liu ZH, Zeng CH, Li SJ, Wang QW, Li LS. Podocyte lesions in patients with obesity-related glomerulopathy. Am J Kidney Dis. Nov 2006;48(5):772–79.

61. Fogo A, Ichikawa I. Evidence for a pathogenic linkage between glomerular hypertrophy and sclerosis. Am J Kidney Dis. Jun 1991;17(6):666–69.

62. Wharram BL, Goyal M, Wiggins JE, et al. Podocyte depletion causes glomerulosclerosis: diphtheria toxin-induced podocyte depletion in rats expressing human diphtheria toxin receptor transgene. J Am Soc Nephrol. Oct 2005;16(10):2941–52.

63. Danilewicz M, Wagrowska-Danielwicz M. Morphometric and immunohistochemical insight into focal segmental glomerulosclerosis in obese and non-obese patients. Nefrologia. 2009;29(1):35–41.

64. Cohen AH. Massive obesity and the kidney. A morphologic and statistical study. Am J Pathol. Oct 1975;81(1):117–30.

65. Rea DJ, Heimbach JK, Grande JP, et al. Glomerular volume and renal histology in obese and non-obese living kidney donors. Kidney Int. Nov 2006;70(9):1636–41.

66. Harp JB, Henry SA, DiGirolamo M. Dietary weight loss decreases serum angiotensin-converting enzyme activity in obese adults. Obes Res. Oct 2002;10(10):985–90.

67. Xu ZG, Lanting L, Vaziri ND, et al. Upregulation of angiotensin II type 1 receptor, inflammatory mediators, and enzymes of arachidonate metabolism in obese Zucker rat kidney: reversal by angiotensin II type 1 receptor blockade. Circulation. 19 Apr 2005;111(15):1962–69.

68. Kim S, Soltani-Bejnood M, Quignard-Boulange A, et al. The adipose renin–angiotensin system modulates systemic markers of insulin sensitivity and activates the intrarenal renin–angiotensin system. J Biomed Biotechnol. 2006;2006(5):27012.

69. Nagase M, Yoshida S, Shibata S, et al. Enhanced aldosterone signaling in the early nephropathy of rats with metabolic syndrome: possible contribution of fat-derived factors. J Am Soc Nephrol. Dec 2006;17(12):3438–46.

70. de Paula RB, da Silva AA, Hall JE. Aldosterone antagonism attenuates obesity-induced hypertension and glomerular hyperfiltration. Hypertension. Jan 2004;43(1):41–47.

71. Bomback AS, Klemmer PJ. Renal injury in extreme obesity: the important role of aldosterone. Kidney Int. Nov 2008;74(9):1216. Author reply 7.

72. Wolf G, Hamann A, Han DC, et al. Leptin stimulates proliferation and TGF-beta expression in renal glomerular endothelial cells: potential role in glomerulosclerosis [see comments]. Kidney Int. Sept 1999;56(3):860–72.

73. Wolf G, Ziyadeh FN. Leptin and renal fibrosis. Contrib Nephrol. 2006;151:175–83.

74. Kumpers P, Gueler F, Rong S, et al. Leptin is a coactivator of TGF-beta in unilateral ureteral obstructive kidney disease. Am J Physiol Renal Physiol. Oct 2007;293(4):F1355–62.

75. Scherer PE. Adipose tissue: from lipid storage compartment to endocrine organ. Diabetes. Jun 2006;55(6):1537–45.

76. Sharma K, Ramachandrarao S, Qiu G, et al. Adiponectin regulates albuminuria and podocyte function in mice. J Clin Invest. May 2008;118(5):1645–56.

77. Ohashi K, Iwatani H, Kihara S, et al. Exacerbation of albuminuria and renal fibrosis in subtotal renal ablation model of adiponectin-knockout mice. Arterioscler Thromb Vasc Biol. Sept 2007;27(9):1910–17.

78. Zoccali C, Mallamaci F. Obesity, diabetes, adiponectin and the kidney: a podocyte affair. Nephrol Dial Transplant. Dec 2008;23(12):3767–70.

79. Wassmann S, Stumpf M, Strehlow K, et al. Interleukin-6 induces oxidative stress and endothelial dysfunction by overexpression of the angiotensin II type 1 receptor. Circ Res. 5 Mar 2004;94(4):534–41.

80. Wu Y, Liu Z, Xiang Z, et al. Obesity-related glomerulopathy: insights from gene expression profiles of the glomeruli derived from renal biopsy samples. Endocrinology. Jan 2006;147(1):44–50.

81. Mohamed-Ali V, Goodrick S, Rawesh A, et al. Subcutaneous adipose tissue releases interleukin-6, but not tumor necrosis factor-alpha, in vivo. J Clin Endocrinol Metab. Dec 1997;82(12):4196–200.
82. Burke AP, Tracy RP, Kolodgie F, et al. Elevated C-reactive protein values and atherosclerosis in sudden coronary death: association with different pathologies. Circulation. 30 Apr 2002;105(17):2019–23.
83. Cindik N, Baskin E, Agras PI, Kinik ST, Turan M, Saatci U. Effect of obesity on inflammatory markers and renal functions. Acta Paediatr. Dec 2005;94(12):1732–37.
84. Pou KM, Massaro JM, Hoffmann U, et al. Visceral and subcutaneous adipose tissue volumes are cross-sectionally related to markers of inflammation and oxidative stress: the Framingham Heart Study. Circulation. 11 Sept 2007;116(11): 1234–41.
85. Jiang T, Wang Z, Proctor G, et al. Diet-induced obesity in C57BL/6 J mice causes increased renal lipid accumulation and glomerulosclerosis via a sterol regulatory element-binding protein-1c-dependent pathway. J Biol Chem. 16 Sept 2005;280(37):32317–25.

17 Sleep-Disordered Breathing and Sleep Duration in Childhood Obesity

Stijn Verhulst

CONTENTS

GENERAL INTRODUCTION
SLEEP-DISORDERED BREATHING AND OBESITY IN CHILDREN
SLEEP DURATION AND CHILDHOOD OBESITY
REFERENCES

Key Words: Obstructive sleep apnea, apnea–hypopnea index, snoring, adenotonsillectomy, CPAP, sleep deprivation

GENERAL INTRODUCTION

The increasing prevalence of childhood obesity during the past generation has been accompanied by profound changes in daily lifestyle. Computer-related activities, video games, cell phones, and other diversions have promoted a more sedentary existence, reducing energy expenditure and facilitating weight gain. Much of the screen and cell time is spent during the evening hours at the expense of sleep. Thus, behaviors that foster the development and progression of obesity in children may disrupt fundamental biological rhythms that are vital to child and adolescent health. Obesity in turn is a major risk factor for sleep-disordered breathing (SDB), which may facilitate further weight gain and promote the development of metabolic and cardiovascular morbidities in obese children as well as adults. This underscores the importance of exploring the relationship between childhood obesity and sleep.

The first part of this chapter will review the evidence that obesity is an anatomical and functional risk factor for SDB in children and discusses its consequences and management. The second part of the chapter discusses the relationship between sleep duration and the development of childhood obesity. Sleep duration may be an important determinant of body weight, as it modulates changes in several obesity-related hormones and affects daytime physical activity and the time available for food consumption. This suggests that good sleep hygiene should be added to the list of measures that may assist in the prevention of childhood obesity.

From: *Contemporary Endocrinology: Pediatric Obesity: Etiology, Pathogenesis, and Treatment*
Edited by: M. Freemark, DOI 10.1007/978-1-60327-874-4_17,
© Springer Science+Business Media, LLC 2010

SLEEP-DISORDERED BREATHING AND OBESITY IN CHILDREN

Introduction

Sleep-disordered breathing (SDB) is defined as a clinically relevant disturbance of breathing during sleep. The two most common respiratory events are apneas and hypopneas, which are documented by a formal sleep study or polysomnography. Apnea is defined as a complete cessation of respiratory airflow for at least two respiratory cycles. Hypopnea is defined as a reduction in respiratory airflow by 50% or more of baseline for at least two respiratory cycles. Apneas and hypopneas are then further classified as central, obstructive, or mixed. A respiratory event is classified as central when there is a cessation of all respiratory efforts (measured at the level of thorax and abdomen). During an obstructive event, there is a continuous or even increased respiratory effort. A mixed event has both central and obstructive components. An example of a sleep study showing some of these respiratory events is presented in Fig. 1.

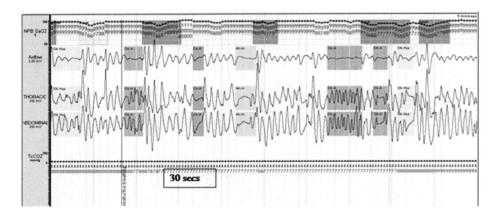

Fig. 1. Screen print of a polysomnography showing an obstructive apnea (*purple box*) and hypopnea (*light blue box*), central apnea (*pink box*), and mixed apnea (*blue box*). Second, following repetitive apneas and hypopneas oxygen saturation intermittently drops (*red box*) which is also referred to as intermittent hypoxia.

Much of the study of SDB has focused on obstructive sleep disorders. Obstructive sleep apnea syndrome (OSAS) is characterized by recurrent events of partial and/or complete upper airway obstruction that disrupt normal ventilation and sleep patterns. The diagnosis of OSAS in children is based on normative data in healthy children without snoring or other symptoms suggesting sleep apnea. Based on these normative data, the current diagnostic threshold is one or more obstructive events per hour of sleep. OSAS is distinguished from primary snoring, a more benign expression of abnormal upper airway resistance that occurs in 3–12% of the general pediatric population. Primary snoring is not associated with obstructive events or desaturations during sleep.

Central sleep apnea has not been studied extensively in children. Reference studies demonstrate that central apneas lasting less than 20 s occur normally in children. These events are rarely accompanied by serious oxygen desaturation; a level of oxygen saturation below 90% following a central apnea event is considered abnormal. We therefore classify children as having central sleep apnea if they present with central events lasting more than 10 s and are accompanied by more than one bradytachycardia event or more than one desaturation below 90%.

Obesity as a Risk Factor of Sleep-Disordered Breathing in Children

Various studies have shown that obese children and adolescents have a higher prevalence of all types of SDB compared to their normal-weight peers. For example, an Italian review of questionnaires from more than 2,000 teenagers found that the frequency of snoring was significantly higher in children with body mass index (BMI) in the 90th percentile or greater. Furthermore, subjects with a BMI exceeding the 95th percentile were 2.6 times more likely to snore than children with a BMI below the 75th percentile *(1)*. Similar findings were noted in a German study which demonstrated that obese children had more than 4 times the risk of snoring when compared to their peers with a BMI in the 75th percentile or less *(2)*.

A number of population-based studies have used nocturnal cardiorespiratory monitoring or polygraphy to delineate factors that predispose to OSAS in children. In the Cleveland Family Study, both African-American race and obesity in children aged 2–18 years were associated with a three- to fivefold higher likelihood of SDB *(3)*. The predisposition of African-Americans to OSAS was confirmed in a follow-up study of 8–11-year-old children; preterm birth was also a significant risk factor but obesity per se was not *(4)*. Sánchez-Armengol found that snoring adolescents, as assessed by questionnaire, expressed higher weights and higher waist-to-hip ratios and were more frequently obese as a group than their non-snoring peers *(5)*.

Various studies have used nocturnal polysomnography in hospital settings to determine the prevalence of OSAS *(6)*. Three general conclusions are warranted.

First, obese children are at greater risk of OSAS. However, there are large variations in observed prevalence rates among studies, ranging from 13 to 59%. The observed differences in prevalence probably reflect a number of factors, including differences in the ethnicity, age, and pubertal status of the studied subjects and, more importantly, the use of different diagnostic criteria for childhood obesity and for childhood OSAS. These factors make the calculation of a pooled estimate for the prevalence of OSAS in childhood obesity very difficult, if not impossible.

Second, in the majority of cases the OSAS is generally mild and non-debilitating.

Finally, not all studies found the expected association between BMI and the apnea–hypopnea index – the classical marker of the severity of OSAS. However, the apnea–hypopnea index may correlate more strongly with the distribution of body fat than with BMI per se. For instance, we reported a significant association between waist-to-hip ratio and the apnea–hypopnea index in one of our studies but failed to find a significant association with BMI.

Moreover, the apnea–hypopnea index is not the only marker of the severity of sleep apnea; various studies have demonstrated that the degree of obesity is associated with other consequences of SDB, such as oxygen desaturation. Our study, for instance, reported a correlation between BMI and the minimal oxygen saturation during sleep; this finding had been described previously by Marcus et al. *(7)*. From a pathophysiological point of view, an association with oxygen desaturation is perhaps more important than a correlation with the number of apneic events, because intermittent hypoxia is the primary mediator of most of the complications associated with sleep apnea.

In contrast to evidence that OSAS is more prevalent in obese children, there are limited data on the prevalence of central apnea. We found that 13% of obese children had central sleep apnea; of all the groups of children we studied, those with central apnea had the most severe oxygen desaturation events *(8)*. Marcus et al. also described three subjects with central apneas associated with desaturation *(7)*. A recent investigation found that high body mass index (BMI) predicted central sleep apnea in a mixed cohort of normal-weight and overweight children *(9)*.

Pathogenesis of Sleep Apnea in Obesity

The classical risk factor for obstructive sleep apnea in normal-weight children is enlargement of the adenoids and/or tonsils. In obese children, both lymphoid hypertrophy and adiposity can compromise the upper airway. For example, obese children with OSAS were 7 times more likely to have enlarged tonsils and 4 times more likely to have enlarged adenoids *(10)*, while subjects without adenotonsillar hypertrophy had a milder spectrum of respiratory abnormalities *(11)*. In a mixed group of normal-weight and overweight subjects, Brooks et al. demonstrated that the degree of obesity was the only predictor of the apnea–hypopnea index but lymphoid hyperplasia affected the duration of the obstructive apneas and the severity of the subsequent desaturation *(12)*. Data from the Cleveland Family Study also showed the importance of both obesity and respiratory disorders (sinusitis and a history of bronchiolitis, bronchitis, or asthma) as risk factors for sleep apnea in children *(3)*.

Numerous studies in adults have shown that waist circumference or visceral fat content correlate strongly with the severity of OSAS, and often more so than BMI *(13–16)*. However, little is known about the importance of fat distribution as a risk factor for sleep apnea in obese children and adolescents. A questionnaire study in children documented that waist circumference correlated with the risk of SDB *(17)*. In a population-based study of 101 adolescents, snoring was associated with a higher waist-to-hip ratio, reflecting a more central body fattening *(5)*. In a study by Li et al., the association between the waist circumference and the presence of OSAS was borderline significant *(18)*.

In our prevalence study, tonsillar hypertrophy was the only significant covariate for obstructive sleep apnea. On the other hand, BMI z-score, waist circumference, waist-to-hip ratio, and percent fat mass predicted central apnea *(8)*. Moreover, abdominal adiposity was associated with increasing values of the "respiratory disturbance index (RDI)," which combines all central and obstructive events (Fig. 2).

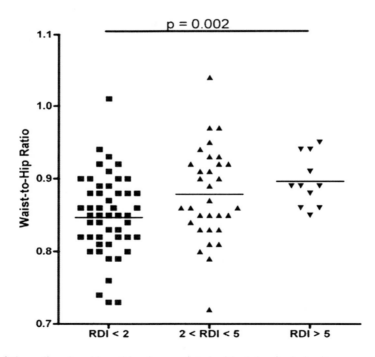

Fig. 2. The severity of sleep-disordered breathing is associated with abdominal obesity, as expressed by the waist-to-hip ratio (RDI = respiratory disturbance index, which is defined as the total number of apneas and hypopneas per hour of sleep) *(6)*.

Although a number of imaging studies in children with SDB have been performed, only one study included overweight subjects. Fregosi et al. failed to find any correlation between BMI and sleep apnea severity, pharyngeal airway dimensions, and soft tissue anatomy (19). However, data from our laboratory (see below) show narrowing of the airway in the region of the adenoids in some obese children with OSAS. It seems likely therefore that the severity of sleep apnea in obese children is mediated both by adenotonsillar hypertrophy and by fat distribution. Recent data suggest that adeno-tonsillar hypertrophy is particularly important in the development of OSAS in young obese children, while progressive upper body fat deposition plays a major role in the obese adolescent. Normal variations in craniofacial anatomy may also contribute to the higher risks of OSAS in certain ethnic groups.

The pathogenesis of central apnea in obese children is unexplained except in children with central nervous system dysfunction following hypothalamic surgery for brain tumors and genetic obesity disorders such as the Prader–Willi syndrome.

Complications of Sleep-Disordered Breathing

The main consequence of repetitive apneas and hypopneas during sleep is intermittent hypoxia, which is a potent trigger of oxidative stress and inflammation (20). Indeed, several studies have documented increased markers of oxidative stress and inflammation in obese children who exhibit sleep apnea (21–23). SDB is also associated with increased sympathetic activity (24), higher serum cortisol levels (25), and other hormonal changes resulting from secondary sleep debt (26–28) (see below).

The neurocognitive and behavioral consequences of SDB in children are the best studied. Common problems include restless sleep, morning headache, and daytime fatigue and sleepiness. Furthermore, children with sleep apnea are at higher risk for concentration problems and learning disabilities, deficits in school performance, and behavioral problems including hyperactivity (29).

In obese children, sleep apnea may augment metabolic and cardiovascular morbidity. Cross-sectional studies indicate that increasing severity of SDB in obese children and adolescents is associated with an increased risk of the metabolic syndrome (30,31), increases in diastolic blood pressure, blunting of the nocturnal fall in blood pressure (32,33), and increases in left ventricular mass and decreases in function (34,35). Moreover, several studies show a positive correlation between sleep apnea and insulin resistance and dyslipidemia in children (30,31,36). However, it must be noted that other studies failed to find a similar relationship (37–39). These conflicting results could be explained by variations in the magnitude of obesity and the ages of study subjects, reflecting varying severity and/or duration of disease; in addition, pubertal status likely plays an important role.

In general, SDB appears to have modest effects on metabolic function in children, and the long-term consequences of childhood sleep apnea on metabolic morbidity in early adulthood remain to be demonstrated in longitudinal investigations. It should be emphasized that no randomized controlled trials of the effects of OSAS treatment on metabolic function have been conducted to date; cross-sectional studies of patients prior to and following treatment have yielded conflicting results (40–42).

Treatment of Sleep-Disordered Breathing in Obese Children and Adolescents

Because obese children have a high prevalence of OSAS, and because OSAS can exacerbate the co-morbidities of obesity, an optimal treatment strategy should target OSAS and obesity simultaneously. A multidisciplinary approach to treatment is essential: an obese child with OSAS should be evaluated by a pediatric sleep physician, an ENT specialist, and a pediatric endocrinologist and should be enrolled in a weight management program staffed by physicians and nutritionists, exercise physiologists, and counselors providing psychological support.

Treatment should be individualized. Adenotonsillectomy can be considered in obese children with adenotonsillar hypertrophy and other signs compatible with chronic upper airway problems, including mouth breathing, chronic rhinitis, recurrent ear infections, and respiratory allergies. In such cases, surgery can provide immediate benefit, though long-term resolution of OSA may depend on concurrent weight loss. Other treatments are preferred when there is little or no obvious upper airway obstruction; these include weight loss for mild cases and continuous positive airway pressure (CPAP) plus weight loss for more severe cases.

Adenotonsillectomy is the first-line treatment for sleep apnea in the child with significant adeno-tonsillar hypertrophy. But a recent meta-analysis showed that adenotonsillectomy reverses OSAS in less than half of obese children with the condition (43). Moreover, several studies indicate that obese children may gain weight after adenotonsillectomy (6). This post-operative weight gain can result in treatment failure and an increase in insulin resistance after surgery (42,44).

This does not imply that adenotonsillectomy should be completely abandoned. However, additional studies are required to identify those children most likely to benefit from adenotonsillectomy. In our center, we have begun to use ultra-low-dose CT scans and functional imaging to identify the subset of obese children who are most likely to benefit from surgery. Figure 3 presents a CT scan from an overweight child with moderate OSAS; it clearly shows that airway narrowing is most severe at the level of the adenoids. Using sophisticated mathematical techniques we can simulate flows through a 3D computer model generated from the CT scan and calculate velocities, pressures, and resistances across the airway. The second part of the figure shows that the pressure drop indeed coincides with narrowing in the region of the adenoids. It is our intention to implement this technique in future clinical practice in order to create an individualized treatment plan for each obese child with OSAS. Should the child undergo adenotonsillectomy, it is mandatory to assess the efficacy of the procedure with a follow-up sleep study.

Systematic studies of the effect of weight loss on the severity of SDB in children are scarce. However, Kalra et al. studied 34 morbidly obese adolescents who underwent bariatric surgery (45). Prior to surgery, 55% of the subjects were diagnosed with OSAS. After surgical weight loss only one subject had sleep apnea.

Our group studied the effect of weight loss on sleep-disordered breathing in 61 obese teenagers enrolled in an inpatient weight loss program (46). Thirty seven subjects were diagnosed with sleep apnea; SDB resolved in 23 of the 37 subjects, but 14 had residual sleep-disordered breathing despite

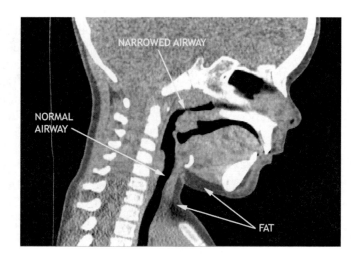

Fig. 3. CT scan and 3D reconstruction with velocity and pressure profile of an overweight child with OSAS.

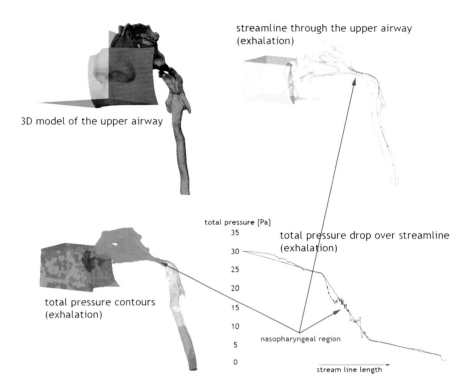

Fig. 3. (continued)

a median weight loss of 24 kg. Interestingly, the apnea–hypopnea index of the baseline screening study correlated significantly with the amount of weight loss that was achieved during the treatment program, suggesting that children with sleep apnea lost more weight than their peers without sleep apnea. Although our weight loss data seem promising, we have no data from obese children less than 10 years of age and no long-term results thus far. Nevertheless, weight loss is an essential component of any treatment regimen for obese children with sleep apnea and represents the first-line approach in those without adenotonsillar obstruction. Whether or not adenotonsillectomy is indicated in subjects resistant to weight loss remains to be determined.

Finally, the use of non-invasive ventilation (CPAP) should be considered in children with severe OSAS. However, CPAP is often poorly tolerated in children. Therefore, children using CPAP should undergo close follow-up to ensure maximal compliance. The additional value of upper airway surgery and/or weight loss in these subjects requires further study.

Conclusions for Daily Practice

1. Childhood obesity is associated with an increased prevalence of all types of sleep-disordered breathing (SDB), including habitual snoring, obstructive sleep apnea, and central sleep apnea. At this moment, there are no valid screening instruments for pediatric SDB. Pediatricians should therefore be aware of its presence in obese children and screen for it through a detailed history, physical examination, and timely referral for polysomnography.
2. The severity of obstructive sleep apnea syndrome (OSAS) in obese children is determined both by adenotonsillar hypertrophy and by adiposity. Future imaging studies are necessary to sort out the individual contribution of these risk factors.

3. Adenotonsillectomy is indicated for adenotonsillary hypertrophy but its success rate is highly variable and there is a risk of a post-operative weight gain.
4. Weight loss seems to be a promising alternative as first-line treatment. However, there are no data on its effects in young obese children and its long-term success rates.
5. CPAP can be considered in children with severe SDB.
6. SDB is associated with the metabolic syndrome. Intervention and longitudinal studies are warranted to assess its effect on long-term metabolic and cardiovascular morbidity.

SLEEP DURATION AND CHILDHOOD OBESITY

Introduction

Calorie intake and energy expenditure are the two fundamental targets in the prevention and treatment of childhood obesity. In recent years, sleep has received much attention since it might affect both energy intake and expenditure. Indeed, sleep plays a major role in the growth and general health of children through its effects on the diurnal rhythms of many hormones related to growth and energy homeostasis. In this section, we review epidemiological evidence suggesting an association between shortened sleep and childhood obesity and discuss possible pathophysiological mechanisms and recommendations for daily clinical practice.

Epidemiological Evidence

A meta-analysis published in 2008 showed that children with shorter sleep duration had a 58% higher risk for overweight or obesity; children with the least sleep had an even higher risk (92%) when compared with children who slept for longer periods of time (47). For each hour increase in sleep, the risk of overweight/obesity was reduced on average by 9%. The study found a significant linear dose–response relationship only in children less than 10 years of age. Boys had a stronger inverse association than girls.

Mechanisms Linking Short Sleep Duration to Obesity

Figure 4 presents a concise overview of possible mechanisms linking sleep curtailment to obesity in children (26,48).

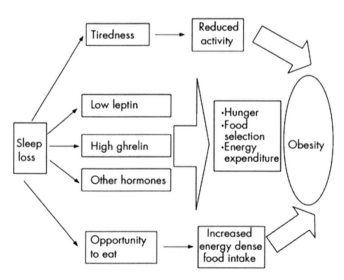

Fig. 4. Possible mechanisms linking sleep restriction with obesity (26,48).

Epidemiological investigations and laboratory studies that subjected young adults to experimental sleep restriction have shown that sleep disruption is associated with adverse changes in several obesity- and appetite-regulating hormones; these include reductions in leptin and growth hormone, and increases in ghrelin, insulin, and cortisol (26,48). The fall in leptin and rise in ghrelin, insulin, and cortisol promote food intake and fat deposition; the fall in growth hormone limits fat breakdown. In concert, these changes might promote the development of obesity and insulin resistance.

Sleep deprivation may also cause emotional distress and daytime fatigue and sleepiness, which may limit daytime physical activity. Interestingly, physical activity has a positive influence on sleep (49), conversely, obesity and emotional distress can disrupt sleep. Thus sleep deprivation may generate a vicious cycle that initiates or perpetuates weight gain.

It is important to note that much of the above evidence originates in studies in adults; little is known about the effects of sleep restriction on hormonal status in children. However, two recent cross-sectional studies in children found that sleep duration was negatively associated with insulin resistance (27,28). It also remains unclear if sleep disruption is a cause or a consequence of obesity; no studies to date have demonstrated that prolongation of sleep can prevent or reverse childhood obesity or reduce its severity (49).

Conclusions for Daily Practice

As noted above, no studies to date have shown that an increase in sleep duration can reduce body weight in obese children; indeed, it is unclear how much a person's sleep would have to be prolonged to exert such an effect. Nevertheless, it seems reasonable to include good sleep hygiene as a preventive measure or as one of the general lifestyle changes necessary to treat childhood obesity. In my opinion this is warranted in view of the consistent epidemiological relationship between sleep duration and obesity in children. General recommendations for good sleep hygiene for children should include: assume a regular bedtime routine; provide a quiet, dark, and relaxing bedroom environment in which there is no place for other activities (television, computer, cell phone); avoid caffeinated drinks during evening hours; avoid bright light in the evening but provide exposure to bright light on awakening in the morning; and finally, do not disrupt the circadian clock by staying up all night and sleeping in during weekends.

Editor's Comments

- As noted by Dr. Verhulst, SDB is associated with deficits in memory, learning, attention, and cognitive function. A recent small study (Kohler et al., 2009) of middle-class Caucasian children (mean age ~7 year) in Australia suggested that SDB is accompanied by a 10-point deficit in IQ relative to age- and gender-matched controls (Controls 110.3, SDB 99.8). The data are difficult to interpret because (a) there was no correlation between intellectual performance and the apnea–hypopnea index either prior to or following surgery; (b) the IQs of the parents and siblings were not measured; and (c) the socioeconomic status of the SDB group was lower than that of the control group.

- Chronic sinusitis/rhinitis, turbinate hypertrophy, and nasal drainage appear to increase the risk of sleep-disordered breathing, particularly in its milder forms [see, for example, Ref. (3) and (Bixler et al., 2009)]. Treatment of nasal congestion with anti-inflammatory agents such as intranasal glucocorticoids and/or montelukast can reduce SDB in mild cases (Goldbart et al., 2005; Kheirandish et al., 2006) but appears to have limited benefit in more severely affected subjects (Kohler et al., 2007).

Bixler EO, et al. Sleep-disordered breathing in children in a general population sample: prevalence and risk factors. SLEEP. 2009;32:731–6.

Goldbart AD, et al. Leukotriene modifier therapy for mild sleep-disordered breathing in children. Am J Respir Crit Care Med. 2005;172:364–70.

Kheirandish L, et al. Intranasal steroids and oral leukotriene modifier therapy in residual sleep-disordered breathing after tonsillectomy and adenoidectom in children. Pediatrics. 2006;117:61–6.

Kohler M, et al. The role of the nose in the pathogenesis of obstructive sleep apnoea and snoring. Eur Respir J. 2007;30:1208–15.

Kohler M, et al. Adenotonsillectomy and neurocognitive deficits in children with sleep disordered breathing. PloS One. 2009;4:e7343.

- Large-scale surveys report that daily sleep duration among American adolescents and adults has declined by 1.5–2 h during the past 40 years (www.sleepfoundation.org). As noted here, severe sleep deprivation can have dramatic effects on human metabolic function: sensitivity to insulin declines, in association with hypercortisolemia and increased sympathetic tone, and a fall in the ratio of leptin to ghrelin may promote excessive daytime caloric intake. This may explain in part the association of night shift work with increased BMI and higher rates of diabetes in adults (see Ruger and Scheer, 2009). Interestingly, sleep deprivation in mice causes weight loss rather than weight gain (Laposky et al., 2008), possibly because forced activity is required to keep the mice awake during the day (when mice normally sleep). Nevertheless, deletion of the circadian Clock gene in mice causes hyperphagia, obesity, glucose intolerance, and fatty liver, findings suggesting a mouse "metabolic syndrome" (Turek et al., 2005). As noted by Dr. Verhulst, it is wise to get yourself and your kids to sleep at a reasonable hour (at least before they go off to college and you have lost all control).

Laposky AD, et al. Sleep and circadian rhythms: key components in the regulation of energy metabolism. FEBS Lett. 2008;582:142–51.

Rüger M, Scheer FA. Effects of circadian disruption on the cardiometabolic system. Rev Endocrinol Metab Disord. 2009 Dec;10(4):245–60.

Turek F, et al. Obesity and metabolic syndrome in circadian Clock mutant mice. Science. 2005;308:1043–5.

REFERENCES

1. Corbo GM, Forastiere F, Agabiti N, Pistelli R, Dell'Orco V, Perucci CA, Valente S. Snoring in 9- to 15-year-old children: risk factors and clinical relevance. Pediatrics. 2001;108:1149–54.

2. Urschitz MS, Guenther A, Eitner S, Urschitz-Duprat PM, Schlaud M, Ipsiroglu OS, Poets CF. Risk factors and natural history of habitual snoring. Chest. 2004;126:790–800.

3. Redline S, Tishler PV, Schluchter M, Aylor J, Clark K, Graham G. Risk factors for sleep-disordered breathing in children. Associations with obesity, race, and respiratory problems. Am J Respir Crit Care Med. 1999;159: 1527–32.

4. Rosen CL, Larkin EK, Kirchner HL, Emancipator JL, Bivins SF, Surovec SA, Martin RJ, Redline S. Prevalence and risk factors for sleep-disordered breathing in 8- to 11-year-old children: association with race and prematurity. J Pediatr. 2003;142:383–9.

5. Sanchez-Armengol A, Fuentes-Pradera MA, Capote-Gil F, Garcia-Diaz E, Cano-Gomez S, Carmona-Bernal C, Castillo-Gomez J. Sleep-related breathing disorders in adolescents aged 12–16 years: clinical and polygraphic findings. Chest. 2001;119:1393–400.

6. Verhulst SL, Van Gaal L, De Backer W, Desager K. The prevalence, anatomical correlates and treatment of sleep-disordered breathing in obese children and adolescents. Sleep Med Rev. 2008;12(5):339–46.

7. Marcus CL, Curtis S, Koerner CB, Joffe A, Serwint JR, Loughlin GM. Evaluation of pulmonary function and polysomnography in obese children and adolescents. Pediatr Pulmonol. 1996;21:176–83.

8. Verhulst SL, Schrauwen N, Haentjens D, Suys B, Rooman RP, Van Gaal L, De Backer W, Desager KN. Sleep-disordered breathing in overweight and obese children and adolescents: prevalence, characteristics and the role of fat distribution. Arch Dis Child. 2007;92:205–8.

9. Kohler, M., Lushington K, Couper R, Martin J, van den Heuvel C, Pamula Y, Kennedy D. Obesity and risk of sleep related upper airway obstruction in Caucasian children. J Clin Sleep Med. 2008;4(2):129–36.

10. Chay OM, Goh A, Abisheganaden J, Tang J, Lim WH, Chan YH, Wee MK, Johan A, John AB, Cheng HK, Lin M, Chee T, Rajan U, Wang S, Machin D. Obstructive sleep apnea syndrome in obese Singapore children. Pediatr Pulmonol. 2000;29:284–90.

11. Silvestri JM, Weese-Mayer DE, Bass MT, Kenny AS, Hauptman SA, Pearsall SM. Polysomnography in obese children with a history of sleep-associated breathing disorders. Pediatr Pulmonol. 1993;16:124–9.

12. Brooks LJ, Stephens BM, Bacevice AM. Adenoid size is related to severity but not the number of episodes of obstructive apnea in children. J Pediatr. 1998;132:682–6.

13. Schafer H, Pauleit D, Sudhop T, Gouni-Berthold I, Ewig S, Berthold HK. Body fat distribution, serum leptin, and cardiovascular risk factors in men with obstructive sleep apnea. Chest. 2002;122:829–39.

14. Grunstein R, Wilcox I, Yang TS, Gould Y, Hedner J. Snoring and sleep apnoea in men: association with central obesity and hypertension. Int J Obes Relat Metab Disord. 1993;17:533–40.

15. Levinson PD, McGarvey ST, Carlisle CC, Eveloff SE, Herbert PN, Millman RP. Adiposity and cardiovascular risk factors in men with obstructive sleep apnea. Chest. 1993;103:1336–42.

16. Vgontzas AN, Papanicolaou DA, Bixler EO, Hopper K, Lotsikas A, Lin HM, Kales A, Chrousos GP. Sleep apnea and daytime sleepiness and fatigue: relation to visceral obesity, insulin resistance, and hypercytokinemia. J Clin Endocrinol Metab. 2000;85:1151–8.

17. Carotenuto M, Bruni O, Santoro N, Del Giudice EM, Perrone L, Pascotto A. Waist circumference predicts the occurrence of sleep-disordered breathing in obese children and adolescents: a questionnaire-based study. Sleep Med. 2006;7: 357–61.

18. Li AM, Chan MH, Chan DF, Lam HS, Wong EM, So HK, Chan IH, Lam CW, Nelson EA. Insulin and obstructive sleep apnea in obese Chinese children. Pediatr Pulmonol. 2006;41:1175–81.

19. Fregosi RF, Quan SF, Kaemingk KL, Morgan WJ, Goodwin JL, Cabrera R, Gmitro A. Sleep-disordered breathing, pharyngeal size and soft tissue anatomy in children. J Appl Physiol. 2003;95:2030–8.

20. Lavie L. Obstructive sleep apnoea syndrome – an oxidative stress disorder. Sleep Med Rev. 2003;7:35–51.

21. Verhulst SL, Van HK, Schrauwen N, Haentjens D, Rooman R, Van GL, De Backer W, Desager KN. Sleep-disordered breathing and uric acid in overweight and obese children and adolescents. Chest. 2007;132:76–80.

22. Tauman R, O'Brien LM, Gozal D. Hypoxemia and obesity modulate plasma C-reactive protein and interleukin-6 levels in sleep-disordered breathing. Sleep Breath. 2007;11:77–84.

23. Larkin EK, Rosen CL, Kirchner HL, Storfer-Isser A, Emancipator JL, Johnson NL, Zambito AM, Tracy RP, Jenny NS, Redline S. Variation of C-reactive protein levels in adolescents: association with sleep-disordered breathing and sleep duration. Circulation. 2005;111:1978–84.

24. Aljadeff G, Gozal D, Schechtman VL, Burrell B, Harper RM, Ward SL. Heart rate variability in children with obstructive sleep apnea. Sleep. 1997;20:151–7.

25. Bratel T, Wennlund A, Carlstrom K. Pituitary reactivity, androgens and catecholamines in obstructive sleep apnoea. Effects of continuous positive airway pressure treatment (CPAP). Respir Med. 1999;93:1–7.

26. Spiegel K, Knutson K, Leproult R, Tasali E, Van Cauter CE. Sleep loss: a novel risk factor for insulin resistance and Type 2 diabetes. J Appl Physiol. 2005;99:2008–19.

27. Flint J, Kothare SV, Zihlif M, Suarez E, Adams R, Legido A, De LF. Association between inadequate sleep and insulin resistance in obese children. J Pediatr. 2007;150:364–9.

28. Verhulst SL, Schrauwen N, Haentjens D, Rooman RP, Van GL, Backer WADE, Desager KN. Sleep duration and metabolic dysregulation in overweight children and adolescents. Arch Dis Child. 2008;93:89–90.

29. Beebe DW. Neurobehavioral morbidity associated with disordered breathing during sleep in children: a comprehensive review. Sleep. 2006;29:1115–34.

30. Verhulst SL, Schrauwen N, Haentjens D, Rooman R, Van Gaal L, De Backer W, Desager K. Sleep-disordered breathing and the metabolic syndrome in overweight and obese children and adolescents. J Pediatr. 2007;150:612–6.

31. Redline S, Storfer-Isser A, Rosen CL, Johnson NL, Kirchner HL, Emancipator J, Kibler AM. Association between metabolic syndrome and sleep disordered breathing in adolescents. Am J Respir Crit Care Med. 2007;176(4):401–8.

32. Amin RS, Carroll JL, Jeffries JL, Grone C, Bean JA, Chini B, Bokulic R, Daniels SR. Twenty-four-hour ambulatory blood pressure in children with sleep-disordered breathing. Am J Respir Crit Care Med. 2004;169:950–6.

33. Marcus CL, Greene MG, Carroll JL. Blood pressure in children with obstructive sleep apnea. Am J Respir Crit Care Med. 1998;157:1098–103.

34. Amin RS, Kimball TR, Bean JA, Jeffries JL, Willging JP, Cotton RT, Witt SA, Glascock BJ, Daniels SR. Left ventricular hypertrophy and abnormal ventricular geometry in children and adolescents with obstructive sleep apnea. Am J Respir Crit Care Med. 2002;165:1395–9.

35. Amin RS, Kimball TR, Kalra M, Jeffries JL, Carroll JL, Bean JA, Witt SA, Glascock BJ, Daniels SR. Left ventricular function in children with sleep-disordered breathing. Am J Cardiol. 2005;95:801–4.

36. Waters KA, Mast BT, Vella S, de la ER, O'Brien LM, Bailey S, Tam CS, Wong M, Baur LA. Structural equation modeling of sleep apnea, inflammation, and metabolic dysfunction in children. J Sleep Res. 2007;16:388–95.

37. Dubern B, Tounian P, Medjadhi N, Maingot L, Girardet JP, Boule M. Pulmonary function and sleep-related breathing disorders in severely obese children. Clin Nutr. 2006;25:803–9.

38. Tauman R, O'Brien LM, Ivanenko A, Gozal D. Obesity rather than severity of sleep-disordered breathing as the major determinant of insulin resistance and altered lipidemia in snoring children. Pediatrics. 2005;116:e66–73.

39. Kaditis AG, Alexopoulos EI, Damani E, Karadonta I, Kostadima E, Tsolakidou A, Gourgoulianis K, Syrogiannopoulos GA. Obstructive sleep-disordered breathing and fasting insulin levels in nonobese children. Pediatr Pulmonol. 2005;40:515–23.

40. Waters KA, Sitha S, O'Brien LM, Bibby S, de Torres C, Vella S, de la ER. Follow-up on metabolic markers in children treated for obstructive sleep apnea. Am J Respir Crit Care Med. 2006;174:455–60.

41. Gozal D, Capdevila OS, Kheirandish-Gozal L. Metabolic Alterations in Obstructive Sleep Apnea among Non-Obese and Obese Prepubertal Children. Am J Respir Crit Care Med. 2008;177(10):1142–9.

42. Apostolidou MT, Alexopoulos EI, Damani E, Liakos N, Chaidas K, Boultadakis E, Apostolidis T, Gourgoulianis K, Kaditis AG. Absence of blood pressure, metabolic, and inflammatory marker changes after adenotonsillectomy for sleep apnea in Greek children. Pediatr Pulmonol. 2008;43:550–60.

43. Costa DJ, Mitchell R. Adenotonsillectomy for obstructive sleep apnea in obese children: a meta-analysis. Otolaryngol Head Neck Surg. 2009;140:455–60.

44. Amin R, Anthony L, Somers V, Fenchel M, McConnell K, Jefferies J, Willging P, Kalra M, Daniels S. Growth velocity predicts recurrence of sleep disordered breathing 1 year after adenotonsillectomy. Am J Respir Crit Care Med. 2008;177:654–9.

45. Kalra M, Inge T, Garcia V, Daniels S, Lawson L, Curti R, Cohen A, Amin R. Obstructive sleep apnea in extremely overweight adolescents undergoing bariatric surgery. Obes Res. 2005;13:1175–9.

46. Verhulst SL, Franckx H, Van GL, De BW, Desager K. The effect of weight loss on sleep-disordered breathing in obese teenagers. Obesity (Silver Spring). 2009;17:1178–83.

47. Chen X, Beydoun MA, Wang Y. Is sleep duration associated with childhood obesity? A systematic review and meta-analysis. Obesity (Silver Spring). 2008;16:265–74.

48. Leproult R, Van Cauter E. Role of sleep and sleep loss in hormonal release and metabolism. Endocr Dev. 2010;17:11–21.

49. Taheri S. The link between short sleep duration and obesity: we should recommend more sleep to prevent obesity. Arch Dis Child. 2006;91:881–4.

18 The Long-Term Metabolic Complications of Childhood Obesity

Charles J. Glueck, John A. Morrison, Muhammad Umar, Naila Goldenberg, and Ping Wang

CONTENTS

Key Words: Insulin resistance, hyperinsulinemia, metabolic syndrome, type 2 diabetes, race, cardiovascular disease, PCOS, diet, metformin

INTRODUCTION

Childhood obesity and associated insulin resistance (IR) and hyperinsulinemia *(1–6)* have broad-ranging metabolic effects that have profound impacts on adult health. They are associated with cardiovascular risk factors, including hypertension, hypertriglyceridemia, low HDL levels, and high cholesterol (HDL-C) levels, which track with time and are central to the long-term development of impaired fasting glucose (IFG), type 2 diabetes mellitus (T2DM), and the metabolic syndrome *(2,7,8)* (Fig. 1).

Sound models are required to predict which children are at increased risk for subsequent glucose intolerance and cardiovascular disease (CVD) *(9)*. An understanding of the joint roles of childhood hyperinsulinemia and obesity on this process should illuminate approaches to deal simultaneously with both, with a goal of preventing or ameliorating metabolic disease in adolescence and adulthood. The studies summarized in this chapter suggest complex interrelationships between obesity and hyperinsulinemia in children and the subsequent development of glucose intolerance and T2DM.

This research was supported in part by American Heart Association (National)-9750129 N, NIH- HL62394, HC55025 and HL48941 (Dr Morrison) and by the Lipoprotein Research Fund of the Jewish Hospital of Cincinnati (Dr Glueck)

From: *Contemporary Endocrinology: Pediatric Obesity: Etiology, Pathogenesis, and Treatment*
Edited by: M. Freemark, DOI 10.1007/978-1-60327-874-4_18,
© Springer Science+Business Media, LLC 2010

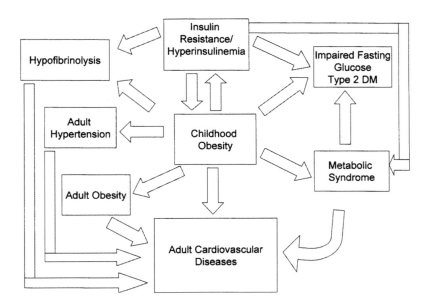

Fig. 1. Centrality of childhood obesity, insulin resistance, and hyperinsulinemia to adult cardiovascular diseases, type 2 diabetes mellitus, and metabolic syndrome.

Obesity and Insulin Resistance (IR) as Chicken and Egg

In response to nutrient-dependent weight gain, humans and experimental animals develop resistance to insulin action in skeletal muscle, liver, and adipose tissue. The insulin resistance triggers a compensatory increase in insulin secretion and reduces hepatic insulin uptake, thereby increasing fasting and post-prandial insulin concentrations (hyperinsulinemia). Insulin resistance also attenuates the lipogenic effect of insulin in white adipose tissue and thereby limits further progression of weight gain. Thus, most investigators have considered insulin resistance and hyperinsulinemia to be *adaptive responses* to adiposity.

On the other hand, several investigators have postulated that hyperinsulinemia may be a primary factor in the *development* of obesity through its induction of fat deposition. The latter hypothesis is supported by four lines of evidence: (1) vagal-dependent hyperinsulinemia appears to play a central role in the development of hypothalamic obesity (see Chapter 2 by Lustig on energy balance); (2) the risks of adult obesity and type 2 diabetes in Pima Indians correlate with plasma insulin concentrations at 5–10 years of age; and (3) the risks of obesity, T2DM, and the metabolic syndrome in black and white American adults correlate with plasma insulin concentrations measured at 9–10 years of age (see below); and (4) there is mounting evidence that the insulin-sensitizing drug metformin manages weight gain in patients taking antipsychotic drugs and in obese adolescents (see below). Given that plasma insulin levels may be determined by familial/genetic and well as environmental factors, it is conceivable that the roles of insulin resistance and hyperinsulinemia in the development or progression of obesity may vary according to racial, ethnic, socioeconomic, and cultural background. A variety of genes have been implicated in the development of obesity in children and adults; studies from our group suggest that polymorphisms in the AGT and CYP11 B2 genes may play roles in white and black youths (unpublished data, 2009).

Tracking of Obesity and IR from Childhood into Adulthood

It is well known that the risk of adult obesity in an obese child correlates with the age of the child; in other words, adolescent obesity is more predictive of adult obesity than obesity in early childhood

(10). Yet childhood BMI does predict adult obesity. The NHLBI Growth and Health Study (NGHS) analyzed a cohort of 9- and 10-year-old black and white girls to study the development of obesity and its effects on CVD risk factors during a 10-year follow-up. The clinical centers in Cincinnati and Washington DC elected to conduct an ancillary project, collecting fasting bloods for the measurement of glucose and insulin in years 1 and 10 in addition to measures of body composition. Data from this ancillary project showed that pre-teen BMI was associated with BMI and HOMA-IR (a measure of insulin resistance) at age 19 *(11)*. Interestingly, high-fat, high-calorie diets led to greater adolescent weight gain, but more so in participants with higher BMI and IR at age 10 *(8)*.

Over the 10-year study period obesity was more persistent in black than white girls: 88.2% of black girls who were obese at ages 9 and 10 were obese at ages 18–19, compared to 61.2% of white girls *(11)*. Importantly, mean BMI was greater in the girls who were obese at both visits (39.8 and 37.1 kg/m^2 in black and white girls, respectively) than in girls who were obese at age 18–19 but not at age 9–10 (34.6 and 33.5 kg/m^2).

A second longitudinal study, The Princeton Follow-up Study (PFS), was designed to assess changes in CVD risk factors from childhood into the fourth and fifth decades of life and changes in the familial lipoprotein correlations from the period of shared households to separate households *(12–16)*. PFS participants included students in grades 1–12 of the public and parochial schools of the Cincinnati Princeton School District (LRC 1,2) and a 50% sample of their parents. The original student population was 73% white and 27% black, 52% male and 48% female (LRC 1). Adult BMI was strongly associated with pediatric BMI, with an overall tracking coefficient of 0.59; 63% of participants at risk of overweight at enrollment were obese at follow-up *(16)*.

Black–White Differences in Plasma Insulin and Obesity and Progression Over Time

It is known that black adolescents have significantly higher insulin levels than their white counterparts *(11,17)*. Interestingly, the association of insulin levels with BMI is similar in black and white children ($r = 0.44$ in both black and white girls at ages 9–10 and $r = 0.48$ and 0.56 respectively at ages 18–19, all $p < 0.0001$), but the insulin distribution is shifted to the right in black girls *(11)*. The 9-year-old black girls in NGHS had significantly higher fasting insulin (11.5 μU/mL vs. 8.7 μU/mL in white girls, $p = 0.002$; HOMA-IR = 2.7 vs. 2.1, $p = 0.01$) prior to puberty and prior to the appearance of racial differences in BMI *(11)*. The median insulin level in black girls equates roughly to the 75th percentile of insulin levels in white girls (Morrison et al. 2009, unpublished data). In both black and white girls, insulin and BMI increase sharply with onset of puberty, but the increase in insulin and BMI is sharper in black girls than white girls *(17)*. Even after pair-matching black and white girls in the cohort by BMI, insulin, and pubertal status at age 9–10 *(8)*, black girls had higher BMI, insulin, and glucose (black girls higher) at age 19. White girls had lower lean body mass and greater adiposity than black girls matched for BMI at ages 9 and 10, but black girls had marginally greater adiposity as well as higher BMI at age 19.

Insulin levels are strongly and positively associated with glucose levels in both black and white girls at ages 9–10 and 18–19 years, but *(11)* the slopes were steeper in black than white girls, showing that at any level of fasting glucose, black girls have higher insulin levels. The hyperinsulinemia in black children may be explained by heightened insulin secretion and reduced hepatic insulin clearance (see also Chapter 6 by Haidet et al., this book) *(18)*. In both black and white girls, there is a stepped increase in fasting insulin levels and HOMA-IR with pubertal maturation, but insulin sensitivity in blacks is lower than that in whites at all time points studied *(19–24)*. The black–white differences in insulin levels and insulin resistance (HOMA-IR) persist after controlling for BMI and pubertal stage *(11)*. Finally, the magnitude of the post-pubertal decrease in IR is less in black than white girls.

Although black girls have higher insulin levels than white girls overall, obese black and white girls have similar insulin levels *(8)*. This finding suggests that when white girls become obese, they attain the same level of IR as black girls. Furthermore, although the interaction of IR and fat calories was a highly significant independent predictor of 10-year change in BMI in both black and white girls, the interaction term accounted for 27% of the variability in the 10-year change in BMI in white girls but only 3.6% of the variability in black girls *(8)*. IR may have less discriminating power in black girls since black girls are more insulin resistant than white girls *(8)*.

Our finding that HOMA-IR at age 10 interacts with fat calories to increase BMI during 10-year follow-up *(8)* is congruent with a report by Mosca et al. *(25)*, whose 14-year longitudinal study in adults showed that weight gain over time was positively associated with fat intake in both insulin-resistant and insulin-sensitive subjects, but the slope of the fat intake–weight gain association was greater in the subjects with IR *(25)*. Kahn and Flier *(26)* have proposed that IR and hyperinsulinemia, in addition to being caused by obesity, can contribute to the development of obesity via an interaction with total and fat calories. Our findings reviewed are consistent with this hypothesis *(8)*.

Long-Term Risks of Childhood Obesity and Insulin Resistance (IR): Impaired Fasting Glucose, Impaired Glucose Tolerance, and T2DM

During the past 25 years, the prevalence of T2DM has increased markedly and its age of onset has declined dramatically, especially in black females *(27,28)*. T2DM now presents in the teenage years with increasing frequency; that this reflects the effects of prolonged obesity and IR in childhood and early adolescence is suggested by older studies in Pima Indians *(28)* and by more recent clinic-based and population-based studies from Yale and from our group reviewed below.

The Pima subjects whose glucose metabolism deteriorated during a 25-year longitudinal study were older, and more obese, and had presented with higher fasting and 2-h glucose and insulin concentrations at the time of enrollment *(29)*. Factors that predicted the progression *from normal to impaired glucose tolerance (IGT)* included age, higher BMI, and increased 2-h plasma glucose and insulin concentrations. Predictors of progression *from IGT to diabetes* included an increased 2-h plasma glucose level and a fall in 2-h plasma insulin concentration. Importantly, higher BMI was not a predictor of progression from carbohydrate intolerance to diabetes, but the duration of obesity was highly correlated with the development of diabetes after adjustment for current BMI *(28)*. Although IR was not identified as a separate stage in this study, the pattern of higher fasting insulin and BMI prior to progression from normal to carbohydrate intolerance supports the existence of IR as a stage preceding carbohydrate intolerance. Biochemical (silent, preclinical) diabetes preceded overt diabetes *(29)*. These longitudinal data document the progression through specific stages in the development of T2DM and identify predictors of progression at each stage of developing diabetes.

More recently, clinic-based studies of obese adolescents by Weiss, Caprio, and colleagues at Yale *(30)* are consistent with the earlier Pima studies. These studies have focused on obesity, insulin, glucose, and inflammatory markers in children and adolescents *(30–32)*. Of particular importance here is the report by Weiss et al. *(32)* on 117 obese white, African-American, and Hispanic youth who were followed over a 2-year period to assess metabolic changes (see also Chapter 13 by Weiss and Caprio et al., this volume). All participants had oral glucose tolerance tests at enrollment and follow-up. Of the 117 youth, 84 youth had normal glucose tolerance (NGT) and 33 had IGT at enrollment. Mean baseline BMI did not differ between the NGT (35.5 kg/m^2) and IGT (36.6 kg/m^2) groups *(32)*. After 2 years, eight subjects had T2DM; all eight had had IGT at baseline. In addition, eight subjects with NGT at baseline had IGT at follow-up and 15 subjects with IGT at baseline had NGT. Analyses focused on factors contributing to the development of T2DM in the cohort. The best predictors of T2DM in the cohort were severe obesity (mean baseline BMI was 44.8 kg/m^2 in the eight subjects that developed T2DM), African-American background (seven of the eight were African-American females and one white case), and IGT (all subjects developing T2DM had IGT at baseline). Baseline insulin was not a significant predictor *(32)*, but it should be noted that all subjects had hyperinsulinemia (fasting mean insulin levels in the NGT and IGT groups were 27 and 42 µU/mL respectively, and 40 µU/mL in the eight T2DM subjects). Since most individuals with insulin resistance do not develop T2DM and all subjects were hyperinsulinemic, the significant predictor of future T2DM in this study was evidence of failing glucose tolerance at enrollment.

The ancillary project of the NGHS study assessing pre-teen fasting insulin and glucose as predictor of subsequent IFG and T2DM (see above) produced epidemiological results that partially support the clinical findings of Weiss et al. (32). The differences in findings can be attributed to a large extent to differences in study design and study populations. NGHS recruited black and white girls with a wide range of BMI. Weiss et al. recruited only obese (BMI > 95th percentile for age and sex) subjects. As a large, epidemiological study, NGHS measured BMI and fasting insulin and glucose, while Weiss et al. in their clinical study conducted oral glucose tolerance tests on subjects recruited from the Yale Pediatric Obesity Clinic. In the NGHS ancillary study, high baseline insulin and elevated glucose predicted the development of T2DM and IFG at age 19. In multivariate analyses there was a sevenfold increase in the risk of T2DM in pre-teens with IFG (8). In the study Weiss et al. (32), in which all subjects were obese and hyperinsulinemic at baseline, static tests of fasting insulin and glucose failed to predict the outcome (T2DM); only the dynamic test of IGT did. In both studies, T2DM predominated in black girls.

Recent population-based cross-sectional studies in general populations have examined the relationship between childhood obesity, IR, and glucose intolerance. Analysis of the NHANES data shows that adolescents with hyperinsulinemia have a fourfold higher prevalence of IFG, IGT, and pre-diabetes than those without hyperinsulinemia. Interestingly, neither overweight nor the number of cardio-metabolic risk factors was significantly associated with pre-diabetes after adjustment for hyperinsulinemia (33). Hyperinsulinemia may therefore account for the association of overweight and clustering of cardio-metabolic risk factors with pre-diabetes (33).

The risk of future T2DM in children with IFG or IGT is likely a graded one as it is in adults, with risk increasing with increasing evidence of glucose dysregulation. A longitudinal follow-up study is that 8.1% of adults with glucose values ranging from 100 to 109 mg/dL progressed to T2DM during a 9-year follow-up period (1.34% per year) compared to 24.3% of subjects with fasting glucose values of 110–125 mg/dL (5.56% per year) (34). The association of IR with T2DM in adolescents, as in adults, depends, in large part, upon a positive family history of diabetes (35). IR is robustly associated with development of T2DM in adult offspring of two parents with T2DM, but not in adults whose parents did not have T2DM. *Thus a strong family history of diabetes is an ominous finding in an obese, insulin-resistant adolescent or child.*

Childhood Obesity, Insulin Resistance (IR), and the Metabolic Syndrome

The concept of a metabolic syndrome (36) as a predictor of future T2DM and CVD in adults grew out of Reaven's 1988 Banting Lecture (37). Reaven (37) showed that a cluster of metabolic risk factors, including obesity, dyslipidemia, hypertension, and glucose intolerance predisposed to cardiovascular disease. Despite widespread use of the phrase "metabolic syndrome," there is considerable variability in its definition (38) and controversy over its theoretical and clinical applicability. Nevertheless, our recent investigations suggest it has utility as an organizing tool for assessment of long-term cardiovascular and diabetes risk in children (2,7,8).

In a series of reports on the PFS and NGHS cohorts and subsequent disease outcomes, we defined pediatric metabolic syndrome using age-specific cutoffs for its various components (39) and calculated a metabolic syndrome z-score that normalized data for triglycerides, HDL-C, glucose, systolic blood pressure, diastolic blood pressure, and waist circumference according to gender and race. Longitudinal follow-up of black and white girls, first seen at ages 9 and 10 years of age, showed that IR interacts with BMI to predict metabolic syndrome 10 years later (2). Subjects in the highest tertiles for both

BMI and HOMA-IR at baseline had the highest mean metabolic syndrome z-score at age 19, while subjects in the lowest tertiles for both BMI and HOMA-IR at ages 9–10 had the lowest aggregate z-score. Within the top BMI tertile, there was a progressive increase in aggregate z-score (reflecting increasing risk of metabolic syndrome) as HOMA-IR increased *(2)*.

Childhood Metabolic Syndrome and Adult T2DM and CVD

In the Princeton Follow-Up Study, described above, we found that metabolic syndrome in childhood predicted adult metabolic syndrome and the development of T2DM *(7)* and CVD during the ensuing 25–30 years *(16)*.

Diabetes in the former students and their parents was determined by report of the participants and/or fasting blood glucose ≥ 126 mg/dl. There were 44 cases of T2DM in the Princeton cohort. The incidence of adult T2DM was 15.6% ($n = 5$) among the 32 subjects who had metabolic syndrome as children, compared to 5% in subjects who did not have metabolic syndrome as children ($p < 0.0001$). In the multivariate model pediatric metabolic syndrome (OR $= 11.5$, $p = 0.005$), parental history of diabetes (OR $= 5.0$, $p = 0.0003$), age at follow-up (OR $= 1.12$, $p = 0.01$), and black race (OR $= 2.2$, $p = 0.03$) were significant explanatory variables; the interaction of pediatric metabolic syndrome and parental history of diabetes was not significant at $p < 0.05$, but was suggestive (OR $= 6.5$, $p = 0.08$). Thus, pediatric metabolic syndrome predicts T2DM in the fourth and fifth decades of life.

CVD in participants and their parents was determined by report of the participants and included myocardial infarction, coronary artery by-pass graft, angioplasty, or stroke. There were 17 cases of CVD in the Princeton sample. The incidence of CVD in subjects who had metabolic syndrome as children was 19.4% ($n = 6$), compared to 1.5% in subjects who did not have metabolic syndrome as children. In multivariate logistic analysis, pediatric metabolic syndrome (OR $= 14.7$, $p < 0.0001$) and age (OR $= 1.2$, $p = 0.03$) were significant predictors of CVD; sex, race, and parental history of CVD were not. When change in BMI percentile was added to the final model, it was not significant. Finally, CVD at follow-up was not associated with a glucose level above 100 or 110 mg/dL in childhood ($p = 0.13$). Thus, pediatric metabolic syndrome, rather than BMI or fasting glucose alone, predicts CVD in the fourth and fifth decades of life.

Obesity is the driving force underlying the metabolic syndrome on a population basis. The prevalence of BMI above the 90th age-specific percentile was 77% in students with metabolic syndrome, with an additional 13% of cases with BMI above the 85th percentile, but below the 90th. Thus 90% of pediatric cases were at risk of obesity or worse. Adult metabolic syndrome was even more strongly associated with BMI at follow-up: 95% of cohort members with adult metabolic syndrome had BMI ≥ 25 kg/m^2 (at risk of obesity) and 72% were obese (BMI ≥ 30 kg/m^2). In multivariate analysis, with adult metabolic syndrome as the dependent variable, pediatric metabolic syndrome (OR $= 9.4$), parental history of diabetes (OR $= 2.4$), age at follow-up (OR $= 1.06$), and the change in weight (age-specific BMI percentile) (OR $= 1.025$) were significant explanatory variables. A positive parental history of diabetes was strongly associated with overweight status in both childhood and adulthood: 24.6% of participants reporting a positive parental history of T2DM had BMI $\geq$ 85th percentile in childhood compared to 11.7% of participants who did not ($p < 0.0001$), and in adulthood the prevalence of overweight (BMI ≥ 25 kg/m^2) was 72.2% in participants who reported parental diabetes compared to 60.6% in those who did not ($p < 0.0004$). The prevalence of adult metabolic syndrome was 69% in subjects with pediatric metabolic syndrome compared to 24% in subjects without metabolic syndrome as children ($p < 0.0001$). Thus, pediatric BMI predicts adult BMI, and pediatric metabolic syndrome predicts adult metabolic syndrome.

Finally, we examined the progression of glucose intolerance in a cohort of 568 black and white school children followed from ages 9–10 to ages 24–25 with nine measures of insulin and glucose. Our recent findings *(Arch Pediatr Adol Med*, in press, 7/09) indicate that metabolic syndrome rarely developed (1.2% of subjects) in the absence of hyperinsulinemia. The combination of hyperinsuline-mia and metabolic syndrome increased the risk of IFG + T2DM almost 3.3-fold compared to girls with normal insulin levels and no metabolic syndrome at ages 9–10 years. Of the five factors defining metabolic syndrome only elevated fasting glucose (100 $\leq$ glucose < 126) and waist circumference were significant predictors of future IFG + T2DM.

Our findings are consistent with those of the Bogalusa Heart Study, which reported that high insulin levels *(40,41)* and overweight were associated with higher levels of the component factors in the metabolic syndrome later in life. The role of familial factors in development of the metabolic syn-drome was explored by Srinivasan et al. *(42)*, who examined the timing and the course of development of the components of the metabolic syndrome from childhood to adulthood in the offspring of parents with diabetes. The study enrolled a community-based cohort with ($n = 303$) and without ($n = 1,136$) a parental history of type 2 diabetes; subjects were followed longitudinally since childhood (aged 4–17 years; mean follow-up period, 15 years) by repeated surveys *(42)*. Relative to offspring with-out parental diabetes, offspring with parental diabetes had excess generalized and truncal adiposity beginning in childhood, higher levels of fasting insulin and glucose and HOMA-IR from adolescence, and higher levels of low-density lipoprotein (LDL) cholesterol and triglycerides, and lower levels of high-density lipoprotein (HDL) cholesterol in adulthood *(42)*. Many of these risk variables changed adversely at an increased rate in offspring of diabetic parents.

In a multivariate analysis, parental diabetes was an independent predictor of longitudinal changes in adiposity, glucose, insulin, HOMA-IR, systolic and diastolic blood pressure, and LDL cholesterol in the offspring, regardless of race and gender *(42)*. As young adults, the offspring of diabetic parents had a higher prevalence of generalized (BMI > 30, 36% vs. 16%), visceral obesity (waist > 100 cm, 15% vs. 6%), hyperinsulinemia (insulin > 18 μU/mL, 15% vs. 8%), hyperglycemia ($\geq$110 mg/dl, 2% vs. 0.5%), high LDL cholesterol ($\geq$160 mg/dl, 11% vs. 7%, $p = 0.02$), low HDL cholesterol (<40 mg/dl for males and <50 mg/dl for females, 40% vs. 31%), high triglycerides ($\geq$150 mg/dl, 23% vs. 15%), and hypertension (>140/90 mmHg, 11% vs. 6%) *(42)*. Thus, the offspring of diabetic parents displayed excess body fatness beginning in childhood and accelerated progression of adverse risk profile characteristics of insulin resistance syndrome from childhood to young adulthood *(42)*.

Polycystic Ovary Syndrome

Polycystic ovary syndrome (PCOS), which affects ~6% of white and 8–10% of black and Hispanic adolescent girls *(43)*, has its genesis in IR and hyperinsulinemia (see also the Chapter 24 by Franks and Joharatnam, this volume). PCOS in adults is strongly associated with obesity, hyperinsulinemia, dys-lipidemia, and glucose intolerance. In addition, obesity may mimic or exacerbate PCOS and increase the likelihood of gestational diabetes both in PCOS and in non-PCOS women.

We compared BMI, fat patterning, insulin, lipids, and blood pressure in 39 adolescent girls with PCOS and 229 schoolgirl controls with normal menses. As expected the PCOS patients had signifi-cantly higher BMI, waist circumference, insulin, systolic and diastolic blood pressure, triglycerides, and free testosterone and lower HDL-C. After matching PCOS patients and controls for BMI or waist circumference, the differences in all risk factors except free testosterone were no longer significant, suggesting that if and when adolescent girls achieve BMI and central adiposity similar to PCOS girls, they acquire similar CVD risk profiles, except for free testosterone *(44)*.

Intervention with Diet, Exercise, and Metformin in Obese, Hyperinsulinemic Children Reduces Metabolic Complications of Childhood Obesity

Given the cumulative findings of studies from our group and others, we consider obese, hyperin-sulinemic children to be at risk for metabolic decompensation, particularly if there is a strong family history of T2DM or early cardiovascular disease. In such cases, we believe that measures to restrict diet, increase physical activity, and decrease insulin and IR (45) may be warranted.

In some cases, lifestyle intervention can have beneficial effects on BMI and metabolic function. For example, supervised exercise in obese Chinese children reduced glucose, insulin, and IR, along with BMI, but 3 months after completion of the exercise program, glucose, insulin, and IR returned to pre-intervention levels (46). Exercise alone can reduce IR in obese children independently of changes in body composition (47) (see also Chapter 21 by Eliakim and Nemet, this volume). Dietary counseling and psychological support may also prove useful and effective in motivated subjects (see Chapter 20 by Wilfley et al.).

On the other hand, an intensive nutrition program combined with strength training failed to produce changes in insulin sensitivity or body composition in obese Latino adolescents (48). Moreover, lifestyle changes did not produce significant weight loss in obese adolescents in Tennessee; however, the combination of metformin and lifestyle intervention caused significant weight loss (49). In a randomized, double-blind, placebo-controlled trial in adolescents with IR, diet–exercise modification did not lead to weight loss, but addition of metformin increased weight loss in girls (50). In Australian obese children, a randomized, double-blind, cross-over trial showed that metformin therapy resulted in significant improvement in body composition and fasting insulin (51). In normo-glycemic morbidly obese adolescents, a randomized double-blind, placebo-controlled trial revealed that combined metformin treatment and low-calorie diet had a significant anti-obesity effect in hyperinsulinemic obese adolescents compared to low-calorie diet alone (52). Freemark and Bursey (53) found that metformin reduced fasting insulin and BMI z-score in obese adolescents. Finally, Glueck et al. (54,55) reported that metformin, when combined with diet, reduces IR and weight in obese, hyperinsulinemic adolescent girls with polycystic ovary syndrome (PCOS). Moreover, Arslanian et al. (56) reported that metformin treatment reduced plasma insulin and androgen concentrations and improved glucose tolerance in obese adolescents with PCOS. We speculate that diet, exercise, and, if needed, metformin have promise in primary prevention of metabolic syndrome if initiated in hyperinsulinemic obese adolescents. This hypothesis is explored in more detail in Chapter 23 by Freemark.

Finally, previous (57) and recent (58–60) reports suggest that metformin may moderate the weight gain that frequently accompanies the use of atypical antipsychotic drugs. Findings suggest that the combination of metformin and lifestyle intervention is more effective than lifestyle intervention alone.

CONCLUSIONS

Childhood obesity promotes development and amplification of obesity, IR, and the metabolic syndrome into young adulthood and increases adult risks of IFG, T2DM, and CVD. Reductions in adiposity and hyperinsulinemia through diet, exercise, and insulin-sensitizing agents may reduce the long-term risks of metabolic disease.

Editor's Question and Authors' Response

- **The use of the term "metabolic syndrome" has generated controversy. However, your findings suggest that the metabolic syndrome in childhood predicts the development of T2DM and CVD later in life. How do you respond to those who argue that the long-term risks of metabolic syndrome are no greater that the sum of the risks of its component parts?**

- Whether diagnosis of the metabolic syndrome has diagnostic implications for development of cardiovascular disease and type 2 diabetes beyond its component parts remains an unanswered question. However, we found that the presence of the metabolic syndrome was an independent risk factor for IFG, T2DM, and CVD, increasing the probability of the outcomes in insulin-resistant and non-insulin-resistant participants alike. Moreover, and most important in our opinion, treating the individual factors one-factor-at-a-time (with prescribed drugs) may constitute a less efficient, less effective approach to the problem than addressing the underlying problem, which, on a population basis, is obesity-related insulin resistance. The success of the lifestyle intervention arm in the Diabetes Prevention Program suggests that a holistic approach is the better way to go.

REFERENCES

1. Berenson GS. Obesity – a critical issue in preventive cardiology: the Bogalusa Heart Study. Prev Cardiol. 2005;8: 234–41; quiz 42–3.
2. Morrison JA, Glueck CJ, Horn PS, Schreiber GB, Wang P. Homeostasis model assessment of insulin resistance*body mass index interactions at ages 9–10 years predict metabolic syndrome risk factor aggregate score at ages 18–19 years: a 10-year prospective study of black and white girls. Metabolism. 2009;58:290–5.
3. Bhardwaj S, Misra A, Khurana L, Gulati S, Shah P, Vikram NK. Childhood obesity in Asian Indians: a burgeoning cause of insulin resistance, diabetes and sub-clinical inflammation. Asia Pac J Clin Nutr. 2008;17(Suppl 1):172–5.
4. Chiarelli F, Marcovecchio ML. Insulin resistance and obesity in childhood. Eur J Endocrinol. 2008;159(Suppl 1): S67–74.
5. Franks PW, Hanson RL, Knowler WC, et al. Childhood predictors of young-onset type 2 diabetes. Diabetes. 2007;56:2964–72.
6. Freedman DS, Dietz WH, Srinivasan SR, Berenson GS. The relation of overweight to cardiovascular risk factors among children and adolescents: the Bogalusa Heart Study. Pediatrics. 1999;103:1175–82.
7. Morrison JA, Friedman LA, Wang P, Glueck CJ. Metabolic syndrome in childhood predicts adult metabolic syndrome and type 2 diabetes mellitus 25–30 years later. J Pediatr. 2008;152:201–6.
8. Morrison JA, Glueck CJ, Horn PS, Schreiber GB, Wang P. Pre-teen insulin resistance predicts weight gain, impaired fasting glucose, and type 2 diabetes at age 18–19 years: a 10-years prospective study of black and white girls. Am J Clin Nutr. 2008;88:778–88.
9. Steinberger J, Daniels SR. Obesity, insulin resistance, diabetes, and cardiovascular risk in children: an American Heart Association scientific statement from the Atherosclerosis, Hypertension, and Obesity in the Young Committee (Council on Cardiovascular Disease in the Young) and the Diabetes Committee (Council on Nutrition, Physical Activity, and Metabolism). Circulation. 2003;107:1448–53.
10. Williams S. Overweight at age 21: the association with body mass index in childhood and adolescence and parents' body mass index. A cohort study of New Zealanders born in 1972–1973. Int J Obes Relat Metab Disord. 2001;25:158–63.
11. Klein DJ, Aronson Friedman L, Harlan WR, et al. Obesity and the development of insulin resistance and impaired fasting glucose in black and white adolescent girls: a longitudinal study. Diabetes Care. 2004;27:378–83.
12. Morrison JA, deGroot I, Edwards BK, et al. Plasma cholesterol and triglyceride levels in 6,775 school children, ages 6–17. Metabolism. 1977;26:1199–211.
13. Morrison JA, deGroot I, Edwards BK, et al. Lipids and lipoproteins in 927 schoolchildren, ages 6–17 years. Pediatrics. 1978;62:990–95.
14. Morrison JA, Namboodiri K, Green P, Martin J, Glueck CJ. Familial aggregation of lipids and lipoproteins and early identification of dyslipoproteinemia. The Collaborative Lipid Research Clinics Family Study. JAMA. 1983;250: 1860–68.
15. Morrison JA, Kelly K, Horvitz R, et al. Parent-offspring and sibling lipid and lipoprotein associations during and after sharing of household environments: the Princeton School District Family Study. Metabolism. 1982;31:158–66.
16. Morrison JA, Friedman LA, Gray-McGuire C. Metabolic syndrome in childhood predicts adult cardiovascular disease 25 years later: the Princeton Lipid Research Clinics Follow-up Study. Pediatrics. 2007;120:340–45.
17. Svec F, Nastasi K, Hilton C, Bao W, Srinivasan SR, Berenson GS. Black-white contrasts in insulin levels during pubertal development. The Bogalusa Heart Study. Diabetes. 1992;41:313–7.
18. Arslanian S, Suprasongsin C, Janosky JE. Insulin secretion and sensitivity in black versus white prepubertal healthy children. J Clin Endocrinol Metab. 1997;82:1923–7.

19. Caprio S, Bronson M, Sherwin RS, Rife F, Tamborlane WV. Co-existence of severe insulin resistance and hyperinsuli-naemia in pre-adolescent obese children. Diabetologia. 1996;39:1489–97.

20. Sinha R, Fisch G, Teague B, et al. Prevalence of impaired glucose tolerance among children and adolescents with marked obesity. N Engl J Med. 2002;346:802–10.

21. Arslanian SA, Saad R, Lewy V, Danadian K, Janosky J. Hyperinsulinemia in African-American children: decreased insulin clearance and increased insulin secretion and its relationship to insulin sensitivity. Diabetes. 2002;51:3014–9.

22. Moran A, Jacobs DR Jr, Steinberger J, et al. Insulin resistance during puberty: results from clamp studies in 357 children. Diabetes. 1999;48:2039–44.

23. Goran MI, Gower BA. Longitudinal study on pubertal insulin resistance. Diabetes. 2001;50:2444–50.

24. Gower BA, Granger WM, Franklin F, Shewchuk RM, Goran MI. Contribution of insulin secretion and clearance to glucose-induced insulin concentration in African-American and Caucasian children. J Clin Endocrinol Metab. 2002;87:2218–24.

25. Mosca CL, Marshall JA, Grunwald GK, Cornier MA, Baxter J. Insulin resistance as a modifier of the relationship between dietary fat intake and weight gain. Int J Obes Relat Metab Disord. 2004;28:803–12.

26. Kahn BB, Flier JS. Obesity and insulin resistance. J Clin Invest. 2000;106:473–81.

27. Mokdad AH, Ford ES, Bowman BA, et al.. Diabetes trends in the US: 1990–1998. Diabetes Care. 2000;23:1278–83.

28. Everhart JE, Pettitt DJ, Bennett PH, Knowler WC. Duration of obesity increases the incidence of NIDDM. Diabetes. 1992;41:235–40.

29. Saad MF, Knowler WC, Pettitt DJ, Nelson RG, Charles MA, Bennett PH. A two-step model for development of non-insulin-dependent diabetes. Am J Med. 1991;90:229–35.

30. Weiss R, Dziura J, Burgert TS, et al. Obesity and the metabolic syndrome in children and adolescents. N Engl J Med. 2004;350:2362–74.

31. Weiss R. Impaired glucose tolerance and risk factors for progression to type 2 diabetes in youth. Pediatr Diabetes. 2007;8(Suppl 9):70–5.

32. Weiss R, Taksali SE, Tamborlane WV, Burgert TS, Savoye M, Caprio S. Predictors of changes in glucose tolerance status in obese youth. Diabetes Care. 2005;28:902–9.

33. Li C, Ford ES, Zhao G, Mokdad AH. Prevalence of pre-diabetes and its association with clustering of cardiometabolic risk factors and hyperinsulinemia among US adolescents: National Health and Nutrition Examination Survey 2005–2006. Diabetes Care. 2009;32:342–7.

34. Nichols GA, Hillier TA, Brown JB. Progression from newly acquired impaired fasting glucose to type 2 diabetes. Diabetes Care. 2007;30:228–33.

35. Goldfine AB, Bouche C, Parker RA, et al. Insulin resistance is a poor predictor of type 2 diabetes in individuals with no family history of disease. Proc Natl Acad Sci USA. 2003;100:2724–9.

36. Executive summary of the third report of the National Cholesterol Education Program (NCEP) expert panel on detection, evaluation, and treatment of high blood cholesterol in adults (Adult Treatment Panel III). JAMA. 2001;285:2486–97.

37. Reaven GM. Banting Lecture 1988. Role of insulin resistance in human disease. Diabetes. 1988;37:1595–607.

38. Ford ES, Li C. Defining the metabolic syndrome in children and adolescents: will the real definition please stand up? J Pediatr. 2008;152:160–4.

39. Cook S, Weitzman M, Auinger P, Nguyen M, Dietz WH. Prevalence of a metabolic syndrome phenotype in adolescents: findings from the third National Health and Nutrition Examination Survey, 1988–1994. Arch Pediatr Adolesc Med. 2003;157:821–7.

40. Deshmukh-Taskar P, Nicklas TA, Morales M, Yang SJ, Zakeri I, Berenson GS. Tracking of overweight status from childhood to young adulthood: the Bogalusa Heart Study. Eur J Clin Nutr. 2006;60:48–57.

41. Bao W, Srinivasan SR, Berenson GS. Persistent elevation of plasma insulin levels is associated with increased cardiovascular risk in children and young adults. The Bogalusa Heart Study. Circulation. 1996;93:54–9.

42. Srinivasan SR, Myers L, Berenson GS. Changes in metabolic syndrome variables since childhood in prehypertensive and hypertensive subjects: the Bogalusa Heart Study. Hypertension. 2006;48:33–9.

43. Knochenhauer ES, Key TJ, Kahsar-Miller M, Waggoner W, Boots LR, Azziz R. Prevalence of the polycystic ovary syndrome in unselected black and white women of the southeastern United States: a prospective study. J Clin Endocrinol Metab. 1998;83:3078–82.

44. Glueck CJ, Morrison JA, Friedman LA, Goldenberg N, Stroop DM, Wang P. Obesity, free testosterone, and cardio-vascular risk factors in adolescents with polycystic ovary syndrome and regularly cycling adolescents. Metabolism. 2006;55:508–14.

45. Caranti DA, de Mello MT, Prado WL, et al. Short- and long-term beneficial effects of a multidisciplinary therapy for the control of metabolic syndrome in obese adolescents. Metabolism. 2007;56:1293–300.

46. Chang C, Liu W, Zhao X, Li S, Yu C. Effect of supervised exercise intervention on metabolic risk factors and physical fitness in Chinese obese children in early puberty. Obes Rev. 2008;9(Suppl 1):135–41.

47. Bell LM, Watts K, Siafarikas A, et al. Exercise alone reduces insulin resistance in obese children independently of changes in body composition. J Clin Endocrinol Metab. 2007;92:4230–5.

48. Davis JN, Kelly LA, Lane CJ, et al. Randomized control trial to improve adiposity and insulin resistance in overweight Latino adolescents. Obesity (Silver Spring). 2009;17(8):1542–8.

49. Harden KA, Cowan PA, Velasquez-Mieyer P, Patton SB. Effects of lifestyle intervention and metformin on weight management and markers of metabolic syndrome in obese adolescents. J Am Acad Nurse Pract. 2007;19:368–77.

50. Love-Osborne K, Sheeder J, Zeitler P. Addition of metformin to a lifestyle modification program in adolescents with insulin resistance. J Pediatr. 2008;152:817–22.

51. Srinivasan S, Ambler GR, Baur LA, et al. Randomized, controlled trial of metformin for obesity and insulin resistance in children and adolescents: improvement in body composition and fasting insulin. J Clin Endocrinol Metab. 2006;91:2074–80.

52. Kay JP, Alemzadeh R, Langley G, D'Angelo L, Smith P, Holshouser S. Beneficial effects of metformin in normoglycemic morbidly obese adolescents. Metabolism. 2001;50:1457–61.

53. Freemark M, Bursey D. The effects of metformin on body mass index and glucose tolerance in obese adolescents with fasting hyperinsulinemia and a family history of type 2 diabetes. Pediatrics. 2001;107:E55.

54. Glueck CJ, Wang P, Fontaine R, Tracy T, Sieve-Smith L. Metformin to restore normal menses in oligo-amenorrheic teenage girls with polycystic ovary syndrome (PCOS). J Adolesc Health. 2001;29:160–9.

55. Glueck CJ, Aregawi D, Winiarska M, et al. Metformin-diet ameliorates coronary heart disease risk factors and facilitates resumption of regular menses in adolescents with polycystic ovary syndrome. J Pediatr Endocrinol Metab. 2006;19:831–42.

56. Arslanian SA, Lewy V, Danadian K, Saad R. Metformin therapy in obese adolescents with polycystic ovary syndrome and impaired glucose tolerance: amelioration of exaggerated adrenal response to adrenocorticotropin with reduction of insulinemia/insulin resistance. J Clin Endocrinol Metab. 2002;87:1555–9.

57. Morrison JA, Cottingham EM, Barton BA. Metformin for weight loss in pediatric patients taking psychotropic drugs. Am J Psychiatry. 2002;159:655–7.

58. Baptista T, Rangel N, Fernandez V, et al. Metformin as an adjunctive treatment to control body weight and metabolic dysfunction during olanzapine administration: a multicentric, double-blind, placebo-controlled trial. Schizophr Res. 2007;93:99–108.

59. Wu RR, Zhao JP, Jin H, et al. Lifestyle intervention and metformin for treatment of antipsychotic-induced weight gain: a randomized controlled trial. J Am Med Assoc. 2008;299:185–93.

60. Klein DJ, Cottingham EM, Sorter M, Barton BA, Morrison JA. A randomized, double-blind, placebo-controlled trial of metformin treatment of weight gain associated with initiation of atypical antipsychotic therapy in children and adolescents. Am J Psychiatry. 2006;163:2072–9.

19 Childhood Obesity, Atherogenesis, and Adult Cardiovascular Disease

Henry C. McGill Jr., C. Alex McMahan, and Samuel S. Gidding

CONTENTS

Key Words: Atherosclerosis, coronary heart disease, risk factors, obesity, endothelial dysfunction, Pathobiological Determinants of Atherosclerosis in Youth (PDAY) Study

PEDIATRIC OBESITY AND ATHEROSCLEROSIS

Atherosclerosis and Cardiovascular Disease

Natural history of atherosclerosis – Atherosclerosis was described as a medical curiosity in human arteries by numerous observers over the last three centuries. Early in the twentieth century, atherosclerosis of the coronary arteries was linked to thrombosis, arterial occlusion, and myocardial infarction *(1)* and is now known to be the arterial lesion underlying most forms of adult cardiovascular disease [coronary heart disease (CHD), stroke, abdominal aortic aneurysm, peripheral arterial disease]. The frequency of cardiovascular disease due to atherosclerosis increased in the United States and in the other industrialized countries until it became the leading cause of disability and death by the 1950s *(2)*.

The natural history of atherosclerosis was established by examining arteries of autopsied individuals of all ages. Atherosclerosis begins in childhood, progresses during adolescence and young adulthood, and results in arterial obstruction and ischemic organ injury in middle age and later. Deposits of cholesterol and its esters, described as *fatty streaks*, appear in the intima of the aorta of the first decade of life (Fig. 1) *(3)* and in the coronary, cerebral, and peripheral arteries in the second and third decades. Lipid continues to accumulate in some fatty streaks, primarily during the third and fourth decades but earlier in some individuals, and the resulting core of extracellular lipid is covered by a cap of smooth muscle and connective tissue to form a *fibrous plaque*. In subsequent years, fibrous plaques undergo various complications. They may continue to increase in thickness and protrude into the arterial lumen, but

From: *Contemporary Endocrinology: Pediatric Obesity: Etiology, Pathogenesis, and Treatment*
Edited by: M. Freemark, DOI 10.1007/978-1-60327-874-4_19,
© Springer Science+Business Media, LLC 2010

NATURAL HISTORY OF ATHEROSCLEROSIS

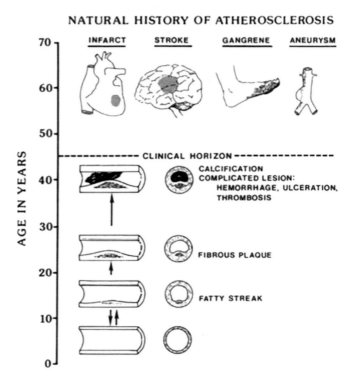

Fig. 1. Natural history of atherosclerosis beginning with the development of the fatty streak in childhood and adolescence. Some fatty streaks accumulate more lipid with age and begin to develop a fibromuscular cap, forming the lesion termed a fibrous plaque. In subsequent years, fibrous plaques enlarge and undergo calcification, hemorrhage, ulceration or rupture, and thrombosis. Thrombotic occlusion precipitates one of the clinical disease, depending on which artery is affected. Reproduced from McGill et al. *(3)*.

usually the artery is simultaneously remodeled and obstruction to blood flow is minimized. Fibrous plaques may become calcified, a change that renders them detectable by X-ray but does not cause obstruction to blood flow. Small vessels may grow into the plaque and rupture, causing hemorrhage, rapid swelling of the plaque, and obstruction to blood flow. The most frequent serious change is rupture of the fibromuscular cap of the plaque, resulting in exposure of blood to the lipid-rich core, thrombosis, and rapid occlusion of the artery. The appearance of the fatty streak early in life led to the suggestion that atherosclerosis was a pediatric problem and that long-range prevention should begin in childhood *(4)*.

The risk factors for cardiovascular disease – Even as the frequency of its clinical manifestations began to increase, atherosclerosis was considered an inevitable consequence of aging, but population comparisons showed large differences in both clinically manifest atherosclerotic disease *(5)* and severity of atherosclerosis *(6)*. Longitudinal epidemiologic studies begun at mid-twentieth century showed that certain conditions called "risk factors" (dyslipoproteinemia, hypertension, smoking, and diabetes mellitus) not only predicted clinical disease *(7)* but were also associated with the extent and severity of atherosclerosis *(8)*. The ability of the risk factors to predict clinical CHD and the association of the risk factors with advanced atherosclerosis were confirmed by the results of similar studies in many different populations. These results led to the concept that atherosclerosis was not inevitable with aging and that advanced atherosclerosis and its clinical sequelae might be prevented by preventing or modifying the risk factors.

Control of the risk factors in order to reduce the incidence of CHD, stroke, and peripheral arterial disease became major objectives of preventive and clinical medicine after clinical trials demonstrated that reducing serum low-density lipoprotein (LDL) cholesterol concentration with cholestyramine *(9)* and simvastatin *(10)* reduced the incidence of CHD. Control of hypertension and cessation of smoking showed similar beneficial effects *(11,12)*.

Obesity as a risk factor – The relation of obesity to atherosclerosis and CHD has a checkered and controversial history. Early reviews *(13,14)* concluded that, except through its contribution to hypertension and type-2 diabetes, obesity had no effect on cardiovascular disease. However, as the prevalence of obesity increased and as the results of long-term (>25 years) follow-up studies became available *(15–17)*, evidence of an independent association emerged (that is, an association that remained statistically significant in multivariable analyses that accounted for the effects of other risk factors) *(18)*. In a meta-analysis of 21 cohort studies involving 300,000 persons, overweight [$25 \leq$ body mass index (BMI) <30] compared to normal weight showed a risk ratio for CHD events (adjusted for age, sex, physical activity, and smoking) of 1.32 (95% CI, 1.24–1.40); and obesity (BMI$\geq$30) compared to normal weight, a risk ratio of 1.81 (95% CI, 1.56–2.10) *(19)*. Adjustment for blood pressure and serum cholesterol concentration reduced the risk ratios to 1.17 (95% CI, 1.11–1.23) for overweight and 1.49 (95% CI, 1.32–1.67) for obesity, indicating a substantial increased risk of CHD due to obesity independent of the other traditional risk factors. Obesity is now firmly established as a contributor to dyslipidemia, hypertension, and diabetes and also as an independent contributor to cardiovascular disease through other yet unrecognized mechanisms.

Cardiovascular risk factors in children and adolescents – In the 1970s, surveys of children and adolescents showed substantial variation among individuals in serum lipid concentrations, blood pressure, smoking status, and adiposity *(20–22)*. In the 1990s, the association of these conditions with the early stages of atherosclerosis and with their progression to advanced lesions was investigated by autopsy and cohort studies of young persons.

Risk Factors and Atherosclerosis in Youth: Autopsy Studies

The Pathobiological Determinants of Atherosclerosis in Youth (PDAY) Study collected arteries, tissue, and selected data from 2,876 individuals 15–34 years of age dying from external causes (accidents, homicide, and suicide) and autopsied in eight medical examiners' laboratories between 1987 and 1994. Central laboratories measured the extent and severity of atherosclerosis in the aorta and coronary arteries; total and high-density lipoprotein (HDL) cholesterol in serum; glycohemoglobin in red blood cells for hyperglycemia and diabetes; and thickness of small renal arteries as an indicator of hypertension (mean arterial blood pressure $\geq$110 mmHg). We calculated BMI from body measurements at autopsy and calculated non-HDL cholesterol by subtraction. Data analyses evaluated the association of each cardiovascular risk factor with the extent (percent intimal surface involvement) of each stage of atherosclerosis in the coronary arteries and the aorta. Fatty streaks were divided into flat fatty streaks, the earliest grossly detectable structural change, and raised fatty streaks, which represent lesions in transition to fibrous plaques. Complicated lesions were not encountered in PDAY cases. Coronary artery lesions were evaluated microscopically using the American Heart Association classification system. The results summarized below were presented in publications between 1990 and 2008 *(23–34)*.

The immutable risk factors: age, sex, and race – Both types of fatty streaks and raised lesions increased with age. Women and men had about the same extent of fatty streaks in the coronary arteries and abdominal aorta as men, but women had about half as extensive raised lesions in the coronary arteries. Women also had about half as frequent advanced microscopic atherosclerotic lesions as did men. Coronary artery lesions in women lagged about 10 years behind lesions in men and corresponded with the lag in rate of CHD among women as compared with men during middle age. There were minor differences in lesions between whites and blacks after adjustment for sex, age, and risk factors, but the relationships of the risk factors to atherosclerosis were similar in both groups.

The mutable risk factors – The extent of both types of fatty streaks and of raised lesions and the frequency of advanced microscopic lesions were associated positively with non-HDL cholesterol concentrations and negatively with HDL cholesterol concentrations. The extent of raised lesions and the frequency of advanced microscopic lesions in the coronary arteries were associated with hypertension. All measures of atherosclerosis were strongly associated with glycohemoglobin levels above 8%, a value approximately equal to a HbA_{1c} level of 7%. Smokers had higher microscopic grades of lesions in the coronary arteries, and more extensive fatty steaks and raised lesions in the abdominal aorta.

Obesity – Fatty streaks, raised lesions, and advanced microscopic lesions were strongly associated with obesity (BMI $\geq$ 30) in men (Fig. 2) *(31)*. The associations were independent of other risk factors in multivariable analyses. There was no association of BMI with extent or quality of atherosclerosis in women, but there was a trend for an association of extent of coronary artery fatty streaks with increasing BMI in women with a thick panniculus adiposus. The lack of association in women was probably due in part to the slower progression of atherosclerosis in women than in men.

Obesity was associated directly with non-HDL cholesterol concentration, inversely with HDL cholesterol concentration, directly with glycohemoglobin, directly with hypertension, and inversely with smoking prevalence. Adjustment for the effects of these risk factors in multivariable analyses accounted for only about 15% of the effect of obesity on atherosclerosis.

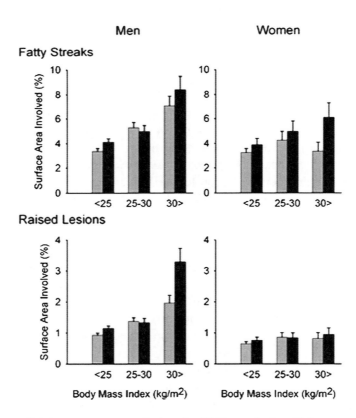

Fig. 2. Mean (+SE) extent of right coronary artery lesions by BMI, panniculus thickness, and sex, adjusted for race and 5-year age group. *Light gray bars* denote panniculus thickness $\leq$ median for sex and BMI. *Black bars* denote panniculus thickness > median for sex and BMI. Reproduced from McGill et al. *(31)*.

Combined risk factor effects – Individuals often had more than one risk factor, and their effects were cumulative. The PDAY study developed a coronary artery risk score which provided a weighted summary of the effects of the risk factors on atherosclerosis (Table 1) *(33)*. Increasing risk score was associated with increasing probability of advanced coronary artery lesions.

Although the PDAY risk score was developed to predict advanced atherosclerotic lesions, it was associated with all stages of lesions including the transition from normal tissue to the earliest detectable anatomic lesion *(34)*.

Table 1
Pathobiological Determinants of Atherosclerosis in Youth (PDAY) Study Risk
Score for Predicting Advanced Atherosclerotic Lesions in the Coronary
Arteries

Risk factor	Category	Risk score Coronary arteries
Age, year	15–19[a]	0
	20–24	5
	25–29	10
	30–34	15
Sex	Male[a]	0
	Female	−1
Non-HDL cholesterol, mg/dl	<130[a]	0
	130–159	2
	160–189	4
	190–219	6
	≥220	8
HDL cholesterol, mg/dl	<40	1
	40–59[a]	0
	≥60	−1
Smoking	Nonsmoker[a]	0
	Smoker	1
Blood pressure	Normotensive[a]	0
	Hypertensive	4
Obesity (BMI, kg/m²) Men	≤30[a]	0
	>30	6
Women	≤30	0
	>30	0
Hyperglycemia (glycohemoglobin, %)	<8[a]	0
	≥8	5

To convert mg/dl to mmol/l, multiply values for non-HDL and HDL cholesterol by 0.0259

[a]Reference category

Reproduced from McMahan et al. *(33)*. Copyright © 2005, American Medical Association. All rights reserved.

The PDAY risk score also predicted the extent of advanced coronary artery lesions in persons 36–55 years of age from another sample of autopsied persons *(35)*. This result was consistent with the concept that atherosclerosis progresses seamlessly from youth through middle age as indicated in Fig. 1 and that the major established CHD risk factors influence the rate of progression.

Risk Factors and Atherosclerosis in Youth: Cohort Studies

Three cohort studies [Muscatine Study *(36)*, Cardiovascular Risk in Young Finns Study *(37)*, Bogalusa Heart Study *(38)*] measured cardiovascular risk factors in childhood or adolescence and followed the subjects into adulthood. All three studies found that the risk factors measured in childhood or adolescence (between 4 and 18 years of age) predicted either carotid artery intima-media thickness (IMT) or coronary artery calcification, both of which are widely accepted as noninvasive markers of atherosclerosis, when the subjects reached 30–40 years of age. Serial measurements of risk factors over a substantial number of years did not predict adult carotid IMT appreciably better than the measurements of risk factors in childhood *(37,38)*. In two cohort studies [Coronary Artery Risk Development in Young Adults (CARDIA) *(39)* and Cardiovascular Risk in Young Finns Study *(40)*], the PDAY risk score predicted atherosclerosis measured 15 years later; and the change in the PDAY risk score over the 15-year interval (both positively and negatively) also predicted atherosclerosis.

Childhood obesity was associated with adult carotid IMT in adulthood independently of adult BMI and the other risk factors *(41)*. Obesity was associated with carotid IMT in 10–24 year-old youth and the relationship was only partially explained by the traditional risk factors *(42)*. Childhood or adolescent BMI has consistently been a strong and independent predictor of markers of atherosclerosis in adults.

A study of 277,000 Danish children showed that BMI measured between 10 and 13 years of age was positively associated with CHD risk in adults >25 years of age *(43)*. Childhood obesity between 2 and 14 years of age predicted a twofold greater risk of CHD mortality after 57 years *(44)*.

Taken together, the results of both autopsy and cohort studies leave little doubt that childhood and adolescent obesity are major contributors to adult CHD through both recognized and unidentified mechanisms and that the epidemic of obesity will lead to higher rates of CHD among adults in the future *(45)*.

Endothelial Dysfunction and Atherosclerosis

In the early 1980s, the role of endothelial cells in relaxation of arterial smooth muscle in response to increased blood flow was discovered *(46)* and traced to release of nitric oxide *(47)*. Intense interest in this endothelial function has led to an enormous number of related publications during the 3 decades since its discovery. As currently measured, the brachial artery is briefly occluded by a pneumatic cuff and released, and dilation of the distal artery and increased blood flow are assessed by ultrasound *(48)*. The percent change in flow after ischemic stress is called *flow-mediated dilation* and diminution of the response is termed *endothelial dysfunction*. A similar phenomenon occurs in the coronary arteries after administration of acetylcholine during coronary angiography *(48)*.

Acetylcholine-induced relaxation was impaired in aortic rings from cholesterol-fed hypercholesterolemic rabbits *(49)* and this effect was confirmed in other animal models. Endothelial dysfunction in adults was associated with the established risk factors for CHD *(50)* and with coronary artery atherosclerosis *(51)*. These observations led to the suggestion that endothelial dysfunction may represent an early stage of atherosclerosis *(52)*. This view was amplified to suggest that endothelial dysfunction summarizes the effects of all the causes of atherosclerosis, known and unknown, and therefore is a comprehensive marker for the progression of atherosclerosis and for the risk of clinically manifest CHD *(53)*. The possibility that an easily performed noninvasive procedure might be a marker for the early stages of atherosclerosis led to many studies of endothelial dysfunction in children and adolescents.

Endothelial dysfunction was associated with hypercholesterolemia and with active and passive smoking in children and adolescents (54–56). Endothelial function was enhanced and serum cholesterol concentrations were lower in 11-year-old children who had consumed a low-saturated-fat diet from infancy (57). Statin therapy restored normal endothelial function in 9–18-year-old children with familial hypercholesterolemia (58). Leisure-time physical activity in adolescent boys (59) and increased physical activity and fitness were associated with improved endothelial function (60–62). However, exercise restored endothelial function with minimal, if any, change in body mass index (60,61,63).

Minimum forearm vascular resistance, which is correlated with endothelial dysfunction, was increased in obese adolescents and was associated with insulin resistance (64). Both variables improved after a 20-week weight loss program. Subsequently, a number of reports described studies of endothelial dysfunction in obese children. A 6-month exercise regimen involving 11–16-year-old obese children reduced body fat mass, improved carotid IMT and endothelial function, and led to favorable changes in blood pressure, blood lipids, and insulin (63). In a survey of children averaging about 14 years of age, obesity was associated with endothelial dysfunction, hypertension, carotid IMT, and markers of endothelial inflammation (65).

A number of studies have examined the association of endothelial dysfunction with carotid artery IMT in children with type-1 diabetes (66), in young adults (67), and in other obese children among whom the association was weaker (63,65,68). These associations constitute the only evidence relating endothelial dysfunction directly to the pre-clinical stages of atherosclerosis in youth.

The major problem in linking endothelial dysfunction with atherosclerosis is the wide variety of conditions with which it is associated, including infections, postmenopause in women, trauma, periodontitis, low birth weight, and many others [reviewed by Félétou (50)]. This lack of specificity is reflected in the weaker relation of endothelial dysfunction to CHD risk factors in generally healthy children (68–71). Thus, there is clearly an association of impaired vascular function with obesity in youth, but this effect may be mediated by both the established CHD risk factors and the other conditions not associated with CHD. Although endothelial dysfunction is associated with carotid IMT, which in turn is associated with atherosclerosis of the coronary arteries, no data relate endothelial dysfunction directly to coronary atherosclerosis in children, adolescents, or young adults. More specifically, no data indicate whether endothelial dysfunction is associated with or precedes the earliest anatomic lesion of atherosclerosis, the fatty streak, or whether it is associated with progression to the fibrous plaque in adolescence and early adulthood. Finally, no data show that endothelial dysfunction measured in childhood predicts arterial lesions years later, as do the traditional risk factors.

In summary, endothelial dysfunction is a complex physiological response to a wide variety of conditions which include obesity and the other established CHD risk factors. It is associated with coronary atherosclerosis in adults, but its relationship to the initial lesions of atherosclerosis in childhood and adolescence is not known. Its usefulness in decision making for individuals has not been established and it should not be used as a surrogate marker of atherosclerosis in young persons (72).

PREVENTION OF ADULT CORONARY HEART DISEASE

Prevention programs for adult CHD – After the demonstration that reducing LDL cholesterol, blood pressure, and smoking in adults reduced the risk of CHD, programs directed almost exclusively at adults were initiated by voluntary and government health agencies. From the peak mortality rates of CHD mortality in 1968, the US CHD mortality rate fell by about 50% by 1990. About half of the decline was attributed to risk factor control and about half to improved treatment of CHD. However, the rate of decline has slowed and some investigators predict that the epidemic of obesity will cause it to rise.

Prevention of adult CHD by risk factor prevention in childhood – As evidence accumulated showing that the adult risk factors were present in children and adolescents and that they tracked into adulthood, suggestions were made that CHD prevention should begin in childhood *(73–76)*. The validity of these recommendations was strengthened when autopsy studies (PDAY and Bogalusa Heart Study) showed the association of the risk factors with all stages of atherosclerosis in youth, a finding indicating that they probably drive progression; when cohort studies showed that the risk factors measured in childhood or adolescence predicted the prevalence of markers of advanced atherosclerosis in adults; and when changes in risk factors also predicted adult atherosclerosis.

Preventive measures adopted in early middle age, as recommended by programs targeting adults, are too late because advanced plaques, vulnerable to rupture and thrombotic occlusion, have already formed by this age and the opportunity for prevention is limited. Not allowing the risk factors to develop would prevent or at least retard progression of the initial lesion, and this expectation supports the concept of *primordial* prevention, that is, not allowing the risk factors to develop in the first place *(77)*.

The 50% myth – A popular objection to the concept of preventing CHD by preventing or modifying risk factors is the belief that the risk factors explain only 50% of CHD. Adults who do not have one or more of the risk factors have a very low probability of developing CHD. Estimates of lifetime CHD risk (to age 95) showed that individuals with no risk factors at age 50 in the Framingham population had a lifetime risk of CHD of 5.2% for men and 8.2% for women compared to 51.7% for men and 39.2% for women in the entire cohort *(78)*. Individuals who attained age 50 without risk factors probably never had risk factors (except possibly smoking). In several longitudinal studies, men without any of the major risk factors and followed for 16–22 years had 77–92% lower CHD mortality, and women, 79% lower CHD mortality *(79)*. On the basis of these results, it should be possible to reduce CHD incidence by 90% (instead of 50%) if we could prevent the appearance of the risk factors in youth or control them if they develop *(80)*.

All risk factors are important – The points assigned to each risk factor in the PDAY risk score indicate the relative effect of each risk factor. No established risk factor can be safely ignored, and more aggressive intervention is indicated for persons with multiple risk factors. The evaluation of "importance" depends on whether it pertains to a population, where importance is determined by a combination of prevalence and effect; or whether it pertains to an individual, where an important risk factor is the one that the person has. Any risk factor present in an individual is important not only because all contribute to atherosclerosis and CHD, but because most of them – particularly obesity – have other adverse effects on health as well. Obesity in youth is an important target for the prevention of CHD in the industrialized societies because of its high prevalence and its effects on the progression of atherosclerosis in addition to its other demonstrated adverse health effects.

CONCLUSIONS

All of the established major risk factors for clinically manifest adult CHD accelerate the progression of atherosclerosis from the initial fatty streaks in childhood and adolescence to the advanced fibrous and complicated plaques of middle age and later. Obesity is a major contributor to accelerated progression and subsequent increased risk of CHD both by predisposing to other risk factors (dyslipidemia, hypertension, and diabetes) and independently by other yet unidentified mechanisms. High risk of future adult CHD can be easily evaluated in children and adolescents by assessment of family history, serum lipoprotein profile, blood pressure, blood glucose, smoking status, and adiposity. Effective prevention of adult CHD must begin by preventing the mutable risk factors or controlling them if they do develop.

Editor's Questions and Authors' Response

- **Why does obesity predict a higher risk of atherosclerosis in men than in women?**

- Many investigators have been intrigued (baffled may be a better word) by the sex differences in atherosclerosis and its clinical manifestations. We can suggest few possible reasons for the differences and fewer possible reasons for the difference in effect of obesity on atherosclerosis between young men and young women. Proving which, if any, of the reasons is true is more difficult. The differential obesity effect is part of the overall problem of the sex differential in atherosclerosis and coronary heart disease.

- In 1979 an extensive review of the topic concluded "It is not possible to extract a single unifying hypothesis out of the numerous observations on the sex difference in coronary heart disease..." and listed nine possible mechanisms, none of which could be definitively supported (McGill and Stern, 1979). Estrogen prevented atherosclerosis in cholesterol-fed chickens (Stamler et al., 1974), but a few years later estrogens given to men led to increased mortality (Coronary Drug Project Research Group, 1973). The heart and arteries contained estrogen and androgen receptors (McGill and Sheridan, 1981) but their presence did not explain the sex differential in atherosclerosis. Results of the Women's Health Initiative overturned the clinical dogma derived from observational studies that postmenopausal estrogen and progesterone prevented coronary heart disease (Nelson et al., 2002). Investigation of this issue continues, but the mechanism of the sex difference in atherosclerosis and coronary heart disease between premenopausal women and men of the same age remains an enigma.

- Atherosclerosis progresses much more rapidly in young men than in young women, independently of the established risk factors. In the PDAY data, the extent of coronary artery fatty streaks is about equal in men and women between 15 and 34 years of age, but the lesions progress more rapidly to fibrous plaques in men than in women so that, by age 30–34 years, men have about twice as extensive fibrous plaques, even when adjusted for the traditional risk factors (McGill et al., 2002). Thus, women lag behind men in the progression of fatty streaks to fibrous plaques by about 10 years, corresponding to the lag in onset of coronary heart disease later in life. Curiously, young women (15–34 years) have more extensive fatty streaks in their abdominal aortas than do men, but they develop an equal extent of fibrous plaques.

- With no explanation for the sex difference in atherosclerosis and with no explanation for the independent effect of obesity on atherosclerosis, we are unable to suggest a credible physiological mechanism for the selective effect of obesity on the early stages of atherosclerosis in young men. Probably young women simply do not have sufficiently advanced atherosclerosis to show an effect of obesity within the 15–34 year age range.

Coronary Drug Project Research Group. The Coronary Drug Project. Findings leading to discontinuation of the 25-mg/day estrogen group. J Am Med Assoc. 1973;226:652–7.

McGill HC, Jr, Stern MP. Sex and atherosclerosis. Atheroscler Rev. 1979;4:157–242.

McGill HC, Jr, Sheridan PJ. Nuclear uptake of sex steroid hormones in the cardiovascular system of the baboon. Circ Res. 1981;48:238–44.

McGill HC, Jr, McMahan CA, Herderick EE, Malcom GT, Tracy RE, Strong JP. Origin of atherosclerosis in childhood and adolescence. Am J Clin Nutr. 2000;72:1307S–15S.

McGill HC, Jr, McMahan CA, Herderick EE, Zieske AW, Malcom GT, Tracy RE, Strong JP; for the Pathobiological Determinants of Atherosclerosis in Youth (PDAY) Research Group. Obesity accelerates the progression of coronary atherosclerosis in young men. Circulation. 2002;105:2712–8.

Nelson HD, Humphrey LL, Nygren P, Teutsch SM, Allan JD. Postmenopausal hormone replacement therapy: scientific review. J Am Med Assoc. 2002;288:872–81.

Stamler J, Pick R, Katz LN. Inhibition of cholesterol-induced coronary atherogenesis in the egg-producing hen. Circulation. 1954;10:251–4.

- **What do we know about the reversibility of fatty streaks or raised lesions in young people? At what point does an atherosclerotic lesion become irreversible?**

- The histologic characteristics of atherosclerotic lesions at various stages suggest that simple fatty streaks, particularly those seen in persons <20 years, should be reversible. Lipid is predominantly in macrophages and smooth muscle cells, there are scattered lipid droplets in the interstitial spaces, and there is little or no fibrosis. In the third decade, fatty streaks accumulate more extracellular lipid deposits and proliferation of fibroblasts and smooth muscle cells increases. These seem partially reversible, and if progression were halted they would leave innocuous stigmata. In subsequent years, fibrous plaques accumulate larger deposits of extracellular lipid and thicker fibromuscular caps and appear to have much less potential for regression. Calcification, which begins in the fourth decade, is probably not reversible (Stary et al., 1995).

- Experiments in cholesterol-fed rabbits, chickens, and dogs yielded conflicting results. In 1970, coronary artery lesions produced by feeding cholesterol to rhesus monkeys were reduced in thickness by 80% after 40 months of cholesterol-free diets, but lesions did not disappear completely (Armstrong et al., 1970). These results were widely hailed at the time as encouraging for the programs aimed at controlling serum cholesterol levels to prevent coronary heart disease. Other regression experiments in monkeys yielded similar results (Clarkson et al., 1984; Strong et al., 1994).

- In the first study of regression of human coronary atherosclerotic lesions, colestipol-niacin treatment reduced LDL cholesterol by 43%, and coronary angiograms showed reductions in atherosclerotic lesions in 16% of treated subjects (Blankenhorn et al., 1987). Intensive statin treatment reduced LDL cholesterol to 60 mg/dL (half the baseline value), and intravascular ultrasound showed a 10% reduction in coronary artery lesion volume (Nissen et al., 2006). There are no data regarding regression of fatty streaks or fibrous plaques in young humans. With development of better non-invasive imaging methods, it may be possible in the future to assess the effects of risk factor modification in young persons.

- In conclusion, fatty streaks and early fibrous plaques in young persons <30 years are probably reversible to a limited degree if the established mutable risk factors are controlled. Complete restoration of normal arterial intimal structure does not seem feasible, but is not essential. Stabilizing lesions in young persons and preventing progression should be effective in reducing risk of adult atherosclerotic disease. The most effective long-range prevention of atherosclerotic disease is to prevent the occurrence of risk factors in childhood.

Armstrong ML, Warner ED, Connor WE. Regression of coronary atheromatosis in rhesus monkeys. Circ Res. 1970;27:59–67.

Blankenhorn DH, Nessim SA, Johnson RL, Sanmarco ME, Azen SP, Cashin-Hemphill L. Beneficial effects of combined colestipol-niacin therapy on coronary atherosclerosis and coronary venous bypass grafts. J Am Med Assoc. 1987;257:3233–40.

Clarkson TB, Bond MG, Bullock BC, McLaughlin KJ, Sawyer JK. A study of atherosclerosis regression in *Macaca mulatta*. V. Changes in abdominal aorta and carotid and coronary arteries from animals with atherosclerosis induced for 38 months and then regressed for 24 or 48 months at plasma cholesterol concentrations of 300 or 200 mg/dl. Exp Mol Pathol. 1984;41:96–118.

Nissen SE, Nicholls SJ, Sipahi I, Libby P, Raichlen JS, Ballantyne CM, Davignon J, Erbel R, Fruchart JC, Tardif JC, Schoenhagen P, Crowe T, Cain V, Wolski K, Goormastic M, Tuzcu EM. Effect of very high-intensity statin therapy on regression of coronary atherosclerosis: the ASTEROID trial. J Am Med Assoc. 2006;295:1556–65.

Stary HC, Chandler AB, Dinsmore RE, Fuster V, Glagov S, Insull W, Jr, Rosenfeld ME, Schwartz CJ, Wagner WD, Wissler RW. A definition of advanced types of atherosclerotic lesions and a histological classification of atherosclerosis: a report from the Committee on Vascular Lesions of the Council on Arteriosclerosis, American Heart Association. Arterioscler Thromb Vasc Biol. 1995;15:1512–1531.

Strong JP, Bhattacharyya AK, Eggen DA, Stary HC, Malcom GT, Newman WP, 3rd, Restrepo C. Long-term induction and regression of diet-induced atherosclerotic lesions in rhesus monkeys. II. Morphometric evaluation of lesions by light microscopy in coronary and carotid arteries. Arterioscler Thromb. 1994;14:2007–16.

REFERENCES

1. Herrick JB. Clinical features of sudden obstruction of the coronary arteries. J Am Med Assoc. 1912;59:2015–20.

2. Moriyama I, Krueger DE, Stamler J. Cardiovascular diseases in the United States. Cambridge, MA: Harvard University Press; 1971.

3. McGill HC Jr, Geer JC, Strong JP. Natural history of human atherosclerotic lesions. In: Sandler M, Bourne GH, editors. Atherosclerosis and its origin. New York, NY: Academic Press; 1963. pp. 39–65.

4. Holman RL. Atherosclerosis – a pediatric nutrition problem? Am J Clin Nutr. 1961;9:565–9.

5. Keys A. Coronary heart disease – the global picture. Atherosclerosis. 1975;22:149–92.

6. Tejada C, Strong JP, Montenegro MR, Restrepo C, Solberg LA. Distribution of coronary and aortic atherosclerosis by geographic location, race, and sex. Lab Invest. 1968;18:509–26.

7. Dawber TR, Moore FE, Mann GV. Coronary heart disease in the Framingham study. Am J Pub Health. 1957;47(April Suppl):4–23.

8. Solberg LA, Strong JP. Risk factors and atherosclerotic lesions: a review of autopsy studies. Arteriosclerosis. 1983;3:187–98.

9. Lipid Research Clinics Program. The Lipid Research Clinics coronary primary prevention trial results. I. Reduction in incidence of coronary heart disease. J Am Med Assoc. 1984;251:351–64.

10. Scandinavian Simvastatin Survival Study Group. Randomised trial of cholesterol lowering in 4,444 patients with coronary heart disease: the Scandinavian Simvastatin Survival Study (4S). Lancet. 1994;344:1383–9.

11. Hypertension Detection and Follow-up Program Cooperative Group. Persistence of reduction in blood pressure and mortality of participants in the hypertension detection and follow-up program. J Am Med Assoc. 1988;259:2113–22.

12. Samet JM. The 1990 report of the surgeon general: the health benefits of smoking cessation. Am Rev Respir Dis. 1990;142:993–4.

13. Heald FP. The natural history of obesity. Adv Psychosom Med. 1972;7:102–15.

14. Mann GV. The influence of obesity on health (two parts). N Engl J Med. 1974;291:178–85.

15. Rabkin SW, Mathewson FAL, Hsu PH. Relation of body weight to development of ischemic heart disease in a cohort of young North American men after a 26 year observation period: the Manitoba Study. Am J Cardiol. 1977;39:452–8.

16. Hubert HB, Feinleib M, McNamara PM, Castelli WP. Obesity as an independent risk factor for cardiovascular disease: a 26-year follow-up of participants in the Framingham Heart Study. Circulation. 1983;67:968–77.

17. Lee IM, Manson JE, Hennekens CH, Paffenbarger RSJ. Body weight and mortality: a 27-year follow-up of middle-aged men. J Am Med Assoc. 1993;270:2823–8.

18. Alexander JK. Obesity and coronary heart disease. Am J Med Sci. 2001;321:215–24.

19. Bogers RP, Bemelmans WJ, Hoogenveen RT, et al. Association of overweight with increased risk of coronary heart disease partly independent of blood pressure and cholesterol levels: a meta-analysis of 21 cohort studies including more than 300,000 persons. Arch Intern Med. 2007;167:1720–8.

20. Berenson GS, Foster TA, Frank GC, et al. Cardiovascular disease risk factor variables at the preschool age. The Bogalusa Heart Study. Circulation. 1978;57:603–12.

21. Lauer RM, Connor WE, Leaverton PE, Reiter MA, Clarke WR. Coronary heart disease risk factors in school children: the Muscatine Study. J Pediatr. 1975;86:697–706.

22. Akerblom HK, Viikari J, Uhari M, et al. Atherosclerosis precursors in Finnish children and adolescents. I. General description of the cross-sectional study of 1980, and an account of the children's and families' state of health. Acta Paediatr Scand Suppl. 1985;318:49–63.

23. PDAY Research Group. Relationship of atherosclerosis in young men to serum lipoprotein cholesterol concentrations and smoking: a preliminary report from the Pathobiological Determinants of Atherosclerosis in Youth (PDAY) Research Group. J Am Med Assoc. 1990;264:3018–24.

24. McGill HC Jr, McMahan CA, Malcom GT, Oalmann MC, Strong JP, for the PDAY Research Group. Effects of serum lipoproteins and smoking on atherosclerosis in young men and women. Arterioscler Thromb Vasc Biol. 1997;17: 95–106.

25. McGill HC Jr, McMahan CA, Tracy RE, et al. Relation of a postmortem renal index of hypertension to atherosclerosis and coronary artery size in young men and women. Arterioscler Thromb Vasc Biol. 1998;18:1108–18.

26. Strong JP, Malcom GT, McMahan CA, et al. Prevalence and extent of atherosclerosis in adolescents and young adults: implications for prevention from the Pathobiological Determinants of Atherosclerosis in Youth Study. J Am Med Assoc. 1999;281:727–35.

27. McGill HC Jr., McMahan CA, Herderick EE, et al. Effects of coronary heart disease risk factors on atherosclerosis of selected regions of the aorta and right coronary artery. Arterioscler Thromb Vasc Biol. 2000;20:836–45.

28. McGill HC Jr, McMahan CA, Zieske AW, et al. Association of coronary heart disease risk factors with microscopic qualities of coronary atherosclerosis in youth. Circulation. 2000;102:374–9.

29. McGill HC Jr, McMahan CA, Zieske AW, et al. Associations of coronary heart disease risk factors with the intermediate lesion of atherosclerosis in youth. Arterioscler Thromb Vasc Biol. 2000;20:1998–2004.

30. McGill HC Jr, McMahan CA, Zieske AW, et al. Effects of nonlipid risk factors on atherosclerosis in youth with a favorable lipoprotein profile. Circulation. 2001;103:1546–50.

31. McGill HC Jr, McMahan CA, Herderick EE, et al. Obesity accelerates the progression of coronary atherosclerosis in young men. Circulation. 2002;105:2712–8.

32. Zieske AW, McMahan CA, McGill HC Jr, et al. Smoking is associated with advanced coronary atherosclerosis in youth. Atherosclerosis. 2005;180:87–92.

33. McMahan CA, Gidding SS, Fayad ZA, et al. Risk scores predict atherosclerotic lesions in young people. Arch Intern Med. 2005;165:883–90.

34. McMahan CA, Gidding SS, Malcom GT, et al. Pathobiological Determinants of Atherosclerosis in Youth risk scores are associated with early and advanced atherosclerosis. Pediatrics. 2006;118:1447–55.

35. McMahan CA, McGill HC, Gidding SS, et al. PDAY risk score predicts advanced coronary artery atherosclerosis in middle-aged persons as well as youth. Atherosclerosis. 2007;190:370–7.

36. Davis PH, Dawson JD, Riley WA, Lauer RM. Carotid intimal-medial thickness is related to cardiovascular risk factors measured from childhood through middle age: the Muscatine Study. Circulation. 2001;104:2815–9.

37. Raitakari O, Juonala M, Kahonen M, et al. Cardiovascular risk factors in childhood and carotid artery intima-media thickness in adulthood. The Cardiovascular Risk in Young Finns Study. J Am Med Assoc. 2003;290:2277–83.

38. Li S, Chen W, Srinivasan SR, et al. Childhood cardiovascular risk factors and carotid vascular changes in adulthood: the Bogalusa Heart Study. J Am Med Assoc. 2003;290:2271–6.

39. Gidding SS, McMahan CA, McGill HC, et al. Prediction of coronary artery calcium in young adults using the Pathobiological Determinants of Atherosclerosis in Youth (PDAY) risk score. Arch Intern Med. 2006;166: 2341–7.

40. McMahan CA, Gidding SS, Vikari JSA, et al. Association of Pathobiological Determinants of Atherosclerosis in Youth risk score and 15-year change in risk score with carotid artery intima-media thickness in young adults (from the Cardiovascular Risk in Young Finns Study). Am J Cardiol. 2007;100:1124–9.

41. Freedman DS, Patel DA, Srinivasan SR, et al. The contribution of childhood obesity to adult carotid intima-media thickness: the Bogalusa Heart Study. Int J Obes. 2008;32:749–56.

42. Urbina EM, Kimball TR, McCoy CE, Khoury PR, Daniels SR, Dolan LM. Youth with obesity and obesity-related type 2 diabetes mellitus demonstrate abnormalities in carotid structure and function. Circulation. 2009;119:2913–9.

43. Baker JL, Olsen LW, Sorensen TI. Childhood body-mass index and the risk of coronary heart disease in adulthood. N Engl J Med. 2007;357:2329–37.

44. Gunnell DJ, Frankel SJ, Nanchahal K, Peters TJ, Smith GD. Childhood obesity and adult cardiovascular mortality: a 57-year follow-up study based on the Boyd Orr cohort. Am J Clin Nutr. 1998;67:1111–8.

45. Bibbins-Domingo K, Coxson P, Pletcher MJ, Lightwood J, Goldman L. Adolescent overweight and future adult coronary heart disease. N Engl J Med. 2007;357:2371–9.

46. Furchgott RF, Zawadzki JV. The obligatory role of endothelial cells in the relaxation of arterial smooth muscle by acetylcholine. Nature. 1980;288:373–5.

47. Palmer RMJ, Ferrige AG, Moncada S. Nitric oxide release accounts for the biological activity of endothelium-derived relaxing factor. Nature. 1987;327:524–6.

48. Deanfield J, Donald A, Ferri C, et al. Endothelial function and dysfunction. Part I: methodological issues for assessment in the different vascular beds: a statement by the Working Group on Endothelin and Endothelial Factors of the European Society of Hypertension. J Hypertens. 2005;23:7–17.

49. Jayakody L, Senaratne M, Thomson A, Kappagoda T. Endothelium-dependent relaxation in experimental atherosclerosis in the rabbit. Circ Res. 1987;60:251–64.

50. Félétou M, Vanhoutte PM. Endothelial dysfunction: a multifaceted disorder (The Wiggers Award Lecture). Am J Physiol Heart Circ Physiol. 2006;291:H985–1002.

51. Cox DA, Vita JA, Treasure CB, et al. Atherosclerosis impairs flow-mediated dilation of coronary arteries in humans. Circulation. 1989;80:458–65.

52. Healy B. Endothelial cell dysfunction: an emerging endocrinopathy linked to coronary disease. J Am Coll Cardiol. 1990;16:357–8.

53. Bonetti PO, Lerman LO, Lerman A. Endothelial dysfunction: a marker of atherosclerotic risk. Arterioscler Thromb Vasc Biol. 2003;23:168–75.

54. Celermajer DS, Sorenden KE, Gooch VM, et al. Non-invasive detection of endothelial dysfunction in children and adults at risk of atherosclerosis. Lancet. 1992;340:1111–5.

55. Celermajer DS, Sorensen KE, Georgakopoulos D, et al. Cigarette smoking is associated with dose-related and potentially reversible impairment of endothelium-dependent dilation in healthy young adults. Circulation. 1993;88:2149–55.

56. Kallio K, Jokinen E, Raitakari OT, et al. Tobacco smoke exposure is associated with attenuated endothelial function in 11-year-old healthy children. Circulation. 2007;115:3205–12.

57. Raitakari OT, Ronnemaa T, Jarvisalo MJ, et al. Endothelial function in healthy 11-year-old children after dietary intervention with onset in infancy: the Special Turku Coronary Risk Factor Intervention Project for children (STRIP). Circulation. 2005;112:3786–94.

58. de Jongh S, Lilien MR, op't Roodt J, et al. Early statin therapy restores endothelial function in children with familial hypercholesterolemia. J Am Coll Cardiol. 2002;40:2117–21.

59. Pahkala K, Heinonen OJ, Lagstrom H, et al. Vascular endothelial function and leisure-time physical activity in adolescents. Circulation. 2008;118:2353–9.

60. Woo KS, Chook P, Yu CW, et al. Effects of diet and exercise on obesity-related vascular dysfunction in children. Circulation. 2004;109:1981–6.

61. Watts K, Beye P, Siafarikas A, et al. Effects of exercise training on vascular function in obese children. J Pediatr. 2004;144:620–5.

62. Hopkins ND, Stratton G, Tinken TM, et al. Relationships between measures of fitness, physical activity, body composition and vascular function in children. Atherosclerosis. 2008;204–49.

63. Meyer AA, Kundt G, Lenschow U, Schuff-Werner P, Kienast W. Improvement of early vascular changes and cardiovascular risk factors in obese children after a 6-month exercise program. J Am Coll Cardiol. 2006;48:1865–70.

64. Rocchini AP, Moorehead C, Katch V, Key J, Finta KM. Forearm resistance vessel abnormalities and insulin resistance in obese adolescents. Hypertension. 1992;19:615–20.

65. Glowinska-Olszewska B, Tolwinska J, Urban M. Relationship between endothelial dysfunction, carotid artery intima media thickness and circulating markers of vascular inflammation in obese hypertensive children and adolescents. J Pediatr Endocrinol Metab. 2007;20:1125–36.

66. Jarvisalo MJ, Raitakari M, Toikka JO, et al. Endothelial dysfunction and increased arterial intima-media thickness in children with type 1 diabetes. Circulation. 2004;109:1750–5.

67. Juonala M, Viikari JS, Laitinen T, et al. Interrelations between brachial endothelial function and carotid intima-media thickness in young adults: the cardiovascular risk in young Finns study. Circulation. 2004;110:2918–23.

68. Woo KS, Chook P, Yu CW, et al. Overweight in children is associated with arterial endothelial dysfunction and intima-media thickening. Int J Obes Relat Metab Disord. 2004;28:852–7.

69. Leeson CP, Whincup PH, Cook DG, et al. Flow-mediated dilation in 9- to 11-year-old children: the influence of intrauterine and childhood factors. Circulation. 1997;96:2233–8.

70. Aggoun Y, Farpour-Lambert NJ, Marchand LM, Golay E, Maggio AB, Beghetti M. Impaired endothelial and smooth muscle functions and arterial stiffness appear before puberty in obese children and are associated with elevated ambulatory blood pressure. Eur Heart J. 2008;29:792–9.

71. Mimoun E, Aggoun Y, Pousset M, et al. Association of arterial stiffness and endothelial dysfunction with metabolic syndrome in obese children. J Pediatr. 2008;153:65–70.

72. Gidding SS. Noninvasive cardiac imaging: implications for risk assessment in adolescents and young adults. Ann Med. 2008;40:506–13.

73. American Academy of Pediatrics. Effects of cigarette-smoking on the fetus and child. Pediatrics. 1976;57:411–3.

74. American Academy of Pediatrics, Committee on Nutrition. Toward a prudent diet for children. Pediatrics. 1983;71: 78–80.

75. American Academy of Pediatrics, Committee on Nutrition. Prudent life-style for children: dietary fat and cholesterol. Pediatrics. 1986;78:521–5.

76. National Cholesterol Education Program. Report of the expert panel on blood cholesterol levels in children and adolescents. Bethesda, MD: US Department of Health and Human Services; 1991. NIH Publication No. 91-2732.

77. Stamler J, Fortmann SP, Levy RI, Prineas RJ, Tell G. Primordial prevention of cardiovascular disease risk factors: panel summary. Prev Med. 1999;29:S130–5.

78. Lloyd-Jones DM, Leip EP, Larson MG, et al. Prediction of lifetime risk for cardiovascular disease by risk factor burden at 50 years of age. Circulation. 2006;113:791–8.

79. Stamler J, Stamler R, Neaton JD, et al. Low risk-factor profile and long-term cardiovascular and noncardiovascular mortality and life expectancy: findings for 5 large cohorts of young adult and middle-aged men and women. J Am Med Assoc. 1999;282:2012–8.

80. McGill HC Jr, McMahan CA, Gidding SS. Preventing heart disease in the 21st century: implications of the Pathobiological Determinants of Atherosclerosis in Youth (PDAY) Study. Circulation. 2008;117:1216–27.

VII TREATMENT OF CHILDHOOD OBESITY: LIFESTYLE INTERVENTION

20 Family-Based Behavioral Interventions

Denise E. Wilfley, Anna Vannucci, and Emily K. White

CONTENTS

Key Words: Behavior, counseling, diet, energy expenditure, weight regain, community, lifestyle intervention, family-based treatment, weight maintenance, parent, youth, obesity, overweight

IMPORTANCE OF EARLY INTERVENTION

The phenomenon of the tracking of pediatric overweight across the lifespan is well documented *(1)*. Elevated childhood height and body mass index (BMI) are robust predictors of young adult BMI *(2)*, as findings show that overweight children (BMI >85th percentile) are more likely to continue to gain weight and to be overweight as adolescents than normal weight children *(3)*. While the popular notion is that children will simply outgrow their overweight status, the reality is that childhood overweight is one of the most compelling risk factors for overweight in adulthood *(1)* and the risk of developing obesity later in life increases progressively with child age and increasing child BMI *(1–3)*. This tendency for overweight status to track into later childhood, adolescence, and adulthood necessitates early intervention, as pediatric overweight clearly does not resolve spontaneously with age.

Childhood is an ideal point of intervention for several reasons. First, adult interventions tend to lead to only modest weight losses *(4)* and it is more difficult to reverse obesity with time, suggesting that overweight becomes more intractable later in life. Second, addressing overweight early in life has the potential to reduce or even reverse the deleterious effects of excess weight and decrease the associated psychosocial and medical sequelae that can persist into adulthood *(5,6)*. Third, weight loss interventions implemented early in life may be more efficacious because younger children's dietary and physical activity habits are not yet fully ingrained and tend to be more amenable to change. Fourth, children can benefit from early intervention due to natural increases in height, which make it easier to

From: *Contemporary Endocrinology: Pediatric Obesity: Etiology, Pathogenesis, and Treatment*
Edited by: M. Freemark, DOI 10.1007/978-1-60327-874-4_20,
© Springer Science+Business Media, LLC 2010

show a reduction in percent overweight even while maintaining the same weight. Finally, traditional, universal prevention programs (e.g., in-school physical activity) for children who are already overweight are not sufficient, as they have shown little efficacy *(7)*. Thus, treating overweight and obese children with a multi-component intervention is a promising avenue to induce weight loss and to slow the weight gain trajectory in youth (ages 1–18) *(7,8)*.

The purpose of this chapter is to review the literature on family-based lifestyle interventions for pediatric obesity, which are currently the most well-established treatments for pediatric obesity to date *(9,10)*. This chapter also explains the specific role of parents as key partners in child weight loss within these interventions, critically reviews the components of family-based behavioral interventions, and finally makes recommendations on how best to expand the current scope, duration, and intensity of treatment to enhance the traditional approaches to losing weight by including weight loss maintenance components within a socio-ecological framework.

FAMILY-BASED BEHAVIORAL INTERVENTIONS

Lifestyle interventions are defined as active treatment approaches that focus on modifying overweight children's daily practices, such as improved dietary intake and increased physical activity. By definition, lifestyle interventions are meant to be compatible with daily living; therefore, associated behavior changes are sustained better over time *(5)*. Family-based behavioral interventions are one example of a lifestyle intervention and are often regarded as the first line of treatment for childhood overweight due to their empirically demonstrated efficacy *(8,11–16)* and for their relative safety, compared to pharmacotherapy or bariatric surgery *(8)*. However, pharmacotherapy or bariatric surgery may be warranted in some cases dependent on child age, severity of obesity, and presence of obesity-related comorbidities *(17)*. Even with severely overweight children, the efficacy of pharmacotherapy or bariatric surgery can be enhanced by implementing these approaches in consort with lifestyle interventions. (For a review of pharmacotherapy and bariatric surgery, see Chapters 12 and 23 by Freemark and Chapter 27 by Yurcisin and Demaria in this volume.)

Numerous randomized controlled trials (RCTs) and meta-analyses have demonstrated that active lifestyle interventions are superior to no-treatment control or education-only conditions *(18)*, the results of which are summarized in Table 1. A recent meta-analysis indicated that lifestyle interventions result in an average decrease in percent overweight of 8.9%, as compared to education-only controls that result in an average increase of 2.7% at follow-up *(18)*. Recent work by Kalarchian and colleagues *(19)* reinforces the need for active intervention for pediatric overweight. Those receiving a targeted, multi-component family-based intervention demonstrated significant decreases in percent overweight, as well as improvements in overweight-related medical comorbidities, while children receiving usual care showed no changes in percent overweight *(19)*. Furthermore, the positive effects of family-based behavioral interventions are not limited to changes in child weight; these approaches produce significant reductions in blood pressure and cholesterol levels *(17)* while producing significant psychosocial health benefits *(6,13,20)*.

Evidence also suggests that usual care is not effective in treating overweight *(21)*. For example, investigators in the LEAP (Live, Eat, and Play) trial offered a brief program, in which children attended visits with their primary care physician and parents received educational materials. This usual care intervention had little to no effect on child BMI or other outcome measures, such as physical activity level or parent BMI *(21)*. Clearly, education-only or usual care is not sufficient to produce significant changes in child weight seen in behavioral interventions. Overall, the existing literature provides support for the use of multi-component lifestyle interventions in the treatment of pediatric obesity.

Table 1
Recent Reviews and Meta-Analyses of Pediatric Weight Loss Studies

Author	Type of review and number of studies	Target population	Conclusions
American Dietetic Association (20)	Review of 29 RCTs and 15 other types of studies	Overweight children (ages 2–12) and adolescents (ages 13–18)	Positive effects for multi-component, family-based programs especially for children ages 5–12
McGovern et al. (72)	Meta-analysis of 61 randomized trials	Overweight children and adolescents (ages 2–18)	Small to moderate treatment effects of combined lifestyle interventions on BMI
Snethen et al. (113)	Meta-analysis of seven interventions	Overweight children (ages 6–16 with an overall mean age not older than 12)	Multi-component lifestyle interventions that include parental involvement can be effective in assisting children to lose weight
Tsiros et al. (114)	Review of 34 RCTs	Overweight or obese adolescents (ages 12–19)	Lifestyle interventions with behavior/cognitive-behavioral components are promising particularly for long-term maintenance
Wilfley et al. (18)	Meta-analysis of 14 RCTs	Overweight youth (ages 19 or younger)	Lifestyle interventions produce significant changes in weight status in the short term with encouraging results for the persistence of effects

Reprinted with permission from TODAY Study Group (34).

The rationale for including parents in lifestyle interventions for overweight children is twofold. First and foremost, parental obesity has been identified as a significant risk factor for childhood obesity (22), with one study reporting that children with obese parents are at a two- to threefold increased risk for being obese themselves (1). This concordance of parent–child weight status, which is likely due to shared genetic and environmental factors, suggests that parents have a strong influence on the weight status of their offspring and could have a powerful positive influence in family-based lifestyle interventions. Second, family-based interventions recognize that the child's weight-related behaviors are developed and maintained within the context of the family (23); therefore, lifestyle interventions aim to capitalize on the influence parents have over the weight-related behaviors of their young children and the structure of the family environment (24,25).

Parents or caregivers are seen as necessary partners in pediatric weight loss (25,26) due to their role as key agents of change and due to the impact of parent behavior change on child weight outcomes. Most commonly, parents are conceptualized in a "helper" or "facilitator" role and are taught to encourage their children to exercise and to make healthy choices as well as modify the shared home environment, utilizing behavioral techniques learned in treatment (24). Parental involvement is supported by behavioral economics theory, which suggests that individuals will choose behaviors that are less effortful and highly reinforcing. Therefore, inducing child behavior change is contingent upon the parent providing healthful, reinforcing alternatives while limiting access to less healthy options. Social cognitive theory (27) also provides a strong argument for including parents in treatment, as it posits that parental modeling is a potent contributor to the success of interventions for pediatric obesity because children learn through observing their parents' behaviors. In addition, the benefits of parents and children modeling healthier behaviors in the shared home environment may generalize to at-risk siblings (16). Overall, harnessing parental influence has the potential to beneficially affect the weight status of the entire family by creating an environment that is supportive of a healthy lifestyle.

In summary, the most effective interventions for childhood overweight incorporate multiple components, and parental involvement is imperative to the success of these interventions. Intensive family-based behavioral interventions can have powerful treatment effects and provide a promising alternative to more invasive procedures.

KEY TREATMENT COMPONENTS OF FAMILY-BASED BEHAVIORAL INTERVENTIONS

The goal of family-based behavioral interventions is either (1) to induce weight loss or (2) to prevent excess weight gain and normalize growth by slowing the trajectory of weight gain relative to height. In order to determine the intensity, duration, and scope of treatment, the child's severity of obesity and age are taken into consideration. Although further research to develop specific treatment algorithms is needed, experts have suggested a staged approach to weight management (28). Within a staged approach, the primary treatment consideration is whether to target weight gain prevention or weight loss. It is recommended that weight gain prevention be used for very young children and youth with lower levels of obesity (i.e., those who are overweight, between the 85th and 95th BMI percentile). Cost-effective interventions such as internet-based prevention psycho-education programs and TV allowance devices, which limit access to screen time, may be sufficient to prevent excess weight gain. Weight loss, achieved through a family-based lifestyle intervention, would be indicated for older children and adolescents, especially those above the 95th percentile. The second treatment consideration is deciding how intensive the intervention should be. In general, interventions that are more intense, longer in duration, and wider in their scope are likely to benefit children with more severe obesity. Children may advance through stages of care to increasingly more comprehensive interventions such as pharmacotherapy or bariatric surgery based on age, as well. For instance, bariatric surgery would not be indicated for a very young obese child, but an adolescent may benefit from bariatric surgery accompanied by an intensive family-based behavioral intervention.

Within family-based behavioral interventions, the energy balance equation is used to conceptualize weight gain, weight loss, and weight maintenance. Positive energy balance, when energy intake exceeds energy expenditure, results in weight gain over an extended period of time. Conversely, negative energy balance occurs when energy expenditure exceeds energy intake, resulting in weight loss. Achieving negative energy balance is the goal of behavioral weight loss interventions; therefore, participants are encouraged to decrease energy intake while increasing energy expenditure. Within weight maintenance and behavioral prevention programs, the primary goal is to prevent excess weight gain and make the child leaner through achieving a stable energy balance. In general, family-based behavioral interventions promote small, successive changes in children's dietary and physical activity behaviors through the use of behavior change strategies and familial support. Specifically, the most efficacious lifestyle treatment approaches include a focus on the following components: dietary modification, changes in energy expenditure, behavior change techniques, and parental involvement at all levels of change *(24)*.

Dietary Modification

Given evidence that obese children have greater daily caloric intake than non-obese peers *(5,29)* (effects of social context), dietary modification (i.e., reducing caloric intake) is fundamental to the weight loss and the prevention of excess weight gain within the context of a lifestyle intervention *(5)*. Effective dietary modification strategies aim to result in an overall negative energy balance; however, it is imperative to ensure that children receive proper nutrition when modifying both the quantity and the quality of food consumed. One strategy to achieve such a caloric deficit is to increase intake of low-energy density (LED) foods (i.e., highly nutritious, low-calorie-dense foods) while simultaneously decreasing intake of high-energy density (HED) foods (i.e., high fat, high sugar foods) *(30–32)*. The most widely studied dietary modification approach of this kind is the Traffic Light Program *(33,34)*, which classifies foods into three categories: red (low in nutrients/HED; STOP), yellow (nutrient-dense, yet HED; CAUTION), and green (nutrient-dense/LED; GO). This strategy enables children and their parents to moderately restrict their caloric and fat intake and gradually replace unhealthy foods in their diets with healthful ones.

Interventions focused on increasing LED foods have been associated with decreased energy intake, successful weight loss outcomes, and the prevention of excess weight gain *(8,30,35)*. Fruits and vegetables are often targeted to decrease energy intake, and it is recommended that children should consume 5 servings of fruits and vegetables daily *(20,30)*. Increased fruit and vegetable intake may also lead to decreased intake of HED foods *(36)*. Additionally, studies have shown that targeting increases in "good" fats (e.g., nuts, fish) and high-fiber foods (e.g., raisins, multi-grain breads) may also be effective for reducing caloric intake *(30,37)*. Such dietary approaches have been found to increase nutrient density (e.g., protein, calcium, iron) and decrease density of fat intake in children aged pre-school to adolescence *(8,30)*. Overall, these types of strategies have been shown to decrease overall energy intake needed to achieve a caloric deficit.

Decreasing HED food intake is the most commonly used strategy in pediatric weight loss programs and is found to be effective in children and adolescents *(8,30)*. In order to reduce the frequency of HED foods, precise, well-defined behavioral targets are used to improve the efficacy of dietary modification strategies *(17)*. These include decreases in sugar-sweetened beverage (SSB) consumption and HED snacking, and fewer meals outside of the home.

Consumption of SSBs has increased dramatically during the past generation, and overweight children get a higher proportion of their caloric intake from SSBs than normal weight peers *(38)*. Research suggests that substituting water in the place of SSBs can decrease average daily caloric intake by as much as 235 kCal *(39)*. Likewise, children and adolescents have increased their energy intake from daily snacking between 1977 and 1996 *(40)*. To avoid HED snacking, dietary interventions recommend that foods containing 5 g or more of fat, sugary cereals, and fast food items be eaten sparingly and limited to no more than 10–15 servings/week *(41)*. The rise in proportion of meals eaten outside the home is one factor that contributes to the higher saturated fat and cholesterol consumption in children *(42)*.

Targeting these specific behaviors through a lifestyle approach has the potential to decrease overall caloric intake, increase the likelihood of meeting pediatric standards of nutrient intake, and result in long-term weight maintenance *(43)*. For example, an on-going weight loss trial *(34)* for overweight adolescents with type-2 diabetes sets adaptable caloric intake goals, typically between 1,200 and 1,500 kCal/day, adjusted based on baseline weight and ensuing weight loss. Limiting portion sizes is also an effective way to gradually reduce caloric intake, as one recent study indicates that children served larger entrees consumed 25% more food than those served smaller portions *(44)*. Dietary modification strategies which employ a more flexible, "free-choice" approach may be effective because interventionists are able to take into account individual taste preferences, beliefs surrounding food, and customs from diverse cultural and ethnic backgrounds (34,45). For example, interventionists can recommend cooking methods to lower the caloric value of preferred foods (e.g., baking chicken rather than frying it) (34). Regardless of the dietary modification strategy employed in the intervention, these recommendations are always complemented by strong behavior change components reinforced by the parent (described in more detail later in this chapter).

Energy Expenditure Modification

Changes in patterns of energy expenditure are critical to inducing an overall negative energy balance needed for sustained success within family-based behavioral interventions. Research indicates that adopting an active lifestyle is an important step that families can take to promote weight loss and prevent excess weight gain (46,47). Targeting changes in activity levels may include increasing physical activity (e.g., walking, sports), reducing sedentary activity, in which a minimal number of calories are burned (e.g., television watching, computer time), or both to achieve successful weight loss or weight management. Consistent with dietary modification strategies, behavior change techniques and parental support are instrumental in promoting sustainable changes in physical activity.

Interventions focusing on increases in physical activity have been associated with significant weight loss in family-based approaches for children and adolescents (48). Current recommended guidelines for physical activity are 60 min/day for children and adolescents (46). Most of this activity should be moderate- to vigorous-intensity (46), such as playing soccer, riding a bike, or running. It is also recommended that youth should include muscle- and bone-strengthening physical activity, which may include activities that involve running or jumping (e.g., basketball), playing on playground equipment, or resistance training, such as push-ups (46). Children and adolescents who are initially inactive need to gradually increase their activity to prevent injuries and work toward maintaining ideal levels. Further, it is important to encourage families to find activities their children enjoy, that are age-appropriate, and that offer variety.

Another method for modifying energy expenditure levels in children is to focus on reducing time spent in sedentary behaviors, which is particularly important given that children find sedentary behaviors more reinforcing than physically active alternatives (36). It is recommended that children should engage in no more than 2 h of sedentary time per day outside of school (49) and should try to reduce overall sedentary behavior time by 50%. Reduced time spent in sedentary behavior leads children to reallocate time to physical activity (41,50–52). Decreased sedentary behavior and increased physical activity in turn lead to long-term reductions in zBMI (50). *Notably*, reducing sedentary behavior *has been shown* to reduce overall energy intake, since many children snack while watching television (53).

Evidence suggests that encouraging increases in lifestyle activity (e.g., taking the stairs instead of the escalator) effectively sustains behavior change and weight maintenance. Findings from one study suggest that unstructured, flexible lifestyle activity is more effective in the long term than structured and higher intensity aerobic or calisthenics exercise (8,54). There were no differences in weight maintenance during the first year of treatment; however, in the second year of follow-up, the lifestyle activity group maintained weight loss and the participants in the calisthenics and aerobic exercise groups gained significant amounts of weight (54). Data also indicate that long-term diet plus increased lifestyle activity is superior to diet plus increased aerobic exercise (8,55).

Behavior Change Techniques

Components of behavior therapy and behavior change are vital to family-based behavioral weight loss interventions. Standard behavioral weight loss methods include goal setting, self-monitoring and logging, family-based reward systems, and stimulus control strategies (8,43,56). It has been shown that interventions that incorporate behavior change strategies are more successful at achieving weight loss and the prevention of excess weight gain than education alone *(41,50,57)*.

Goal setting includes setting specific targets for eating and activity behaviors and is central for the achievement of behavioral goals in effective behavioral interventions *(41,58)*. Sample goals include consuming less than 15 servings of HED foods per week, engaging in 60 min of activity per day, reducing time spent in sedentary behavior by 50%, or achieving projected weight loss or weight maintenance. Over the course of an intervention, goals change gradually to accommodate participant progress. Findings suggest that the frequency of goal setting – both during treatment and after treatment cessation – predicts the use of behavioral strategies and is associated with sustained behavior change and weight maintenance *(58)*.

Self-monitoring and logging approaches teach parents and children to pay close attention to their dietary and activity behaviors and to record their daily patterns in a diary. Logging is a simple way to determine if behavioral goals are being met (i.e., "Did I consume more than 15 servings of HED foods this week?"). Mastering both behavioral techniques is imperative for families in the short and long term, as data suggest that regular self-monitoring and logging help parents and children to become more aware of their energy balance behaviors and are associated with successful weight outcomes *(59)*. Both caregivers and children are instructed to self-monitor and log various aspects of their eating (e.g., daily intake of fruits, vegetables, and calorie-dense foods) and activity (e.g., time spent in moderate to vigorous activity, television and computer time). Additionally, through weekly weight monitoring, children are taught to learn the association between their eating and activity behaviors and changes in their weight.

Research also suggests that it is helpful to reinforce behaviors with a family-based incentive system (Fig. 1), in which parents develop a list of acceptable reward items/privileges and provide contingent rewards to their children for goal achievement (e.g., giving stickers for improvements in self-monitoring). Rewards may include contracting and incentives (e.g., spending time with parent playing a game), which are provided as reinforcement for having met goals. It is strongly recommended that parents do not use food as a reward and instead try to increase the reinforcing value of physical activity or peer interactions.

Stimulus control is defined as restructuring the home and environment to increase the likelihood of engaging in desired behaviors. Parents play particularly important roles in enforcing stimulus control strategies by controlling the availability of healthful foods, the access to unhealthy foods, and the amount of physical activity and screen time in which children engage. Specifically, parents can promote healthy energy balance behaviors by encouraging and facilitating physical activity, limiting screen time (which reduces snacking and sedentary behavior), reducing home/school availability of, or access to, nutrient-poor, energy-dense foods, and providing ready access to low-energy, nutrient-rich foods including fruits and vegetables. These are discussed in more detail below.

Family Involvement and Support

Parental and family involvement in pediatric obesity interventions is considered crucial, as several studies suggest that a greater degree of parental involvement leads to greater child weight loss and management outcomes *(15,60–64)*. Targeting both the parent and the child has been shown to be more effective than targeting the child alone *(60,65,66)*. In addition, parent weight loss is an independent predictor of child weight loss, suggesting that youth benefit from more intensive targeting and commitment of the parents. The relationship between child and parent outcomes likely operates through the following mechanisms. Primarily, parents can effect change through shaping the home environment, modeling healthy eating and activity behaviors, and using enhanced parenting skills acquired through family-based intervention. See Table 2 for a summary of specific ways that parents can support their children in changing their energy balance behaviors.

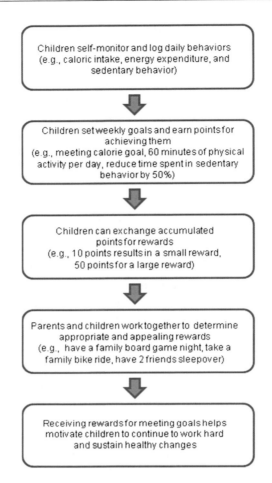

Fig. 1. Family-based incentive system.

Parents play an important role in laying a foundation for sustaining health-promoting eating and activity behaviors by building a home environment where healthy eating and activity are the norms. They can do so by monitoring healthful lifestyles in themselves and their children (as described above) and by utilizing stimulus control strategies (as described above) to provide sufficient opportunities and motivation for the consumption of low-energy-dense foods and participation in active events for their families within the home environment.

In addition, modeling healthy eating and activity behaviors and attitudes for their children likely contributes to the effectiveness of parental involvement *(68,69)*. Parents who model healthful behaviors, such as regular engagement in physical activity, low levels of sedentary behavior, high fruit and vegetable intake, and low fat and sweet intake, accordingly influence the behaviors of their children *(68,69)*. Promoting weight loss in parents is likely to be an effective behavior change strategy in addition to modeling, with data demonstrating a high concordance between parent and weight outcomes *(67,70,71)*.

Familial support for the overweight child is also imperative to sustaining healthful behavior change and to improving weight loss outcomes, and so parenting skills training is a common component of treatment *(10,24,72)*. During this training, parents learn and practice skills needed to support their overweight child to ensure that behavior change has occurred and is maintained (see Table 2 for a description of parental involvement). Parents are taught to provide consistency within the home and to

Table 2
Parental Involvement in Family-Based Behavioral Interventions

Supporting healthy eating behaviors	Supporting physical and lifestyle activity	Supporting healthful behavior change
Increase low-energy density foods • Plan for healthy meals • Shop for fruits and vegetables and nutritious foods with "good" fats and high fiber • Prepare healthy meals • Serve fruits and vegetables at meals and for snacks	*Increase physical activity* • Make a weekly activity schedule • Provide equipment and clothing for exercise • Set up active play dates with child's peer group • Join a local community recreation center • Make use of local parks and playgrounds	*Use behavior modification strategies* • Set goals for weight and behavioral change targets • Create a family-based rewards system • Engage in self-monitoring and logging • Use stimulus control strategies in the shared home environment
Decrease high-energy density foods • Limit high-energy density foods in the home • Limit access to fast food restaurants • Limit eating away from the kitchen and dining room • Replace sugar-sweetened beverages with water or serve low-fat milk products at home	*Increase lifestyle activity* • Plan fun activities for the family • Model for and encourage their children to take the stairs instead of escalators or elevators • Walk instead of drive with family, when possible	*Target changes in the parent* • Focus on weight loss in parents • Model healthful behaviors for child *Provide support for child* • Hold family meetings • Review self-monitoring logs • Praise healthy behaviors • Encourage healthy behaviors, and minimize attention to unhealthy behaviors • Explain the family-based behavioral intervention to family and friends
Use a lifestyle approach • Serve healthy portion sizes • Involve child in preparing meals • Cook traditionally unhealthy foods in a healthier way	*Decrease time spent in sedentary behaviors* • Limit child's TV and computer time to 2 h/day	

establish stable meal and snack times for their children *(43)*. Parents are also taught to identify common barriers to behavior change (e.g., gatherings/parties with unhealthy food) *(43)* and to acquire skills to overcome these challenges *(56,73)*. Furthermore, parents learn to provide positive reinforcement by praising and encouraging healthy, desired behaviors while simultaneously minimizing attention to unhealthy, negative behaviors *(43,50,74)*.

PROBLEM OF WEIGHT REGAIN

While weight loss during family-based behavioral interventions has been clearly demonstrated, weight regain after lifestyle change is a common phenomenon among adults and is a challenge for children as well (8,62,75). Studies have tracked long-term weight change in families in intervals as long as 10 years and found that children lose significant weight during the initial family-based behavioral intervention but have difficulty with weight loss maintenance; thus the magnitude of treatment effect declines over time (13,14,73). Findings also suggest that parents show weight change, but their maintenance is not as strong, so the majority of parents return to baseline levels of adiposity by the 10-year follow-up (13,14).

Contextual learning laboratory research sheds light on the potential behavioral mechanisms of weight regain, indicating that previously learned behaviors are not replaced by newly learned behaviors, but rather coexist with them (76). In addition, newly learned behaviors are less generalizable across contexts, and old, previously learned behaviors are particularly susceptible to contextual cues for activation (76). This coexistence of new learning with old behavior patterns creates an ambiguous situation for individuals when faced with a behavior choice, and this ambiguity results in increased likelihood that old obesity-related behaviors (e.g., poor eating habits, sedentary behaviors) will be activated, especially in novel contexts (77,78). Therefore, concerted efforts must be made to ensure that new learning is practiced across most or all relevant contexts, that appropriate support and cues for healthful behaviors are in place, and that there is sufficient time devoted to the mastery and practice of these strategies.

There is also mounting evidence that behavior change may be particularly challenging for a certain subset of genetically susceptible individuals that possess particular obesogenic genotypes (79–82). Evidence has illustrated the impact of genes on the metabolic and physiological aspects of obesity. Only recently research has indicated that behavioral phenotypes are also genetically influenced. These phenotypes are often expressed as appetitive traits, including satiety responsiveness (82), motivation to eat (80,83,84), and binge eating (79,81,85,86). These appetitive traits are highly heritable and have been shown to be strongly related to increases in energy intake and predictive of obesity risk. Behavioral phenotypes interact with obesogenic genotypes to determine one's weight status, thus rendering a subset of the population particularly susceptible to developing and maintaining obesity within the pervasive obesogenic environment (87). In other words, obese individuals with these high-risk genotypes and behavioral phenotypes may be more vulnerable to relapse in environmental contexts that promote obesity-related behaviors. Although it is not possible to alter an individual's genetic makeup after birth, it is possible to change one's immediate surrounding environment (e.g., the home environment) through interventions designed to decrease the likelihood of the phenotypic expression of obesity-related behaviors.

Given the difficulty of establishing new eating and activity behaviors, likely even more so for genetically susceptible individuals, it is not surprising that weight regain occurs following the end of brief (i.e., 4–6 months) family-based behavioral interventions; there is little time available for the intensive practice across contexts necessary for enduring change. One approach to preventing weight regain in the long term is to expand the scope, intensity, and duration of family-based interventions to enhance the generalization of newly acquired behaviors across contexts. Generalization of new habits to multiple contexts increases the likelihood that weight loss maintenance will continue after contact with the treatment provider ends.

FAMILY-BASED WEIGHT LOSS MAINTENANCE TREATMENT

In order to overcome the problem of weight regain, it is critical to extend the focus of family-based behavioral interventions to sustaining weight maintenance behaviors and extending the length of treatment. Maintenance approaches build on what is learned in family-based behavioral interventions, but assume that the skills needed to lose weight are distinct from those required to maintain weight. Weight maintenance among both adults *(4,62,88–90)* and children *(13,14)* is associated with long-term adherence to healthy eating behaviors and regular physical activity. In addition, a meta-analysis of adult behavioral weight loss interventions *(91)* and a review of pediatric weight loss treatment *(92)* indicated that duration of treatment is the most important predictor of weight change in the short and long terms *(91)*. Thus, an extended treatment plan which promotes weight maintenance behaviors across multiple contexts should significantly reduce the number of children who relapse into old behaviors and gain weight following weight loss interventions.

Wilfley and colleagues *(18)* were the first to target weight loss maintenance in children through extended contact following traditional family-based treatment. Two distinct approaches, behavioral skills maintenance treatment (BSM) and social facilitation maintenance treatment (SFM), were compared to a control condition, which consisted of a written plan for continuing healthy behaviors learned in family-based treatment with no further contact. BSM emphasizes maintaining healthful changes within the individual context and focuses on self-regulation behaviors and relapse-prevention strategies (e.g., self-monitoring weight status and returning to weight loss behaviors if weight gain occurs, cognitive restructuring, coping with high-risk situations). SFM extends the scope of the intervention to the family's social context; it uses empirically supported techniques to help parents bolster child peer networks that support health behaviors and targets peer (e.g., teasing) and self-perceptual (e.g., body image) factors *(18,93)*. Both maintenance approaches highlight the importance of the family treatment milieu, as parents have great potential to increase the generalizability of new behaviors learned in the clinic by making changes across multiple contexts (e.g., the home, school lunches, play dates).

Findings indicate that children receiving either BSM or SFM maintain relative weight significantly better than the control group in the short term *(18)*; however, BSM was no more effective than control at long-term follow-up. *These results suggest that attention to multiple contexts (familial, social, environmental) and extension of treatment duration may be imperative for achieving sustainable weight loss outcomes and behavior change.* Further, long-term results of this trial indicate that children receiving SFM demonstrated significantly greater improvements in their ability to cope with teasing and to enlist friends to support physical activity over the short and long term, compared to both BSM and control *(18)*. There was also a specificity of effect, suggesting that children with few social problems (e.g., ability to get along with others, no participation in bullying or teasing, obedience at home or school) particularly benefited from the SFM approach of focusing on gaining and maintaining social support for maintenance behaviors *(18)*. However, children with higher levels of social problems may need more intensive treatment to achieve long-term weight maintenance *(18)*. Clearly, weight loss maintenance approaches like SFM are effective ways to promote sustainable behavior change; however, improvements are needed to further enhance their long-term efficacy *(78)*.

Expanding the Scope of Maintenance Treatment: A Multi-Level Approach

One promising approach for enhancing long-term childhood weight loss maintenance is to utilize a socio-ecological framework of health behavior change that extends the scope of treatment into additional socio-environmental settings. Socio-ecological models acknowledge the multiple contexts within which weight-related behaviors are fostered and constrained *(94)* and posits that obesity is the result of individual/family, peer/social, and community factors that interact dynamically with genetic susceptibilities *(94,95)*. According to the socio-ecological model *(78)*, weight regain (Fig. 2) occurs following the conclusion of traditional family-based behavioral interventions because the contextual stimuli that set the occasion for previously learned, obesity-related behaviors are not modified, cuing the child and caregiver to relapse into old behavior patterns *(78)*. Family-based maintenance interventions with a socio-ecological focus are thought to produce sustainable behavior modifications by

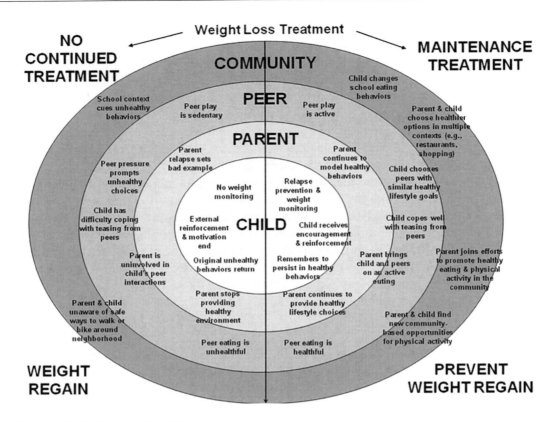

Fig. 2. Socio-ecological model of weight regain.

effecting change across multiple contexts (see Fig. 2), thus enhancing the efficacy of treatment in the long term *(78)*.

Wilfley and colleagues *(78)* have applied this theory in the design of an enhanced version of SFM, which expands its interpersonal focus at the peer/social level, includes additional self-regulation strategies at the individual/family level, and promotes environmental change at the community level (see following text and Fig. 3 for a more comprehensive description of treatment components). The projected efficacy of enhanced SFM is based upon computer simulation models of change in child percent overweight over time. Using data from the original RCT *(18)*, including weight loss outcome, weight maintenance, and follow-up, results of biosimulation analysis indicate an anticipated decrease of 12.9% overweight at the most distal timepoint (30-month follow-up) *(78)*. Ultimately, this simulated approach supports the use of an intervention that is longer in duration, higher in intensity, and extended further into the environmental context, which should further enhance long-term weight maintenance outcomes. Enhanced SFM, with its focus on social ecology and multiple behavioral contexts, is a promising approach for improving weight maintenance treatment outcomes and is currently being evaluated in an on-going randomized controlled trial.

Components of a Family-Based, Multi-Level Maintenance Intervention

In order to successfully implement family-based, multi-level maintenance interventions, interventionists need to focus on both the parent and the child and their ability to sustain newly learned eating and activity behaviors. Factors on the individual/family, peer/social, and community levels all impact the family's ability to adhere to treatment components and to maintain these changes after

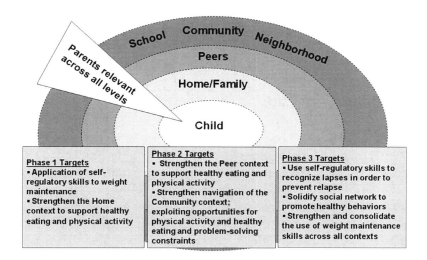

Fig. 3. Enhanced social facilitation maintenance treatment: a social-ecological model.

treatment cessation. Attention to these factors will create a more tailored treatment approach; promising treatment components at each level are described below. In particular, individuals with obesogenic genotypes and associated behavioral phenotypes may benefit from a multi-level approach because altering the obesogenic environment across multiple contexts can constrain the expression of these traits and therefore decrease the risk of relapsing into old behaviors.

At the *individual/family level*, persistent self-regulation is required to maintain long-term adherence to healthy eating behaviors and regular physical activity associated with successful weight maintenance in both adults *(4,88)* and children *(13,96,97)*. Specific self-regulation behaviors are distinct from weight loss skills and include comparing one's current weight with a maintenance weight (through regular self-weighing and using a weight graph), adhering to healthy eating and activity behaviors, planning for high-risk situations, and returning to weight loss behaviors if needed *(97)*. These self-regulation behaviors have consistently shown to help with weight maintenance in children *(18)* and adults *(97)*, while failure to maintain these behaviors is associated with weight regain *(96)*. It is important for the caregivers and children to engage in these behaviors, particularly in light of the evidence indicating that parent weight outcomes are strongly associated with child weight outcomes *(67,71)*.

At the *peer/social level*, expanding the contexts that support, reward, and encourage healthy behaviors can have a powerful influence on whether or not healthful behaviors are sustained *(98,99)*. Peer factors, such as a lack of social support for physical activity and healthy eating *(14,93)* and teasing related to physical activity *(100)*, are likely to contribute to weight regain. However, peers can also reinforce behaviors that prevent weight regain. For example, overweight youth make healthier eating and activity choices in the presence of supportive peers than when they are alone *(29,101,102)*. In addition, social connectedness (i.e., being satisfied with one's social network) among children and adolescents is positively correlated with greater physical activity *(103)* and healthy dietary practices *(104)*.

Thus, the nature or choice of one's peers is a critical factor in long-term weight control. The overarching goal of a peer/social component is to increase the ratio of individuals that are supportive of a healthier lifestyle rather than to change the attitudes and behaviors of all individuals within the social network (e.g., a grandmother who is unwilling to change) *(105)*. Family-based approaches are an obvious source of social support for healthful behaviors, and incorporating an interpersonal focus can help families create a supportive health-oriented social network. Parents can also foster healthful peer networks by organizing active play dates for children and exposing them to healthful events within their communities. Overall, the data suggest that family and peer support of healthful behaviors are critical targets for long-term weight loss maintenance in children.

At the *community level*, aspects of the built environment may affect an individual's choice to engage in energy balance behaviors *(106)*. Environmental features of one's neighborhood are associated with rates of obesity and physical activity in children *(107,108)*. Important environmental factors include access to healthy foods, proximity to fast food restaurants, relative cost of healthy and unhealthy foods, perceived safety and neighborhood walkability, and access to community recreation facilities and local parks *(95,106)*. For example, access to parks is a strong predictor of children's physical activity *(108,109)*, and distance to the nearest food store is significantly associated with a greater preference for vegetables *(110)*. Within a family-based, multi-level maintenance treatment, parents are encouraged to practice self-regulatory skills in high-risk environmental contexts (e.g., school parties). It is also important that families learn to create a lifestyle that capitalizes on healthful environmental opportunities (e.g., local parks) while limiting access to obesity-promoting aspects of the environment (e.g., fast food restaurants). Families can develop lists of community resources and events that are supportive of weight maintenance behaviors and make plans to increase the utilization of those resources. Overall, weight loss maintenance treatment would be enhanced by encouraging parents and children to modify, where possible, the stimuli present in the contexts of school, neighborhood, and community that facilitate or constrain their use of newly acquired weight maintenance skills.

CONCLUSIONS AND FUTURE DIRECTIONS

Obesity is a major public health threat to society that requires a multi-pronged approach. Family-based behavioral interventions are the current gold-standard treatment for pediatric obesity, and it is clear from the extant literature that parents should be used as partners to enact and support healthful behavior change in their children. To enhance the long-term intervention effects, it is necessary to expand the intensity, duration, and scope of treatment. Preliminary evidence suggests that extending the length and amount of contact produces better long-term weight outcomes in children. To further improve intervention efficacy, it is crucial that future researches identify the treatment components associated with the most broad-based and persistent effects as well as the biological, social, environmental characteristics and factors that constrain or prompt weight-regulating behaviors. Focusing on weight loss maintenance and the practice of new behaviors across multiple contexts has been shown to be effective. In particular, socio-ecological approaches are promising and merit further evaluation.

There is also a need for more personalized, tailored intervention approaches with particular attention given to individual vulnerabilities, including: (1) genotypes and associated behavioral phenotypes such as satiety responsiveness *(82)*, motivation to eat *(16,84)*, and binge eating *(79,81,85,86,111,112)*; (2) severity of obesity status; (3) age of the child; (4) risk factors such as having an overweight parent, race/ethnicity, or socioeconomic status; and (5) co-morbid problems such as type-2 diabetes *(34)*. Future research evaluating a range of delivery options, such as the Internet, Smartphone, or residential treatment, for behavioral approaches is warranted. Finally, further investigation of cost-effective methods for dissemination of family-based behavioral interventions into community settings and primary care practices is sorely needed, given the vast numbers of children suffering from pediatric obesity.

ACKNOWLEDGMENTS

Funding sources to be acknowledged: K24MH070446; R01HD36904; R01DK065757; R01MH081125; R01MH064153. The authors wish to thank Dr. Dorothy Van Buren and Rachel Goldstein in their invaluable assistance in the preparation of this chapter.

Editor's Comments

- The findings summarized in your chapter dovetail quite nicely with the conclusions reached by other authors in this volume. Your focus on energy density in dietary *treatment* complements the findings of Johnson and Debb, who note the central role of energy density in the *development* of childhood obesity. Likewise, your review of the long-term benefits of lifestyle activity (as opposed to formal exercise) complements the views of Lanningham-Foster and Levine, who postulate a critical role for non-exercise activity thermogenesis in obesity development and maintenance. Your focus on the parents and family strengthens and extends the findings of genetic investigations and of studies (summarized by Mayer) implicating a critical role for maternal health and behavior prior to, during, and after pregnancy. And your emphasis on positive reinforcement and reward as critical components of behavior change recapitulates the central role of reward mechanisms in appetite control, as noted by Lustig. It is interesting that the paths of family counseling and public health have now converged in a therapeutic approach that focuses on social ecology and multiple behavioral contexts. School/community programs for obesity prevention are discussed in more detail in Chapter 22 by Gittelsohn and Park.

- Intensive treatment for obesity is discussed in the chapters on exercise (Nemet and Eliakim), pharmacotherapy, and bariatric surgery. I agree with your opinion about the value of *intensive dietary approaches*. Studies in adults show that low-carbohydrate diets are most effective for short-term (≤ 6 months) weight loss. However, long-term studies suggest that the major determinants of weight control are total caloric intake and dietary compliance, not macronutrient composition; a comparison of low-fat, low-carb, and low-glycemic diets showed few or no differences after 12 months (Dansinger et al., 2005; Gardner et al., 2007) Similar observations have been made in children (Demol et al., 2008).

Dansinger ML, Gleason JA, Griffith JL, Selker HP, Schaefer EJ. Comparison of the Atkins, Ornish, Weight Watchers, and Zone diets for weight loss and heart disease risk reduction: a randomized trial. *JAMA*. 2005;293: 43–53

Demol S, Yackobovitch-Gavan M, Shalitin S, Nagelberg N, Gillon-Keren M, Phillip M. Low-carbohydrate (low & high-fat) versus high-carbohydrate low-fat diets in the treatment of obesity in adolescents. Acta Paediatr. 2009;98 2:346–51; Sondike SB, Kay GA, Emmett MK. Weight loss regimens that control for carbohydrate quality or quantity: a review. Pediatr Diabetes. 2008;9 3 Pt 2:33–45.

Gardner CD, Kiazand A, Alhassan S, Kim S, Stafford RS, Balise RR, Kraemer HC, King AC. Comparison of the Atkins, Zone, Ornish, and LEARN diets for change in weight and related risk factors among overweight premenopausal women: the A to Z weight loss study: a randomized trial. JAMA. 2007;297:969–77.

Editor's Question and Authors' Response

- **What is your opinion of alternative dietary regimens including low-carbohydrate, vegetarian, and very low calorie diets, for the management of obese children?**

- The recent popularity of several alternative diets focused on making changes in macronutrient intake [including high protein, low carbohydrate, Mediterranean, and vegetarian] among adults has raised the question of whether such intensive dietary modification approaches are appropriate for children. Studies with obese adults adhering to either high-protein, low-carbohydrate, low-fat or Mediterranean diets suggest that altering the specific macronutrient content alone does not seem to have a differential impact on weight in the long term (Due et al., 2004; Shai et al., 2008; Sondike et al., 2008; Sacks et al., 2009). However, preliminary evidence suggests that vegetarian or vegan diets may be effective: in one trial, women randomized to a vegan diet lost more weight than women on a low-cholesterol diet, and this weight loss was maintained over 2-year follow-up (Turner-McGrievy et al., 2007). Long-term success is predicted by the ability to maintain compliance to a specific diet (Sacks et al., 2009; Dansinger et al., 2005), and many adult participants are unable to adhere to the recommended macronutrient guidelines after treatment cessation (Katan, 2009). Thus, it appears that a long-term reduction of total energy intake, rather than adhering to alternative diets targeted at drastically altering macronutrient content, is the key determinant of weight loss in adults.

- Although the majority of research in this area has been conducted with adults, recent studies have begun to evaluate differential interventions with alternative dietary regimens for youth. Similar to findings in adults, research with obese youth comparing diets that reduce overall caloric intake but have distinct dietary regimens is successful, but do not result in significant long-term differences in weight (Demol et al., 2009; Epstein et al., 1998) or waist circumference (Sacks et al., 2009). In line with this, Epstein and colleagues' (1998) systematic review found that total energy intake is the key determinant of weight loss, rather than macronutrient content. It is noteworthy, however, that obese adolescents adhering to a low-carbohydrate diet demonstrated a significant drop in insulin levels and homeostasis model assessment in the long term (HOMA) as compared to a low-fat, high-carbohydrate diet (Demol et al., 2009). These preliminary results suggest that it may be important to tailor dietary interventions based on metabolic considerations, and further research is needed to determine the impact of specific dietary regimens altering macronutrient content in obese and insulin-resistant youth.

- Given the dearth of evidence in support of dietary regimens altering macronutrient content, it is important to consider the feasibility of intensive dietary interventions that emphasize extreme over-all reductions in energy intake (i.e., very low calorie, *VLC,* diets) for obese children and adolescents. Such dietary approaches have been shown to lead to significant short-term reductions in percent overweight (Demol et al., 2009; Epstein et al., 1994; Amador et al., 1990) and other improvements in health indicators (Sothern et al, 2009; Due et al., 2004; Shai et al., 2008). However, the long-term sustainability of these intensive dietary strategies has yet to be determined (Gibson et al., 2006). Data from randomized controlled trials have also indicated that the presence of a controlled environment (e.g., weight loss camps), which includes a VLC dietary component, can lead to greater sustainability of behavior change and better weight outcomes in children and adolescents in the long term (Kirschenbaum et al., 2009). Another key consideration while implementing VLC diets is ensuring that children continue to receive adequate vitamins and nutrients, especially when daily caloric intake is so minimal. VLC diets may be sufficient to produce initial weight loss in youth, yet a lifestyle approach in the weight loss maintenance phase of treatment warrants evaluation as a method for prolonging the benefits of dietary modification.

- Encouraging lifestyle dietary changes, which emphasize an overall reduction in caloric intake, appears to be a more sustainable approach to reducing child overweight rather than aiming for a specific macronutrient composition or extreme reductions in energy intake. Utilizing a dietary system, such as the Traffic Light diet, that broadly divides foods (with appropriate serving sizes) into easily recognizable "green," "yellow," and "red" categories allows children to understand the nutritional value of food and reduce their overall caloric intake. Moreover, this system may encourage greater flexibility with food selection and does not require parents and children to vigilantly track calorie counts and fat content, which likely increases adherence to dietary changes in the long term. In conclusion, achieving negative or stable energy balance, regardless of the specific dietary method used, is the key to producing sustained reductions in child overweight while attending to a child's nutrition for overall growth and development.

Amador M, Ramos LT, Morono M, Hermelo MP. Growth rate reduction during energy restriction in obese adolescents. Exp Clin Endocrinol. 1990;96:73–82.

Dansinger ML, Gleason JA, Griffith JL, Selker HP, Schaefer EJ. Comparison of the Atkins, Ornish, Weight Watchers, and Zone diets for weight loss and heart disease risk reduction: a randomized trial. JAMA. 2005;29(3):43–53.

Demol S, Yackobovitch-Gavan M, Shalitin S, Nagelberg N, Gillon-Keren M, Phillip M. Low-carbohydrate (low & high-fat) versus high-carbohydrate low-fat diets in the treatment of obesity in adolescents. Acta Paediatr. 2009;98(2): 346–51.

Due A, Toubro S, Skov AR, Astrup A. Effect of normal-fat diets, either medium or high in protein, on body weight in overweight subjects: a randomized 1-year trial. Int J Obes Relat Metab Disord. 2004;28:1283–90.

Epstein LH, Valoski AM, Wing RR, McCurley J. Ten-year outcomes of behavioral family based treatment for childhood obesity. Health Psychol. 1994;13:373–83.

Epstein LH, Myers MD, Raynor HA, Saelens BE. Treatment of pediatric obesity. Pediatrics. 1998;101(3):S554–70.

Gibson LJ, Peto J, Warren JM, dos Santos Silva I. Lack of evidence on diets for obesity for children: a systematic review. Int J Epidemiol. 2006;35(6):1544–52.

Katan MB. Weight-loss diets for the prevention and treatment of obesity. N Engl J Med. 2009;360(9):923–5.

Kirschenbaum DS, Craig RD, Decker TM, Germann JN. The remarkable potential of scientifically based immersion programs for the treatment of childhood and adolescent obesity: Wellspring camps demonstrate substantial weight loss even during a follow-up period. Obes Res. 2010. under review.

Sacks FM, Bray GA, Carey VJ, Smith SR, Ryan DH, Anton SD, McManus K, Champagne CM, Bishop LM, Laranjo N, Leboff MS, Rood JC, de Jonge L, Greenway FL, Loria CM, Obarzanek E, Williamson DA. Comparison of weight-loss diets with different compositions of fat, protein, and carbohydrates. N Engl J Med. 2009;360(9):859–73.

Shai I, Schwarzfuchs D, Henkin Y, Shahar DR, Witkow S, Greenberg I, Golan R, Fraser D, Bolotin A, Vardi H, Tangi-Rozental O, Zuk-Ramot R, Sarusi B, Brickner D, Schwartz Z, Sheiner E, Marko R, Katorza E, Thiery J, Fiedler GM, Bluher M, Stumvoll M, Stampfer MJ; for the DIRECT GROUP. Weight loss with a low-carbohydrate, Mediterranean, or low-fat diet. N Engl J Med. 2008;359(3):229–41.

Sondike SB, Kay GA, Emmett MK. Weight loss regimens that control for carbohydrate quality or quantity: a review. Pediatr Diabetes. 2008;9(3 Pt 2):33–45.

Sothern MS, Udall JN, Suskind RM, Vargas A, Blecker U. Weight loss and growth velocity in obese children after very low calorie diet, exercise, and behavior modification. Act Pediatr. 2000;89:1036–43.

Turner-McGrievy GM, Barnard ND, Scialli AR. A 2-year randomized weight loss trial comparing a vegan diet to a more moderate low-fat diet. Obesity. 2007;15(9):2276–81.

REFERENCES

1. Whitaker RC, Wright JA, Pepe MS, Seidel KD, Dietz WH. Predicting obesity in young adulthood from childhood and parental obesity. N Engl J Med. 1997;337(13):869–73.

2. Stovitz SD, Pereira MA, Vazquez G, Lytle LA, Himes JH. The interaction of childhood height and childhood BMI in the prediction of young adult BMI. Obesity. 2008;16(10):2336–41.

3. Nader PR, O'Brien M, Houts R, et al. Identifying risk for obesity in early childhood. Pediatrics. Sept 2006;118(3):e594–601.

4. Perri MG. The maintenance of treatment effects in the long-term management of obesity. Clin Psychol. 1998;5(4): 526–43.

5. Faith MS, Saelens BE, Wilfley DE, Allison DB. Behavioral treatment of childhood and adolescent obesity: current status, challenges, and future directions. In: Thompson JK, Smolak L, editors. Body image, eating disorders, and obesity in youth: assessment, prevention, and treatment. Washington, DC: American Psychological Association; 2001. pp. 313–39.

6. Tanofsky-Kraff MH, Hayden-Wade HA, Cavazos P, Wilfley DE. Pediatric overweight treatment and prevention. In: Anderson R, editor. Overweight: etiology, assessment, treatment and prevention. Champaign, IL: Human Kinetics; 2003. pp. 155–76.

7. Simon C, Schweitzer B, Oujaa M, et al. Successful overweight prevention in adolescents by increasing physical activity: a 4-year randomized controlled intervention. Int J Obes. 2008;32:1489–98.

8. Epstein LH, Myers MD, Raynor HA, Saelens BE. Treatment of pediatric obesity. Pediatrics. 1998;101(3): S554–70.

9. Jelalian E, Saelens BE. Empirically supported treatment in pediatric psychology: pediatric obesity. J Pediatr Psychol. 1999;24(3):223–48.

10. Nowicka P, Flodmark C. Family in pediatric obesity management: a literature review. Int J Pediatr Obes. 2008;3:44–50.

11. Epstein LH. Family-based behavioral intervention for obese children. Int J Obes Relat Metab Disord. 1996;20:14–21.

12. Epstein LH, Valoski AM, Koeske R, Wing RR. Family-based behavioral weight control in obese young children. J Am Diet Assoc. 1986;86:481–4.

13. Epstein LH, Valoski AM, Wing RR, McCurley J. Ten-year follow-up of behavioral, family-based treatment for obese children. J Am Med Assoc. 1990;264:2519–23.

14. Epstein LH, Valoski AM, Wing RR, McCurley J. Ten-year outcomes of behavioral family based treatment for childhood obesity. Health Psychol. 1994;13:373–83.

15. Epstein LH, Wing RR, Koeske R, Valoski A. A comparison of lifestyle exercise, aerobic exercise, and calisthenics on weight loss in obese children. Behav Ther. 1985;16(4):345–56.

16. Epstein LH, Paluch R, Roemmich JN, Beecher MD. Family-based obesity treatment: then and now. Twenty-five years of pediatric obesity treatment. Health Psychol. 2007;26(4):381–91.

17. Pratt CA, Stevens J, Daniels S. Childhood obesity prevention and treatment: recommendations for future research. Am J Prev Med. Sept 2008;35(3):249–52.

18. Wilfley DE, Stein RI, Saelens BE, et al. Efficacy of maintenance treatment approaches for childhood overweight: a randomized controlled trial. J Am Med Assoc. 2007;298(14):1661–73.

19. Kalarchian M, Levine MD, Arslanian SA, et al. Family-based treatment of severe pediatric obesity: randomized, controlled trial. Pediatrics. 2009;124:1060–8.

20. ADA. Position of the American Dietetic Association: individual-, family-, school-, and community-based interventions for pediatric overweight. J Am Diet Assoc. 2006;106(6):925–45.

21. Wake MW, Baur LA, Gerner B, et al. Outcomes and costs of primary care surveillance and intervention for overweight or obese children: the LEAP 2 randomised controlled trial. BMJ. 2009;339:1–8.

22. Hunt MS, Katzmarzyk PT, Perusse L, Rice T, Rao DC, Bouchard C. Familial resemblance of 7-year changes in body mass and adiposity. Obes Res. 2002;10:507–17.

23. Golan M, Weizman A. Familial approach to the treatment of childhood obesity: conceptual model. J Nutr Educ. 2001;33(2):102–7.

24. Young KM, Northern JJ, Lister KM, Drummond JA, O'Brien WH. A meta-analysis of family-behavioral weight-loss treatments for children. Clin Psychol Rev. 2007;27:240–9.

25. Davison KK, Birch LL. Childhood overweight: a contextual model and recommendations for future research. Obes Rev. 2001;2:159–71.

26. Kitzmann KM, Beech BM. Family-based interventions for pediatric obesity: methodological and conceptual challenges from family psychology. J Fam Psychol. 2006;20(2):175–89.

27. Bandura A. Social foundations of thought and action: a social cognitive theory. Englewood Cliffs, NJ: Prentice-Hall; 1986.

28. Spear BA, Barlow SE, Ervin C, et al. Recommendations for treatment of child and adolescent overweight and obesity. Pediatrics. 2007;120:S254–88.

29. Salvy S, Coelho JS, Kieffer E, Epstein LH. Effects of social context on overweight and normal-weight children's food intake. Physiol Behav. 2007;92(5):840–6.

30. Epstein LH, Paluch RA, Beecher MD, Roemmich JN. Increasing healthy eating vs. reducing high energy-dense foods to treat pediatric obesity. Obesity. 2008;16(2):318–26.

31. Katan MB. Weight-loss diets for the prevention and treatment of obesity. N Engl J Med. 2009;360(9):923–5.

32. Sacks FM, Bray GA, Carey VJ, et al. Comparison of weight-loss diets with different compositions of fat, protein, and carbohydrates. N Engl J Med. 2009;360(9):859–73.

33. Epstein LH, Squires S. The stoplight diet for children. Boston, MA: Little, Brown and Co; 1988.

34. TODAY Study Group. Design of a family-based lifestyle intervention for youth with type 2 diabetes: The TODAY Study. Int J Obes. 2010;34(2):217–26.

35. de Oliveira MC, Sichieri R, Venturim MR. A low-energy-dense diet adding fruit reduces weight and energy intake in women. Appetite. 2008;51:291–5.

36. Epstein LH, Gordy CC, Raynor HA, Beddome M, Kilanowski CK, Paluch R. Increasing fruit and vegetable intake and decreasing fat and sugar intake in families at risk for childhood obesity. Obes Res. 2001;9(3):171–8.

37. Ebbeling CB, Leidig MM, Feldman HA, Lovesky MM, Ludwig DS. Effects of a low-glycemic load vs low-fat diet in obese young adults: a randomized trial. J Am Med Assoc. May 2007;297(19):2092–102.

38. Troiano RP, Briefel RR, Carroll MD, Bialostosky K. Energy and fat intakes of children and adolescents in the United States: data from the National Health and Nutrition Examination Surveys. Am J Clin Nutr. Nov 2000;72(5):1343–53S.

39. Wang YC, Ludwig DS, Sonneville K, Gortmaker SL. Impact of change in sweetened caloric beverage consumption on energy intake among children and adolescents. Arch Pediatr Adolesc Med. 2009;163(4):336–43.

40. Jahns L, Siega-Riz AM, Popkin BM. The increasing prevalence of snacking among US children from 1977 to 1996. J Pediatr. 2001;138:493–8.

41. Epstein LH, Paluch R, Kilanowski CK, Raynor HA. The effect of reinforcement or stimulus control to reduce sedentary behavior in the treatment of pediatric obesity. Health Psychol. 2004;23:371–80.

42. Lin B-H, Frazao E. Away-from-home foods increasingly important to quality of American diet. Agric Inf Bull. 1999;AIB749:1–32.

43. Barlow SE, Dietz WH. Obesity evaluation and treatment: expert committee recommendations. Pediatrics. 1998;102(3):e29–39.

44. Orlet Fisher J, Rolls BJ, Birch LL. Children's bite size and intake of an entree are greater with large portions than with age-appropriate or self-selected portions. Am J Clin Nutr. 2003;77:1164–70.

45. Williams JH, Auslander WF, de Groot M, Robinson AD, Houston C, Haire-Joshu D. Cultural relevancy of a diabetes prevention nutrition program for African American women. Health Promot Pract. Jan 2006;7(1):56–67.

46. U.S. Department of Health and Human Services. Physical activity guidelines advisory committee report. Washington, DC: Department of Health and Human Services; 2008.

47. Epstein LH, Goldfield GS. Physical activity in the treatment of childhood overweight and obesity: current evidence and research issues. Med Sci Sports Exerc. 1999;31(11):S553–9.

48. Epstein LH, Kilanowski CK, Consalvi AR, Paluch RA. Reinforcing value of physical activity as a determinant of child activity level. Health Psychol. 1999;18(6):599–603.

49. American Academy of Pediatrics Committee on Public Education. Children, adolescents, and television. Pediatrics. 2001;107:423–6.

50. Epstein LH, Paluch R, Gordy CC, Dorn J. Decreasing sedentary behaviors in treating pediatric obesity. Arch Pediatr Adolesc Med. 2000;154:220–6.

51. Epstein LH, Paluch RA, Consalvi A, Riordan K, Scholl T. Effects of manipulating sedentary behavior on physical activity and food intake. J Pediatr. 2002;140(3):334–9.

52. Gortmaker SL, Must A, Sobol AM, Peterson K, Colditz GA, Dietz WH. Television viewing as a cause of increasing obesity among children in the United States, 1986–1990. Arch Pediatr Adolesc Med. 1996;150(4):356–62.

53. Coon KA, Goldberg J, Rogers BL, Tucker KL. Relationships between use of television during meals and children's food consumption patterns. Pediatrics. 2001;107(1):1–9.

54. Epstein LH, Wing RR, Woodall K, Penner BC, Kress MJ, Koeske R. Effects of family-based behavioral treatment on obese 5–8 year old children. Behav Ther. 1985;16:205–12.

55. Epstein LH, Wing RR, Koeske R, Valoski AM. Effects of diet plus exercise on weight change in parents and children. J Consult Clin Psychol. 1984;52:429–37.

56. Graves T, Meyers AW, Clark L. An evaluation of parental problem solving training in the behavioral treatment of childhood obesity. J Consult Clin Psychol. 1988;56(2):246–50.

57. Golan M, Fainaru M, Weizman A. Role of behavior modification in the treatment of childhood obesity with the parents as the exclusive agents of change. Int J Obes. 1998;22:1217–24.

58. Nothwehr F, Yang JZ. Goal setting frequency and the use of behavioral strategies related to diet and physical activity. Health Educ Res. 2007;22(4):532–8.

59. Wilfley DE, Saelens BE. Behavioral weight control for overweight adolescents initiated in primary care. Obesity. 2001;10:22–32.

60. Epstein LH, Wing RR, Koeske R, Andrasik F, Ossip DJ. Child and parent weight loss in family-based behavior modification programs. J Consult Clin Psychol. 1981;49:672–85.

61. Kirschenbaum DS, Harris ES, Tomarken AJ. Effects of parental involvement in behavioral weight-loss therapy for preadolescents. Behav Ther. 1984;15:485–500.

62. Wadden TA, Butryn M, Byrne K. Efficacy of lifestyle modification for long-term weight control. Obes Res. 2004;12:151–62S.

63. White MA, Martin PD, Newton RL, et al. Mediators of weight loss in a family-based intervention presented over the internet. Obes Res. 2004;12:1050–9.

64. Israel AC, Stolmaker L, Sharp JP, Silverman WK, Simon LG. An evaluation of two methods of parental involvement in treating obese children. Behav Ther. 1984;15:266–72.

65. Golan M, Crow S. Parents are key players in the prevention and treatment of weight-related problems. Nutr Rev. 2004;62(1):39–50.

66. Golan M, Crow S. Targeting parents exclusively in the treatment of childhood obesity: long-term results. Obes Res. 2004;12(2):357–61.

67. Wrotniak BH, Epstein LH, Roemmich JN, Paluch R, Pak Y. The relationship between parent weight change and child weight change from 6 months to 10 years in family-based behavioral weight control treatment. Obes Res. 2005;13(6):1089–96.

68. Perry RP, LeBow MD, Buser MM. An exploration of obese observational learning in modifying selected eating responses of obese children. Int J Obes. 1979;3(3):193–9.

69. Ritchie LD, Welk G, Styne D, Gerstein DE, Crawford PB. Family environment and pediatric overweight: what is a parent to do? J Am Diet Assoc. 2005;105(5):70–9.

70. Wrotniak BH, Epstein LH, Paluch R, Roemmich JN. The relationship between parent and child self-reported adherence and weight loss. Obes Res. 2005;13:1089–96.

71. Wrotniak BH, Epstein LH, Paluch RA, Roemmich JN. Parent weight change as a predictor of child weight change in family-based behavioral obesity treatment. Arch Pediatr Adolesc Med. 2004;158:342–7.

72. McGovern L, Johnson JN, Paulo R, et al. Treatment of pediatric obesity: a systematic review and meta-analysis of randomized trials. J Clin Endocrinol Metab. 2008;93(12):4600–5.

73. Duffy G, Spence SH. The effectiveness of cognitive self-management as an adjunct to a behavioural intervention for childhood obesity: a research note. J Child Psychol Psychiatry. 1993;34(6):1043–50.

74. McLean N, Griffin S, Toney K, Hardeman W. Family involvement in weight control, weight maintenance and weight-loss interventions: a systematic review of randomized trials. Int J Obes Relat Metab Disord. 2003;27:987–1005.

75. Jeffery RW, Drewnowski A, Epstein LH, et al. Long-term maintenance of weight loss: current status. Health Psychol. 2000;19(1 Suppl):5–16.

76. Bouton ME. Context, ambiguity, and unlearning: sources of relapse after behavioral extinction. Biol Psychiatry. 2002;52(10):976–86.

77. Kumanyika SK. Cultural differences as influences in obesity treatment. In: Bray GA, Bouchard C, editors. Handbook of obesity: clinical applications, vol. 1, 3rd ed. New York, NY: Informa Health Care; 2008. pp. 45–68.

78. Wilfley DE, Van Buren DJ, Theim KR, et al. The use of biosimulation in the design of a novel multi-level weight loss maintenance program for overweight children. Obesity. 2010;18(1 Suppl):S91–8.

79. Davis CA, Levitan RD, Reid C, et al. Dopamine for "wanting" and opioids for "liking": a comparison of obese adults with and without binge eating. Obesity. 2009;17(6):1220–5.

80. Epstein LH, Temple JL, Neaderhiser BJ, Salis RJ, Erbe RW, Leddy JJ. Food reinforcement, the dopamine D2 receptor genotype, and energy intake in obese and nonobese humans. Behav Neurosci. 2007;121(5):877–86.

81. Tanofsky-Kraff M, Han JC, Anandalingam K, et al. The FTO gene rs9939609 obesity-risk allele and loss of control over eating. Am J Clin Nutr. 2009;90(6):1483–8.

82. Wardle J, Carnell S. Appetite is a heritable phenotype associated with adiposity. Ann Behav Med. 2009;38(1 Suppl):25–30.

83. Hill JO. Can a small-changes approach help address the obesity epidemic? A report of the Joint Task Force of the American Society for Nutrition, Institute of Food Technologists, and International Food Information Council. Am J Clin Nutr. 2009;89(2):477–84.

84. Hill C, Saxton J, Webber L, Blundell J, Wardle J. The relative reinforcing value of food predicts weight gain in a longitudinal study of 7–10-years-old children. Am J Clin Nutr. 2009;90(2):276–81.

85. Goldschmidt AB, Jones M, Manwaring JL, et al. The clinical significance of loss of control over eating in overweight adolescents. Int J Eat Disord. 2008;41:153–8.

86. Goldschmidt AB, Aspen VP, Sinton MM, Tanofsky-Kraff M, Wilfley DE. Disordered eating attitudes and behaviors in overweight youth. Obesity. 2008;16(2):257–64.

87. Wardle J. The triple whammy. Psychologist. 2005;18(4):216–9.

88. Haus G, Hoerr SL, Mavis B, Robinson J. Key modifiable factors in weight maintenance: fat intake, exercise, and weight cycling. J Am Diet Assoc. 1994;94(4):409–13.

89. Perri MG. Improving maintenance of weight loss following treatment by diet and lifestyle modification. In: Wadden TA, Van Itallie TB, editors. Treatment of the seriously obese patient. New York, NY: The Guilford Press; 1993. pp. 456–77.

90. Wadden TA, Vogt RA, Foster GD, Anderson DA. Exercise and the maintenance of weight loss: 1-year follow-up of a controlled clinical trial. J Consult Clin Psychol. Apr 1998;66(2):429–33.

91. Bennett GA. Behavior therapy for obesity: a quantitative review of the effects of selected treatment characteristics on outcome. Behav Ther. 1986;17(5):554–62.

92. Epstein LH. Development of evidence-based treatments for pediatric obesity. In: Kazdin AE, Weisz JR, editors. Evidence-based psychotherapies for children and adolescents. New York, NY: Guilford Press; 2003.

93. Zabinski MF, Saelens BE, Stein RI, Hayden-Wade HA, Wilfley DE. Overweight children's barriers to and support for physical activity. Obes Res. 2003;11(2):238–46.

94. Glass TA, McAtee MJ. Behavioral science at the crossroads in public health: extending horizons, envisioning the future. Soc Sci Med. 2006;62(7):1650–71.

95. Huang TT, Drenowski A, Kumanyika SK, Glass TA. A systems-oriented multilevel framework for addressing obesity in the 21st century. Prev Chronic Dis. 2009;6(3):1–10.

96. McGuire MT, Wing RR, Klem ML, Lang W, Hill JO. What predicts weight regain in a group of successful weight losers? J Consult Clin Psychol. 1999;67(2):177–85.

97. Wing RR, Tate AA, Gorin HA, Raynor HA, Fava JL. A self-regulation program for maintenance of weight loss. N Engl J Med. 2006;355(15):1563–71.

98. Christakis NA, Fowler JH. The spread of obesity in a large social network over 32 years. N Engl J Med. 2007;357(4):370–9.

99. Hill JO, Wyatt HR, Reed GW, Peters JC. Obesity and the environment: where do we go from here? Science. 2003;299:853–5.

100. Hayden-Wade HA, Stein RI, Ghaderi A, Saelens BE, Zabinski MF, Wilfley DE. Prevalence, characteristics, and correlates of teasing experiences among overweight children vs. non-overweight peers. Obes Res. 2005;13(8):1381–92.

101. Salvy S, Romero N, Paluch R, Epstein LH. Peer influence on pre-adolescent girls snack intake: effects of weight status. Appetite. 2007;49(1):177–82.

102. Salvy SJ, Bowker JW, Roemmich JN, et al. Peer influence on children's physical activity: an experience sampling study. J Pediatr Psychol. 2008;33(1):39–49.

103. Smith AL. Perceptions of peer relationships and physical activity participation in early adolescence. J Sport Exerc Psychol. 1999;21(4):329–50.

104. Neumark-Sztainer D, Wall M, Perry CL, Story M. Correlates of fruit and vegetable intake among adolescents. Findings from project EAT. Prev Med. 2003;37(3):198–208.

105. Litt MD, Kadden RM, Kabela-Cormier E, Petry N. Changing network support for drinking: initial findings from the network support project. J Consult Clin Psychol. 2007;75:542–55.

106. Sallis JF, Glanz K. The role of built environments in physical activity, eating, and obesity in childhood. Future Child. 2006;16(1):89–108.

107. Epstein LH, Raja S, Gold SS, Paluch RA, Roemmich JN. The neighborhood built environment influences substitution of physical activity for sedentary behavior in youth. Psych Sci. 2006;17:654–9.

108. Roemmich JN, Epstein LH, Raja S, Yin L, Robinson J, Winiewicz D. Association of access to parks and recreational facilities with the physical activity of young children. Prev Med. 2006;43(6):437–41.

109. Roemmich JN, Epstein LH, Raja S, Yin L. The neighborhood and home environments: disparate relationships with physical activity and sedentary behaviors in youth. Ann Behav Med. 2007;33(1):29–38.

110. Jago R, Baranowski T, Baranowski JC, Cullen KW, Thompson D. Distance to food stores & adolescent male fruit and vegetable consumption: mediation effects. Int J Behav Nutr Phys Act. 2007;4:35.

111. Tanofsky-Kraff M, Wilfley DE. Interpersonal psychotherapy for the treatment of eating disorders. In: Agras WS, editor. Oxford handbook of eating disorders. New York, NY: Oxford University Press (in press).

112. Tanofsky-Kraff M, Wilfley DE, Young JF et al. A pilot study of interpersonal psychotherapy for preventing excess weight gain in adolescent girls at-risk for obesity. Int J Eat Disord 2009. [epub ahead of print].

113. Snethen JA, Broome ME, Cashin SE. Effective weight loss for overweight children: a meta-analysis of intervention studies. J Pediatr Nurs. 2006;21(1):45–56.

114. Tsiros MD, Sinn N, Coates AM, Howe PR, Buckley JD. Treatment of adolescent overweight and obesity. Eur J Pediatr. 2008;167(1):9–16.

21 Exercise and Childhood Obesity

Alon Eliakim and Dan Nemet

CONTENTS

Key Words: Nutrition, physical activity, fitness, growth hormone, catecholamines, training

INTRODUCTION

The mechanisms responsible for the increasing prevalence of childhood obesity are not entirely understood, yet lifestyle changes associated with increased caloric intake and decreased energy expenditure probably play central roles, especially in genetically predisposed populations *(1–3)*. This indicates that preventive health education and therapeutic programs for childhood obesity require a multi-disciplinary approach that includes lifestyle/behavioral modification, nutritional education, and changes in physical activity patterns *(4,5)*. In this chapter we will focus on the relationships between children's exercise knowledge and preferences and obesity; habitual activity and fitness level of obese children; the effect of exercise on appetite and nutritional preferences; the hormonal effects of exercise in obese children; and the role of exercise training as part of a multi-disciplinary approach to treat childhood obesity.

WHAT DO YOUNG CHILDREN KNOW ABOUT NUTRITION AND EXERCISE AND HOW DOES THIS AFFECT THEIR PREFERENCES?

Intervention programs for the treatment of childhood obesity must take into account the existing nutritional and physical activity knowledge and preferences of children. In light of the fact that the roots of obesity begin early in children's lives, it is interesting that only a few studies have examined the nutritional and physical activity knowledge of elementary school-aged and kindergarten children.

From: *Contemporary Endocrinology: Pediatric Obesity: Etiology, Pathogenesis, and Treatment*
Edited by: M. Freemark, DOI 10.1007/978-1-60327-874-4_21,
© Springer Science+Business Media, LLC 2010

Two older studies in schoolchildren raised concerns regarding lack of knowledge about food composition; findings noted their inability to choose foods low in fat and/or saturated fat and their limited understanding of fiber *(6,7)*. A third investigation *(8)* in kindergartners assessed nutritional and physical activity knowledge and preferences using a photo-pair food and exercise questionnaire developed by Calfas et al. *(9)*. Physical activity knowledge scores were found to be significantly lower than nutrition knowledge scores. However, while food preferences were not consistent with food knowledge in kindergarten children, physical activity knowledge and preference were concordant (Fig. 1).

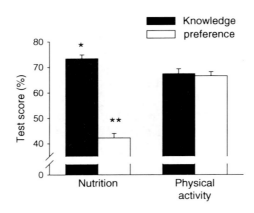

Fig. 1. Nutrition and physical activity knowledge and preferences of kindergarten children [data from Nemet et al. *(8)*]. *$p < 0.0001$ nutrition knowledge vs. preference. ** $p < 0.006$ nutrition knowledge vs. physical activity knowledge.

Previous studies in kindergarten children also reported that food preferences were not consistent with knowledge of dietary guidelines *(10)*. This suggests that dietary education should not only focus on delivering nutritional information to children; rather it should develop new ways to reinforce existing nutritional knowledge so that children can make better and healthier food choices.

Nutritional intervention studies in kindergarten children have been associated with positive effects on food selection *(11,12)*. In order to promote physical activity, efforts should concentrate on increasing children's knowledge about the importance of physical activity and fitness on health. Since exercise knowledge correlates positively with exercise preference, the expansion of exercise knowledge will probably beget more active lives. Promoting physical activity in kindergartens and schools may limit the frequency and/or severity of common childhood diseases (obesity, diabetes, lipid abnormalities, asthma, etc.) and might also be associated with increased academic performance and improved quality of life *(13,14)*.

Interestingly, gender differences were found in the kindergartners' nutritional and physical activity knowledge and preference scores. Nutritional knowledge and preference scores were significantly higher in females, while physical activity preferences were significantly higher in males. This finding indicates that the development of gender-specific favorite interests and inclinations occurs as early as the pre-school and kindergarten years. Therefore, health-care providers should concentrate on developing new methods to increase nutritional knowledge in young boys and to improve physical activity preferences and the motivation to exercise in young girls.

Finally, there were no differences in nutritional and physical activity knowledge and preferences scores between overweight (BMI > 85 percentile) and normal weight kindergarten children. This suggests that there might still be a gap between knowledge or preference and its actual implementation in overweight youth. Therefore, efforts should be made to create environments that will encourage obese pre-school and kindergarten children to eat healthier foods and exercise. Strategies might include additional physical exercise classes for children and/or homework that includes physical activity.

However, since obese children may feel embarrassed to exercise with their normal weight peers, and since obese children tend to increase their physical activity and improve their fitness when trained in small groups of only obese partners (15), referral to structured programs for obese children might be required.

OBESITY AND HABITUAL PHYSICAL ACTIVITY

The increased prevalence of childhood obesity in recent decades occurred despite little or no change in overall energy intake and a decrease in fat consumption, suggesting that reduced energy expenditure probably plays a major role. Increased sedentary behaviors such as television viewing and computer games no doubt contribute to this trend (16); the likelihood of developing overweight increases dramatically as a function of hours of television watching (five times higher for watcher of >5 h/day compared to <2 h/day) (17). Moreover, Viner et al. demonstrated that television viewing in early childhood can predict adult body mass index (18): each additional daily hour of television viewing (mainly during the weekends) at the age of 5 years increased by 7% the risk of having BMI above 30 kg/m^2 at the age of 30 years. The cause for these relationships is reduced energy expenditure during TV watching and enhanced intake of high-caloric foods, which rises in proportion to the number of food-related commercials (19,20).

There is some evidence to support the idea that obese children are usually less active when compared to normal weight children; one well-cited investigation of a small number of subjects found that obese children spent more time sitting, standing, and walking during the day while normal weight children spent far more time running (21). Yet the total energy expenditure of obese children, estimated by oxygen cost or the doubly labeled water technique, is not reduced when measured in absolute terms; however, it is lower when normalized to body mass (21,22), consistent with normal or increased basal metabolic rate (reflecting muscle metabolism) and an excess of body fat.

There are a number of possible explanations for these findings. First, it is likely that apparent or observed activity patterns do not accurately reflect energy expenditure. Second, it is possible that the link between reduced physical activity and obesity is indirect, mediated by other factors that promote obesity such as increased food intake. Third, measurements of energy expenditure in obese children would not detect prior reductions in energy expenditure that led to the development of obesity in the first place. In this regard, Roberts et al. demonstrated that total energy expenditure (TEE), but not resting energy expenditure, of 12-month-old overweight infants of obese mothers was lower at the age of 3 months (23). However, other studies in normal weight mothers failed to demonstrate a relationship between TEE at the age of 3 months and obesity at 2–3 years (24). Finally, measurements of energy expenditure in obese children (and adults) reflect in part the body's adaptive responses to weight change (see the Chapter 4 by Lustig and Chapter 28 by Lechan and Fekete) and therefore cannot determine if hypoactivity is a cause or consequence of obesity.

Recently, Ischander et al. (25). assessed patterns of daily life (e.g., participation in high school sports) in a group of normal weight adolescent girls to determine whether or not levels of habitual physical activity per se influenced anatomic indices of body composition, circulating inflammatory mediators, and growth factors. Sedentary and physically active girls were matched for BMI (mean 58.7 percentile, none > 85th percentile); as expected from the recruitment/selection strategy, the two groups differed substantially in habitual physical activity (sedentary: ≤ three 20-min bouts of vigorous physical activity per week and ≤ five 30-min bouts of moderate physical activity per week; active: ≥60 min of moderate-to-vigorous physical activity per day). Lower levels of inflammatory mediators and leptin and higher levels of adiponectin and fitness were found in the active girls. Moreover, active girls had significantly higher lean body mass and reduced fat mass. These data demonstrate that habitual levels of physical activity influence inflammatory and growth mediators in adolescent girls and can alter body composition in a way that is not detectable by measuring BMI alone. As there is mounting evidence that a variety of adult diseases originate from lifestyle patterns during childhood and adolescence *(26)*, the beneficial effects of exercise-associated reduced inflammatory mediators and increased adiponectin levels in this important period must be appreciated.

OBESITY AND FITNESS

Many (but not all *(29)*) laboratory and field-based studies report that the fitness level of obese children is lower than that of non-obese children, and that reduced fitness is related to the degree of obesity. For example, maximal oxygen consumption (VO_2max) normalized to body weight, an indicator of aerobic fitness, correlated inversely with percent body fat estimated either by skinfold measurements or by abdominal and thigh MRI *(27)*. However, variability in the relative proportion of fat and muscle can confound the determination of fitness when VO_2max is normalized to body weight. This is because VO_2max is determined primarily by the metabolically active exercising muscle, while body weight includes both muscle and fat.

To interpret this data it is useful to consider two separate components of fitness: muscle size *dependent* and muscle size *independent*. In the former, training-induced increases in measurements like VO_2max are mediated by increases in muscle mass; in the latter, increases result from other factors such as greater muscle tissue capillary or mitochondrial density and/or alterations in muscle fiber type. To evaluate the roles of muscle and fat mass in body fitness we assessed the relationship between VO_2max/kg body weight and thigh muscle volume and fat content in adolescents during cycle ergometry. As shown in Fig. 2, aerobic fitness as measured by VO_2max/kg body weight was inversely related to thigh (and abdominal) fat content; however, this relationship was abolished when VO_2max/kg body weight was normalized for thigh muscle volume. Moreover, VO_2max scaled *directly* (i.e., a scaling factor not different from 1.0) with muscle volume in this population.

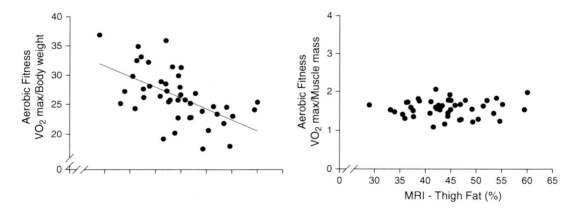

Fig. 2. Cross-sectional relationship between fitness determined by VO_2max normalized to body weight and mean thigh fat percent assessed by MRI *(upper panel, r = –0.57, p < 0.002)*. Cross-sectional relationship between VO_2max normalized to thigh muscle volume and mean thigh fat percent *(lower panel, r = 0.06, NS)*. Size-independent components of VO_2max were not related to adiposity [data from Eliakim et al. *(27)*].

These observations suggested that size-*independent* components of VO_2max are not related to fatness. The decrease in VO_2max/kg with increasing fatness occurred because the proportion of muscle volume to fat volume in the thigh decreases as weight increases. Simply put, while obese children might have an increased muscle mass, this mass is not great enough to support and carry their increased body weight. The same applies for muscle strength. No differences were found in isokinetic muscle force per muscle cross-sectional area, and there were no differences in contractile characteristics except for lower activated motor unit percentage during maximal voluntary contraction *(28)*. Therefore, the reduced performance of obese children in tasks that require lifting/carrying their own bodies does not result from reduced muscle contractile ability but from reduced muscle mass relative to excess body mass.

Another reason for the decreased performance of obese children during aerobic tasks is reduced economy of movement (higher O_2 uptake during sub-maximal effort). Reduced economy of movement is evident mainly during weight bearing activities (e.g., walking) and at high speeds. The cause for the high cost of locomotion in obese children is the higher fat mass and a "wasteful activity pattern" accompanied by gait asymmetry, longer gait cycle and stance duration, and reduced velocity *(29,30)*.

Finally, obese children and adolescents rate the intensity of exercise higher than normal weight peers *(31)*. A higher rating of perceived exertion may result in reluctance to pursue intense or prolonged exercise activities.

HORMONAL EFFECTS OF EXERCISE IN OBESE CHILDREN

Very few studies have examined the hormonal effects of exercise in obese children and adolescents. A recent investigation *(32)* assessed the effects of intense exercise on the growth hormone (GH)/IGF axis and neuroadrenergic hormones in obese compared with normal weight children and adolescents. The exercise consisted of ten 2-min bouts of constant work rate cycle ergometry at a level 50% between the anaerobic threshold and maximal oxygen consumption, with a 1-min rest interval between each of the 10 exercise bouts. The major finding of the study was that GH and catecholamine responses to exercise were attenuated in obese subjects (Fig. 3). In contrast, peak heart rate, respiratory exchange ratio,

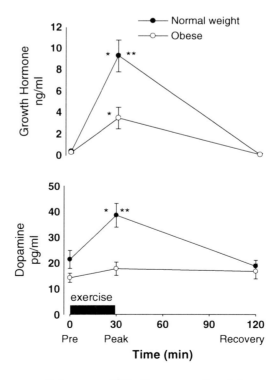

Fig. 3. The effect of exercise on growth hormone (GH, *Upper panel*) and dopamine (*Lower panel*) in obese and normal weight children. Peak levels of both GH and dopamine were significantly reduced in obese children [data from Eliakim *(32)*]. * Within group differences ($p < 0.05$). ** Between group differences ($p < 0.05$).

serum lactate levels, and peak VO_2 normalized to lean body mass were comparable to those of normal weight subjects, indicating that the cardiovascular responses to maximal exercise were equivalent in the two groups.

The mechanisms underlying the blunted GH response to exercise in obese children are not completely understood, but may reflect baseline reductions in ghrelin, increases in insulin and free IGF-1, and the general attenuation of GH responses to stimulation characteristic of obesity. The reduced epinephrine and norepinephrine responses and the absent dopamine response to exercise in obese subjects suggest the possibility of a centrally mediated attenuation of sympathetic adrenomedullary function. Reduced central dopaminergic tone could explain the blunted catecholamine and GH responses to exercise in obese subjects. There are indirect data suggesting that dopamine-2 receptor (D2) gene expression may be abnormal in obese subjects (33); in theory, this could lead to reduced central dopaminergic tone.

Several investigators (e.g., Kanaley and coworkers (34)) speculate that the attenuation of GH responses in obese subjects might limit the benefits derived from exercise. However, it is now well established that many of the effects of exercise training are mediated by IGF-I and are GH independent (35,36). Despite the reduced GH response to exercise in obese subjects, levels of total IGF-I did not differ between the two groups, and IGF-I increased significantly with exercise in the obese as well as the normal weight subjects. Thus, the attenuated GH response to exercise in obesity appears to be compensated by other hormonal mechanisms. Nevertheless, exercise might have less impact in obese children with true GH deficiency, low baseline IGF-I levels, and low IGF-I responses to exercise (as, for example, in children with Prader–Willi syndrome (37)). Such children might benefit from an intensive approach that includes both exercise and exogenous GH.

Interestingly, both pre- and post-exercise insulin levels were significantly elevated in obese children. The combination of hyperinsulinemia with suppressed GH and catecholamine responses could in theory increase the risk of hypoglycemia during and after exercise. Hypoglycemia is rare in this setting, but the lower GH and catecholamine levels in obese children may reduce carbohydrate and fat utilization during exercise and thereby increase protein utilization (38–44). This may explain, at least partially, the difficulty in reducing fat stores and increasing muscle mass in obese subjects through exercise alone. Consistent with this hypothesis, previous studies demonstrated that elevated BMI was associated with reduced responses to prolonged resistance training (39). It is possible that the baseline GH and catecholamine responses to exercise might predict the response to weight reduction interventions; an insufficient GH or catecholamine response might presage a need for more intense intervention. Further studies are needed to clarify the extent to which these hormonal abnormalities persist after weight loss and/or exercise training programs in obese children and adolescents.

Finally, the relationship between pre-exercise food consumption and hormonal responses was recently examined in children (40). The GH response to exercise was severely attenuated when children were given a fatty meal 45 min before exercise. Therefore, exercise intervention programs for obese children should account for the content of pre-exercise meals.

OBESITY AND EXERCISE-RELATED FOOD CHOICES

Animal and human adult studies suggest that appetite is suppressed and total energy intake reduced immediately after strenuous exercise (41,42). However, macronutrient choices are also modulated by exercise. Exercise-induced increases in catecholamines, growth hormone, and free fatty acids acutely increase carbohydrate intake and decrease fat intake (43).

Very few studies have examined the relationships between physical activity and nutrition in childhood obesity. The effects of different types of physical activity (e.g., aerobic, resistance and swimming) on appetite and food choices were recently studied in normal weight and obese pre-pubertal children (44). The immediate effects of exercise on macronutrient choices were found to differ significantly between normal weight and overweight pre-pubertal children. Total energy intake was reduced following resistance-type exercise in the normal weight children. Moreover, all forms of exercise were associated with increased relative consumption of carbohydrate and decreased consumption of fat in the normal weight children. In contrast, all types of exercise increased the relative consumption of protein in overweight children, and total energy intake normalized to body mass was significantly increased in the obese children following the swimming practice. This suggests that swimming might be less effective than other forms of aerobic exercise in achieving negative energy balance and reducing body weight in obese children.

The mechanisms controlling the post-exercise increase in energy and protein intake in obese children are not known. As noted previously, the blunted GH and catecholamine responses to exercise may reduce carbohydrate and fat utilization and increase protein utilization; this may explain why appetite was not suppressed in the obese children immediately following exercise and why protein intake increased.

It is important to point out that our study tested only the *immediate* effects of a single bout of exercise on food intake. It is possible that the various forms of exercise have intermediate or long-term effects as well or that both the normal weight and the obese children compensate for immediate effects during the rest of the day.

Very little is known about the effects of chronic exercise training on food and macronutrient consumption. It was thought that an increase in physical activity would be accompanied by increases in appetite and food intake. However, the few studies of obese children found that increased activity was accompanied by a decrease in energy intake; even if intake increases with exercise, negative energy balance persists *(45)*. It is speculated that increased appetite occurs only above a threshold level of physical activity. The activity level of obese children in exercise intervention programs is probably below this threshold *(46)*.

EXERCISE TRAINING AND TREATMENT OF CHILDHOOD OBESITY

The short- and long-term effects of lifestyle behavioral, nutritional, and physical activity interventions for the treatment of childhood obesity were recently assessed in a Cochrane review *(47)*. Only randomized, controlled trials were selected for evaluation, with a minimum of 6 months follow-up. The primary outcome of the review was BMI standard deviation scores (SDS) and percentage overweight. Sixty-four studies were included in the review, and only 12 studied the effect of lifestyle interventions that focused on physical activity and sedentary behavior. Nine of the interventions were performed in pre-pubertal children (defined as <12-year-old) and were compared to standard care. Of these, some *(48,49)* found beneficial effects on adiposity and pedometer walking with no significant between group differences. Weintraub et al. *(50)* compared an after school soccer program to an active placebo (health and nutrition education program) and found that the subsequent increase in BMI was significantly smaller in the soccer group. Three studies compared an experimental activity program to an active placebo or control intervention for the treatment of adolescent obesity (defined as >12-year-old). The authors *(51–53)* found that an after school activity program had no effect on BMI-SDS compared to an active placebo or control group. The conclusion of the Cochrane review authors was that "... a combined dietary, physical activity and behavioral intervention appears effective. Family-based, lifestyle interventions with a behavioral program aimed at changing diet and physical activity thinking patterns provide significant and clinically meaningful decrease in overweight in both children and adolescents compared to standard care or self help in the short and long-term."

We recently demonstrated *(15)* the short (3 months) and longer term (1 year) beneficial effects of a combined nutritional–behavioral–physical activity intervention in obese children and adolescents. The 3-month intervention included four evening lectures (childhood obesity, general nutrition, therapeutic nutritional approach for childhood obesity, and exercise and childhood obesity) for the children and their parents. Participants met with the dietitian six times during the program and received a balanced hypocaloric diet. The diet consisted of 1,200–2,000 kcal depending on the age and weight of the child; this equated to a caloric intake 30% below reported intake or 15% less than estimated daily required intake. In addition participants received dietary information by working sheets/flyers on important nutritional issues.

All intervention subjects participated in a twice-weekly, endurance type training program (1 h/training session). Subjects were instructed to include an additional 30–45 min of walking/other weight bearing sport activities at least once a week. Subjects were encouraged throughout the program by the physicians, nutritionist, and coaches to reduce sedentary activities (e.g., television viewing, video games, use stairs instead of elevators, play outside instead of inside).

The intervention was associated with significant weight loss, reduced BMI, reduced body fat, increased habitual physical activity and improved fitness, and reduced total and LDL-cholesterol (Fig. 4). In contrast, obese children who received standard of care treatment gained weight, increased their body fat percent, did not change their habitual physical activity level, and had a lesser improvement in fitness. More importantly, the favorable effects on body weight, BMI, body fat, and habitual physical activity and fitness were maintained in the intervention participants compared to the control subjects after a 1-year follow-up. These results highlight the importance of *multi-disciplinary* programs for the treatment of childhood obesity and emphasize the value of long-term studies to assess success.

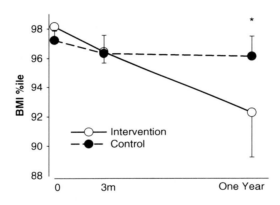

Fig. 4. The short- (3 m) and long (12 m)-term effects of a 3-month multi-disciplinary program for the treatment of childhood obesity. There was a significant reduction in BMI percentile in the intervention group compared to control [data from Nemet et al. *(15)*]. *$p < 0.05$.

The mean decrease of 5–6% in age-adjusted BMI percentiles observed in this study is impressive; some of the obese children and adolescents were no longer categorized as overweight at the 1-year follow-up, and many with marked obesity (BMI > 95%) were reclassified as overweight (BMI 85–95%). Moreover, serum cholesterol and LDL levels declined, and the level of fitness improved. This is of great importance, since increased physical fitness, even without weight loss, can improve insulin sensitivity and lipid profiles, reduce blood pressure, and reduce the risk of coronary heart disease later in life *(54)*.

Although not measured in our study, an important, often neglected, effect of exercise interventions in obese children and adolescent is psychological in nature. Training-related changes include improvement in self-esteem, body image, self-confidence, and ability to adjust to peer society *(52)*.

In summary, childhood obesity has reached epidemic proportions worldwide despite major efforts to promote weight reduction. The mechanisms responsible for the increasing prevalence of childhood obesity are not completely understood, but lifestyle changes associated with increased caloric intake and decreased energy expenditure likely play critical roles. In the future we will need to better understand the knowledge, preferences, and capabilities of young children and must delineate the relative roles of food intake and habitual physical activity in childhood weight gain and fitness. This will require a more comprehensive understanding of the hormonal effects of exercise in obese children and the role of exercise training in treatment. New information will help us to optimize exercise interventions for obese children and to select the best exercise protocols to achieve the desired energy balance.

Editor's Comment

- Winston Churchill once attributed his success in life to "conservation of energy: never stand up when you can sit down, and never sit down when you can lie down." Nevertheless, exercise reduces visceral fat mass and increases lean body mass, thereby augmenting resting energy expenditure. Aerobic training increases insulin sensitivity, reduces fasting and post-prandial glucose, free fatty acid, and TG concentrations, and increases plasma HDL levels. Muscle oxidative enzyme activity is induced, possibly via increases in mitochondrial size, the resulting induction of AMP-activated protein kinase (AMPK) promotes Glut-4-dependent glucose uptake. In the aggregate, these effects improve fitness, which in adults is related inversely to cardiovascular mortality (Jakicic, 2009).

Editor's Question and Authors' Response

- **In concert with dietary modification, exercise can promote and maintain weight loss in obese patients (Klem et al., 1997; Jakicic et al., 2008) and may help to prevent weight gain in high-risk subjects. Yet there is controversy regarding the ability of exercise per se to reduce body weight. This is because the effects of physical activity in isolation on BMI are modest and can be neutralized by subsequent food intake (see, for example, Jakicic, 2009; Melanson et al., 2009). Your studies of the effects of swimming on food intake in children are therefore of interest. Can the differential effects of swimming and other forms of aerobic exercise on food intake be explained?**

- It is a popular belief that swimming stimulates appetite and energy intake. Interestingly, our results supported this notion, but only in obese children. Although high adiposity makes floating easier and may lead to less energy expenditure in overweight children, we found that energy intake was significantly greater in the overweight compared to the normal weight children even after normalization to body weight. Previous studies suggested that a possible mechanism for the increased energy intake immediately post-swimming is related to the effects of cold immersion. This, however, cannot explain why only obese children overeat after swimming. Other studies suggested that the post-swimming increase in energy intake may be related to changes in leptin, catecholamines and dopamine. This requires additional study.

Jakicic JM, et al. Effect of exercise on 24-month weight loss maintenance in overweight women. Arch Int Med. 2008;168:1550–9.

Jakicic JM. The effect of physical activity on body weight. Obesity (Silver Spring). 2009 Dec;17 Suppl 3:S34–8.

Klem ML, Wing RR, McGuire MT, Seagle HM, Hill JO. A descriptive study of individuals successful at long-term maintenance of substantial weight loss. Am J Clin Nutr. 1997 Aug;66(2):239–46.

Melanson EL, Gozansky WS, Barry DW, Maclean PS, Grunwald GK, Hill JO. When energy balance is maintained, exercise does not induce negative fat balance in lean sedentary, obese sedentary, or lean endurance-trained individuals. J Appl Physiol. 2009 Dec;107(6):1847–56.

REFERENCES

1. Hancox RJ, Milne BJ, Poulton R. Association between child and adolescent television viewing and adult health: a longitudinal birth cohort study. Lancet. 17 Jul 2004 ;364(9430):257–62.
2. Dietz WH. Overweight in Childhood and Adolescence. N Engl J Med. 26 Feb 2004;350(9):855–7.
3. Clement K, Ferre P. Genetics and the pathophysiology of obesity. Pediatr Res. May 2003;53(5):721–5.
4. Goran MI, Reynolds KD, Lindquist CH. Role of physical activity in the prevention of obesity in children. Int J Obes Relat Metab Disord. 1999 Apr;23(Suppl 3):S18–33.
5. Williams CL, Campanaro LA, Squillace M, Bollella M. Management of childhood obesity in pediatric practice. Ann N Y Acad Sci. May 1997;28(817):225–40.
6. Zemel P, Brokaw S, Huntsinger D, McMichael C. What do teachers use and what do they need to teach healthful eating in schools? Sch Food Serv Res Rev. 1993;77(1):41–5.
7. Resnicow K, Reinhardt J. What do children know about fat, fiber, and cholesterol? A survey of primary and secondary school students. J Nutr Educ. 1991;23(3):65–71.
8. Nemet D, Perez S, Reges O, Eliakim A. Physical activity and nutrition knowledge and preferences in kindergarten children. Int J Sports Med. Oct 2007;28(10):887–90.
9. Calfas KJ, Sallis JF, Nader PR. The development of scales to measure knowledge and preference for diet and physical activity behavior in 4- to 8-year-old children. J Dev Behav Pediatr. Jun 1991;12(3):185–90.
10. Murphy AS, Youatt JP, Hoerr SL, Sawyer CA, Andrews SL. Kindergarten students' food preferences are not consistent with their knowledge of the Dietary Guidelines. J Am Diet Assoc. Feb 1995;95(2):219–23.
11. Graves K, Shannon B, Sims L, Johnson S. Nutrition knowledge and attitudes of elementary school students after receiving nutrition education. J Am Diet Assoc. Oct 1982;81(4):422–7.
12. Shannon B, Graves K, Hart M. Food behavior of elementary school students after receiving nutrition education. J Am Diet Assoc. Oct 1982;81(4):428–34.
13. Strong WB, Malina RM, Blimkie CJR, et al. Evidence based physical activity for school-age youth. J Pediatr. Jun 2005;146(6):732–7.
14. Datar A, Sturm R, Magnabosco JL. Childhood overweight and academic performance: national study of kindergartners and first-graders. Obes Res. Jan 2004;12(1):58–68.
15. Nemet D, Barkan S, Epstein Y, Friedland O, Kowen G, Eliakim A. Short- and long-term beneficial effects of a combined dietary-behavioral-physical activity intervention for the treatment of childhood obesity. Pediatrics. Apr 2005;115(4):e443–9.
16. Cheng TO. Television viewing as a global risk factor for childhood obesity. Int J Cardiol. 1 Sept 2005;103(3):344.
17. Gortmaker SL, Must A, Sobol AM, Peterson K, Colditz GA, Dietz WH. Television viewing as a cause of increasing obesity among children in the United States, 1986–1990. Arch Pediatr Adolesc Med. Apr 1996;150(4):356–62.
18. Viner RM, Cole TJ. Television viewing in early childhood predicts adult body mass index. J Pediatr. Oct 2005;147(4):429–35.
19. Klesges RC, Shelton ML, Klesges LM. Effects of television on metabolic rate: potential implications for childhood obesity. Pediatrics. Feb 1993;91(2):281–6.
20. Robinson TN. Television viewing and childhood obesity. Pediatr Clin North Am. Aug 2001;48(4):1017–25.
21. Waxman M, Stunkard AJ. Caloric intake and expenditure of obese boys. J Pediatr. Feb 1980;96(2):187–93.
22. Bandini LG, Schoeller DA, Dietz WH. Energy expenditure in obese and nonobese adolescents. Pediatr Res. Feb 1990;27(2):198–203.
23. Roberts SB, Savage J, Coward WA, Chew B, Lucas A. Energy expenditure and intake in infants born to lean and overweight mothers. N Engl J Med. 25 Feb 1988;318(8):461–6.
24. Wells JC, Stanley M, Laidlaw AS, Day JM, Davies PS. The relationship between components of infant energy expenditure and childhood body fatness. Int J Obes Relat Metab Disord. Sept 1996;20(9):848–53.
25. Ischander M, Zaldivar F Jr, Eliakim A, et al. Physical activity, growth, and inflammatory mediators in BMI-matched female adolescents. Med Sci Sports Exerc. Jul 2007;39(7):1131–8.
26. Cooper C, Westlake S, Harvey N, Javaid K, Dennison E, Hanson M. Review: developmental origins of osteoporotic fracture. Osteoporos Int. Dec 2005;6.
27. Eliakim A, Burke GS, Cooper DM. Fitness, fatness, and the effect of training assessed by magnetic resonance imaging and skinfold-thickness measurements in healthy adolescent females. Am J Clin Nutr. Aug 1997;66(2):223–31.
28. Blimkie CJ, Sale DG, Bar-Or O. Voluntary strength, evoked twitch contractile properties and motor unit activation of knee extensors in obese and non-obese adolescent males. Eur J Appl Physiol Occup Physiol. 1990;61(3–4):313–8.
29. Hills AP, Parker AW. Locomotor characteristics of obese children. Child Care Health Dev. Jan 1992;18(1):29–34.
30. Shultz SP, Anner J, Hills AP. Paediatric obesity, physical activity and the musculoskeletal system. Obes Rev. 12 May 2009;10(5):576–82.

31. Ward DS, Bar-Or O. Use of the Borg scale in exercise prescription for overweight youth. Can J Sport Sci. Jun 1990;15(2):120–5.
32. Eliakim A, Nemet D, Zaldivar F, et al. Reduced exercise-associated response of the GH-IGF-I axis and catecholamines in obese children and adolescents. J Appl Physiol. May 2006;100(5):1630–7.
33. Pijl H. Reduced dopaminergic tone in hypothalamic neural circuits: expression of a "thrifty" genotype underlying the metabolic syndrome? Eur J Pharmacol. 7 Nov 2003;480(1–3):125–31.
34. Kanaley JA, Weatherup-Dentes MM, Jaynes EB, Hartman ML. Obesity attenuates the growth hormone response to exercise. J Clin Endocrinol Metab. Sept 1999;84(9):3156–61.
35. DeVol DL, Rotwein P, Sadow JL, Novakofski J, Bechtel PJ. Activation of insulin-like growth factor gene expression during work-induced skeletal muscle growth. Am J Physiol. 1990;259:E89–95.
36. Zanconato S, Moromisato DY, Moromisato MY, et al. Effect of training and growth hormone suppression on insulin-like growth factor-I mRNA in young rats. J Appl Physiol. 1994;76:2204–9.
37. van Mil EGAH, Westerterp KR, Gerver WJ, Van Marken Lichtenbelt WD, Kester ADM, Saris WHM. Body composition in Prader-Willi syndrome compared with nonsyndromal obesity: relationship to physical activity and growth hormone function. J Pediatr. Nov 2001;139(5):708–14.
38. Lopes IM, Forga L, Martinez JA. Effects of leptin resistance on acute fuel metabolism after a high carbohydrate load in lean and overweight young men. J Am Coll Nutr. Dec 2001;20(6):643–8.
39. Falk B, Sadres E, Constantini N, Zigel L, Lidor R, Eliakim A. The association between adiposity and the response to resistance training among pre- and early-pubertal boys. J Pediatr Endocrinol Metab. May 2002;15(5):597–606.
40. Galassetti P, Larson J, Iwanaga K, Salsberg SL, Eliakim A, Pontello A. Effect of a high-fat meal on the growth hormone response to exercise in children. J Pediatr Endocrinol Metab. Jun 2006;19(6):777–86.
41. King NA, Burley VJ, Blundell JE. Exercise-induced suppression of appetite: effects on food intake and implications for energy balance. Eur J Clin Nutr. Oct 1994;48(10):715–24.
42. Blundell JE, King NA. Physical activity and regulation of food intake: current evidence. Med Sci Sports Exerc. Nov 1999;31(11 Suppl):S573–83.
43. Verger P, Lanteaume MT, Louis-Sylvestre J. Human intake and choice of foods at intervals after exercise. Appetite. Apr 1992;18(2):93–9.
44. Nemet D, Arieli R, Meckel Y, Eliakim A. Immediate post exercise energy intake and macronutrient preferences in normal weight and overweight pre-pubertal children. Int J Pediatr Obes. 2010;5:221–9.
45. Owens S, Gutin B, Allison J, et al. Effect of physical training on total and visceral fat in obese children. Med Sci Sports Exerc. Jan 1999;31(1):143–8.
46. Ambler C, Eliakim A, Brasel JA, Lee WN, Burke G, Cooper DM. Fitness and the effect of exercise training on the dietary intake of healthy adolescents. Int J Obes Relat Metab Disord. Apr 1998;22(4):354–62.
47. Oude LH, Baur L, Jansen H, et al. Interventions for treating obesity in children. Cochrane Database Syst Rev. 2009;1:CD001872.
48. Rodearmel SJ, Wyatt HR, Stroebele N, Smith SM, Ogden LG, Hill JO. Small changes in dietary sugar and physical activity as an approach to preventing excessive weight gain: the America on the Move Family study. Pediatrics. Oct 2007;120(4):e869–79.
49. Epstein LH, Paluch RA, Gordy CC, Dorn J. Decreasing sedentary behaviors in treating pediatric obesity. Arch Pediatr Adolesc Med. Mar 2000;154(3):220–6.
50. Weintraub DL, Tirumalai EC, Haydel KF, Fujimoto M, Fulton JE, Robinson TN. Team sports for overweight children: the Stanford Sports to Prevent Obesity Randomized Trial (SPORT). Arch Pediatr Adolesc Med. Mar 2008;162(3):232–7.
51. Carrel AL, Clark RR, Peterson SE, Nemeth BA, Sullivan J, Allen DB. Improvement of fitness, body composition, and insulin sensitivity in overweight children in a school-based exercise program: a randomized, controlled study. Arch Pediatr Adolesc Med. Oct 2005;159(10):963–8.
52. Daley AJ, Copeland RJ, Wright NP, Roalfe A, Wales JK. Exercise therapy as a treatment for psychopathologic conditions in obese and morbidly obese adolescents: a randomized, controlled trial. Pediatrics. Nov 2006;118(5):2126–34.
53. Gutin B, Barbeau P, Owens S, et al. Effects of exercise intensity on cardiovascular fitness, total body composition, and visceral adiposity of obese adolescents. Am J Clin Nutr. May 2002;75(5):818–26.
54. Carnethon MR, Gidding SS, Nehgme R, Sidney S, Jacobs DR Jr, Liu K. Cardiorespiratory fitness in young adulthood and the development of cardiovascular disease risk factors. J Am Med Assoc. 17 Dec 2003;290(23):3092–100.

22 School- and Community-Based Interventions

Joel Gittelsohn and Sohyun Park

CONTENTS

INTRODUCTION
SUMMARY OF THE LITERATURE
STUDY RESULTS
DISCUSSION
REFERENCES

Key Words: School, community, obesity prevention

INTRODUCTION

For decades, school-based programs have constituted the primary approach for addressing the childhood obesity epidemic at the population level. School programs have the potential to reach many children and affect many factors in the causal path to obesity (i.e., diet, physical activity, knowledge, and other psychosocial factors); in theory, they have great promise for long-term sustainability through institutionalization of intervention components *(1–4)*.

On the other hand, the effectiveness of school-based interventions has for the most part been disappointing. Most school programs have been associated with only modest impacts on childhood behavior and weight gain *(5–8)*. Some success has been observed in school intervention trials that have had strong program champions, but the beneficial effects in children are often reversed if staff members who championed the program leave the school *(9,10)*. These findings have led us and other investigators to question the school-centered approach to child obesity prevention *(11–15)*. One of the primary critiques has been that school-centered programs are unlikely to be successful if not heavily reinforced by strong interventions in the community.

Children are influenced by the wide range of choices and factors that constitute the food and physical activity environments outside of schools; these include the presence and proximity of retail food stores, the availability of prepared and "fast" foods, the variety and quantity of foods available and served within the home, and the accessibility of parks and recreation centers. Parents and other caregivers can influence greatly the foods consumed by their children, particularly at a young age *(16,17)*. In recent years, a growing number of school-based intervention trials have sought to expand beyond the confines of the school to engage the broader community. We term these interventions "school–community programs." In addition to school-based interventions, they include community and family components that invoke community involvement, nutrition environment intervention near schools, and

From: *Contemporary Endocrinology: Pediatric Obesity: Etiology, Pathogenesis, and Treatment*
Edited by: M. Freemark, DOI 10.1007/978-1-60327-874-4_22,
© Springer Science+Business Media, LLC 2010

family education and participation. Here we review the literature on "school–community" intervention trials to answer three questions:

(1) What types of "school–community intervention trials" are found in the literature? How do these programs vary in terms of program components, emphasis on school versus community, strategies, and study size, etc?
(2) How successful have "school–community" programs been? What components appear to be most successful overall?
(3) What are future directions for school-based and school–community programs to prevent childhood obesity?

To identify the relevant literature for school–community programs, we conducted a literature search for the years from 1990 to 2009 using Medline, PubMed, PsycINFO, and the Cochrane Database of Systematic Reviews. The following inclusion criteria were used to select articles for the review: (1) selected studies should have both school-based intervention programs and substantial components outside the school aimed at preventing childhood obesity; (2) the overall goal of studies should be preventing unhealthy weight gain or obesity among children through increased physical activity, better nutrition, and/or environmental policy changes in schools and communities; (3) evaluation outcomes must include obesity, physical activity, and/or energy intake to be included in this review. We excluded studies that sent home materials and/or had activities within the school for family members as their primary form of community engagement (e.g., Pathways (18), CATCH (19)). In addition, recent review articles (2000–2007) on school-based and community-based childhood obesity prevention program were manually checked to be sure that any studies mentioned in the reviews would meet the inclusion criteria for this study. A total of eight intervention studies were found matching these criteria and 22 articles were reviewed. Additional searches were performed to identify the relevant literature for school–community-based diabetes prevention studies. Two additional studies were reviewed and included in the tables.

Therefore, a total of ten intervention studies were reviewed. In addition to reference to published articles, we contacted the lead authors when information was missing and included the information provided by the authors to provide a more complete description of the studies.

SUMMARY OF THE LITERATURE

Summary of Articles of School–Community Programs for Obesity Prevention

Tables 1 and 2 summarize our findings from the review of the literature. Table 1 describes the background, target population, and intervention approach of each program. Table 2 outlines the methods of evaluation used and the primary results and recommendations.

General Description of the Intervention Trials

Of ten studies reviewed, six were implemented in the USA, one in Canada, one in Australia, one in New Zealand, and one in France. The intervention periods ranged from 1 to 3 years, with two exceptions (9,28). With the exception of one study by Perman and colleagues (27), all interventions were controlled trials with comparison groups; three of the studies (TAAG (10), SNPI (34), Switch (38)) randomly assigned schools as intervention and control.

One study conducted in France, titled Fleurbaix-Laventie Ville Santé (FLVS (26)), has a different approach than others included here. Unlike the other studies, which were designed as school–community interventions, the French study was initiated in 1992 as a school-based nutrition education intervention and evolved into a school–community intervention beginning in 1999. The program was

Table 1
Theory and Intervention Strategies Used in the Ten School–Community Intervention Trials

Study title, duration	Theory used	Preparatory work	Main intervention components		Outside of school
			School based		
The Apple Project (A Pilot Programme for Lifestyle and Exercise) (20,21,22,23,24)	"ANGELO" (Analysis Grid for Environments Linked to Obesity)	Community Activity Coordinators (ACs); interviews with community stakeholders and school personnel	*Curriculum*: science/health lessons and an interactive card game on nutrition *Policy/Env*: non-curricular activity at recess, lunchtimes, and after-school; teachers to facilitate short bursts of activity in class and after-school		*Family*: increased parental involvement *Community Links*: physical activity classes; community-based healthy eating resource and free fruit for 6 months
Be Active Eat Well (BAEW) (25)	Capacity-building approach	Community involvement in planning activities	*Curriculum*: a 2-week curriculum for reducing screen time *Policy/Env*: school dietitian and nutrition policies; after-school activities		*Family*: healthy families program *Community Links*: community garden; fruit shop displays; activity programs *Policy*: Municipal Public Health Plan
Fleurbaix-Laventie Ville Sante Study (FLVS) (26)	Not reported	Not reported	*Curriculum*: nutrition education program for all grades *Activities in schools*: cooking classes, visits to farms, family breakfast in schools *Policy/Env*: school cafeterias to increase affordable and diversified food		*Family*: health checkup and clinical examination, targeted counseling *Community Links*: dietitians and sport educators; town councils for sporting activities/facilities

(Continued)

Table 1
(continued)

Study title, duration	Theory used	Preparatory work	Main intervention components	
			School based	Outside of school
Jumpin' Jaguars: Community-Driven Obesity Prevention and Intervention in an Elementary School (27)	Universal, targeted	Academic, community partners, school teachers	*Curriculum:* behavior modification to all children in the school *Policy/Env:* not reported *After-school:* targeting activity and counseling	*Family:* evening classes on healthy cooking and lifestyle changes *Community Links:* free healthy snacks by local NGO; scholarship incentives
Kahnawake School Diabetes Prevention Project (KSDPP) (28,29,30,31–33)	Social learning theory, behavior change theory, native learning styles, health promotion	Community Advisory Board	*Curriculum:* structured school health education program *Policy/Env:* healthy nutrition policy; teacher training	*Family:* healthy breakfasts *Community links:* Community Advisory Board; research ethics code; conferences
School Nutrition Policy Initiative (SNPI) (34)	Social learning theory	Community-based organization; Nutrition Advisory Group	*Curriculum:* nutrition education *Policy/Env:* staff training to change in-school nutrition environment	*Family:* parent meetings and weekly nutrition workshops *Community links:* community-based organization with Family Resource Network Coordinators and Parent Teacher organizations

Intervention	Theory	Formative research/community involvement	Intervention components
Shape up Somerville: Eat Smart, Play Hard (SUS) (35,36,37)	Social-ecological approach	Meetings, focus groups, interviews, advisory councils	*Curriculum*: classroom curriculum *Policy/Env*: breakfast program; walk to school; staff development; school food service; enhanced recess after-school curriculum *Family*: parent outreach and education; family events; nutrition forums; "Health Report Card" *Community links*: Community Advisory Council; Ethnic-minority group collaborations; pedestrian training; wellness campaign; farmers markets; physician and clinic staff training
Switch what you Do, View, and Chew (Switch) (38,39)	Social-ecological model	Community events	*Curriculum*: monthly teacher's packet *Policy/Env*: school-wide kickoff *Family*: materials on physical activity, nutrition and screen time. *Community links*: a community wide event; public service advertising campaign
Trial for Activity for Adolescent Girls (TAAG) (10,40–44,45,46,47,48)	Social-ecological theory, operant learning theory, social cognitive theory, social marketing, organizational change theory	Formative research with adolescent girls, parents, school personnel, and community members	*Curriculum*: physical education, health education *Policy/Env*: teacher workshop and materials; school champions *Community links*: collaboration between schools, community agencies and university staff; after-school programs; social marketing efforts

(Continued)

Table 1
(continued)

Study title, duration	Theory used	Preparatory work	Main intervention components		
			School based	Outside of school	
Zuni Diabetes Prevention Program (ZDPP) (9)	Social cognitive theory	Focus group, interviews, dietary survey	Curriculum: diabetes education in school curricula Policy/Env: workshop with school administrators, teachers, employees; modification of food supply; wellness facility	Family: meetings with Parent–Teacher Organizations (PTOs) Community links: supportive social networks; teen task force	

Table 2

Study Design, Results, and Main Conclusions of the Ten School–Community Intervention Trials

Study title	Study design; evaluation methods used	Results	Main conclusions/recommendations
The Apple Project	*Treatment*: semi-rural community in Otago, New Zealand. Elementary schools ($n = 4$, 5–12 years; 381 children) *Control*: one community in same area. Elementary schools ($n = 3$, 5–12 years; 346 children) *Ethnicity*: mostly white, middle-class (17.3% Maori, 0.9% Pacific Island)	*Process evaluation*: not reported *Behaviors*: higher activity level with intervention; lower consumption of carbonated beverages and more fruit *Health*: *Year 1*: BMI z-score −0.11 ($p < 0.05$). No difference in the risk of being overweight or obese, waist circumference, blood pressure or pulse rate *Year 2*: BMI z-score −0.26 ($p < 0.05$). WC −1 cm ($p < 0.05$) *Follow-up after ~2 year*: BMI z-score −0.17 ($p < 0.05$) and less likely to be overweight	Increased activity and slowed unhealthy weight gain in primary school children *Sustainability*: after the discontinuation benefits in BMI remained apparent in intervention children
BAEW	*Treatment*: Colac, Australia (pop 11,000). All preschools ($n = 4$, 4 years) and primary schools ($n = 6$, 5–12 years) *Control*: random samples from the region of Victoria (pop 323,000) *Ethnicity*: mostly white	*Process evaluation*: 6,789 person-hours *Psychosocial*: no harm in body image *Health*: intervention group gained less weight (−0.92 kg), smaller increases in waist circumference (−3.14 cm), BMI z-score (−0.11), and waist/height ratio (−0.02, all $p < 0.05$); no difference in prevalence and incidence of overweight and obesity	Effective at slowing rate of weight gain

(Continued)

Table 2
(continued)

Study title	Study design; evaluation methods used	Results	Main conclusions/recommendations
FLVS study	*Treatment:* two communities in northern France, elementary school children 5–12 years; analysis sample 633 children in 2004 *Control:* two communities in same area with similar SES as T *Ethnicity:* not reported	*Process evaluation:* not reported *Behaviors:* not reported *Health:* decrease in prevalence of overweight between 2000 and 2004: boys from 10.2 to 7.4% and girls from 18.6 to 10.4% (2000–2004). Adjusted OR for overweight was 0.72 (boys) and 0.52 (girls). Lower prevalence of overweight with treatment 8.8% vs. 17.8%	Low SES population may benefit from nutritional and health-related interventions
Jumpin' Jaguars	*Treatment:* elementary school in Kentucky ($n = 1$; 166 children for universal school program, 40 children for the targeted after-school program) *Control:* elementary school with similar demographics selected upon completion in the project school's first year (184 children) *Ethnicity/SES:* 57% of annual household incomes < \$10,000; 80% of participants AA or Hispanic	*Process evaluation:* 27/40 participated in 80% or more of sessions; parental participation low *Health:* BMI percentile lower ($T = 68.57 \pm 31.62$, $C = 75.49 \pm 26.11$, $p = 0.027$) No significant differences in mean BMI percentile for after-school participants	Easily implemented at reasonably low cost

| KSDPP | *Treatment*: Kahnawake (Mohawk), Canada; 458 students in grades 1–6
 Control: Tyendinaga; 199 students in grades 1–6
 Ethnicity/SES: first nations | *Behaviors*: no significant differences in mean intake of energy, fat, and sucrose after 4 years of intervention; significant decrease in the frequency of consumption of high-fat foods ($p < 0.05$) and fruits ($p < 0.001$); significant increase in energy contribution of white sugar ($p < 0.05$). Consumption of high-fat and high-sugar foods and fruits and vegetables decreased after 8 years of intervention. Activity and TV watching favorable trends 1994–1999; not sustained in 2002
 Health: increases in skinfold thickness and BMI from repeated cross-sectional measures. Fitness showed favorable trends from 1994 to 1999 that were not sustained in 2002 | Early results showed some successes; benefits not maintained over 8 years |

(Continued)

Table 2
(continued)

Study title	Study design; evaluation methods used	Results	Main conclusions/recommendations
SNPI	*Treatment and control*: elementary school in Pennsylvania ($n = 10$; 1,349 children in 4–6 grades) *Ethnicity/SES*: >=50% of children eligible for free or reduced lunch; 44% African American, 17% Asian, 22% Hispanic	*Process evaluation*: teachers and support staff averaged 10.4 and 8.4 h of training, respectively, and devoted 48.0 and 44.0 h to each year of intervention *Behaviors*: no difference in dietary intake, activity change before and after the program but less sedentary behavior *Psychosocial*: no harm in body image *Health*: predicted odds of overweight ~33% lower for T. No difference in incidence of obesity; Effect strongest for black students (OR: 0.59)	A multicomponent school-based intervention can be effective in children in grades 4–6 but stronger or additional interventions are needed
SUS	*Treatment*: Somerville, MA public elementary schools ($n = 10$, grades 1–3; 631 children) *Control*: two communities that matched by SES ($n = 20$ schools; 1,065 children) *Ethnicity*: mixed (7.5% AA, 18.2% Hispanic, 9.1% Asian)	*Health*: BMI z-score decreased −0.1005 ($p = 0.001$); expected to decrease weight gain by 1 pound for a child at the 75th percentile BMI z-score and 50th percentile for height	It is possible to address childhood obesity through a multifaceted environmental change approach that involves the community, schools, families, and students.

SWITCH	*Treatment*: two communities from Lakeville, MN, and Cedar Rapids, IA, USA (*n* = 5 schools, grades 3–5; 685 children) *Control*: two nearby communities (*n* = 5 schools, grades 3–5; 674 children) *Ethnicity/SES*: 90% white	*Behaviors*: decreased screen time (1.38 h/week at 6-months post-intervention); increased fruit and veg consumption (1 serving/week); no difference in activity *Psychosocial*: positive perceptions on target behaviors *Health*: no difference in mean BMI	Positive effect on child-reported screen time was greatest for obese children
TAAG	*Treatment*: 18 schools in six US areas *Control*: 18 schools 6th graders in 2003 (*n* = 1,721), 8th graders in 2005 (*n* = 3,504) and 8th graders in 2006 (*n* = 3,502); Girls the focus of intervention; however, both boys and girls received health and physical education classes *Ethnicity*: mixed	*Behaviors*: no differences in adjusted MET-weighted minutes of moderate-to-vigorous physical activity Girls in intervention schools were more physically active (mean difference 10.9 MET-weighted minutes of MVPA, 95% CI = 0.52–21.2). *Health*: no differences in fitness or % body fat	Modestly improved physical activity in girls
ZDPP	*Treatment*: Zuni Indian reservation (western New Mexico) High school (*n* = 2, 119 students in year 1, 9–12 grades) *Control*: Anglo females and males of same age in Tuscon area *Ethnicity/SES*: Native American	*Behaviors*: decreased consumption of sugared beverages *Health*: increase in glucose/insulin ratios No comparison group and statistical analysis was done between 1 and 3 years	Cross-sectional analysis limits conclusions

still ongoing in 2007 when the evaluation paper was published; the reviewed paper summarized the intervention effect through 2004.

Target Populations

Most of the studies reviewed here targeted elementary school students, most of whom ranged from 4 to 12 years of age. SNPI study targeted 4th–6th graders, whereas, SUS mainly focused on 1st–3rd graders. TAAG worked mainly with middle school girls and ZDPP study targeted high school students.

The trials included in this review included children from a wide range of ethnic groups. Many of the studies focused on low-income populations; for example, the two studies designed to reduce diabetes risk factors were conducted in American Indian and First Nation children (9,29). Of the remaining seven investigations, two specifically targeted populations with relatively lower socio-economic status. Jumpin' Jaguars worked with one elementary school in a community in which 57% of households earned less than $10,000 annually; among participating children, 80% were either African-American or Hispanic (27). Similarly, more than 50% of the SNPI participants were eligible for federally subsidized, free, or reduced-price meals. The majority were ethnic minorities: 44% African-American, 17% Asian, and 22% Hispanic children (34). On the other hand, the BAEW study population (Australia) and the Switch population were mostly white (25,39).

Theoretical and Participatory Approaches

Not surprisingly, all ten studies mentioned community engagement as a key component of the formative phase of the intervention. The TAAG study obtained detailed information on formative research with community and school members as well as youth and family members (40–44). The SUS and the SNPI formed advisory councils to assist in assessing community needs and designing the program (34,35). The community-based intervention components in the FLVS study were proposed by community members and organizations that had previously participated in an earlier school-based nutrition education intervention in the community. The communities themselves suggested and organized events for increasing physical activity levels targeting whole communities (26). Lastly, all the diabetes prevention studies in native communities emphasized partnership between research teams and community leaders for a successful intervention; this is well documented in KSDPP (28,30,49).

Intervention Components Inside and Outside Schools

All the studies included in this review have both school-based and out-of-school components (Table 3). While studies that solely emphasized family materials/workshops were not considered sufficient for inclusion, most investigations included parent outreach programs and events (except TAAG (10)). Most of the studies (7/10) included policy and environmental changes as components of school-based programs. For example, the SNPI study (34) used a coalition of community-based organizations to focus on changing food and nutrition environments in schools. After-school programs were incorporated to increase physical activity levels [BAEW (25), SUS (35), TAAG (10), and APPLE (20)] and to target overweight or obese children by collaborating with other local agencies [Jumpin' Jaguars (27)].

The types and intensities of community programs varied considerably (Table 3). However, more than half of the studies (6/10) endeavored to change the food environments in their communities. For example, the SUS study devoted a substantial part of the intervention to developing community gardens and farmers' markets and recruiting SUS "approved" restaurants in the city (35). SNPI also worked with local food stores to help customers identify healthier food options by providing point of purchase information (34). Half of the studies (5/10) focused on environmental factors that encourage physical activity in communities. With the support of the town councils, the FLVS study led

Table 3
Types of Intervention Strategies Used in the Studies Included in This Review

	APPLE	BAEW	FLVS	JJ	KSDPP	SNPI	SUS	SWITCH	TAAG	ZDPP
Classroom curriculum	x	x	x	x	x	x	x	x	x	x
School policy development[a]	x	x			x	x	x			x
Before school program[b]		x	x			x	x		x	
After-school program	x	x		x			x		x	
Parent outreach	x	x	x	x	x	x	x	x		x
Community components										
Participatory research	x	x		x	x	x	x		x	x
Advisory council formed					x	x	x			
Changing food environments[c]	x	x	x		x	x	x			
Changing PA environments		x	x		x		x		x	
Working with various local stakeholders[d]		x	x	x	x	x	x	x	x	x
Collaboration with local health offices		x	x				x			
Community events	x	x	x		x		x	x		
Mass media campaigns	x	x	x		x		x	x		

[a]Including a wide variety of school policies with regard to better nutrition and higher physical activities (school food service, vending machines, cooled water filters, improvement of school physical activity facilities, etc).
[b]Including breakfast program, walk to school campaign.
[c]Including farmers market, community gardening, working with local food stores and restaurants.
[d]Including local physician, clinic staff and city employers training, and involvement of other community-based organizations.

to the construction of new sporting facilities; new sport educators were employed as a part of the intervention (26). The KSDPP study held various promotional events on increasing physical activities targeting the whole community (28). The SUS study worked closely with the city government to increase walkability and bikeability in the community (35).

Most of the interventions (8/10) worked closely with various local stakeholders. The TAAG study implemented intervention components for increasing physical activity among girls both on and off school property, working with small advisory groups of school staff and community organizations and members. Community organizations, such as the YMCA or YWCA, local health clubs, and community recreation centers, were identified in intervention schools and invited to plan and implement programs and events. Moreover, the study recruited and trained Program Champions from intervention schools and communities to take ownership of the program for the purpose of sustainability after researchers from outside the community leave the study *(10)*. The Jumpin' Jaguars study enlisted the support of various local community-based organizations (e.g. YMCA, Community Trust Bank, and God's pantry) for their after-school program *(27)*. Lastly, the SNPI study worked with local food stores to promote intake of healthy foods *(34)*. The SUS trained local physicians and clinic staff to increase awareness of childhood obesity and formed collaborations with ethnic-minority group in the community *(35)*. The Zuni Diabetes Prevention Program (ZDPP) developed supportive social networks by forming a Teen Task Force, which helped to recruit youth participants into the study and served as peer mentors for other students *(9)*. Three of ten studies included collaboration with local health offices or support from government organizations. For example, the BAEW strategies were incorporated into the Municipal Public Health Plan and Integrated Health Promotion Plan *(25)*. Most studies (7/10) reported that the intervention attempted to reach the whole community in order to increase awareness of the programs through various mass media campaigns.

Process Evaluation

Most of the studies (8/10) collected process evaluation data [except *(27,26)*], with great variation in methods and documentation. Process evaluation measures included changes in schools' and in communities' environments as well as dose, reach, and fidelities of intervention activities *(28,35,45)*. Two papers from the SUS study presented the results of food environment modification efforts in the community, focusing on food service at schools and local restaurants *(36,37)*.

Psychosocial Measures and Behavioral Impacts

We compared the forms of evaluation used by the different trials. Psychosocial factors were measured in more than half of the studies reviewed. The BAEW *(25)* and the SNPI *(34)* studies administered body dissatisfaction questionnaires to monitor adverse effects of the interventions. The KSDPP *(28)*, Switch *(39)*, TAAG *(46)*, and ZDPP *(9)* studies measured psychosocial factors such as self-efficacy, outcome expectations, knowledge, perceptions, and/or attitudes.

Seven studies measured both dietary intake and physical activity. The TAAG study measured only physical activity levels among participating girls using accelerometers and observations *(10)*. FLVS and Jumpin' Jaguars did not include behavioral assessments *(27,26)*. Most of the studies of physical activity level and dietary intake used self-reported questionnaires. Some specific behaviors, such as intake of fruits and vegetables or screen time, were reported separately in some studies [KSDPP *(29)*, Switch *(39)*, and ZDPP *(9)*].

Health Outcomes

BMI and BMI *z*-scores were the most common health outcomes measured. In addition, some studies included other anthropometric measures such as waist–hip ratio, percent body fat, and physiological measures such as blood pressure and pulse rate. Overweight or obesity prevalence and incidence were also reported in some studies [FLVS *(26)*, SNPI *(34)*].

Community Measures

Impacts at the community level were assessed in some trials. One study measured sustainability of the program effect after 2 years of program completion by interviewing school principals [APPLE (22)]. Other studies (28,45,36) mentioned environmental and policy changes as a measure of the impact of intervention. The Switch study performed community surveys before and after the intervention to measure the changes on community awareness of the study's target healthy behaviors (38). The SUS study team described efforts to change food environments in restaurants and schools. The compliance rate of restaurants that followed approval criteria was not high (~50%); however, school food environments improved after implementation, with increased availability of fruits, vegetables, whole grains, and low fat dairy products (36,37).

STUDY RESULTS

Impact on Psychosocial Factors and Behavior

Three studies assessed the psychosocial impacts of intervention: two studies found no increase in body dissatisfaction or eating disorders among participants [BAEW (25), SNPI (34)], and one study reported that participants perceived positive changes in their behaviors (39).

Among five studies that reported nutrition-related behavioral changes, three had positive results (9,20,39) while two found no changes in dietary intake (34,29). The APPLE project documented lower consumption of carbonated beverages and higher consumption of fruit among intervention children and the ZDPP noted lower consumption of sugared beverages. Lastly, the parents of children from the Switch intervention communities reported higher consumption of fruits and vegetables (39). Only one study reported dietary results at the nutrient level (KSDPP); no significant impacts were observed.

Among five studies that reported effects on physical activity, four had a positive impact. The APPLE intervention increased physical activity level (20), SNPI and Switch reduced sedentary behavior (34,39), and the TAAG study increased the activity levels of adolescent girls (10). The KSDPP study showed increases in physical activity during the initial study period (1994–1999); however, these changes were not sustained in a 3-year follow-up (29).

Impact on BMI and Anthropometric Measures

Six of the ten studies demonstrated positive albeit small impacts on BMI and related anthropometric measures (Table 4). Children undergoing the BAEW intervention gained less weight and had smaller increases in waist circumference, BMI z-score, and waist–hip ratio than children in the comparison group. Even though the program did not analyze changes in the prevalence and incidence of overweight and obesity between intervention and comparison groups, the changes in BMI and other anthropometric measures are encouraging (25). The SUS (35) and the APPLE project also showed promising outcomes (20,22): mean BMI z-scores were reduced. Moreover, BMI z-scores and the prevalence of overweight remained lower in the APPLE intervention group for 2 years. The SNPI program (34), which focuses on changing nutrition environment at schools, showed that the predicted odds of incidence and prevalence of overweight were lower for the intervention group. The KSDPP showed some early positive effects on skinfold thickness but not on BMI or fitness (29). Glucose/insulin ratios were increased in the ZDPP study; the significance of this finding is unclear without proper comparison groups and without controlling for other factors in the analysis (9).

Impact on Community

Most of the studies sought to work with community groups to reduce unhealthy weight gain or diabetes risk factors; however, little information on how the intervention changed communities was found

Table 4
Study Impact and Target Age Summary

Study	Age (years)	Effect on BMI z or rates of overweight/obesity
APPLE	5–12	–0.11 to –0.26
BAEW	4–12	–0.11
FLVS	5–12	Odds Ratio overweight: 0.72 boys, 0.52 girls
Jumpin' Jaguars	Elementary school	Mean BMI percentile lowered in T
KSDPP	6–12 (1st–6th graders)	None
SNPI	9–12 (4th–6th graders)	Odds ratio overweight 0.67/No effect on obesity
SUS	6–9 (1st–3rd graders)	–0.10
SWITCH	8–11 (3rd–5th graders)	None in BMI mean value
TAAG	11–14 (6th–8th grade girls)	None
ZDPP	14–18 (9th–12th graders)	None (lowered BMI post-intervention but NS)

NS: Not statistically significant, T: Treatment group.

in the papers. One follow-up study of APPLE explicitly addressed sustainability issues: whether the intervention components in schools and communities were still in place 2 years after program cessation *(50)*. Some studies mentioned that they followed environmental and policy changes in communities as part of process evaluation but results were not documented [e.g., KSDPP *(38)*, TAAG *(26)*].

DISCUSSION

Our review of the literature identified a limited number of school-based obesity prevention programs that had a substantial community component. It is clear that a great deal of work remains to expand this area of intervention research as a means of addressing the child obesity epidemic. Some large-scale interventions with extensive community involvement are underway: the SUS study is being replicated in six urban communities in the USA (renamed BALANCE) and is being adapted and implemented in eight rural communities in the USA (renamed CHANGE) *(51)*. We expect to see more evaluation results in a few years; this should provide more definitive information regarding the effectiveness of school–community intervention programs. Nevertheless, on the basis of the work reviewed, some limited conclusions can be drawn.

In general, the school–community trials reviewed in this chapter have had a limited but significant impact in reducing BMI z-scores or obesity rates in children. Limited success has also been achieved with efforts to change food and physical activity environments in order to increase the choices available to children and their caregivers, such as working with food stores to increase the availability of healthy foods. However, more work needs to be done to tie these school-external changes to those that have been made to curriculum and to activities within the schools so that children and their adult caregivers are aware of the changes made.

It should be noted that eight of the ten studies we reviewed were conducted in *elementary school children*; the two studies of teenagers found no effect on weight gain or fat mass, although the TAAG intervention increased activity levels in adolescent girls. The preferential responses of prepubertal children to a lifestyle intervention likely reflect greater parental supervision and tighter control of food intake and selection. Other studies have noted the difficulty in changing weight-related behaviors in obese adolescents *(50,52,53)*.

Changing the environment around schools and in communities is enormously challenging and requires a great deal of focused effort and community support and engagement. Community engagement and participatory approaches are central features of the successful "school–community" intervention trials reviewed in this chapter. No single approach appears to have been highly effective, and in fact the level of engagement ranged considerably.

Many of the programs reviewed stressed and incorporated policy changes both inside and outside schools *(34,25,35,20)*. Policy changes may be viewed as another form of community engagement. Policy changes would lead to institutionalization of program activities in schools and community settings, which may lead to long-term sustainability.

Serious deficiencies exist for most of the intervention trials reviewed in terms of evaluation methodologies. While the studies included community intervention components, there is significant room for improvement in assessing change at the community and environmental levels pre- and post-intervention. A further weakness is the lack of substantial process evaluation of each component of the intervention implemented in the community. These are major gaps that should be addressed in future trials of school–community programs. Furthermore, most of the studies did not provide data on the impact of their programs on dietary intake at the nutrient level. Behavioral outcomes like diet and physical activity are required to explain the mechanisms for change in weight status or lack thereof.

In addition, it is important to document and disseminate information regarding costs for future assessment of trials in this area. Only one study conducted a cost analysis *(23)*; a second mentioned the total cost of intervention implementation *(27)*. We contacted the original authors of the studies to gather more information on cost (Table 5). Due to the complex nature of school–community-based interventions, including variation in study size, geographical differences, and evaluation methods, it was challenging to make any comprehensive comparisons using the data provided by the authors. The variation that we observed was substantial: costs of intervention ranged from 2 euro ($\sim$ 2.9 USD) to 429 USD per child per year. This can be explained by program differences. One was an intensive 2-year intervention beginning with building partnership with other stakeholders in the community to working with school cafeterias to alter food choices *(23)*; the other capitalized on an established collaboration with the community and did not require many external resources *(26)*.

Table 5
Intervention Cost Summary

Study	Total cost
APPLE	$239,518 for 2 years; $429/children/year
BAEW	$326,806 for 4 years
FLVS	$2.84/person/year
Jumpin' Jaguars	$14,000–16,000/school/year
KSDPP	N/A
SNPI	$30,000/school/year
SUS	N/A
SWITCH	$1.2 million for the whole program; $35–40/family
TAAG	N/A
ZDPP	N/A

Two studies found no adverse effects on children's psychological health. Stigmatization of children in school-based programs is a potential concern and led to the termination of one reportedly successful approach that targeted overweight children (54,55). Only one of the ten studies reported here (Jumpin' Jaguars) included a specific intervention for overweight children. On the one hand, the inclusion of the entire school population represents a strength of school–community programs. On the other hand, the lack of targeting may limit the effectiveness of school-based obesity interventions for overweight or high-risk children. More detailed investigation will be required to resolve this conundrum.

An additional challenge lies in the area of study design. We emphasized intervention strategy as the primary criterion by which we selected studies for this review; this enabled us to include many studies with various forms of school–community interventions. However, limitations in design of some of the studies (such as lack of a control group) weaken our ability to draw firm conclusions. In addition, many school-based studies, such as CATCH (19) and Pathways (18), took the unit of analysis and randomization as the school itself. This is not possible when extensive community engagement and changes become an additional focus of the intervention. Instead the unit of analysis becomes the community. Rigorous statistical analytical methods are needed to capture the unique aspects of community involvement and social engagement.

As noted, the reductions in mean BMI z observed in these studies were modest and variable, and the interventions are time consuming and, in some cases, expensive. Should we then abandon our efforts with school and communities and focus on targeting families and children at the highest risk for obesity and its complications? Strong evidence indicates that these targeted efforts can be effective (56,57). We would argue, however, that the sheer size, scope, and progression of the obesity epidemic will not permit us to focus our efforts solely on the small number at greatest risk.

To conclude, the experience with *school-based interventions* has been discouraging, and an emerging body of literature reveals strong associations between the obesogenic environment and the prevalence of childhood obesity. Our findings suggest that *school–community interventions* provide one possible solution to the problem. Ongoing studies with strong design and evaluation plans will provide more information regarding the efficacy and costs of school–community programs for prevention (and management) of childhood obesity. In the meantime, the positive trends noted in our review provide support for continued and expanded research trials that intervene in both schools and the communities that surround them.

REFERENCES

1. Pyle S, Sharkey J, Yetter G, Felix E, Furlong M. Fighting an epidemic: the role of schools in reducing childhood obesity. Psychol Sch. 2006;43(3):361.
2. Caballero B. Obesity prevention in children: opportunities and challenges. Int J Obes Relat Metab Disord. Nov 2004;28(Suppl 3):S90–5.
3. Budd GM, Volpe SL. School-based obesity prevention: research, challenges, and recommendations. J Sch Health. Dec 2006;76(10):485–95.
4. Naylor PJ, McKay HA. Prevention in the first place: schools a setting for action on physical inactivity. Br J Sports Med. Jan 2009;43(1):10–3.
5. Brown T, Summerbell C. Systematic review of school-based interventions that focus on changing dietary intake and physical activity levels to prevent childhood obesity: an update to the obesity guidance produced by the National Institute for Health and Clinical Excellence. Obes Rev. Jan 2009;10(1):110–41.
6. Kropski JA, Keckley PH, Jensen GL. School-based obesity prevention programs: an evidence-based review. Obesity (Silver Spring). May 2008;16(5):1009–18.
7. Shaya FT, Flores D, Gbarayor CM, Wang J. School-based obesity interventions: a literature review. J Sch Health. Apr 2008;78(4):189–96.

8. Sharma M. School-based interventions for childhood and adolescent obesity. Obes Rev. Aug 2006;7(3):261–9.

9. Teufel NI, Ritenbaugh CK. Development of a primary prevention program: insight gained in the Zuni Diabetes Prevention Program. Clin Pediatr (Phila). Feb 1998;37(2):131–41.

10. Webber LS, Catellier DJ, Lytle LA, Murray DM, Pratt CA, Young DR, et al. Promoting physical activity in middle school girls: trial of activity for adolescent girls. Am J Prev Med. Mar 2008;34(3):173–84.

11. Gittelsohn J, Kumar MB. Preventing childhood obesity and diabetes: is it time to move out of the school? Pediatr Diabetes. Dec 2007;8(Suppl 9):55–69.

12. Peterson KE, Fox MK. Addressing the epidemic of childhood obesity through school-based interventions: what has been done and where do we go from here? J Law Med Ethics. Spring 2007;35(1):113–30.

13. Thomas H. Obesity prevention programs for children and youth: why are their results so modest? Health Educ Res. Dec 2006;21(6):783–95.

14. Lytle LA. School-based interventions: where do we go next? Arch Pediatr Adolesc Med. Apr 2009;163(4):388–9.

15. Lee A. Health-promoting schools: evidence for a holistic approach to promoting health and improving health literacy. Appl Health Econ Health Policy. 2009;7(1):11–7.

16. Savage JS, Fisher JO, Birch LL. Parental influence on eating behavior: conception to adolescence. J Law Med Ethics. Spring 2007;35(1):22–34.

17. Arcan C, Neumark-Sztainer D, Hannan P, van den Berg P, Story M, Larson N. Parental eating behaviours, home food environment and adolescent intakes of fruits, vegetables and dairy foods: longitudinal findings from Project EAT. Public Health Nutr. Nov 2007;10(11):1257–65.

18. Caballero B, Clay T, Davis SM, Ethelbah B, Rock BH, Lohman T, et al. Pathways: a school-based, randomized controlled trial for the prevention of obesity in American Indian schoolchildren. Am J Clin Nutr. Nov 2003;78(5):1030–8.

19. Edmundson E, Parcel GS, Feldman HA, Elder J, Perry CL, Johnson CC, et al. The effects of the Child and Adolescent Trial for Cardiovascular Health upon psychosocial determinants of diet and physical activity behavior. Prev Med. Jul–Aug 1996;25(4):442–54.

20. Taylor RW, McAuley KA, Barbezat W, Strong A, Williams SM, Mann JI. APPLE Project: 2-year findings of a community-based obesity prevention program in primary school age children. Am J Clin Nutr. Sept 2007;86(3):735–42.

21. Taylor RW, Mcauley KA, Williams SM, Barbezat W, Nielsen G, Mann JI. Reducing weight gain in children through enhancing physical activity and nutrition: the APPLE project. Int J Pediatr Obes. 2006;1(3):146–52.

22. Taylor RW, McAuley KA, Barbezat W, Farmer VL, Williams SM, Mann JI, et al. Two-year follow-up of an obesity prevention initiative in children: the APPLE project. Am J Clin Nutr. Nov 2008;88(5):1371–7.

23. Williden M, Taylor RW, McAuley KA, Simpson JC, Oakley M, Mann JI. The APPLE project: an investigation of the barriers and promoters of healthy eating and physical activity in New Zealand children aged 5–12 years. Health Educ J. 2006;65(2):135–48.

24. McAuley KA, Taylor RW, Farmer VL, Hansen P, Williams SM, Booker CS, et al. Economic evaluation of a community-based obesity prevention program in children: the APPLE project. Obesity (Silver Spring). Jan 2010;18(1):131–6.

25. Sanigorski AM, Bell AC, Kremer PJ, Cuttler R, Swinburn BA. Reducing unhealthy weight gain in children through community capacity-building: results of a quasi-experimental intervention program, Be Active Eat Well. Int J Obes (London). Jul 2008;32(7):1060–7.

26. Romon M, Lommez A, Tafflet M, Basdevant A, Oppert JM, Bresson JL, et al. Downward trends in the prevalence of childhood overweight in the setting of 12-year school- and community-based programmes. Public Health Nutr. Dec 2008;23:1–8.

27. Perman JA, Young TL, Stines E, Hamon J, Turner LM, Rowe MG. A community-driven obesity prevention and intervention in an elementary school. J Ky Med Assoc. Mar 2008;106(3):104–8.

28. Macaulay AC, Paradis G, Potvin L, Cross EJ, Saad-Haddad C, McComber A, et al. The Kahnawake Schools Diabetes Prevention Project: intervention, evaluation, and baseline results of a diabetes primary prevention program with a native community in Canada. Prev Med. Nov–Dec 1997;26(6):779–90.

29. Paradis G, Levesque L, Macaulay AC, Cargo M, McComber A, Kirby R, et al. Impact of a diabetes prevention program on body size, physical activity, and diet among Kanien'keha:ka (Mohawk) children 6–11 years old: 8-year results from the Kahnawake Schools Diabetes Prevention Project. Pediatrics. Feb 2005;115(2):333–9.

30. Potvin L, Cargo M, McComber AM, Delormier T, Macaulay AC. Implementing participatory intervention and research in communities: lessons from the Kahnawake Schools Diabetes Prevention Project in Canada. Soc Sci Med. Mar 2003;56(6):1295–305.

31. McComber AM, Macaulay AC, Kirby R, Desrosiers S, Cross EJ, Saad-Haddad C. The Kahnawake Schools Diabetes Prevention Project: community participation in a diabetes primary prevention research project. Int J Circumpolar Health. 1998;57(Suppl 1):370–4.

32. Jimenez MM, Receveur O, Trifonopoulos M, Kuhnlein H, Paradis G, Macaulay AC. Comparison of the dietary intakes of two different groups of children (grades 4–6) before and after the Kahnawake Schools Diabetes Prevention Project. J Am Diet Assoc. Sept 2003;103(9):1191–4.

33. Levesque L, Guilbault G, Delormier T, Potvin L. Unpacking the black box: a deconstruction of the programming approach and physical activity interventions implemented in the Kahnawake Schools Diabetes Prevention Project. Health Promot Pract. Jan 2005;6(1):64–71.

34. Foster GD, Sherman S, Borradaile KE, Grundy KM, Vander Veur SS, Nachmani J, et al. A policy-based school intervention to prevent overweight and obesity. Pediatrics. Apr 2008;121(4):e794–802.

35. Economos CD, Hyatt RR, Goldberg JP, Must A, Naumova EN, Collins JJ, et al. A community intervention reduces BMI z-score in children: shape Up Somerville first year results. Obesity (Silver Spring). May 2007;15(5):1325–36.

36. Economos CD, Folta SC, Goldberg J, Hudson D, Collins J, Baker Z, et al. A community-based restaurant initiative to increase availability of healthy menu options in Somerville, Massachusetts: shape Up Somerville. Prev Chronic Dis. Jul 2009;6(3):A102.

37. Goldberg JP, Collins JJ, Folta SC, McLarney MJ, Kozower C, Kuder J, et al. Retooling food service for early elementary school students in Somerville, Massachusetts: the Shape Up Somerville experience. Prev Chronic Dis. Jul 2009;6(3):A103.

38. Eisenmann JC, Gentile DA, Welk GJ, Callahan R, Strickland S, Walsh M, et al. SWITCH: rationale, design, and implementation of a community, school, and family-based intervention to modify behaviors related to childhood obesity. BMC Public Health. Jun 2008;29(8):223.

39. Gentile DA, Wlk G, Eisenmann JC, Reimer RA, Walsh DA, Russell DW, Callahan R, Walsh M, Strickland S, Fritz K. Evaluation of a multiple ecological level child obesity prevention program: switch what you Do, View, and Chew. BMC Med. Sept 2009;7(18):49.

40. Gittelsohn J, Steckler A, Johnson CC, Pratt C, Grieser M, Pickrel J, et al. Formative research in school and community-based health programs and studies: "state of the art" and the TAAG approach. Health Educ Behav. Feb 2006;33(1):25–39.

41. Moe SG, Pickrel J, McKenzie TL, Strikmiller PK, Coombs D, Murrie D. Using school-level interviews to develop a Multisite PE intervention program. Health Educ Behav. Feb 2006;33(1):52–65.

42. Saunders RP, Moody J. Community agency survey formative research results from the TAAG study. Health Educ Behav. Feb 2006;33(1):12–24.

43. Vu MB, Murrie D, Gonzalez V, Jobe JB. Listening to girls and boys talk about girls' physical activity behaviors. Health Educ Behav. Feb 2006;33(1):81–96.

44. Young DR, Johnson CC, Steckler A, Gittelsohn J, Saunders RP, Saksvig BI, et al. Data to action: using formative research to develop intervention programs to increase physical activity in adolescent girls. Health Educ Behav. Feb 2006;33(1):97–111.

45. Young DR, Steckler A, Cohen S, Pratt C, Felton G, Moe SG, et al. Process evaluation results from a school- and community-linked intervention: the Trial of Activity for Adolescent Girls (TAAG). Health Educ Res. Dec 2008;23(6):976–86.

46. Stevens J, Murray DM, Catellier DJ, Hannan PJ, Lytle LA, Elder JP, et al. Design of the Trial of Activity in Adolescent Girls (TAAG). Contemp Clin Trials. Apr 2005;26(2):223–33.

47. Treuth MS, Baggett CD, Pratt CA, Going SB, Elder JP, Charneco EY, et al. A longitudinal study of sedentary behavior and overweight in adolescent girls. Obesity (Silver Spring). May 2009; 17(5):1003–8.

48. McKenzie TL, Catellier DJ, Conway T, Lytle LA, Grieser M, Webber LA, et al. Girls' activity levels and lesson contexts in middle school PE: TAAG baseline. Med Sci Sports Exerc. Jul 2006;38(7):1229–35.

49. Cargo M, Levesque L, Macaulay AC, McComber A, Desrosiers S, Delormier T, et al. Community governance of the Kahnawake Schools Diabetes Prevention Project, Kahnawake Territory, Mohawk Nation, Canada. Health Promot Int. Sept 2003;18(3):177–87.

50. Whitlock EA, O'Connor EP, Williams SB, Beil TL, Lutz KW. Effectiveness of weight management programs in children and adolescents. Evid Rep Technol Assess (Full Rep). Sept 2008;170:1–308.

51. Children in Balance. Research and Projects. Available at: http://www.childreninbalance.org (2009). Accessed 20 Aug 2009.

52. Oude Luttikhuis H, Baur L, Jansen H, Shrewsbury VA, O'Malley C, Stolk RP, et al. Interventions for treating obesity in children. Cochrane Database Syst Rev. 21 Jan 2009;1:CD001872.

53. Summerbell CD, Waters E, Edmunds LD, Kelly S, Brown T, Campbell KJ. Interventions for preventing obesity in children. Cochrane Database Syst Rev. 20 Jul 2005;3:CD001871.

54. Toh CM, Cutter J, Chew SK. School based intervention has reduced obesity in Singapore. BMJ. 16 Feb 2002;324(7334):427.

55. Agence France Presse. Schools making fat students thin, but emotional burden is heavy. Feb 2005.
56. Brandou F, Savy-Pacaux AM, Marie J, Bauloz M, Maret-Fleuret I, Borrocoso S, et al. Impact of high- and low-intensity targeted exercise training on the type of substrate utilization in obese boys submitted to a hypocaloric diet. Diabetes Metab. Sept 2005;31(4 Pt 1):327–35.
57. Reinehr T, Widhalm K, l'Allemand D, Wiegand S, Wabitsch M, Holl RW, et al. Two-year follow-up in 21,784 overweight children and adolescents with lifestyle intervention. Obesity (Silver Spring). Jun 2009;17(6):1196–9.

VIII

MANAGEMENT OF OBESITY WITH COMPLICATIONS: PHARMACOTHERAPY AND BARIATRIC SURGERY

23 Pharmacotherapy of Childhood Obesity and Pre-diabetes

Michael Freemark

CONTENTS

Key Words: Type 2 diabetes, cardiovascular disease, cancer, Diabetes Prevention Program, sibutramine, orlistat, metformin, incretins

BACKGROUND

The use of pharmacologic agents for treatment of obesity has a checkered history. A variety of drugs and hormones have been shown to cause short-term weight loss in obese adults; however, attempts to reduce body weight with powerful stimulants and appetite suppressants – examples include amphetamines, phenmetrazine, thyroid hormone, dexfenfluramine, and rimonabant – ultimately proved disastrous when the drugs were found to cause life-threatening cardiovascular complications and/or psychological decompensation *(1)*.

Yet, the pediatric community faces a serious challenge: The obesity epidemic has generated a rising tide of major metabolic complications, including impaired glucose tolerance (IGT) and type 2 diabetes, hypertension, dyslipidemia, ovarian hyperandrogenism, hepatic steatosis, and sleep apnea

From: *Contemporary Endocrinology: Pediatric Obesity: Etiology, Pathogenesis, and Treatment*
Edited by: M. Freemark, DOI 10.1007/978-1-60327-874-4_23,
© Springer Science+Business Media, LLC 2010

in adolescents and young adults; yet the traditional approaches to weight reduction, in the form of diet and exercise counseling, have been inconsistently or marginally effective. This has renewed interest in "safer" pharmacologic approaches that might complement the effects of lifestyle intervention and thereby reduce the incidence or severity of co-morbidities. This chapter assesses the benefits and potential risks of pharmacologic agents for treatment of childhood obesity and presents a conceptual approach to patient and drug selection, timing of intervention, and the setting of short- and long-term therapeutic goals.

THE RATIONALE FOR PHARMACOTHERAPY

The Limits of Lifestyle Intervention

The classic approach to reducing body weight in obese subjects consists of diet and exercise counseling (so-called lifestyle intervention). Lifestyle intervention can reduce rates of weight gain and fat deposition in children [see *(2)* and Chapter 20 by Wilfley et al. and Chapter 21 by Eliakim and Nemet, this volume] and delay or prevent the development of type 2 diabetes in obese adults during trial periods lasting as long as 4 years (see below). However, lifestyle intervention is effective only if applied intensively and continuously in highly motivated subjects. Indeed, a recent Cochrane analysis *(3)* of 62 investigations showed that responses of children and adolescents to diet and exercise counseling have been highly variable and often disappointing: The mean reductions in BMI *z* score were 0.05 and 0.14 in pre-adolescents and adolescents, respectively. The Cochrane data are representative, but comparisons among studies must be interpreted with caution because of variations in patient populations and study designs. In general, "intensive" lifestyle intervention, with obligatory caloric restriction, multiple individual and/or group counseling sessions, daily exercise, and numerous clinic visits, reduces body weight by as much as 4.3–7 kg (~4.5–6.5% of body weight) during the first year, while the standard lifestyle approaches delivered to nearly all obese people, namely dietary recommendations and regular clinic visits, have little benefit for the majority of kids *(2,3)*.

Most studies demonstrating clinical benefit of lifestyle intervention in children have been short-term (6 months to 2 years) investigations, and rebound weight gain has in some cases obliterated prior weight loss *(2)*. Nevertheless, at least one controlled trial provides evidence for long-term (5–10 years) weight maintenance in children who received intensive intervention, including dietary, exercise, and family counseling [see *(4)* and Chapter 20 by Wilfley et al.].

It should be noted that published studies of the benefits of lifestyle intervention have selected for highly motivated families and children willing (and often eager) to participate in investigational protocols. On the other hand, children *referred* by their general pediatricians to specialty clinics for "obesity treatment" may lack the motivation and/or resources necessary to achieve weight control; many (if not most) such people have difficulty losing weight or sustaining weight loss. Time commitments and the costs of lifestyle changes may play important roles *(5)* in treatment failure, and some people may simply tire of living with, or may rebel against, dietary restrictions. However, there are also important biological considerations: As noted in Chapter 26 by Lustig and Chapter 28 by Lechan and Fekete, weight loss is accompanied by reductions in plasma leptin, insulin, and tri-iodothyronine and increases in plasma ghrelin, adiponectin, and insulin sensitivity. These adaptations stimulate appetite and promote food craving, reduce sympathetic tone and energy expenditure, and enhance lipogenesis, thereby facilitating rebound weight gain. Consequently, short-term weight loss cannot be sustained without considerable effort. Many will fail.

What Happens if Lifestyle Intervention Fails and Obesity Persists or Worsens Over Time?

As described in detail in various chapters in this volume, progressive obesity in children and adolescents is associated with impaired glucose tolerance (IGT), hypertension, dyslipidemia, ovarian hyperandrogenism, hepatic steatosis, and sleep apnea. Long-term risks include type 2 diabetes (T2D), cardiovascular disease, and malignancy.

T2D is a progressive condition that appears to begin with insulin resistance. Progression to glucose intolerance is associated with expansion of body (particularly visceral) fat mass, declining insulin sensitivity, and a reduction in glucose-stimulated insulin secretion.

What are the long-term risks of T2D in people who were obese as children? In markedly obese adolescents studied at Yale Medical Center (6), the prevalence of T2D rose from 2 to 6% within a 20-month period between the ages of 12.5 and 14.5 years. In the Bogalusa study (7), the prevalence of T2D was 13.5% by age 32 years in subjects who were obese at age 9–11 years; in the Princeton (Cincinnati) study (8), the prevalence of T2D was 15.6% by age 37 years in those who had metabolic syndrome as children.

But those data tell only a part of the story. The prevalence of T2D in young American blacks is more than twice as high as that in whites, and in African-American children with preexisting co-morbidities, the rates of development of T2D are impressive. In the Princeton study (8), diabetes developed in more than one in four African-American young adults (25.8%) who had metabolic syndrome as children; the rates were even higher in those who had a family history of the disease. In the group studied at Yale (6), 7 of 10 African-American tweens (mean age 12.5 years) who had marked obesity *and* impaired glucose tolerance developed diabetes within a 20-month period. So, severe obesity, insulin resistance, and impaired glucose tolerance are prone to progress to frank T2D in high-risk groups. Failure to intervene in a timely and effective manner may therefore have serious long-term metabolic consequences.

Insulin resistance and impaired glucose tolerance increase the risk for development of cardiovascular disease as well as diabetes. As discussed in Chapter 19 by McGill et al., obesity and insulin resistance are associated with carotid intimal medial thickness (CIMT) in 5- to 14-year-old children and with CIMT, arterial fatty streaks, right carotid atherosclerosis (PDAY study), and coronary artery fibrous plaques (Bogalusa study) in 15- to 24-year-old young men. This explains why the risk of coronary artery disease in adults increases 10–15% for every 1 unit increase in BMI z in childhood (9,10).

Finally, severe obesity in adults predisposes to malignancies of the liver, colon, pancreas, and breast. Whether or not childhood obesity predisposes to adult malignancy is unclear. One long-term follow-up study (10) showed that middle-aged men (not women) who had been obese as children were at higher risk for colon cancer; the odds ratios were highly variable (OR 9.1, CI 1.1–77.5). A more recent investigation (11) found a twofold increase in the rates of pancreatic cancer in adults who had been obese between the ages of 14 and 29 years.

Thus, intensive lifestyle counseling may be successful in some children referred to pediatricians or pediatric specialists for treatment; but those with persistent obesity, severe insulin resistance, and impaired glucose tolerance (IGT) who fail to respond to lifestyle intervention are at risk for life-threatening complications as adults. This has stimulated interest in pharmacologic and surgical approaches for treatment of childhood obesity and prevention or reversal of complications. In a subsequent chapter (Chapter 27) Drs. Yurcisin and DeMaria discuss the benefits and risks of surgical intervention in obese adolescents. Here I analyze the benefits and risks of pharmacologic agents for obese children and teenagers and present a conceptual approach to tailored drug selection and timing of intervention.

EFFECTS OF PHARMACOLOGIC AGENTS IN OBESE SUBJECTS

Can pharmacologic agents complement the effects of lifestyle intervention and reduce the risks of complications in those who fail to respond adequately to lifestyle change? This review focuses on three major classes of medications used to treat obesity and its complications. The drugs have differential mechanisms of actions and, as will be seen, differential benefits and adverse effects. *Sibutramine* acts centrally to inhibit reuptake of serotonin, norepinephrine, and, to a lesser extent, dopamine. It reduces hunger and increases satiety *(12)*. *Orlistat* inhibits intestinal lipases and reduces by 25–30% the gastrointestinal absorption of fat *(12)*. Finally, through activation of AMP-activated protein kinase (AMPK), *metformin* reduces hepatic glucose production and fasting insulin concentrations and inhibits fat cell lipogenesis *(13)*. It can increase peripheral insulin sensitivity and may reduce food intake by raising levels of glucagon-like peptide 1 and/or reducing hypothalamic expression of neuropeptide Y *(14–16)*. Newer drugs that may prove useful for obesity treatment in the future are discussed briefly at the end of the chapter.

SIBUTRAMINE

Sibutramine ((±)-1-[1-(4- chlorophenyl) cyclobutyl]-*N,N*,3-trimethylbutan-1-amine, Figs. 1 and 2) is approved by the FDA for treatment of obese adolescents (≥16 years) and adults. Following oral administration the medication is metabolized (CYP3A4) by the liver; peak plasma levels of the drug and its two active metabolites are achieved at 1 and 3–4 h, respectively. The active metabolites have half-lives of 14–16 h; inactive metabolites are excreted in the urine.

Sibutramine acts centrally to reduce appetite and increase satiety; these effects are mediated in part by serotonergic (5-HT$_{2c}$ receptor) activation of POMC neurons and release of α-MSH, an anorexigenic peptide, in the hypothalamic arcuate nucleus. In addition, binding of serotonin to 5-HT$_{1B}$ receptors inhibits the release of the orexigenic peptide AgRP and (possibly) neuropeptide Y *(17)*; see also Chapter 2 by Lustig and Chapter 28 by Lechan and Fekete. Weight reduction is facilitated by increases in energy expenditure, mediated in part by sympathetic induction of brown adipose tissue thermogenesis *(18)*.

In overweight and obese adults, sibutramine reduces BMI and waist circumference; in combination with a low-calorie diet, the drug can reduce body weight as much as 10–12 kg within the first 6 months of treatment. The effect of the drug tends to plateau thereafter; discontinuation of medication leads to

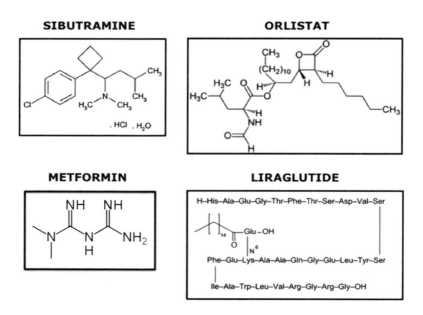

Fig. 1. Chemical structures of anti-obesity agents.

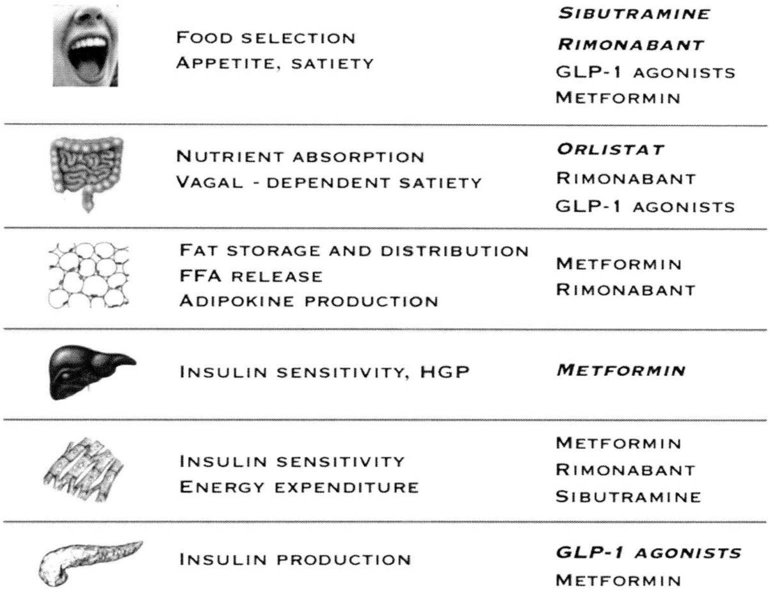

	FOOD SELECTION APPETITE, SATIETY	*SIBUTRAMINE* *RIMONABANT* GLP-1 AGONISTS METFORMIN
	NUTRIENT ABSORPTION VAGAL - DEPENDENT SATIETY	*ORLISTAT* RIMONABANT GLP-1 AGONISTS
	FAT STORAGE AND DISTRIBUTION FFA RELEASE ADIPOKINE PRODUCTION	METFORMIN RIMONABANT
	INSULIN SENSITIVITY, HGP	*METFORMIN*
	INSULIN SENSITIVITY ENERGY EXPENDITURE	METFORMIN RIMONABANT SIBUTRAMINE
	INSULIN PRODUCTION	*GLP-1 AGONISTS* METFORMIN

Fig. 2. Mechanisms of action of anti-obesity agents. Major sites of action are indicated in *italics*. GLP-1, glucagon-like peptide 1; FFA, free fatty acids; HGP, hepatic glucose production.

rebound weight gain within 2 months *(19)*. Meta-analyses of trials lasting 1–2 years show a mean weight loss ranging from 3 to 5 kg. Waist circumference declines by 4 cm, with reductions in visceral fat *(20)*.

The drug is most effective when combined with behavior therapy and caloric restriction; a 12-month randomized study in obese adults *(21)* showed that sibutramine alone was as effective as intensive lifestyle intervention in reducing weight (mean ± SD weight loss for sibutramine alone 5.0 ± 7.4 kg, amounting to 4.6% of body weight; intensive lifestyle 6.7 ± 7.9 kg, 6.4% of body weight); the addition of so-called brief lifestyle intervention to sibutramine therapy provided no additional benefit, while the effects of sibutramine plus intensive lifestyle intervention (12.1 ± 9.8 kg, 11.4% of body weight) exceeded the benefits of either intervention alone. These findings suggest that lifestyle change plus pharmacotherapy may act in concert when lifestyle intervention is pursued with resolve. Recent reviews suggest that the combination of sibutramine and lifestyle intervention can limit weight regain after weight reduction.

Factors in adults that predict weight loss in response to sibutramine include higher baseline BMI, younger age, lower depression scores, and lower energy intake at baseline *(17)*. Moreover, certain genes may influence the response to the drug; in obese women, the GG and AA genotypes of the phenylethanolamine *N*-methyltransferase gene (the rate-limiting enzyme in catecholamine biosynthesis) were associated with greater weight loss with sibutramine than the AG genotype. Other studies suggest possible effects of polymorphisms of the GNβ3 gene, which encodes the β3 subunit of the G-proteins, the α2A adrenoreceptor, and the serotonin transporter protein *(17)*.

Sibutramine-induced weight loss in adults is accompanied by variable increases (2.5–11%) in HDL-cholesterol (HDL-C) levels and small reductions in serum triglycerides *(17)*. Improvements in insulin sensitivity and liver fat content tend to parallel the magnitude of weight loss. Effects on serum leptin and adiponectin levels are inconsistent; HbA1c levels were not reduced in adults with type 2 diabetes *(17)*.

The effects of sibutramine in obese adolescents are consistent with those in adults. A placebo-controlled trial (22) in 82 obese adolescents receiving behavior therapy demonstrated that sibutramine reduced body weight by 4.6 kg relative to placebo after 6–12 months. In a second study (23) of 60 obese teens, sibutramine reduced body weight and BMI by 7.9 kg and 2.7 kg/m^2, respectively, relative to placebo. There were no effects of the drug on serum lipids or insulin sensitivity in either study. A recent 12-month investigation (24) in 498 obese adolescents receiving behavior therapy showed that sibutramine (10–15 mg/day) reduced body weight by 8.4 kg, BMI by 2.9 kg/m^2, and waist circumference by 6.4 cm relative to placebo; HDL levels increased 3.1 mg%, triglyceride levels declined 25.2 mg%, fasting insulin levels fell (–7 μU/ml), and insulin sensitivity improved. A recent meta-analysis (25) demonstrated that the drug reduced mean BMI in obese teens by 2.4 kg/m^2.

No studies to date have demonstrated that treatment with sibutramine can reduce the prevalence or severity of obesity co-morbidities. Indeed, long-term use of sibutramine may be problematic, because medication use is associated with a number of adverse effects. Meta-analyses show that sibutramine increases pulse rate by 4–8 bpm and blood pressure by 1–3 mmHg in adult subjects (12,25–27). In a major placebo-controlled study of sibutramine in obese adolescents (22), hypertension forced 19 of 43 subjects to reduce the dose of the drug and 5 of 43 (11.6%) to discontinue the medication altogether. The follow-up multicenter study (24) excluded subjects with baseline systolic and/or diastolic blood pressures exceeding 130 and 85 mmHg, respectively. Nevertheless, sibutramine increased mean systolic and diastolic blood pressure by 1 mm and 1.7 mmHg, respectively, and 2.1% of patients developed hypertension during treatment. A total of 6.3% of patients became tachycardic, and mean pulse rate increased by 2.5 bpm. No patients developed arrhythmias, but there are reports of ventricular ectopy and prolonged QT syndrome in a few patients treated with sibutramine (28). The drug may interfere with the metabolism of erythromycin and ketoconazole. Sibutramine can also cause insomnia (3.2% of adolescents), dizziness (4%), dry mouth, and constipation and *must not be used in combination with monoamine oxidase inhibitors, selective serotonin reuptake inhibitors (SSRIs), ergot alkaloids, or a variety of other medications that can cause the serotonin syndrome (29)* The long-term effects of sibutramine on behavior and cognition are unknown.

ORLISTAT

Orlistat [(1S)-1-[(2S,3S)-3-hexyl-4-oxo-oxetan-2-yl]methyldodecyl] (2S)-2-formamido-4-methyl-pentanoate, Figs. 1 and 2] is approved by the FDA for treatment of obese teenagers (>12 years of age) and adults. An over-the-counter preparation (60 mg capsules) contains half the dose of the usual prescription regimen. The drug has a short half-life (~1–2 h) and must be administered three times per day with meals. Gastrointestinal absorption is negligible; the drug is excreted in the stool.

Orlistat inhibits intestinal lipases and thereby blocks hydrolysis of triglycerides; intestinal absorption of fatty acids and monoglycerides is reduced by 25–30%. In adults, the drug reduces body weight by a mean of 2.7 kg (~2.9%) relative to placebo; there are variable reductions (0.7–3.4 cm) in waist circumference (30). The response to treatment and compliance with therapy are highly variable; approximately one in five subjects achieves weight loss >5%. Nevertheless, the effect may persist for as long as 4 years in compliant patients (31), and drug treatment may limit weight regain (32,33).

Orlistat therapy in adults is associated with reductions in total cholesterol (–12.7 mg%) and LDL-cholesterol (–10.4 mg%) and only minimal reductions in HDL-cholesterol (–0.8 mg%); consequently, the cholesterol/HDL and LDL/HDL ratios decline. There are small reductions in systolic and diastolic pressure (~1.5–2 mmHg) and insignificant reductions in fasting glucose (–1.8 mg%) and insulin (1.8 μU/ml). HbA1c declined 0.5% in adults with type 2 diabetes but not in non-diabetic patients (34). Preliminary studies suggest that serum ALT levels may decline in patients with fatty liver disease (35).

The effects of orlistat in obese adolescents appear to be similar to those in obese adults. A yearlong multi-center trial (36) comparing orlistat (N = 357) to placebo (N = 182) in obese teens showed that

BMI decreased in both groups at 3 months and then stabilized in orlistat-treated patients but increased in the placebo-treated group. At study completion, BMI decreased by 0.55 kg/m² in those treated with orlistat and increased by 0.31 kg/m² in those in the placebo group, and waist circumference declined with orlistat but increased with placebo. However, a subsequent 6-month randomized trial in 40 obese adolescents showed no effect of orlistat on BMI *(37)*. Orlistat had no effects on fasting glucose, insulin, or lipids in either study.

No studies to date have examined the effect of long-term orlistat treatment on the development or severity of cardiovascular disease. However, three reports suggest that orlistat may reduce the rate of development of type 2 diabetes mellitus in high-risk adults. The first *(38)*, a post hoc analysis of 675 obese adults with impaired glucose tolerance, showed that the combination of orlistat and a low-energy diet was associated with a reduction in the rate of development of type 2 diabetes (orlistat 3%, placebo 7.6%). The subsequent prospective XENDOS study *(31)* compared the effect of orlistat plus lifestyle changes (800 kcal deficit + daily physical activity) with that of lifestyle modification alone in 3,305 Swedish adults with BMI >30 kg/m². Over the 4-year study period, orlistat reduced the incidence of new-onset type 2 diabetes by 37.3% in the group as a whole and by 45% in those with impaired glucose tolerance at baseline. The reductions in diabetes were accompanied by relative reductions in body weight (~2 kg more than placebo) and visceral fat mass. These findings were confirmed in a follow-up investigation *(39)*, which showed that orlistat reduced by ~50% the incidence of new-onset type 2 diabetes in obese adults (*n* = 309) who had lost weight previously on a very low-calorie diet (8/153 cases with orlistat vs. 17/156 cases with placebo). Drug-dependent reductions in diabetes prevalence could reflect reductions in body fat mass and/or increases in post-prandial levels of glucagon-like peptide 1 (GLP-1), which promotes glucose-stimulated insulin secretion and reduces food intake *(40)*. Orlistat is considered safe because it is minimally absorbed. It can, however, cause flatulence, fecal incontinence, diarrhea, and malabsorptive stools. This limits its acceptability, particularly in adolescents. The drug may reduce vitamin A, D, E, and K levels and increase bone turnover in some patients *(12,41)*. Serum 25OH vitamin D levels should be monitored during treatment; a multivitamin (administered 2 h before or after orlistat) may help to prevent osteopenia. The lower dose over-the-counter preparation of orlistat may have fewer side effects but may also have less potent effects on body weight and associated co-morbidities.

Of possible concern was the development of seven new cases of gall bladder disease among the 357 children who took orlistat for a single year *(36)*. One of these children required cholecystectomy. Among the placebo-treated patients, only 1 of 182 developed new gall bladder disease. Since cholecystitis occurs more commonly even in untreated obese individuals *(42)*, it is unclear whether orlistat increases the risk of gall bladder disease or whether long-term use of the drug should be discouraged for patients with preexisting gall stones.

In theory, delivery of free fatty acids to the lower gastrointestinal tract may increase oxalate absorption and heighten the risk of kidney stones *(43)*. Preliminary research in rats showing that orlistat increases colonic preneoplastic markers *(44)* must be confirmed in humans.

Finally, orlistat may reduce absorption of thyroxine, amiodarone, and cyclosporine. Malabsorption of vitamin K may potentiate the anti-coagulant effect of warfarin.

METFORMIN

Metformin (*N,N*-dimethylimidodicarbonimidic diamide, Figs. 1 and 2) is an oral hypoglycemic agent approved for treatment of type 2 diabetes in children and adults. Peak plasma levels are achieved 1–3 h after oral administration of immediate-release metformin and 4–8 h after intake of extended-release formulations. The drug is not *metabolized*; with a half-life approximating 6 h, it is excreted in the urine. The clinical response to metformin may be modulated by genetic variation in the organic cation transporter Oct 1, which transports metformin into hepatocytes *(45)*.

Metformin reduces hepatic glucose production by inhibition of gluconeogenesis and (to a lesser extent) glycogenolysis. These effects are mediated by induction of 5′-AMP-activated protein kinase (AMPK), a metabolic sensor of energy deficit. AMPK activation triggers a cascade of events which include phosphorylation and activation of an atypical protein kinase c, phosphorylation and nuclear exclusion (inactivation) of CREB binding protein and the forkhead protein FoxO1, suppression of PGC1α and the gluconeogenic enzymes phosphoenolpyruvate carboxykinase and glucose 6-phosphatase, and induction of hepatic fatty acid oxidation *(46)*. Activation of AMPK requires the upstream serine–threonine kinase LKB1 (STK11) *(47)*. Small increases in skeletal muscle glucose uptake and peripheral insulin sensitivity may reflect changes in hepatic metabolism rather than direct effects of metformin on skeletal myocytes; in contrast to the thiazolidinediones, metformin causes only slight (and in some cases no) increase in plasma adiponectin levels and has no effect on plasma visfatin or the levels of inflammatory cytokines *(48,49)*. Nevertheless, reductions in hepatic glucose production decrease fasting and post-prandial glucose concentrations, facilitating glycemic control, and reduce fasting insulin levels. Together with a reduction in food intake *(50)*, the relative hypoinsulinemia reduces lipogenesis and limits fat deposition. Preliminary evidence suggests that metformin suppression of food intake may be mediated by increases in plasma GLP-1 or PYY levels and/or suppression of hypothalamic NPY expression *(13–16)*.

Metformin is not approved by the FDA for the treatment of obese non-diabetic children or adults. Yet numerous studies demonstrate that the drug has beneficial effects on weight and metabolic function in obese subjects *(2)*. A recent meta-analysis *(51)* of studies of a total of 4,570 non-diabetic obese adults showed that metformin caused significant reductions in BMI (–5.3%), fasting glucose (–4.3%), fasting insulin (–14.4%), serum LDL (–5.6%), and serum triglycerides (–5.3%); serum HDL levels rose 5.0%.

The results of studies in obese children and teenagers are similar to those in adults. The literature records 10 randomized, controlled trials *(52–61)* of metformin in a total of 534 obese non-diabetic children and adolescents; at 4–12 months the drug reduced BMI by a mean 1.4 kg/m^2 relative to lifestyle and placebo alone. Waist circumference was reduced by 2–6 cm, and fasting insulin levels and/or HbA1c declined in the majority of studies in which they were measured. There were variable (and small) reductions in serum lipids.

Although not dramatic, these effects appear to confer long-term therapeutic benefit and defense against the development and progression of metabolic and cardiovascular disease, at least in adults. Two major studies demonstrate that metformin reduces the rate of progression to type 2 diabetes in obese subjects. The Diabetes Prevention Program *(62)* was a randomized, double-blind, placebo-controlled trial comparing intensive lifestyle intervention and metformin for the prevention of type 2 diabetes in an ethnically mixed group of obese adults with impaired glucose tolerance (total $n =$ 3,234, mean age 51 years, BMI 34, 68% women, 45% minorities). The intensive lifestyle intervention included 16 clinic visits during the first 6 months and additional clinic visits every 1–8 weeks thereafter. Patients received personal supervision from lifestyle coaches and attended an additional four to eight group educational/counseling sessions per year. They were also strongly encouraged to attend physical activity sessions twice per week. Finally they received small monetary supplements (mean $100) for books and food vouchers. Patients in the metformin group received metformin 850 mg bid (blinded to placebo) and "standard" lifestyle counseling. The control group received standard counseling plus placebo.

The trial lasted 3 years. At study end, intensive lifestyle intervention and metformin had reduced body weight by 5.5 and 2.0 kg, respectively, relative to the placebo (standard lifestyle) control. The rates of progression to new-onset type 2 diabetes were reduced 57% by intensive lifestyle intervention and 31% by metformin. Thus intensive lifestyle change was more effective than metformin overall. However, metformin was as effective as intensive lifestyle intervention in the youngest (25–44 years) and heaviest (BMI > 34.9) patients and in women who had a previous history of gestational diabetes *(62,63)*; in these groups metformin reduced the rate of progression to type 2 diabetes by ~50%. Reductions in body weight during metformin therapy were comparable among the men and women of the various racial groups studied; in contrast, black women responded less well than white women to intensive lifestyle intervention *(64)*.

The results of the 3-year Indian Diabetes Prevention Program *(65)* were similar to those of the Diabetes Prevention Program. A low dose (250 mg bid) of metformin reduced by 26% the rate of progression to type 2 diabetes in Asian Indian adults with impaired glucose tolerance (total $n = 531$). The trial lasted 3 years; the cumulative incidence of diabetes was 55% in the control group and 39–40% in the intensive lifestyle and metformin groups. Body weight increased 0.5–1 kg in the control and intensive lifestyle groups but not in patients taking metformin. The effect of metformin was not potentiated by dietary counseling.

A recent 10-year follow-up *(66)* of the DPP (Diabetes Prevention Program Outcomes Study, DPPOS) showed long-term clinical benefits of intensive lifestyle intervention and metformin treatment in obese adults with IGT. After a 2-week medication washout at the end of the DPP, the lifestyle, metformin, and placebo groups were monitored for an additional 5.7 years; the dose of metformin was 850 mg bid. During that time, the intensive lifestyle intervention was maintained, while the metformin and placebo groups were offered group educational sessions every 3 months. Patients in the lifestyle group regained most of the weight lost (~7 kg) during the first year of the DPP; in contrast, the less dramatic weight loss (~2.5 kg) in the metformin group was maintained. By the end of the 10-year study period, the lifestyle and metformin groups had lost approximately 2 and 1.7 kg of weight, respectively, from baseline; weight loss in the placebo group approximated 0.6 kg. The rates of development of T2D *during the DPPOS* were comparable in the three groups (5.9, 4.9, and 5.6 cases/100 person years in the lifestyle, metformin, and placebo groups, respectively); the overall 10-year cumulative rates of type 2 diabetes (*DPP + DPPOS*) were 5.3, 6.4, and 7.8 cases/100 person years in the lifestyle, metformin, and placebo groups, respectively. Thus long-term lifestyle intervention and metformin reduced the 10-year incidence of T2D by 34 and 18%, respectively. Metformin did not reduce overall rates of diabetes in older patients (>60 years at initial enrollment); however, as in the DPP, metformin was as effective as intensive lifestyle intervention in those enrolled at age 25–44 years. At study end, overall mean fasting glucose levels approximated 6.18, 6.33, and 6.40 mM in the metformin, lifestyle, and placebo groups, respectively; overall HbA1c levels in the metformin, lifestyle, and placebo groups were 5.90, 5.96, and 6.02, respectively. Blood pressure and serum triglycerides did not differ among the three groups at study end.

Does metformin therapy defend against the development of cardiovascular disease? We do not know. The UKPDS study of adults with diabetes *(67)* showed that metformin reduced all-cause mortality and stroke by 32–42% relative to treatment with placebo (diet), sulfonylureas, or insulin. In a study of 12,272 Canadian diabetic adults treated only with oral agents, the rate of all-cause mortality with metformin was 40% lower than that with sulfonylureas *(68)*; moreover, patients treated with a combination of metformin and sulfonylurea had mortality rates comparable to that of metformin alone. Finally, the addition of metformin to insulin treatment reduced by 39% the incidence of macrovascular disease in diabetic adults after a follow-up period of 4.3 years *(69)*. The effect was explained in part by weight reduction (–3.1 kg relative to placebo), but preliminary evidence suggests that metformin may also protect against cardiac hypoxia/ischemia through AMPK activation and induction of endothelial cell nitric oxide synthesis *(70)*.

As discussed in Chapter 24 by Franks and Joharatnam, a number of studies show that metformin reduces free testosterone levels and increases ovulation rates in adolescents and adults with PCOS, most of whom are obese. Metformin also decreases blood pressure and LDL levels in adults with PCOS and decreased BMI and insulin resistance in hyperandrogenic girls *(71,72)*. A series of studies *(73)* by

Ibanez and deZegher in Spanish girls with precocious adrenarche and a history of intrauterine growth retardation showed that metformin can reduce pubertal weight gain, visceral fat deposition, glucose intolerance, and hyperandrogenemia. A recent pilot study ($n = 22$) found that metformin treatment of low birth weight girls for 36 months beginning at the onset of puberty (age 8–9 years) reduced BMI z score and abdominal fat mass, increased insulin sensitivity, delayed the onset of menarche, and increased adult height prediction (74,75).

Finally, there is tantalizing evidence, requiring confirmation, that metformin may reduce the risks of malignancy in obese adults with type 2 diabetes. A meta-analysis of 62,809 diabetic adults showed that treatment with insulin or sulfonylureas was associated with a 40% higher rate of total malignancies than treatment with metformin. Moreover, the addition of metformin appeared to reverse the effect of sulfonylureas on rates of total solid tumors, pancreatic cancer, and possibly colon cancer (76,77). It has been proposed, but not established, that induction of AMPK may inhibit tumor development or progression. However, it is unclear if metformin treatment of obese or diabetic children or teenagers would reduce their subsequent risks of malignancy as adults.

Metformin is generally well tolerated but the drug may have adverse side effects. Ten to fifteen percent of patients develop nausea or diarrhea; these may resolve within the first 2 weeks if the drug is given with meals. Persistent GI distress may respond to a reduction in dose. Metformin can also limit gastrointestinal absorption of B vitamins; a daily multivitamin should be administered to patients taking the drug. Liver function studies should be monitored during therapy.

Lactic acidosis occurs rarely in diabetic adults treated with metformin; there were no cases of lactic acidosis in 7,227 patient years in the COSMIC study and one episode of lactic acidosis in an HMO study of 9,875 patients followed for 20 months (78). Baseline lactate levels do not predict the development of disease. Lactic acidosis has not been described in children; nevertheless, *the drug should not be used in pediatric patients with renal insufficiency, hepatic disease, cardiac disease, chronic respiratory insufficiency, or severe infection and should be discontinued during IV contrast studies.*

NEW DEVELOPMENTS IN OBESITY PHARMACOLOGY: INCRETIN MIMETICS AND SELECTIVE SEROTONIN RECEPTOR AGONISTS

Exenatide and liraglutide. In response to a meal, the gastrointestinal tract releases a number of peptides that play roles in nutrient intake and utilization. These include cholecystokinin, peptide YY, oxyntomodulin, glucose-dependent insulinotropic peptide (GIP), and glucagon-like peptide 1 (GLP-1). GLP-1 is produced by the L-cells of the terminal ileum. In rodents and humans it promotes glucose-stimulated insulin secretion, delays gastric emptying, and reduces appetite and energy intake, possibly through binding to GLP-1 receptors expressed in brainstem nuclei (Figs. 1 and 2). However, the native peptide has a circulating half-life of only 1–2 min. GLP-1 mimetics with longer half-lives have been used for the treatment of type 2 diabetes and obesity in adults. Exenatide, which has 53% homology with native GLP-1, causes modest reductions in body mass index in diabetic adults (79); a dose of 10 μg bid reduced weight by an average of 1.25 kg in four large placebo-controlled trials (80). More significant, though variable, weight loss (3–5 kg) has been observed in uncontrolled trials. A pilot investigation (total $n = 60$) found that exenatide reduced BMI and increased insulin sensitivity and ovulation rates in women with PCOS; interestingly the combination of metformin and exenatide was more effective than either drug alone (81).

Liraglutide (Arg^{34}Lys^{26}-(N-ϵ-(γ-Glu(N-α-hexadecanoyl)))-GLP-1 (7–37)) is a synthetic peptide with 97% homology with native GLP-1; following subcutaneous injection it has a half-life of 13 h and can be administered once daily. A recent randomized 20-week trial (82) in obese non-diabetic adults ($n = 564$) showed that the combination of liraglutide and mild caloric restriction (500 kcal deficit) reduced body weight 2.1–4.4 kg relative to caloric restriction alone. Waist circumference and blood pressure declined and the percentage of subjects with metabolic syndrome and pre-diabetes decreased significantly. There were no changes in serum lipids or measures of insulin resistance and only minimal reductions in HbA1c.

The most common side effects of the GLP-1 agonists are nausea (10–47%) and vomiting (4–14%). The frequency and duration of these effects are dose dependent *(82)*. Other possible complications include insomnia and palpitations; scattered reports of pancreatitis in patients treated with exenatide require further study, *but GLP-1 agonists should be discontinued if patients develop unexplained abdominal pain.*

Oxyntomodulin and peptide YY are released from intestinal enteroendocrine cells in response to a meal. They reduce food intake, fat deposition, and body weight and increase energy expenditure in rodents; thus they appear to serve as satiety signals. The effects of oxyntomodulin are mediated through binding to GLP-1 and glucagon receptors. Short-term studies in small numbers of human subjects suggest that their effects in humans *(83,84)* are similar to those in rodents, but the long-term efficacy and safety of these preparations are unknown.

Lorcaserin is a selective serotonin 5-HT$_{2c}$ receptor agonist; preliminary short-term studies in adults *(85)* showed that it can reduce body weight by 1.8–3.6 kg. Side effects include headaches, nausea, and dizziness; no cardiac valvulopathy was noted during a 12-week investigation.

OTHER DRUGS/HORMONES THAT HAVE BEEN USED TO TREAT OBESITY

Phentermine, mazindol, ephedrine, and diethylpropion are sympathomimetic agents approved for short-term (several weeks) weight reduction in adolescents (>16 years) and adults. Chronic use can lead to dependence; adverse side effects include insomnia, palpitations, hypertension, irritability, nervousness, seizures, diarrhea, and dry mouth. *The drugs should not be used in patients with cardiac or psychiatric disorders, hyperthyroidism, or hypertension or in those taking MAO inhibitors or serotonergic agents.*

Rimonabant is a selective inhibitor of cannabinoid receptor 1. In a recent series of studies in obese adults *(2)*, the drug caused significant reductions in body weight and increased HDL levels and reduced serum triglycerides. However, rimonabant was removed from the US commercial market because its use was associated with psychiatric and nervous system disorders including anxiety, depression, and insomnia.

Topiramate is an anti-epileptic that reduces appetite and weight gain. It should not be used to treat obesity in non-epileptic patients because it can cause paresthesias, concentration/attention problems, depression, memory difficulties, language problems, nervousness, and psychomotor slowing.

Finally, *growth hormone, octreotide, and leptin* have been used to limit weight gain in patients with Prader–Willi syndrome, hypothalamic obesity, and leptin deficiency, respectively; their use is discussed in other chapters in this volume.

SUMMARY OF THE BENEFITS AND RISKS OF PHARMACOLOGIC AGENTS

In summary, pharmacologic agents provide modest to moderate, short-term reduction in body weight and (in some cases) cardiovascular risk factors. The effects of the drugs appear to be facilitated by lifestyle change. Their efficacy appears highly variable among individuals, which may reflect genetic influences, perinatal programming, parental motivation, and past and current behavior. The medications have differential effects on weight and metabolic function. Adverse effects are concerning in a subset of patients, and attrition rates from experimental studies are high. The length of time required for treatment is unclear, and the long-term risks of anorectic agents are unknown. Importantly, certain agents (metformin and orlistat) delay the development of type 2 diabetes in high-risk adults, but the long-term benefits for cardiovascular disease or malignancy remain unclear.

CAN WE IDENTIFY PEDIATRIC CANDIDATES FOR PHARMACOLOGICAL THERAPY?

The major goals of any intervention or treatment for childhood obesity are (1) to prevent or reverse metabolic co-morbidities, (2) to reduce the risk of long-term complications including cardiovascular disease and malignancy, and (3) to improve psychosocial function and quality of life. Thus the author believes that prevention and treatment of *co-morbidities* supersedes the treatment of obesity per se. Accordingly *pharmacotherapy should be considered if obesity and co-morbidities persist or worsen despite formal counseling and a good faith effort at diet and exercise.* In general, *anti-obesity drugs should be reserved for peripubertal children and adolescents with BMI equal to or exceeding the 95th percentile for age and gender and should be avoided in young children.*

The risk of metabolic complications correlates with the severity of obesity and insulin resistance *(42,86,87)* and with the presence of abdominal adiposity and/or ovarian hyperandrogenism/PCOS, which predispose to glucose intolerance. A family history of maternal gestational diabetes or of early-onset glucose intolerance or cardiovascular disease also bodes poorly *(2,86). Consequently, the author believes that peripubertal children and adolescents with impaired fasting glucose (IFG), impaired glucose tolerance (IGT), HbA1c $\geq$6.0%, the metabolic syndrome, and/or ovarian hyper-androgenism/PCOS are potential candidates for pharmacotherapy, particularly if there is marked abdominal adiposity and/or a strong family history of gestational diabetes, early-onset type 2 diabetes, myocardial infarction, or stroke.* No absolute guidelines can be provided for the selection of pediatric patients for pharmacologic therapy; the decision to begin medication(s) should be undertaken only after a comprehensive evaluation of the child's metabolic status and family history and an assessment of the current and previous responses to lifestyle intervention. An open and sympathetic discussion with the parents or caretakers is obligatory.

WHEN SHOULD WE INTERVENE?

Lifestyle intervention represents the core treatment for obese and insulin-resistant children and adults. In the opinion of the author and many other clinicians, *lifestyle changes should be undertaken before pharmacotherapy and maintained during pharmacotherapy* (Fig. 3). The addition of a pharmacologic agent may be considered if diet and exercise fail to achieve the medical objectives established by the health-care professional and family. The use of medication early in the course of adiposity might in theory prevent the progression to severe obesity and metabolic complications; nevertheless, such an approach would likely treat many children without due cause or benefit, raise the rates of "unwarranted" side effects, and increase the costs to individuals and to society. On the other hand, initiation of medication very late in the course of obesity may run the risk of irreversible weight gain and long-term morbidity. One approach that reconciles these difficulties is to begin pharmacotherapy when the risk of co-morbidities is very high or soon after complications emerge (denoted by the dotted vertical line in Fig. 3). Such complications include impaired fasting glucose (IFG), IGT, and the metabolic syndrome. The timing of pharmaco-intervention could in theory be moved to the left (in other words slightly sooner) if the family history of a major co-morbidity such as type 2 diabetes is particularly strong.

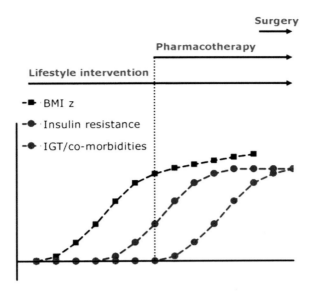

Fig. 3. Timing of intervention with pharmacotherapy and bariatric surgery. IGT, impaired glucose tolerance.

WHICH MEDICATION SHOULD BE USED?

The available evidence suggests that drug selection should be tailored to the individual patient, with strong attention paid to the family history and potential adverse effects.

Metformin reduces the rates of type 2 diabetes (and possibly cardiovascular disease and malignancy) in high-risk adults and increases ovulation rates in patients with ovarian hyperandrogenism; thus the author considers metformin a valuable adjunct to the treatment of obese patients with severe insulin resistance, IFG, IGT, the metabolic syndrome, or PCOS. Metformin is tolerated by the majority of patients and is the least costly of currently used pharmacologic agents. The incretin mimetics, which reduce food intake and increase glucose-stimulated insulin secretion, may (in the future) also prove useful for treatment of obese adolescents with pre-diabetes. Like metformin, orlistat reduces rates of adult-onset diabetes and might prove beneficial in obese children with glucose intolerance. Dyslipidemic patients may benefit from orlistat or metformin, which reduce LDL levels and the LDL-to-HDL ratio in adults.

Of the medications tested thus far in children, sibutramine is most effective at reducing body weight, at least in the short term. However, its tendencies to raise blood pressure and pulse are concerning, given the high rates of systolic hypertension among obese adolescents. Sibutramine should not be used in children with poorly controlled hypertension or cardiovascular disease and is contraindicated in adolescents with preexisting psychiatric disorders. The long-term safety of anorectic agents in children has not been established, and, in the author's opinion, sibutramine remains an experimental approach for the treatment of pediatric obesity, requiring long-term study in carefully controlled clinical trials.

In the future, other classes of pharmacologic agents (e.g., centrally/vagally active melanocortin 4 receptor agonists, ghrelin antagonists) may be used for the treatment of obesity or maintenance of weight loss in adolescents or adults. All such drugs will require systematic investigation and careful consideration of their potential risks, as well as benefits, before they can be used in the general pediatric population.

HOW LONG DO WE NEED TO TREAT?

Obesity is a chronic, and in many cases lifelong, condition. Yet, pharmacotherapy might be discontinued or the dose of medication reduced significantly if short-term objectives of treatment are achieved, i.e., reduction in BMI z score and normalization of blood pressure, plasma lipids, and hepatic and renal function and, in girls with PCOS, reduction in hirsutism scores and restoration of ovulatory menses.

A recent investigation *(61)* in obese adolescents showed that discontinuation of metformin was accompanied by partial weight regain during the subsequent 6 months. Weight regain has also been observed following discontinuation of sibutramine and rimonabant *(88)*. Thus, some patients may require long-term pharmacotherapy for long-lasting benefit. If an anti-obesity medication is discontinued or its dose reduced, it is essential that lifestyle intervention be maintained throughout; this may limit rebound weight gain and might prevent relapse of co-morbidities.

REFERENCES

1. Colman E. Anorectics on trial: a half-century of federal regulation of prescription appetite suppressants. Ann Int Med. 2005;143:380–5.
2. Freemark M. Pharmacotherapy of childhood obesity: an evidence-based, conceptual approach. Diabetes Care. 2007;30:395–402.
3. Luttikhuis HO, Baur L, Jansen H, et al. Interventions for treating obesity in children. Cochrane Database Syst Rev. 2009;1:CD001872.
4. Epstein LH, Valoski A, Wing RR, McCurley J. Ten-year outcomes of behavioral family-based treatment for childhood obesity. Health Psychol. 1994;13:373–83.
5. Turrell G, Kavanagh AM. Socio-economic pathways to diet: modeling the association between socio-economic position and food purchasing behaviour. Public Health Nutr. 2006;9:375–83.
6. Weiss R, Taksali SE, Tamborlane WV, Burgert TS, Savoye M, Caprio S. Predictors of changes in glucose tolerance status in obese youth. Diabetes Care. 2005;28:902–9.
7. Nguyen QM, Srinivasan SR, Xu JH, Chen W, Berenson GS. Changes in risk variables of metabolic syndrome since childhood in pre-diabetic and type 2 diabetic subjects: the Bogalusa Heart Study. Diabetes Care. 2008;31:2044–9.
8. Morrison JA, Friedman LA, Wang P, Glueck CJ. Metabolic syndrome in childhood predicts adult metabolic syndrome and type 2 diabetes mellitus 25–30 years later. J Pediatr. 2008;152:201–6.
9. Baker JL, Olsen LW, Sorensen TIA. Childhood body mass index and the risk of coronary heart disease in adulthood. N Eng J Med. 2007;357:2329–37.
10. Must A, Jacques PF, Dallal GE, Bajema CJ, Dietz WH. Long-term morbidity and mortality of overweight adolescents: a follow-up of the Harvard Growth Study of 1922–1935. N Engl J Med. 1992;327:1350–5.
11. Li D, Morris JS, Liu J, Hassan MM, Day RS, Bondy ML, Abbruzzese JL. Body mass index and risk, age of onset, and survival in patients with pancreatic cancer. JAMA. 2009;301:2553–62.
12. Leung WYS, Thomas N, Chan JCN, Tomlinson B. Weight management and current options in pharmacotherapy: orlistat and sibutramine. Clin Ther. 2003;25:58–80.
13. Zhou G, Myers R, Li Y, Chen Y, Shen X, Fenyk-Melody J, Wu M, Ventre J, Doebber T, Fujii N, Musi N, Hirshman MF, Goodyear LJ, Moller DE. Role of AMP-activated protein kinase in mechanism of metformin action. J Clin Invest. 2001;108:1167–74.
14. Lindsay JR, Duffy NA, McKillop AM, Ardill J, O'Harte FP, Flatt PR, Bell PM. Inhibition of dipeptidyl peptidase IV activity by oral metformin in type 2 diabetes. Diabet Med. 2005;22:654–7.
15. Tsilchorozidou T, Batterham RL, Conway GS. Metformin increases fasting plasma peptide tyrosine tyrosine (PYY) in women with polycystic ovarian syndrome (PCOS). Clin Endocrinol. 2008;69:936–42.
16. Chau-Van C, Gamba M, Salvi R, Gaillard RC, Pralong FP. Metformin inhibits adenosine 5'-monophosphate-activated kinase activation and prevents increases in neuropeptide Y expression in cultured hypothalamic neurons. Endocrinology. 2007;148(2):507–11.
17. Halford JC, Harrold JA, Boyland EJ, Lawton CL, Blundell JE. Serotonergic drugs : effects on appetite expression and use for the treatment of obesity. Drugs. 2007;67(1):27–55.
18. Connoley IP, Liu YL, Frost I, Reckless IP, Heal DJ, Stock MJ. Thermogenic effects of sibutramine and its metabolites. Br J Pharmacol. 1999;126(6):1487–95.

19. Hansen D, Astrup A, Toubro S, et al; Goulder For The STORM Study Group M. Predictors of weight loss and maintenance during 2 years of treatment by sibutramine in obesity. Results from the European multi-centre STORM trial. Sibutramine Trial of Obesity Reduction and Maintenance. Int J Obes Relat Metab Disord. 2001;25(4):496–501.

20. Rucker D, Padwal R, Li SK, Curioni C, Lau DC. Long term pharmacotherapy for obesity and overweight: updated meta-analysis. BMJ. 2007;35:1194–9.

21. Wadden TA, Berkowitz RI, Womble LG, Sarwer DB, Phelan S, Cato RK, Hesson LA, Osei SY, Kaplan R, Stunkard A. Randomized trial of lifestyle modification and pharmacotherapy for obesity. N Engl J Med. 2005;353:2111–20.

22. Berkowitz RI, Wadden TA, Tershakovec AM, Cronquist JL. Behavior therapy and sibutramine for the treatment of adolescent obesity: a randomized controlled trial. JAMA. 2003;289(14):1805–12.

23. Godoy-Matos A, Carraro L, Vieira A, Oliveira J, Guedes EP, Mattos L, Rangel C, Moreira RO, Coutinho W, Appolinario JC. Treatment of obese adolescents with sibutramine: a randomized, double-blind controlled study. J Clin Endocrinol Metab. 2005;90:1460–65.

24. Berkowitz RI, Fujioka K, Daniels SR, Hoppin AG, Owen S, Perry AC, Sothern MS, Renz CL, Pirner MA, Walsh JK, Jasinsky O, Hewkin AC, Blakesley VA. Effects of sibutramine treatment in obese adolescents: a randomized trial. Ann Int Med. 2006;145:81–90.

25. McGovern L, Johnson JN, Paulo R, et al. Treatment of pediatric obesity. A systematic review and meta-analysis of randomized trials. J Clin Endocrinol Metab. 2008;93(12):4600–5.

26. Padwal R, Li SK, Lau DCW. Long-term pharmacotherapy for overweight and obesity: a systematic review and meta-analysis of randomized controlled trials. Int J Obes. 2003;27:1437–46.

27. Ioannides-Demos LL, Proietto J, McNeil JJ. Pharmacotherapy for obesity. Drugs. 2005;65:1391–1418.

28. Harrison-Woolrych M, Clark DWJ, Hill GR, Rees MI, Skinner JR. QT interval prolongation associated with sibutramine treatment. Br J Clin Pharmacol. 2006;61:464–69.

29. Basu D, Gillman PK, Gnanadesigan N, Espinoza RT, Smith RL, Claassen JAHR, Gelissen HPMM, Boyer EW, Shannon M. The serotonin syndrome. N Engl J Med. 2005;352:2454–6.

30. Drew BS, Dixon AF, Dixon JB. Obesity management: update on orlistat. Vasc Health Risk Manag. 2007;3(6):817–82.

31. Torgersen JS, Hauptman J, Boldrin MN, Sjostrom L. XENical in the prevention of Diabetes in Obese Subjects (XENDOS) Study: a randomized study of orlistat as an adjunct to lifestyle changes for the prevention of type 2 diabetes in obese patients. Diabetes Care. 2004;27:155–61.

32. Padwal RS, Majumdar SR. Drug treatments for obesity: orlistat, sibutramine, and rimonabant. Lancet. 2007;369:71–7.

33. Richelsen B, Tonstad S, Rossner S. Effect of orlistat on weight regain and cardiovascular risk factors following a very-low-energy diet in abdominally obese patients: a 3-year randomized, placebo-controlled study. Diabetes Care. 2007;30:27–32.

34. Norris SL, Zhang X, Avenell A, et al. Long-term non-pharmacologic weight loss interventions for adults with type 2 diabetes. Cochrane Database Syst Rev. 2005;2:CD004095. Also Norris SL, Zhang X, Avenell A, et al. Pharmacotherapy for weight loss in adults with type 2 diabetes mellitus. Cochrane Database Syst Rev. 2005;1:CD004096.

35. Zelber-Sagi S, Kessler A, Brazowsky E, et al. A double-blind randomized placebo-controlled trial of orlistat for the treatment of nonalcoholic fatty liver disease. Clin Gastroenterol Hepatol. 2006;4:639–44.

36. Chanoine J-P, Hampl S, Jensen C, Boldrin M, Hauptman J. Effects of orlistat on weight and body composition in obese adolescents: a randomized controlled trial. JAMA. 2005;293:2873–83.

37. Maahs D, de Serna DG, Kolotkin RL, et al. Randomized, double- blind, placebo-controlled trial of orlistat for weight loss in adolescents. Endocr Pract. 2006;12:18–28.

38. Heymsfield SB, Segal KR, Hauptman J, et al. Effects of weight loss with orlistat on glucose tolerance and progression to type 2 diabetes in obese adults. Arch Intern Med. 2000;160:1321–26.

39. Richelsen B, Tonstad S, Rössner S, et al. Effect of orlistat on weight regain and cardiovascular risk factors following a very-low-energy diet in abdominally obese patients: a 3-year randomized, placebo-controlled study. Diabetes Care. 2007;30:27–32.

40. Damci T, Yalin S, Balci H, Osar Z, Korugan U, Ozyazar M, Ilkova H. Orlistat augments postprandial increases in glucagon-like peptide 1 in obese type 2 diabetic patients. Diabetes Care. 2004;27(5):1077–80.

41. Gotfredsen A, Westergren Hendel H, Andersen T. Influence of orlistat on bone turnover and body composition. Int J Obes Relat Metab Disord. 2001;25:1154–60.

42. Artz E, Haqq A, Freemark M. Hormonal and metabolic consequences of childhood obesity. Endocrinol Metab Clin North Am. 2005;34:643–58.

43. Singh A, Sarkar SR, Gaber LW, et al. Acute oxalate nephropathy associated with orlistat, a gastrointestinal lipase inhibitor. Am J Kidney Dis. 2007;49:153–7.

44. Garcia SB, Barros LT, Turatti A, et al. The anti-obesity agent Orlistat is associated to increase in colonic preneoplastic markers in rats treated with a chemical carcinogen. Cancer Lett. 2006;240:221–4.

45. Shu Y, Sheardown SA, Brown C, Owen RP, Zhang S, Castro RA, Ianculescu AG, Yue L, Lo JC, Burchard EG, Brett CM, Giacomini KM. Effect of genetic variation in the organic cation transporter (Oct-1) on metformin. J Clin Invest. 2007;117:1422–31.

46. White MF. Metformin and insulin meet in a most atypical way. Cell Metab. 2009;9(6):485–7.

47. Shaw RJ, Lamia KA, Vasquez D, Koo SH, Bardeesy N, Depinho RA, Montminy M, Cantley LC. The kinase LKB1 mediates glucose homeostasis in liver and therapeutic effects of metformin. Science. 2005;310(5754): 1642–6.

48. Tiikkainen M, Hakkinen AM, Korsheninnikova E, Nyman T, Makimattila S, Yki-Jarvinen H. Effects of rosiglitazone and metformin on liver fat content, hepatic insulin resistance, insulin clearance, and gene expression in adipose tissue in patients with type 2 diabetes. Diabetes. 2004;53:2169–76. See also Orchard TJ, Temprosa M, Goldberg R, Haffner S, Ratner R, Marcovina S, Fowler S. The effect of metformin and intensive lifestyle intervention on the metabolic syndrome: the Diabetes Prevention Program randomized trial. Ann Int Med. 2005;142:611–9.

49. Erdem G, Dogru T, Tasci I, Bozoglu E, Muhsiroglu O, Tapan S, Ercin CN, Sonmez A. The effects of pioglitazone and metformin on plasma visfatin levels in patients with treatment-naïve type 2 diabetes mellitus. Diabetes Res Clin Pract. 2008;82(2):214–8.

50. Paolisso G, Amato L, Eccellente R, Gambardella A, Tagliamonte MR, Varricchio G, Carella C, Giugliano D, D'Onofrio F. Effect of metformin on food intake in obese subjects. Eur J Clin Invest. 1998;28(6):441–6.

51. Salpeter SR, Buckley NS, Kahn JA, Salpeter EE. Meta-analysis: metformin treatment in persons at risk for diabetes mellitus. Am J Med. 2008;121:149–57.

52. Freemark M, Bursey D. The effects of metformin on body mass index and glucose tolerance in obese adolescents with fasting hyperinsulinemia and a family history of type 2 diabetes. Pediatrics. 2001;107:e55–67.

53. Kay JP, Alemzadeh R, Langley G, D'Angelo L, Smith P, Holshouser S. Beneficial effects of metformin in normo-glycemic morbidly obese adolescents. Metabolism. 2001;50:1457–61.

54. Srinivasan S, Ambler GR, Baur LA, Garnett SP, Tepsa M, Yap F, Ward GM, Cowell CT. Randomized, controlled trial of metformin for obesity and insulin resistance in children and adolescents: improvement in body composition and fasting insulin. J Clin Endocrinol Metab. 2006;91:2074–80.

55. Burgert TS, Duran EJ, Goldberg-Gell R, Dziura J, Yeckel CW, Katz S, Tamborlane WV, Caprio S. Short term metabolic and cardiovascular effects of metformin in morbidly obese adolescents with normal glucose tolerance. Pediatr Diabetes. 2008;9(6):567–76.

56. Klein DJ, Cottingham EM, Sorter M, Barton BA, Morrison JA. A randomized, double-blind, placebo-controlled trial of metformin treatment of weight gain associated with initiation of atypical antipsychotic therapy in children and adolescents. Am J Psychiatry. 2006;163(12):2072–9.

57. Love-Osborne K, Sheeder J, Zeitler P. Addition of metformin to a lifestyle modification program in adolescents with insulin resistance. J Pediatr. 2008;152(6):817–22.

58. Atabek ME, Pirgon O. Use of metformin in obese adolescents with hyperinsulinemia: a 6-month, randomized, double-blind, placebo-controlled clinical trial. J Pediatr Endocrinol Metab. 2008;21(4):339–48.

59. Clarson CL, Mahmud FH, Baker JE, Clark HE, McKay WM, Schauteet VD, Hill DJ. Metformin in combination with structured lifestyle intervention improved body mass index in obese adolescents, but did not improve insulin resistance. Endocrine. 2009;36(1):141–6.

60. Yanovski JA, Sorg RA, Krakoff J, Kozlosky M, Sebring NG, Salaita CG, Keil M, McDuffie JR, Calis KA. A randomized, placebo-controlled trial of the effects of metformin on body weight and body composition in children with insulin resistance. Abstract presented at the 90th annual meeting of the Endocrine Society, San Francisco, CA. 2008

61. Wilson DM, Abrams SH, Aye T, Lee PD, Lenders C, Lustig RH, Osganian SV, Feldman HA; Glaser Pediatric Research Network Obesity Study Group. Metformin extended release treatment of adolescent obesity: a 48-week randomized, double-blind, placebo-controlled trial with 48-week follow-up. Arch Pediatr Adolesc Med. 2010 Feb;164(2):116–23.

62. Knowler WC, Barrett-Connor E, Fowler SE, Hamman RF, Lachin JM, Walker EA, Nathan DM. Reduction in the incidence of type 2 diabetes with lifestyle intervention or metformin. N Engl J Med. 2002;346:393–403.

63. Ratner RE, Christophi CA, Metzger BE, Dabelea D, Bennett PH, Pi-Sunyer X, Fowler S, Kahn SE; Diabetes Prevention Program Research Group. Prevention of diabetes in women with a history of gestational diabetes: effects of metformin and lifestyle interventions. J Clin Endocrinol Metab. 2008;93(12):4774–9.

64. West DS, Elaine Prewitt T, Bursac Z, Felix HC. Weight loss of black, white, and Hispanic men and women in the Diabetes Prevention Program. Obesity (Silver Spring). 2008;16(6):1413–20.

65. Ramachandran A, Snehalatha C, Mary S, Mukesh B, Bhaskar AD, Vijay V. The Indian Diabetes Prevention Programme shows that lifestyle modification and metformin prevent type 2 diabetes in Asian Indian subjects with impaired glucose tolerance (IDPP-1). Diabetologia. 2006;49:289–97.

66. Diabetes Prevention Program Research Group; Knowler WC, Fowler SE, Hamman RF, Christophi CA, Hoffman HJ, Brenneman AT, Brown-Friday JO, Goldberg R, Venditti E, Nathan DM. 10-year follow-up of diabetes incidence and weight loss in the Diabetes Prevention Program Outcomes Study. Lancet. 2009;374(9702):1677–86.

67. UKPDS Group. Effect of intensive blood-glucose control with metformin on complications in overweight patients with type 2 diabetes (UKPDS 34): UK Prospective Diabetes Study (UKPDS) Group. Lancet. 1998;352:854–65.

68. Johnson JA, Majumdar SR, Simpson SH, Toth EL. Decreased mortality associated with the use of metformin compared with sulfonylurea monotherapy in type 2 diabetes. Diabetes Care. 2002;25:2244–8.

69. Kooy A, de Jager J, Lehert P, Bets D, Wulffelé MG, Donker AJ, Stehouwer CD. Long-term effects of metformin on metabolism and microvascular and macrovascular disease in patients with type 2 diabetes mellitus. Arch Int Med. 2009;169:616–25.

70. Calvert JW, Gundewar S, Jha S, Greer JJ, Bestermann WH, Tian R, Lefer DJ. Acute metformin therapy confers cardioprotection against myocardial infarction via AMPK-eNOS-mediated signaling. Diabetes. 2008;57:696–705.

71. La Marca A, Artensio AC, Stabile G, Volpe A. Metformin treatment of PCOS during adolescence and the reproductive period. Eur J Obstet Gynecol Reprod Biol. 2005;12:3–7.

72. Arslanian SA, Lewy V, Danadian K, Saad R. Metformin therapy in obese adolescents with polycystic ovary syndrome and impaired glucose tolerance: amelioration of exaggerated adrenal response to adrenocorticotropin with reduction of insulinemia/insulin resistance. J Clin Endocrinol Metab. 2002;87(4):1555–9.

73. Ibanez L, Lopez-Bermejo A, Diaz M, Marcos MV, de Zegher F. Pubertal metformin therapy to reduce total, visceral, and hepatic adiposity. J Pediatr. 2010;156(1):98–102.

74. Ibanez L, Valls C, Ong K, Dunger DB, deZegher F. Metformin therapy during puberty delays menarche, prolongs pubertal growth, and augments adult height: a randomized study in low-birth-weight girls with early-normal onset of puberty. J Clin Endocrinol Metab. 2006;91:2068–73.

75. Ong K, deZegher F, Vallis C, Dunger DB, Ibanez L. Persisting benefits 12–18 months after discontinuation of pubertal metformin therapy in low birthweight girls. Clin Endocrinol. 2007;67:468–71.

76. Currie CJ, Poole CD, Gale EA. The influence of glucose-lowering therapies on cancer risk in type 2 diabetes. Diabetologia. Sept 2009;52(9):1766–77.

77. Libby G, Donnelly LA, Donnan PT, Alessi DR, Morris AD, Evans JM. New users of metformin are at low risk of incident cancer: a cohort study of people with type 2 diabetes. Diabetes Care. Sept 2009;32(9):1620–5.

78. Cryer DR, Nicholas SP, Henry DH, Mills DJ, Stadel BV. Comparative outcomes study of metformin intervention versus conventional approach: the COSMIC Approach Study. Diabetes Care. 2005;28:539–43. See also Selby JV, Ettinger B, Swain BE, Brown JB. First 20 months' experience with use of metformin for type 2 diabetes in a large health maintenance organization. Diabetes Care. 1999;22:38–44.

79. Pi-Sunyer FX. The effects of pharmacologic agents for type 2 diabetes mellitus on body weight. Postgrad Med. 2008;120(2):5–17.

80. Norris SL, Lee N, Thakurta S, Chan BKS. Exenatide efficacy and safety: a systematic review. Diabetic Med. 2009;26:837–46.

81. Elkind-Hirsch K, Marrioneaux O, Bhushan M, Vernor D, Bhushan R. Comparison of single and combined treatment with exenatide and metformin on menstrual cyclicity in overweight women with polycystic ovary syndrome. J Clin Endocrinol Metab. 2008;93(7):2670–8.

82. Astrup A, Rossner S, Van Gaal L, Rissanen A, Niskanen L, Al Hakim M, Madsen J, Rasmussen MF, Lean ME. Effects of liraglutide in the treatment of obesity: a randomized, double-blind, placebo-controlled study. Lancet. 2009;374:1606–16.

83. Pocai A, Carrington PE, Adams JR, Wright M, Eiermann G, Zhu L, Du X, Petrov A, Lassman ME, Jiang G, Liu F, Miller C, Tota LM, Zhou G, Zhang X, Sountis MM, Santoprete A, Capito' E, Chicchi GG, Thornberry N, Bianchi E, Pessi A, Marsh DJ, SinhaRoy R. Glucagon-like peptide 1/glucagon receptor dual agonism reverses obesity in mice. Diabetes. 2009;58(10):2258–66.

84. Wynne K, Park AJ, Small CJ, Meeran K, Ghatei MA, Frost GS, Bloom SR. Oxyntomodulin increases energy expenditure in addition to decreasing energy intake in overweight and obese humans: a randomised controlled trial. Int J Obes (London). 2006;30(12):1729–36.

85. Smith SR, Prosser WA, Donahue DJ, Morgan ME, Anderson CM, Shanahan WR; APD356-004 Study Group. Lorcaserin (APD356), a selective 5-HT(2C) agonist, reduces body weight in obese men and women. Obesity (Silver Spring). 2009;17(3):494–503.

86. Freemark M. Pharmacologic approaches to the prevention of type 2 diabetes in high-risk pediatric patients. J Clin Endocrinol Metab. 2003;88:3–13.

87. Nguyen QM, Srinivasan SR, Xu J-H, Chen W, Kieltyka L, Berenson GS. Utility of childhood glucose homeostasis variables in predicting adult diabetes and related cardiometabolic risk factors: the Bogalusa Heart Study. Diabetes Care. 2010;33(3):670–5.

88. Pi-Sunyer F, Aronne LJ, Heshmati HM, Devin J, Rosenstock J. Effect of rimonabant, a cannabinoid-1 receptor blocker, on weight and cardiometabolic risk factors in overweight or obese patients: RIO-North America. JAMA. 2006;295:761–75.

24 Pathogenesis and Management of Adiposity and Insulin Resistance in PCOS: Prevention and Treatment of the Metabolic Disease Components

Stephen Franks and Jalini Joharatnam

CONTENTS

Key Words: Free androgen, testosterone, hirsutism, anovulation, insulin resistance, metabolic syndrome, oral contraceptives, spironolactone, cyproterone

INTRODUCTION: POLYCYSTIC OVARY SYNDROME (PCOS)

PCOS is the commonest endocrine disorder of women; it affects 5–10% of the female population and typically presents during adolescence. It is a heterogeneous syndrome, but the classic features are anovulation (irregular menstrual cycles) and symptoms of androgen excess such as hirsutism, acne, and alopecia. The most consistent biochemical abnormality is hyperandrogenaemia, as most commonly defined by higher than normal serum concentrations of testosterone (or androstenedione) and/or an elevated-free androgen index (see below). Many subjects with PCOS also have elevated serum levels of LH but normal FSH levels. Importantly, PCOS is also associated with metabolic abnormalities, notably insulin resistance and hyperinsulinaemia, which are associated with a high risk developing type 2 diabetes in later life (1). Obesity is of course an important amplifier of metabolic disturbance

From: *Contemporary Endocrinology: Pediatric Obesity: Etiology, Pathogenesis, and Treatment*
Edited by: M. Freemark, DOI 10.1007/978-1-60327-874-4_24,
© Springer Science+Business Media, LLC 2010

and worryingly, the escalating incidence of childhood obesity means that an increasing number of adolescents with PCOS have metabolic dysfunction.

The diagnostic criteria for PCOS are somewhat controversial. The NIH multi-disciplinary "consensus" conference of 1990 recommended that the diagnosis be based on the classic combination of oligo- or anovulation and hyperandrogenism (2). However, the recognition that many hyperandrogenemic women with polycystic ovaries have regular, ovulatory cycles led to a reappraisal of the diagnostic criteria at the 2003 consensus conference sponsored jointly by the American Society for Reproductive Medicine (ASRM) and the European Society for Human Reproduction & Embryology (ESHRE). The so-called Rotterdam criteria require two of the following three criteria for diagnosis: clinical or biochemical hyperandrogenism, polycystic ovaries on ultrasonography, and menstrual irregularities (3). This classification has the advantage of highlighting the heterogeneity of the disorder but has been controversial because, by definition, women with polycystic ovaries and anovulation who have no obvious evidence of androgen excess can be labelled as having PCOS. Whilst there is good evidence that this subset of women with polycystic ovaries are indeed part of this syndrome (4), it is clear that the women who are most at risk of metabolic sequelae of PCOS are those with both anovulation and hyperandrogenism (5–7). It is primarily for this reason that the Androgen Excess Society (AES) criteria for definition of the syndrome emphasize that androgen excess is the foundation of PCOS (8).

DEVELOPMENTAL ORIGIN OF PCOS AND ITS EVOLUTION DURING CHILDHOOD

There is plentiful evidence that the etiology of PCOS involves a major genetic component (see below) but environmental factors, particularly diet, play an important part (9). The fact that PCOS presents in adolescence suggests that the origins of the disorder occur in childhood, perhaps even in foetal life. Animal models of PCOS support this hypothesis. Female Rhesus monkeys exposed to high concentrations of testosterone in utero develop many of the features of human PCOS as adults, such as high LH levels, ovarian hyperandrogenism, and anovulation in association with increased body weight and insulin resistance (10,11). Similar findings apply to the prenatally androgenized sheep model of PCOS (12,13), and even rodents exposed to excess androgen during early development show a characteristic metabolic phenotype (14,15). This suggests that the PCOS phenotype could be a direct result of androgen exposure, which "programmes" the foetal hypothalamic-pituitary-ovarian (HPO) axis as well as fat deposition and function in utero (16). With regard to the possible effects of androgen programming on reproductive hormones, there is emerging evidence that the high LH levels seen in many women with PCOS may be influenced by androgen. Defects in negative feedback of progesterone and oestrogen on gonadotropins have been described (17) and, importantly, these abnormalities can be reversed by treatment with the anti-androgen flutamide. This highlights the role of hyperandrogenaemia in sustaining this abnormal hypothalamic sensitivity to feedback inhibition (18).

In the case of the Rhesus monkey model of PCOS, it is important to note that the doses of androgen that were used were high enough to exceed two normally very efficient physiological barriers: first, placental aromatase, which converts excess androgen to oestrogens, and second, high circulating sex hormone binding globulin (SHBG) which binds testosterone and prevents placental transfer. It is therefore unlikely that, in pregnant women with PCOS, any excess maternal androgen would be able to cross the placenta in significant amounts (19). So "vertical transmission" of PCOS from mother to foetus probably does not occur. It is therefore suggested that the source of excess androgen is the foetal ovary (and/or adrenal) which may either be actively secreting excess androgen in utero or, perhaps more plausibly, be genetically predisposed to produce high ovarian androgen levels at the time of activation of the hypothalamic-pituitary-ovarian axis in infancy or at puberty (16). If the adrenal is contributing to excess androgen in PCOS, the normal burst of androgen secretion at adrenarche may be advanced or enhanced; indeed, there is indeed evidence for links between premature adrenarche, premature pubarche, and the appearance of PCOS in adolescence *(20)*.

It is not surprising that symptoms of PCOS appear in adolescents. Normal pubertal development is characterized by activation of the hypothalamic-pituitary-ovarian axis and is associated with physiological reductions in insulin sensitivity. In girls with a predisposition to PCOS, these changes are exaggerated by higher than normal levels of LH and, significantly, by hyperinsulinaemia that is further amplified by obesity.

GENES AND PCOS

The etiology of PCOS is unknown but heritability studies suggest a strong genetic susceptibility *(9,21)*. Familial clustering has been noted *(22,23)* and greater concordance in features of PCOS is observed between monozygotic than dizygotic twins *(24)*. Studying complex endocrine diseases such as PCOS and diabetes is difficult due to their likely genetic heterogeneity *(25)*. Several genes are likely to be implicated in the etiology of PCOS, but despite a plethora of candidate gene (mostly case-control) studies, few loci have been convincingly shown to be associated with the condition. Methodological problems have contributed to the confusion since many of the published studies have paid insufficient attention to the importance of having large enough and ethnically homogeneous populations.

However, two genes have recently been highlighted as potentially important. It is known that common variants in a 47 kb region of the first intron of the fat mass and obesity-associated gene (FTO) influence susceptibility to type 2 diabetes, via a substantial effect on BMI and fat mass *(26)*. Barber et al. showed a significant link between the FTO genotype and PCOS status in a UK case–control analysis *(27)*. The association was most evident in obese PCOS patients. Using linkage analysis, an association has also been found between PCOS and a dinucleotide repeat marker D19S884 (close to, but not in linkage disequilibrium with, the insulin receptor gene) on chromosome 19p13.2 *(28)*. Fine mapping places this polymorphism in the region of intron 55 of the fibrillin 3 gene (FBN3) *(25)*. Moreover this locus is associated with metabolic features of the syndrome in reproductive age women and their brothers *(21)*. The function of FBN3 is not clear but fibrillins are transforming growth factor beta (TGFβ) binding proteins, and growth factors in the TGFβ family have been implicated in early follicle development and theca formation in the ovary *(29)*. The poor yield of well-characterized, plausible susceptibility loci, using the candidate gene approach, has been disappointing and there is likely now to be greater focus on genome-wide association studies of the sort undertaken for identification of genes contributing to type II diabetes and other endocrine/metabolic traits *(30)*.

METABOLIC DYSFUNCTION IN PCOS

The central metabolic abnormality in PCOS is impaired insulin sensitivity and its associated hyperinsulinaemia *(31)*. Insulin sensitivity is reduced when compared with weight-matched controls without PCOS and there is an important interaction of insulin sensitivity with BMI so that there is a steeper decline with increasing BMI when compared to control women. The increased insulin resistance accounts for the high prevalence of impaired glucose tolerance in obese women with PCOS and the increased risk *(32)* (probably 3–4 fold) of developing type 2 diabetes *(33–35)*. Dyslipidaemia has also been reported in women with PCOS and may be a factor in the presumed increase in risk of cardiovascular disease *(36)*. At the moment, however, there is no clear evidence that these risk factors translate into an increase in cardiovascular *events* in PCOS. Insulin resistance in PCOS is also related to an abnormality of energy balance, notably reduced post-prandial thermogenesis *(37)*, which itself may have an impact on the development of obesity (see below).

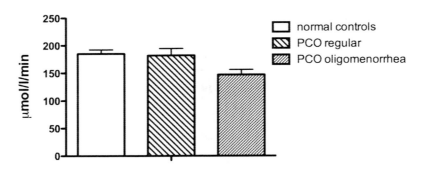

Fig. 1. Insulin sensitivity in BMI-matched groups of women with oligomenorrhea and PCOS ($n = 53$) or in hirsute women with polycystic ovaries and regular cycles ($n = 19$), compared with values in BMI-matched normal controls ($n = 31$). The two groups of women with PCO were equally hyperandrogenemic. Only the group with PCO and oligomenorrhea was insulin resistant ($p < 0.01$ compared with controls). Values shown are means + SEM. Data from Robinson et al. *(32)*.

It is important to emphasize that metabolic abnormalities in PCOS are a feature of women who have both anovulation and androgen excess, whereas weight-matched and equally hyperandrogenemic women with polycystic ovaries, but who have regular menses, have normal insulin sensitivity and serum insulin concentrations *(32)* (Fig. 1). This has implications for prediction of women at risk of long-term metabolic sequelae *(7)*. Another implication of the association between anovulation and metabolic dysfunction is that insulin resistance may be involved in the mechanism of anovulation in hyperandrogenemic women with PCOS; indeed, there is evidence, from both in vitro and clinical studies, that this is the case *(38)*. For example, therapies that lower insulin levels such as weight loss and insulin sensitizing drugs significantly improve menstrual cyclicity, fertility, and hyperandrogenism *(39–41)*.

MECHANISM OF INSULIN RESISTANCE IN PCOS

The cause(s) of reduced insulin sensitivity in PCOS remains unclear. Abnormalities of the insulin receptor itself are rare causes of PCOS and the weight of evidence points to a post-receptor defect in insulin signalling pathways *(31,42,43)*. It is likely that the signalling defect is located proximally in the pathway, involving serine phosphorylation of the insulin receptor (IR) and/or insulin receptor substrates 1 and 2 (IRS1/2) *(31,43)*. In about 50% of women with PCOS who had insulin resistance documented by euglycaemic clamp studies, there appeared to be constitutive activation of serine phosphorylation of the insulin receptor in skin fibroblasts that, in turn, inhibited insulin-stimulated tyrosine phosphorylation and hence normal insulin signalling *(44)*.

In cultures of skeletal muscle in obese women with PCOS, IRS-1 protein abundance was found to be significantly increased, resulting in decreased activity of phosphotidyl inositol 3-kinase (PI3K) *(43)*. Phosphorylation of IRS-1 Ser (312) (equivalent to Ser (307) in rat) was increased in PCOS, but despite these defects, cultured myotubules showed normal insulin responsiveness. No differences in IR tyrosine phosphorylation were seen between women with PCOS and controls. Thus, in contrast to skin fibroblasts, the defects in skeletal muscle seen in vivo are not reproduced in culture, suggesting that the in vivo environment is the major determinant of muscle insulin resistance in PCOS. However, certain defects in insulin signalling persist *(43)*. Serine phosphorylation of IRS1 inhibits its tyrosine phosphorylation and therefore its ability to recruit PI3K *(45)*. Another feature of insulin target tissues in women with PCOS is that expression of the insulin-dependent glucose transporter GLUT4 is abnormally low. This has been shown in adipocytes from subjects with PCOS *(46)* as well as in skeletal muscle from type 2 diabetics *(47)*.

The mechanism of insulin resistance in the ovary also appears to involve a post-receptor abnormality leading to a selective signalling defect. The effect of insulin on glucose metabolism in granulosa-lutein cells from women with anovulatory PCOS is attenuated whilst the steroidogenic response to insulin is preserved *(48)*. Glucose metabolism is needed for efficient oocyte maturation and function *(49)*, and this defect may contribute to infertility seen in PCOS patients.

ADIPOSITY IN PCOS

The relationship between adiposity and PCOS is complex. It is legitimate to pose the questions: (1) Are females with PCOS more likely to gain weight and deposit adipose tissue than those without PCOS? (2) Is there preferential deposition of visceral (i.e. more metabolically active) fat in women with PCOS? and (3) Does excess androgen affect the accumulation and site of adipose deposition? There is some evidence to support the notion that adolescents or adults with PCOS are relatively more prone to gain weight for any given calorie intake. The difference in post-prandial thermogenesis between obese subjects with and without PCOS was 42 kJ; we calculated that if this difference in energy expenditure was maintained daily for 1 year, it would be equivalent to an excess of 735, 000 kJ or 1.9 kg of fat for the same calorie intake *(37)*. Nevertheless, this effect is unlikely to represent a major factor in the genesis of obesity in PCOS.

In comparison with women with normal ovaries and regular cycles, women with PCOS have been thought to be prone to central adiposity, i.e. preferential accumulation of visceral fat deposits. However, results of our recent studies have cast doubt upon this "accepted" view. Barber et al. used systematic magnetic resonance imaging (MRI) to quantify visceral and subcutaneous fat accumulation in women with normal and polycystic ovaries, across a wide range of BMI *(50)*. Surprisingly, it was found that visceral fat depots increased similarly with increasing total body fat in both PCOS patients and controls (Fig. 2) despite clear differences between the groups in indices of androgenicity and insulin sensitivity. Intriguingly, although the relationship between visceral fat and total body fat was similar in the two groups, the relationship of insulin sensitivity to visceral fat area was different between normal and PCOS, suggesting that insulin resistance in PCOS cannot be attributed simply to altered body fat distribution.

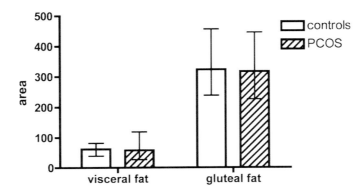

Fig. 2. Area of visceral and gluteal subcutaneous fat (cm^2) (geometric mean and SD) as measured by MRI in 44 BMI-matched obese women with PCOS ($n = 22$) or controls ($n = 22$). Note similar relationship of visceral to subcutaneous fat in both groups. Data from Barber et al. *(50)*.

The best evidence that exposure to excess androgen leads to adiposity comes from the studies of prenatally androgenized animals, as discussed above. Correlations between serum androgen concentrations and body fat mass (or truncal fat) can be found in women with PCOS but such an association does not establish cause and effect. The most consistent relationship is between fat mass and free testosterone index but this phenomenon is most likely to reflect the impact of obesity (via hyperinsulinaemia) on suppression of SHBG, as detailed below.

Whether or not women with PCOS are more likely to accumulate fat, it is quite clear that weight gain and increased fat deposition are associated with a worsening of clinical and biochemical features of PCOS (51,52). Thus, women who are overweight or obese are more likely to have anovulatory cycles or amenorrhea and have a greater degree of hirsutism. Total and, particularly, non-SHBG-bound testosterone concentrations are elevated. The increase in the so-called free testosterone index (calculated by T/SHBG x100) is mainly a function of lowered SHBG concentrations. Serum levels of SHBG are inversely related to BMI and to fasting insulin concentrations and there is evidence for a direct inhibitory effect of insulin on hepatic production of SHBG (53,54).

METABOLIC SYNDROME IN ADOLESCENTS WITH PCOS

Metabolic syndrome (MBS) is associated with increased cardiovascular risk. It is defined by the presence of a cluster of features derived from measurements including waist circumference, blood pressure, fasting glucose, and lipid profile. The prevalence of metabolic syndrome in obese adults with PCOS has been reported to be between 30 and 45% (7,55–58). There are few such studies in adolescent girls with adequate numbers of subjects but a recent publication from Rossi and colleagues has reported the prevalence and features of metabolic syndrome in a group of 43 obese girls (mean age 15.6 years) with PCOS and compared their results with a group of 31 control girls with similar BMI (59). Using adult criteria for diagnosis of MBS, 26% of the PCOS group and 29% of controls had MBS. The authors therefore concluded that obesity, rather than PCOS per se, was the major determinant of MBS in adolescents.

DIAGNOSTIC INVESTIGATION

The diagnosis of PCOS is largely made clinically, but in adolescents with symptoms of hyperandrogenism, measurements of total and free testosterone and adrenal androgens may help to exclude other, more severe causes of androgen excess. Serum 17OH progesterone levels can differentiate patients with non-virilizing 21OHase deficiency from those with PCOS. In those with oligo- or amenorrhea, measurements of LH, FSH, and prolactin should be undertaken. A trans-abdominal ultrasound is useful in some cases; however, some clinicians argue that girls with both hyperandrogenism and menstrual disturbance are likely to have PCOS and that a scan is not essential in further management (3). In patients with BMI exceeding 30 kg/m^2 an oral glucose tolerance test should be performed.

MANAGEMENT OF ADOLESCENTS WITH PCOS

The management of adolescents with PCOS has two main objectives: first to control symptoms of androgen excess and/or anovulation and second to reduce the risk of long-term complications such as type 2 diabetes. It is very important to make an early diagnosis of PCOS so that girls who are symptomatic, but of normal weight, can be given advice about keeping their body weight under control. This is the best way to prevent symptoms of androgen excess and anovulation from escalating and to limit the risk of metabolic complications.

Treatment is tailored to the needs of the patient. Hirsutism and acne cause deep distress in adolescent girls, as does weight gain. Treatment of cutaneous problems should be instituted without delay. Treatment of infertility is, of course, rarely an issue in this age group, although many girls will wish to be reassured about the future prospects of fertility. The preferred and most effective method of treatment for obese adolescents with PCOS is lifestyle modification. It produces an improvement in all the features of PCOS *(39,60)*. This approach is safe and non-pharmacological; unfortunately, weight loss programmes in children are notoriously unsuccessful *(61)*.

Treatment of menstrual irregularities in adolescents centres on re-establishing a predictable cycle of menstruation. This can be attained with the combined oral contraceptive pill (COCP), which is considered first-line therapy for adolescent PCOS by most paediatric endocrinologists *(62)* or by cyclical progestogens. In addition to regulating the cycle, which will prevent future complications resulting from endometrial hyperplasia, the COCP has an anti-androgenic effect by elevating SHBG levels and reducing LH-driven ovarian androgen production. In the overweight or obese population, education about the beneficial effects of weight loss on the menstrual cycle (as well as on future long-term health) should be stressed, and practical advice on diet and exercise should be given.

Symptoms of androgen excess are best treated with a combination of cosmetic management and, if necessary, anti-androgen therapy *(63)*. Cosmetic management includes shaving (very efficient but not popular), waxing, and epilation by electrolysis or laser. The most commonly used anti-androgen in the UK is cyproterone acetate, often used in combination with ethinylestradiol (as in co-cyprindiol: ethinylestradiol 35 µg + cyproterone acetate 2 mg, often prescribed as Dianette in the UK). If necessary, additional cyproterone acetate (25–50 mg daily) can be combined with co-cyprindiol.

Cyproterone acetate is not available in the United States, where the pharmacologically similar spironolactone is preferred. Spironolactone is an equally effective anti-androgen; doses as low as 50 mg daily have produced efficient reduction in hyperandrogenism in adolescents *(64)*. Flutamide is a potent, non-steroidal anti-androgen that is not routinely used in the UK, but is effective in the treatment of hyperandrogenism in adolescents *(65,66)*. Its high cost and potential hepatotoxicity preclude its widepread use; although there is little evidence for liver damage at chronic low doses, it is probably best avoided *(67)*. Acne can be treated with both topical and oral antibiotics. Those with more severe disease often respond to anti-androgen therapy. In resistant cases, treatment with retinoic acid derivatives under the supervision of a dermatologist is recommended.

Treatment with the COCP and/or anti-androgens corrects hyperandrogenism and menstrual irregularities but these agents have little effect on insulin resistance and its metabolic consequences. If lifestyle modification is unsuccessful, drugs which improve insulin sensitivity and lower insulin levels can be useful. Metformin has been shown to reduce central adiposity and free testosterone levels and to increase insulin sensitivity and menstrual regularity in obese adolescents with PCOS *(66,68–70)*. The recommended starting dose is 500 mg daily, increasing to a maximum of 2 g daily in divided doses. However, there are few adequately powered short-term studies of efficacy and a serious lack of data on the long-term effects of metformin on the metabolic complications of PCOS in adults. There are even fewer such studies in adolescents. Recently, a large and well-conducted randomized controlled trial comparing metformin and clomiphene (either alone or in combination) showed no benefit of metformin on ovulation induction *(71)*, which although not usually relevant in adolescents, highlights the importance of large randomized trials in clarifying the potential benefits of metformin. Thiazolidinediones, although successful in adults in improving androgen levels, insulin resistance, and lipid profiles, are not likely to overtake metformin in their use in adolescents due to their side effect profile. They cause weight gain and may have adverse long-term effects on the cardiovascular system and bone development *(72,73)*.

SUMMARY

PCOS is very common and typically presents in adolescent girls. It is the major cause of hirsutism and menstrual abnormalities but is also an important risk factor for development of metabolic abnormalities. Insulin resistance and hyperinsulinaemia are more prevalent in girls with PCOS than in the general population and these metabolic abnormalities are amplified by obesity. Women with PCOS are at higher than normal risk of developing metabolic syndrome (MBS) and type 2 diabetes but in adolescents the risk of MBS appears to be mainly related to obesity rather than PCOS per se. Prevention or treatment of metabolic complications in PCOS is ideally best achieved by modification of diet and lifestyle but this is not easy in teenagers. Insulin sensitizing agents may have a part to play in managing metabolic sequelae of PCOS but there have been, as yet, few large-scale, controlled trials to help guide clinical practice.

Editor's Questions and Authors' Response

- **Precocious adrenarche and/or obesity in childhood predisposes to PCOS in adolescent girls and young women (see, for example, Rosenfield, 2007; Kousta, 2006; Chapter 18 by Glueck and Morrison and Chapters 12 and 23 by Freemark, this volume). How much (or what percent) weight loss is required to reverse anovulation and hirsutism in PCOS?**

- Weight loss in excess of 5% is usually enough to improve ovulation rate. Impact on hirsutism is there but less easily defined – no very good long-term studies.

  Kousta E. Premature adrenarche leads to polycystic ovary syndrome? Long-term consequences. Ann NY Acad Sci. 2006;1092:148–57.
  Rosenfield RL. Identifying children at risk for polycystic ovary syndrome. J Clin Endocrinol Metab. 2007;92:787–96.

- **What are the long-term prospects for fertility in an adolescent with PCOS?**

- Prospects for fertility are generally pretty good. In our studies using clomiphene (or FSH in clomiphene non-responders) the overall pregnancy rate is in excess of 80%. Obesity is a major barrier, so weight loss is important.

Editor's Comment

- PCOS may be accompanied by dyslipidaemia, hypertension, impaired fibrinolysis, arterial stiffness, and endothelial dysfunction, and decreased insulin-mediated vasodilatation (e.g. see Glueck et al., 2008). In theory (not yet demonstrated in PCOS), these may increase the long-term risks of cardiovascular disease. Preliminary studies suggest that metformin may reduce arterial stiffness and improve endothelial function in young women with PCOS (e.g. see Agarwal et al., 2010). These effects may be mediated in part by weight loss, since similar changes can be demonstrated following weight reduction in type 2 diabetes (Barinas-Mitchell et al., 2006).

  Agarwal N, Rice SP, Bolusani H, Luzio SD, Dunseath G, Ludgate M, Rees DA. Metformin reduces arterial stiffness and improves endothelial function in young women with polycystic ovary syndrome: a randomized, placebo-controlled, crossover trial. J Clin Endocrinol Metab. 2010 Feb;95(2):722–30.
  Barinas-Mitchell E, Kuller LH, Sutton-Tyrrell K, Hegazi R, Harper P, Mancino J, Kelley DE. Effect of Weight Loss and Nutritional Intervention on Arterial Stiffness in Type 2 Diabetes. Diabetes Care. 2006;29:2218–22.

Glueck CJ, Morrison JA, Wang P. Insulin resistance, obesity, hypofibrinolysis, hyperandrogenism, and coronary heart disease risk factors in 25 pre-perimenarchal girls age < or =14 years, 13 with precocious puberty, 23 with a first-degree relative with polycystic ovary syndrome. J Pediatr Endocrinol Metab. 2008 Oct;21(10):973–84.

REFERENCES

1. Franks S. Polycystic ovary syndrome. N Engl J Med. 1995;333(13):853–61.
2. Zawadzki J, Dunaif A. Diagnostic criteria for polycystic ovary syndrome: towards a rational approach. In: Dunaif A, Givens JR, Haseltine FP, Merriam GR, editors. Polycystic ovary syndrome. Oxford: Blackwell Scientific Publications. 1992. pp. 377–84.
3. Rotterdam1. Revised 2003 consensus on diagnostic criteria and long-term health risks related to polycystic ovary syndrome (PCOS). Hum Reprod. Jan 2004;19(1):41–7.
4. Franks S. Controversy in clinical endocrinology: diagnosis of polycystic ovarian syndrome: in defense of the Rotterdam criteria. J Clin Endocrinol Metab. Mar 2006;91(3):786–9.
5. Welt CK, Gudmundsson JA, Arason G, et al. Characterizing discrete subsets of polycystic ovary syndrome as defined by the Rotterdam criteria: the impact of weight on phenotype and metabolic features. J Clin Endocrinol Metab. Dec 2006;91(12):4842–8.
6. Dewailly D, Catteau-Jonard S, Reyss AC, Leroy M, Pigny P. Oligoanovulation with polycystic ovaries but not overt hyperandrogenism. J Clin Endocrinol Metab. Oct 2006;91(10):3922–7.
7. Barber TM, Wass JA, McCarthy MI, Franks S. Metabolic characteristics of women with polycystic ovaries and oligo-amenorrhoea but normal androgen levels: implications for the management of polycystic ovary syndrome. Clin Endocrinol. 2007;66(4):513–7.
8. Azziz R, Carmina E, Dewailly D, et al. Positions statement: criteria for defining polycystic ovary syndrome as a predominantly hyperandrogenic syndrome: an Androgen Excess Society guideline. J Clin Endocrinol Metab. Nov 2006;91(11):4237–45.
9. Franks S. Polycystic ovary syndrome in adolescents. Int J Obes (Lond). Jul 2008;32(7):1035–41.
10. Eisner JR, Dumesic DA, Kemnitz JW, Abbott DH. Timing of prenatal androgen excess determines differential impairment in insulin secretion and action in adult female rhesus monkeys. J Clin Endocrinol Metab. Mar 2000;85(3):1206–10.
11. Eisner JR, Barnett MA, Dumesic DA, Abbott DH. Ovarian hyperandrogenism in adult female rhesus monkeys exposed to prenatal androgen excess. Fertil Steril. Jan 2002;77(1):167–72.
12. Padmanabhan V, Manikkam M, Recabarren S, Foster D. Prenatal testosterone excess programs reproductive and metabolic dysfunction in the female. Mol Cell Endocrinol. 26 Feb 2006;246(1–2):165–74.
13. Abbott DH, Zhou R, Bird IM, Dumesic DA, Conley AJ. Fetal programming of adrenal androgen excess: lessons from a nonhuman primate model of polycystic ovary syndrome. Endocr Dev. 2008;13:145–58.
14. Manneras L, Cajander S, Holmang A, et al. A new rat model exhibiting both ovarian and metabolic characteristics of polycystic ovary syndrome. Endocrinology. Aug 2007;148(8):3781–91.
15. Demissie M, Lazic M, Foecking EM, Aird F, Dunaif A, Levine JE. Transient prenatal androgen exposure produces metabolic syndrome in adult female rats. Am J Physiol Endocrinol Metab. Aug 2008;295(2):E262–8.
16. Abbott DH, Dumesic DA, Franks S. Developmental origin of polycystic ovary syndrome – a hypothesis. J Endocrinol. Jul 2002;174(1):1–5.
17. Pastor CL, Griffin-Korf ML, Aloi JA, Evans WS, Marshall JC. Polycystic ovary syndrome: evidence for reduced sensitivity of the gonadotropin-releasing hormone pulse generator to inhibition by estradiol and progesterone. J Clin Endocrinol Metab. Feb 1998;83(2):582–90.
18. Eagleson CA, Gingrich MB, Pastor CL, et al. Polycystic ovarian syndrome: evidence that flutamide restores sensitivity of the gonadotropin-releasing hormone pulse generator to inhibition by estradiol and progesterone. J Clin Endocrinol Metab. Nov 2000;85(11):4047–52.
19. McClamrock HD, Adashi EY. Gestational hyperandrogenism. Fertil Steril. Feb 1992;57(2):257–74.
20. Ibanez L, Jaramillo A, Enriquez G, et al. Polycystic ovaries after precocious pubarche: relation to prenatal growth. Hum Reprod. Feb 2007;22(2):395–400.
21. Urbanek M. The genetics of the polycystic ovary syndrome. Nat Clin Pract Endocrinol Metab. Feb 2007;3(2):103–11.
22. Franks S, Gharani N, Waterworth D, et al. The genetic basis of polycystic ovary syndrome. Hum Reprod. Dec 1997;12(12):2641–8.

23. Legro RS, Driscoll D, Strauss JF 3rd, Fox J, Dunaif A. Evidence for a genetic basis for hyperandrogenemia in polycystic ovary syndrome. Proc Natl Acad Sci USA. 8 Dec 1998;95(25):14956–60.

24. Vink JM, Sadrzadeh S, Lambalk CB, Boomsma DI. Heritability of polycystic ovary syndrome (PCOS) in a Dutch twin-family study. J Clin Endocrinol Metab. 11 Oct 2006;91:2100–4.

25. Stewart DR, Dombroski BA, Urbanek M, et al. Fine mapping of genetic susceptibility to polycystic ovary syndrome on chromosome 19p13.2 and tests for regulatory activity. J Clin Endocrinol Metab. Oct 2006;91(10):4112–7.

26. Frayling TM, Timpson NJ, Weedon MN, et al. A common variant in the FTO gene is associated with body mass index and predisposes to childhood and adult obesity. Science. 11 May 2007;316(5826):889–94.

27. Barber TM, Bennett AJ, Groves CJ, et al. Association of variants in the fat mass and obesity associated (FTO) gene with polycystic ovary syndrome. Diabetologia. Jul 2008;51(7):1153–8.

28. Urbanek M, Woodroffe A, Ewens KG, et al. Candidate gene region for polycystic ovary syndrome (PCOS) on chromosome 19p13.2. J Clin Endocrinol Metab. Dec 2005;90(12):6623–9.

29. Matzuk MM. Revelations of ovarian follicle biology from gene knockout mice [In Process Citation]. Mol Cell Endocrinol. 2000;163(1–2):61–6.

30. Zeggini E, Weedon MN, Lindgren CM, et al. Replication of genome-wide association signals in UK samples reveals risk loci for type 2 diabetes. Science. 1 Jun 2007;316(5829):1336–41.

31. Dunaif A. Insulin resistance and the polycystic ovary syndrome: mechanism and implications for pathogenesis. Endocr Rev. Dec 1997;18(6):774–800.

32. Robinson S, Kiddy D, Gelding SV, et al. The relationship of insulin insensitivity to menstrual pattern in women with hyperandrogenism and polycystic ovaries. Clin Endocrinol (Oxf). 1993;39(3):351–5.

33. Dahlgren E, Johansson S, Lindstedt G, et al. Women with polycystic ovary syndrome wedge resected in 1956–1965: a long-term follow-up focusing on natural history and circulating hormones. Fertil Steril. Mar 1992;57(3):505–13.

34. Wild S, Pierpoint T, Jacobs H, McKeigue P. Long-term consequences of polycystic ovary syndrome: results of a 31 year follow-up study. Hum Fertil (Camb). 2000;3(2):101–5.

35. Solomon CG, Hu FB, Dunaif A, et al. Long or highly irregular menstrual cycles as a marker for risk of type 2 diabetes mellitus. Jama. 21 Nov 2001;286(19):2421–6.

36. Robinson S, Henderson AD, Gelding SV, et al. Dyslipidaemia is associated with insulin resistance in women with polycystic ovaries. Clin Endocrinol (Oxf). Mar 1996;44(3):277–84.

37. Robinson S, Chan SP, Spacey S, Anyaoku V, Johnston DG, Franks S. Postprandial thermogenesis is reduced in polycystic ovary syndrome and is associated with increased insulin resistance. Clin Endocrinol (Oxf). Jun 1992;36(6):537–43.

38. Franks S, Gilling-Smith C, Watson H, Willis D. Insulin action in the normal and polycystic ovary. Endocrinol Metab Clin North Am. Jun 1999;28(2):361–78.

39. Pasquali R, Antenucci D, Casimirri F, et al. Clinical and hormonal characteristics of obese amenorrheic hyperandrogenic women before and after weight loss. J Clin Endocrinol Metab. Jan 1989;68(1):173–9.

40. Ehrmann DA. Polycystic ovary syndrome. N Engl J Med. 24 Mar 2005;352(12):1223–36.

41. Pasquali R, Gambineri A. Insulin-sensitizing agents in polycystic ovary syndrome. Eur J Endocrinol. Jun 2006; 154(6):763–75.

42. Venkatesan AM, Dunaif A, Corbould A. Insulin resistance in polycystic ovary syndrome: progress and paradoxes. Recent Prog Horm Res. 2001;56:295–308.

43. Corbould A, Kim YB, Youngren JF, et al. Insulin resistance in the skeletal muscle of women with PCOS involves intrinsic and acquired defects in insulin signaling. Am J Physiol Endocrinol Metab. May 2005;288(5): E1047–54.

44. Dunaif A, Xia J, Book CB, Schenker E, Tang Z. Excessive insulin receptor serine phosphorylation in cultured fibroblasts and in skeletal muscle. A potential mechanism for insulin resistance in the polycystic ovary syndrome. J Clin Invest. Aug 1995;96(2):801–10.

45. Cohen P. Protein kinases–the major drug targets of the twenty-first century? Nat Rev Drug Discov. Apr 2002;1(4): 309–15.

46. Rosenbaum D, Haber RS, Dunaif A. Insulin resistance in polycystic ovary syndrome: decreased expression of GLUT-4 glucose transporters in adipocytes. Am J Physiol. Feb 1993;264(2 Pt 1):E197–202.

47. Gaster M, Staehr P, Beck-Nielsen H, Schroder HD, Handberg A. GLUT4 is reduced in slow muscle fibers of type 2 diabetic patients: is insulin resistance in type 2 diabetes a slow, type 1 fiber disease? Diabetes. Jun 2001;50(6):1324–9.

48. Rice S, Christoforidis N, Gadd C, et al. Impaired insulin-dependent glucose metabolism in granulosa-lutein cells from anovulatory women with polycystic ovaries. Hum Reprod. Feb 2005;20(2):373–81.

49. Roberts R, Stark J, Iatropoulou A, Becker DL, Franks S, Hardy K. Energy substrate metabolism of mouse cumulus-oocyte complexes: response to follicle-stimulating hormone is mediated by the phosphatidylinositol 3-kinase pathway and is associated with oocyte maturation. Biol Reprod. Jul 2004;71(1):199–209.

50. Barber TM, Golding SJ, Alvey C, et al. Global adiposity rather than abnormal regional fat distribution characterizes women with polycystic ovary syndrome. J Clin Endocrinol Metab. Mar 2008;93(3):999–1004.

51. Kiddy DS, Sharp PS, White DM, et al. Differences in clinical and endocrine features between obese and non-obese subjects with polycystic ovary syndrome: an analysis of 263 consecutive cases. Clin Endocrinol (Oxf). Feb 1990;32(2):213–20.

52. Barber TM, McCarthy MI, Wass JA, Franks S. Obesity and polycystic ovary syndrome. Clin Endocrinol (Oxf). Aug 2006;65(2):137–45.

53. Plymate SR, Matej LA, Jones RE, Friedl KE. Inhibition of sex hormone-binding globulin production in the human hepatoma (Hep G2) cell line by insulin and prolactin. J Clin Endocrinol Metab. Sept 1988;67(3):460–4.

54. Singh A, Hamilton-Fairley D, Koistinen R, et al. Effect of insulin-like growth factor-type I (IGF-I) and insulin on the secretion of sex hormone binding globulin and IGF-I binding protein (IBP-I) by human hepatoma cells. J Endocrinol. Feb 1990;124(2):R1–R3.

55. Glueck CJ, Papanna R, Wang P, Goldenberg N, Sieve-Smith L. Incidence and treatment of metabolic syndrome in newly referred women with confirmed polycystic ovarian syndrome. Metabolism. Jul 2003;52(7):908–15.

56. Dokras A, Bochner M, Hollinrake E, Markham S, Vanvoorhis B, Jagasia DH. Screening women with polycystic ovary syndrome for metabolic syndrome. Obstet Gynecol. Jul 2005;106(1):131–7.

57. Apridonidze T, Essah PA, Iuorno MJ, Nestler JE. Prevalence and characteristics of the metabolic syndrome in women with polycystic ovary syndrome. J Clin Endocrinol Metab. Apr 2005;90(4):1929–35.

58. Ehrmann DA, Liljenquist DR, Kasza K, Azziz R, Legro RS, Ghazzi MN. Prevalence and predictors of the metabolic syndrome in women with polycystic ovary syndrome. J Clin Endocrinol Metab. Jan 2006;91(1):48–53.

59. Rossi B, Sukalich S, Droz J, et al. Prevalence of metabolic syndrome and related characteristics in obese adolescents with and without polycystic ovary syndrome. J Clin Endocrinol Metab. Dec 2008;93(12):4780–6.

60. Kiddy DS, Hamilton-Fairley D, Bush A, et al. Improvement in endocrine and ovarian function during dietary treatment of obese women with polycystic ovary syndrome. Clin Endocrinol (Oxf). Jan 1992;36(1):105–11.

61. Summerbell CD, Ashton V, Campbell KJ, Edmunds L, Kelly S, Waters E. Interventions for treating obesity in children. Cochrane Database Syst Rev. 2003;3:CD001872.

62. Guttmann-Bauman I. Approach to adolescent polycystic ovary syndrome (PCOS) in the pediatric endocrine community in the USA. J Pediatr Endocrinol Metab. May 2005;18(5):499–506.

63. Koulouri O, Conway GS. A systematic review of commonly used medical treatments for hirsutism in women. Clin Endocrinol (Oxf). May 2008;68(5):800–5.

64. Ganie MA, Khurana ML, Eunice M, et al. Comparison of efficacy of spironolactone with metformin in the management of polycystic ovary syndrome: an open-labeled study. J Clin Endocrinol Metab. Jun 2004;89(6):2756–62.

65. Ibanez L, Potau N, Marcos MV, de Zegher F. Treatment of hirsutism, hyperandrogenism, oligomenorrhea, dyslipidemia, and hyperinsulinism in nonobese, adolescent girls: effect of flutamide. J Clin Endocrinol Metab. Sept 2000;85(9):3251–5.

66. Ibanez L, de Zegher F. Low-dose flutamide-metformin therapy for hyperinsulinemic hyperandrogenism in non-obese adolescents and women. Hum Reprod Update. May–Jun 2006;12(3):243–52.

67. Legro RS. Long-term, low-dose flutamide does not cause hepatotoxicity in hyperandrogenic women. Nat Clin Pract Endocrinol Metab. Apr 2006;2(4):188–9.

68. Allen HF, Mazzoni C, Heptulla RA, et al. Randomized controlled trial evaluating response to metformin versus standard therapy in the treatment of adolescents with polycystic ovary syndrome. J Pediatr Endocrinol Metab. Aug 2005;18(8):761–8.

69. Hoeger K, Davidson K, Kochman L, Cherry T, Kopin L, Guzick D. The impact of metformin, oral contraceptives, and lifestyle modification on polycystic ovary syndrome in obese adolescent women in two randomized, placebo-controlled clinical trials. J Clin Endocrinol Metab. 2008;93:4299–306.

70. Arslanian SA, Lewy V, Danadian K, Saad R. Metformin therapy in obese adolescents with polycystic ovary syndrome and impaired glucose tolerance: amelioration of exaggerated adrenal response to adrenocorticotropin with reduction of insulinemia/insulin resistance. J Clin Endocrinol Metab. Apr 2002;87(4):1555–9.

71. Legro RS, Barnhart HX, Schlaff WD, et al. Clomiphene, metformin, or both for infertility in the polycystic ovary syndrome. N Engl J Med. 8 Feb 2007;356(6):551–66.

72. Nissen SE. Perspective: effect of rosiglitazone on cardiovascular outcomes. Curr Cardiol Rep. Sept 2007;9(5):343–4.

73. Grey A, Bolland M, Gamble G, et al. The peroxisome proliferator-activated receptor-gamma agonist rosiglitazone decreases bone formation and bone mineral density in healthy postmenopausal women: a randomized, controlled trial. J Clin Endocrinol Metab. Apr 2007;92(4):1305–10.

25 Obesity and Metabolic Dysfunction in the Child with a Major Behavioral Disorder: Atypical Antipsychotics

Lauren Shin and David C. Henderson

CONTENTS

INTRODUCTION
EFFECTS OF PSYCHOTROPIC MEDICATIONS AND OTHER DRUGS
    ON BODY WEIGHT AND METABOLIC FUNCTION
MANAGEMENT OF EXCESS WEIGHT GAIN IN PATIENTS TREATED
    WITH ATYPICAL ANTIPSYCHOTICS
CONCLUSION
REFERENCES

Key Words: Psychotropic, psychiatric, orlistat, metformin

INTRODUCTION

Obesity in childhood increases the risks of adult obesity and predisposes to metabolic complications including glucose intolerance, type 2 diabetes mellitus, hypertension, dyslipidemia, and the development of cardiovascular disease *(1–4)*. Obesity also impacts physical appearance and may have profound psychosocial consequences including low self-esteem, lack of self-confidence, and social alienation. It is also associated with depressive symptoms and experiences of shame *(1)*. Obese children are often diagnosed with anxiety disorders *(2)* and are more likely to become victims or perpetrators of bullying behavior than their normal-weight peers *(3)*.

Conversely, psychologic and psychiatric disorders can predispose to obesity and metabolic complications. For example, adults with schizophrenia have higher rates of obesity, type 2 diabetes, hypertension, and coronary artery disease than those without psychiatric illness *(4,5–7)*. Three major factors appear to contribute to obesity and co-morbidities in patients with psychiatric disease. First, social isolation and demoralization can lead to poor dietary habits and lack of physical activity. Second, medication-related increases in appetite, especially carbohydrate craving, boost caloric intake while sedating drugs reduce baseline energy expenditure *(8)*. Finally, access to medical care and use of medical resources is often inadequate (and in some cases, non-existent).

From: *Contemporary Endocrinology: Pediatric Obesity: Etiology, Pathogenesis, and Treatment*
Edited by: M. Freemark, DOI 10.1007/978-1-60327-874-4_25,
© Springer Science+Business Media, LLC 2010

EFFECTS OF PSYCHOTROPIC MEDICATIONS AND OTHER DRUGS ON BODY WEIGHT AND METABOLIC FUNCTION

A variety of medications are associated with weight gain in children as well as adults. These are listed in Table 1 and include the so-called "atypical" antispychotic agents. Psychotropic medications have traditionally been used to treat a wide-range of psychologic and psychiatric illnesses including mood, anxiety, externalizing, and psychotic disorders. To those ends, psychotropic drugs have been used with increasing frequency in young patients in the United States (9). But newer "atypical" antipsychotic agents are increasingly employed to treat a widening array of neurologic and psychiatric disorders such as autism (10), tic disorders (11), and obsessive-compulsive disorders (12) as well as schizophrenia and bipolar disease (13). Indeed, in 1992 only 4% of all antipsychotic prescriptions in the United States were for atypical antipsychotics; the percentage now approximates 70% (14). Thus the use of atypical antipsychotics by children and teenagers has considerable impact on public health.

Table 1
Drugs Commonly Associated with Weight Gain

- Atypical antipsychotics
- Glucocorticoids (including high-dose inhaled)
- Sex steroids: medroxyprogesterone, oral contraceptives
- Hypoglycemic agents: insulin, sulfonylureas, and thiazolidinediones
- Tricyclic antidepressants
- Anti-epileptics: valproate, gabapentin

Although studies suggest that atypical antipsychotics may exert beneficial effects on mood, cognition, and behavior in various psychiatric and neurologic conditions, there is increasing concern regarding tolerability and long-term adverse effects of these agents, particularly in young patients (15,16). Indeed, children and adults are at risk for antipsychotic-related adverse complications including excess weight gain, insulin resistance, glucose intolerance, and dyslipidemia (5–7,17). These effects are mediated, at least in part, through central induction of appetite and inhibition of satiety, manifest as food craving, binge eating, and, ultimately, fat deposition. The actions in the central nervous system are exerted through antagonism of hypothalamic histaminergic H1 receptors and (possibly) serotoninergic 5HT2c receptors, which normally suppress appetite, food intake, and weight gain and increase energy expenditure (18). The risks of glucose intolerance and type 2 diabetes correlate best with the ability of the atypical antipsychotics to antagonize pancreatic beta cell muscarinic M3 receptors and thereby reduce glucose-stimulated insulin secretion (18).

Newer antipsychotics generally cause more weight gain than the older agents. Case reports and clinical trials have linked olanzapine and clozapine in particular with significant weight gain in adults (19–23). A meta-analysis estimated that the average increase in weight of subjects treated with antipsychotic agents over a 10-week period ranged from 0.04 kg with ziprasidone and 0.39 kg with molindone to 2.10 kg with risperidone, 2.92 kg with sertindole, 3.19 kg with thioridazine, 4.15 kg with olanzapine, and 4.45 kg with clozapine (4). In comparison, placebo-treated subjects gained an average of 0.74 kg. In a 5-year natural history study, some patients treated with clozapine continued to gain weight for up to 46 months (24). Data from the CATIE trial showed that olanzapine-treated subjects experienced the greatest amount of weight gain, with the highest percentage of subjects gaining 7% or more of their total body weight (25).

Atypical antipsychotics that produce the greatest weight gain in adults are associated with the highest rates of glucose intolerance and type 2 diabetes *(26)*. Combination of antipsychotics may have additive or synergistic effects; compared with antipsychotic monotherapy, polytherapy is associated with elevated rates of obesity and the metabolic syndrome *(27)*. Weight gain in turn is an emotionally distressing side effect that contributes to nonadherence with antipsychotic agents *(5–7)*. Antipsychotic-treated patients who have experienced weight gain have a reduced quality of life, poorer self-reported general health, and decreased vitality *(5)*.

As in adults, weight gain and metabolic complications are common in pediatric patients treated with atypical antipsychotics. Antipsychotic-naïve children and teenagers appear to be at highest risk *(28,47)*. Although larger, longer term studies are clearly needed to better define the relative risks of weight gain in children and adolescents, available data suggest that clozapine, olanzapine, and risperidone are most potent in their ability to promote weight gain and development of the metabolic syndrome. For example, a randomized, double-blind trial in adolescents showed that while 90% gained weight on antipsychotics, the largest increases were noted with olanzapine (0.99 kg/week) and risperidone (0.77 kg/week) *(29)*. Quetiapine has less dramatic effects, followed by aripiprazole and ziprasidone *(29)*. Correll et al. *(30)* reported that 14% (of 131) of antipsychotic-naïve adolescents treated with new atypical antipsychotic agents developed hyperlipidemia, while 22% developed hyperinsulinemia, and 33% developed insulin resistance, which in some cases progresses to type 2 diabetes *(31,32)*. A South Carolina Medicaid database study of 4,140 antipsychotic-treated children and adolescents showed that treatment increased the risks of obesity (OR: 2.13), T2DM (OR: 3.23), and cardiovascular complications (OR: 1.64) *(33)*. Polytherapy was associated with increased prevalence of weight gain and obesity, dyslipidemia, and T2DM.

Weight gain causes significant emotional distress in adolescents and often results in medication discontinuation and relapse. A linear relationship exists between weight status and nonadherence, with patients reporting weight gain as the second most predominant life problem *(34)*. Therefore, weight gain poses a dual risk: it increases symptom relapse through nonadherence and exposes patients to medical and emotional problems.

MANAGEMENT OF EXCESS WEIGHT GAIN IN PATIENTS TREATED WITH ATYPICAL ANTIPSYCHOTICS

The standard of obesity treatment is a lifestyle modification designed to encourage healthy eating behaviors, reduce a sedentary lifestyle, and increase physical activity. Patient management involves a delicate balance between stabilizing psychiatric symptoms, improving functioning, and preventing and managing medication side effects such as obesity and obesity-related complications. Initially, consideration is given to conservative approaches toward weight control – providing education on healthy lifestyle changes and encouraging diet and exercise *(35)*. If these measures prove inadequate, more intensive strategies must be explored. Before and during any intervention for obesity, it is recommended that anthropometrics and metabolic profile be carefully assessed.

Nonpharmacologic Interventions

Most pediatric obesity intervention studies in psychiatric patients are not randomized controlled trials. Few, if any, psychosocial intervention studies exist for obese, mentally ill children and adolescents. Consequently, no standardized educational, nutritional, family-based, multi-modal, or behavioral intervention studies have been established for this population of pediatric patients.

Most weight loss programs for the general population have weight loss as the specific goal of the intervention, and sessions focus on learning and adapting healthy diets and increasing activity levels. Managing stress and enhancing motivation to maintain lifestyle modifications is a critical component.

Self-regulation skills, such as self-observation, self-instruction, self-evaluation, and self-reward, can be learned and utilized. Designing a personal plan for managing eating habits can be helpful *(36)*. The goals are modest lifelong lifestyle modifications. However, the effectiveness may be limited in children receiving medications that cause sedation and increase appetite. Additionally, the struggles of dealing with typical issues of childhood and adolescence along with those of a psychiatric illness may limit the time and energy necessary to participate in such a program.

Group programs for obese children may sometimes be helpful. For example, in a school-based exercise program of 9-month duration, improvement of body composition and insulin sensitivity was noted in a group of middle school children who were randomized to a fitness-oriented gym class compared to a group taking regular gym class *(37)*. However, as stated above, it may be difficult for children and adolescents with psychiatric illness to successfully participate in such programs.

On the other hand, drastic changes in diet or exercise are generally not recommended. Data on the use of a very low-calorie diet *(38)* (400–800 kcal/day) in morbidly obese adolescents *without* psychiatric illness indicate that weight improvement lasts less than 12 months. Most weight loss occurs early; but over time, weight is usually regained toward baseline levels or even higher. Short-term interventions, discontinuation of treatment, or withdrawal from the treatment likely results in subsequent weight increases *(39)*. Severe dietary restriction is even less likely to be successful in children with psychiatric illness because they often have eating disorders and food cravings.

No bariatric surgery data are available for obese pediatric patients with mental illness. Any surgery can potentially lead to significant adverse consequences, and it remains debatable whether an obese youth with a psychiatric illness (especially if symptoms are unstable) should undergo this procedure. The safety and success of the surgery is dependent on the individual's ability to comply with the post-surgery aftercare recommendations, which include eating small meals at a slow pace, chewing each bite dozens of times before swallowing, avoiding certain foods, and taking a complex array of vitamins.

Pharmacologic Interventions

Pharmacologic intervention for medication-induced weight gain begins first with evaluating the risks and benefits of continuing the medication being used to treat the psychiatric disorder. *When there is significant weight gain on a medication, consideration should be given to discontinuing the agent or switching to another medication.*

There is increased interest in prescribing anti-obesity agents to prevent or reverse excess weight gain in patients treated with atypical antipsychotics. The results are summarized in Miller et al. *(40)*. Brief (3–24 week), small ($n = 12$–50) trials found that the histamine 2 receptor antagonists *Nizatidine* and *Amantadine* or the histamine 1 receptor agonist *Modafinil* can reduce body weight in olanzapine-treated adults. However, Amantadine is known to exacerbate mood disorders in patients with schizophrenia, and Modafinil can cause insomnia, headache, nausea, nervousness, hypertension and, rarely, severe dermatologic reactions. Likewise, the anti-convulsant *Topiramate* reduced BMI in adults taking various atypical antipsychotics but caused paresthesias and memory disturbances. The serotonin reuptake inhibitor *Fluoxetine* had no benefit in adults treated with olanzapine. None of these drugs is approved for the treatment of obesity in children.

Currently, only orlistat and sibutramine have been approved by the United States Food and Drug Administration for long-term weight control in adolescents *(41)*. *Orlistat* is a reversible inhibitor of gastric and pancreatic lipases which blocks absorption of digestive lipids *(42)*. Limited evidence suggests that orlistat can reduce BMI in obese adolescents when combined with diet and exercise *(43)* (see Chapter 23 by Freemark), but no studies have examined the effects of the drug in children with psychiatric disease. A 4-month trial showed that orlistat reduced body weight by 1.7 kg in adult males (not females) taking clozapine *(44)*. Diarrhea and flatulence are major side effects. Fatty foods must be avoided, making its use in many psychiatric patients problematic.

Sibutramine is a selective inhibitor of serotonin and noradrenaline reuptake *(45)*. A number of studies show that sibutramine can reduce BMI in obese teenagers without psychiatric disease; for example, a 6-month randomized, double-blind, placebo-controlled trial ($N = 60$, 14–17 years old) found that sibutramine (10 mg daily) combined with diet and exercise led to weight loss on average of 10.3 ± 6.6 kg; in comparison, the placebo group lost 2.4 ± 2.5 kg ($p < 0.001$) *(46)* (see Chapter 23 by Freemark). A double-blind, placebo-controlled trial *(45)* in adult schizophrenia patients found that sibutramine was an effective and well-tolerated adjunct to behavior modification for olanzapine-associated weight gain. At week 12, the sibutramine group had significantly greater weight loss than the placebo group (mean $= 8.3 \pm 2.4$ lb versus mean $= 1.8 \pm 1.6$ lb). However, sibutramine raises mean heart rate and blood pressure and can cause insomnia and dry mouth; in combination with other drugs, sibutramine may also cause the serotonin syndrome.

Metformin, a biguanide oral hypoglycemic, decreases endogenous hepatic glucose production and intestinal glucose absorption, thereby lowering fasting glucose and insulin concentrations; it may also increase insulin sensitivity *(47)*. It is approved for the treatment of type 2 diabetes mellitus in pediatric and adult patients *(48)*. Recent studies show that metformin may reduce BMI and fasting glucose and insulin levels in non-diabetic obese adolescents and adults with insulin resistance and the polycystic ovary syndrome (see Chapters 12 and 23 by Freemark and Chapter 24 by Franks and Joharatnam).

There are a total of 6 double-blind, placebo-controlled studies (total $n = 353$) of the effects of metformin on weight gain in adults treated with atypical antipsychotics; in 4 of the 6 studies metformin had no effect on body weight. However, the two largest studies (total $n = 208$) found that metformin reduced body weight relative to placebo in patients taking olanzapine or another atypical antipsychotic agent *(40)*.

Three studies constitute the pediatric literature on the subject *(40)*. In the first, Morrison and associates *(49)* studied the effects of metformin (500 mg three times daily) in a 12-week, open-label investigation in patients (10–18 years old, $n = 19$) who had more that 10% weight gain during treatment with an atypical antipsychotic. The mean weight loss on metformin was 2.93 ± 3.13 kg and mean BMI decrease was 2.22 ± 1.98 kg/m^2 ($p = 0.003$). The effect was achieved after only 4 weeks. In a 16-week, add-on, parallel-design study in 39 adolescents (10–17 years old) under treatment with an atypical antipsychotic agent, Klein and associates *(50)* found that those assigned to placebo gained an average of 0.31 ± 0.44 kg per week (total 4.01 ± 6.23 kg) and had a BMI increase of 1.12 ± 2.02, compared to no change in weight and an average BMI decline of 0.43 ± 1.07 ($p = 0.0006$) in patients treated with metformin (up to 850 mg twice daily). Because the study was conducted in growing children, there was a reduction in z scores for weight and BMI. Metformin also reduced waist circumference 2.51 cm; in contrast, waist circumference increased 3.64 cm in the placebo group. Finally, a 12-week, placebo-controlled trial in 49 teenagers taking risperidone for schizophrenia or schizoaffective disorder found no effect of metformin on body weight. Common side effects (10–15%) of metformin include nausea and mild-to-moderate gastrointestinal distress; lactic acidosis is rare and has not been described in children (see Chapter 23 by Freemark).

CONCLUSION

The introduction of atypical antipsychotic agents represents a major advance in the management of psychiatric illnesses. However, the weight gain associated with most of these medications is contributing to an increased rate of obesity in this patient population. With rising prescription rates for atypical antipsychotics, an even higher incidence of obesity in patients on these agents may be expected in the future. Given the limited availability of clearly effective means of managing antipsychotic-induced weight gain, it is important to balance the risks and benefits carefully prior to initiating antipsychotic treatment. Once treatment is started, careful monitoring of body weight, BMI, blood pressure, glucose tolerance, and serum lipids is obligatory. From the onset of treatment, healthy lifestyle counseling and interventions should be initiated. A risk assessment (such as previous treatment and side effect experiences, current weight and metabolic state, family history, population-based risk) should be conducted and the medication with the lowest possible risk should be considered first. If unsuccessful, then the next lowest risk medication should be considered. If an adverse event, such as significant weight gain, occurs, then more intensive healthy lifestyle counseling and interventions should be initiated, and one should consider switching the medication. More targeted weight loss interventions, including the use of adjuvant medications, may be considered in certain cases.

The anthropometric and metabolic profile should be integrated into the patient's psychiatric and medical management. Appropriate monitoring will help determine whether it is better to postpone or initiate immediately an intervention, especially one that is intensive. Preventing obesity involves promoting healthy eating behaviors and regular physical activity, enabling patients to achieve and maintain appropriate energy balance. Treatment of obesity should be realistic, as psychiatric patients may not be able to control weight fluctuations as tightly as individuals in the general population.

Finally, the use of pharmacologic interventions may be warranted in only certain individual patients. Given the insufficient and inconsistent data, these agents should not be used as preventive or first-line treatment. Such interventions should be undertaken with caution and close monitoring until further studies are reported in youth with psychiatric illness taking atypical antipsychotics. Communication between the psychiatric treatment team and the pediatric treatment team is essential for prevention and early intervention.

REFERENCES

1. Sjoberg RL, Nilsson KW, Leppert J. Obesity, shame, and depression in school-aged children: a population-based study. Pediatrics. Sept 2005;116(3):e389–92.
2. Vila G, Zipper E, Dabbas M, et al. Mental disorders in obese children and adolescents. Psychosom Med. May–Jun 2004;66(3):387–94.
3. Janssen I, Craig WM, Boyce WF, Pickett W. Associations between overweight and obesity with bullying behaviors in school-aged children. Pediatrics. May 2004;113(5):1187–94.
4. Allison DB, Mentore JL, Heo M, et al. Antipsychotic-induced weight gain: a comprehensive research synthesis. Am J Psychiatry. Nov 1999;156(11):1686–96.
5. Allison DB, Mackell JA, McDonnell DD. The impact of weight gain on quality of life among persons with schizophrenia. Psychiatr Serv. Apr 2003;54(4):565–7.
6. Perkins DO. Adherence to antipsychotic medications. J Clin Psychiatry. 1999;60(Suppl 21):25–30.
7. Perkins DO. Predictors of noncompliance in patients with schizophrenia. J Clin Psychiatry. Dec 2002;63(12):1121–28.
8. Jones B, Basson BR, Walker DJ, Crawford AM, Kinon BJ. Weight change and atypical antipsychotic treatment in patients with schizophrenia. J Clin Psychiatry. 2001;62(Suppl 2):41–4.
9. Cooper WO, Arbogast PG, Ding H. Trends in prescribing of antipsychotic medications for US children. Ambul Pediatr. 2006;6:79–83.
10. Malone RP, Maislin G, Choudhury MS, Gifford C, Delaney MA. Risperidone treatment in children and adolescents with autism: short- and long-term safety and effectiveness. J Am Acad Child Adolesc Psychiatry. Feb 2002;41(2):140–7.
11. Bruun RD, Budman CL. Risperidone as a treatment for Tourette's syndrome. J Clin Psychiatry. Jan 1996;57(1):29–31.
12. Fitzgerald KD, Stewart CM, Tawile V, Rosenberg DR. Risperidone augmentation of serotonin reuptake inhibitor treatment of pediatric obsessive compulsive disorder. J Child Adolesc Psychopharmacol. 1999;9(2):115–23.
13. Armenteros JL, Whitaker AH, Welikson M, Stedge DJ, Gorman J. Risperidone in adolescents with schizophrenia: an open pilot study. J Am Acad Child Adolesc Psychiatry. May 1997;36(5):694–700.
14. Tandon R, Jibson MD. Efficacy of newer generation antipsychotics in the treatment of schizophrenia. Psychoneuroendocrinology. Jan 2003;28(Suppl 1):9–26.

15. Cesena M, Gonzalez-Heydrich J, Szigethy E, Kohlenberg TM, DeMaso DR. A case series of eight aggressive young children treated with risperidone. J Child Adolesc Psychopharmacol. Winter 2002;12(4):337–45.

16. Shaw JA, Lewis JE, Pascal S, et al. A study of quetiapine: efficacy and tolerability in psychotic adolescents. J Child Adolesc Psychopharmacol. Winter 2001;11(4):415–24.

17. Correll CU, Carlson HE. Endocrine and metabolic adverse effects of psychotropic medications in children and adolescents. J Am Acad Child Adolesc Psychiatry. Jul 2006;45(7):771–91.

18. Starrenburg FC, Bogers JP. How can antipsychotics cause Diabetes Mellitus? Insights based on receptor-binding profiles, humoral factors and transporter proteins. Eur Psychiatry. Apr 2009;24(3):164–70.

19. Beasley CM Jr., Hamilton SH, Crawford AM, et al. Olanzapine versus haloperidol: acute phase results of the international double-blind olanzapine trial. Eur Neuropsychopharmacol. May 1997;7(2):125–37.

20. Beasley CM Jr., Tollefson GD, Tran PV. Safety of olanzapine. J Clin Psychiatry. 1997;58(Suppl 10):13–7.

21. Baptista T, Beaulieu S. Body weight gain, insulin, and leptin in olanzapine-treated patients. J Clin Psychiatry. Nov 2001;62(11):902–4.

22. Osser DN, Najarian DM, Dufresne RL. Olanzapine increases weight and serum triglyceride levels. J Clin Psychiatry. 1999;60(11):767–70.

23. Wirshing DA, Wirshing WC, Kysar L, et al. Novel antipsychotics: comparison of weight gain liabilities. J Clin Psychiatry. 1999;60(6):358–63.

24. Henderson DC, Cagliero E, Gray C, et al. Clozapine, diabetes mellitus, weight gain, and lipid abnormalities: a 5-year naturalistic study. Am J Psychiatry. 2000;157:975–81.

25. Lieberman JA, Stroup TS, McEvoy JP, et al. Effectiveness of antipsychotic drugs in patients with chronic schizophrenia. N Engl J Med. 22 Sept 2005;353(12):1209–23.

26. Jin H, Meyer JM, Jeste DV. Phenomenology of and risk factors for new-onset diabetes mellitus and diabetic ketoacidosis associated with atypical antipsychotics: an analysis of 45 published cases. Ann Clin Psychiatry. Mar 2002;14(1):59–64.

27. Correll CU, Frederickson AM, Kane JM, Manu P. Does antipsychotic polypharmacy increase the risk for metabolic syndrome? Schizophr Res. Jan 2007;89(1–3):91–100.

28. Correll CU, Penzner JB, Parikh UH, et al. Recognizing and monitoring adverse events of second-generation antipsychotics in children and adolescents. Child Adolesc Psychiatr Clin N Am. Jan 2006;15(1):177–206.

29. Sikich L, Hamer RM, Bashford RA, Sheitman BB, Lieberman JA. A pilot study of risperidone, olanzapine, and haloperidol in psychotic youth: a double-blind, randomized, 8-week trial. Neuropsychopharmacology. Jan 2004;29(1):133–45.

30. Correll C, Parikh U, Mugahl T, Olshanskiy V, Moroff M, Pleak R. Body composition changes associated with second-generation antipsychotics. Biol Psychiatry. 2005;57:36.

31. Saito E, Kafantaris V. Can diabetes mellitus be induced by medication? J Child Adolesc Psychopharmacol. Fall 2002;12(3):231–6.

32. Bloch Y, Vardi O, Mendlovic S, Levkovitz Y, Gothelf D, Ratzoni G. Hyperglycemia from olanzapine treatment in adolescents. J Child Adolesc Psychopharmacol. Spring 2003;13(1):97–102.

33. McIntyre RS, Jerrell JM. Metabolic and cardiovascular adverse events associated with antipsychotic treatment in children and adolescents. Arch Pediatr Adolesc Med. Oct 2008;162(10):929–35.

34. Weiden PJ, Mackell JA, McDonnell DD. Obesity as a risk factor for antipsychotic noncompliance. Schizophr Res. 1 Jan 2004;66(1):51–7.

35. O'Brien SH, Holubkov R, Reis EC. Identification, evaluation, and management of obesity in an academic primary care center. Pediatrics. Aug 2004;114(2):e154–9.

36. Braet C, Tanghe A, Decaluwe V, Moens E, Rosseel Y. Inpatient treatment for children with obesity: weight loss, psychological well-being, and eating behavior. J Pediatr Psychol. Oct 2004;29(7):519–29.

37. Carrell A, Clark R, Peterson S, Nemeth B, Sullivan J, Allen D. Improvement of fitness, body composition, and insulin sensitivity in overweight children in a school-based exercise program. Arch Pediatr Adolesc Med. 2005;259:963–8.

38. Saris WH. Very-low-calorie diets and sustained weight loss. Obes Res. Nov 2001;9(Suppl 4):295S–301S.

39. Durant N, Cox J. Current treatment approaches to overweight in adolescents. Curr Opin Pediatr. Aug 2005;17(4):454–9.

40. Miller LJ. Management of atypical antipsychotic drug-induced weight gain: focus on metformin. Pharmacotherapy. Jun 2009;29(6):725–35.

41. Molnar D. New drug policy in childhood obesity. Int J Obes (Lond). Sept 2005;29(Suppl 2):S62–5.

42. Henness S, Perry CM. Orlistat: a review of its use in the management of obesity. Drugs. 2006;66(12):1625–56.

43. Chanoine JP, Hampl S, Jensen C, Boldrin M, Hauptman J. Effect of orlistat on weight and body composition in obese adolescents: a randomized controlled trial. JAMA. 15 Jun 2005;293(23):2873–83.

44. Baptista T, Kin NM, Beaulieu S, de Baptista EA. Obesity and related metabolic abnormalities during antipsychotic drug administration: mechanisms, management and research perspectives. Pharmacopsychiatry. Nov 2002;35(6):205–19.

45. Poston WS, Foreyt JP. Sibutramine and the management of obesity. Expert Opin Pharmacother. Mar 2004;5(3):633–42.

46. Godoy-Matos A, Carraro L, Vieira A, et al. Treatment of obese adolescents with sibutramine: a randomized, double-blind, controlled study. J Clin Endocrinol Metab. Mar 2005;90(3):1460–5.

47. Webb E, Viner R. Should metformin be prescribed to overweight adolescents in whom dietary/behavioural modifications have not helped? Arch Dis Child. Sept 2006;91(9):793–4.

48. Jones KL, Arslanian S, Peterokova VA, Park JS, Tomlinson MJ. Effect of metformin in pediatric patients with type 2 diabetes: a randomized controlled trial. Diabetes Care. Jan 2002;25(1):89–94.

49. Morrison JA, Cottingham EM, Barton BA. Metformin for weight loss in pediatric patients taking psychotropic drugs. Am J Psychiatry. Apr 2002;159(4):655–7.

50. Klein DJ, Cottingham EM, Sorter M, Barton BA, Morrison JA. A randomized, double-blind, placebo-controlled trial of metformin treatment of weight gain associated with initiation of atypical antipsychotic therapy in children and adolescents. Am J Psychiatry. Dec 2006;163(12):2072–9.

26 Hypothalamic Obesity

Robert H. Lustig

CONTENTS

Key Words: Sympathetic nervous system, vagus, prolactin, craniopharyngioma, CNS tumor, octreotide

INTRODUCTION

The ventromedial hypothalamus (VMH; consisting of the arcuate and ventromedial nuclei) is the anatomic seat of control of energy balance (see Chapter 2 by Lustig, this volume). When the VMH is damaged, a syndrome of intractable weight gain ensues. This syndrome, termed "hypothalamic obesity," originally described by Babinski (1) and Frohlich (2) at the turn of the twentieth century, is a prime example of the "organicity" of obesity; that is, a pathophysiologic weight gain that is neurally and biochemically driven, rather than driven by dysfunctional behavior.

Hypothalamic obesity occurs most commonly as a sequel of cranial insult due to supra/parasellar brain tumors, surgery, or radiation (3–5). Less commonly, severe obesity manifests in children following surgery and/or radiation therapy for tumors localized to the posterior fossa (6). Rarely, hypothalamic obesity can manifest after blunt head trauma or in association with hypothalamic granulomatous, infectious, or vascular disorders.

INCIDENCE AND RISK FACTORS

Numerous assessments of late effects following cancer therapy in children document an increased incidence of obesity (7). Most of these evaluations have been performed in the acute lymphoblastic leukemia (ALL) survivor population (8–15), in which obesity may be due to several factors (16),

From: *Contemporary Endocrinology: Pediatric Obesity: Etiology, Pathogenesis, and Treatment*
Edited by: M. Freemark, DOI 10.1007/978-1-60327-874-4_26,
© Springer Science+Business Media, LLC 2010

Table 1
Obesity in Acute Lymphoblastic Leukemia (ALL) Survivors

Author, year, journal	Patient population, n	Percent obese, definition	Risk factors, comments
Sainsbury et al. *(14)*	ALL, n = 86	Increased weight/height within 1 year of therapy	Did not standardize for treatment, CrXRT, steroids
Zee et al. *(13)*	ALL, n = 414	30% with BMI > 80th percentile	Correlated with CrXRT. No controls
Odame et al. *(11)*	ALL, n = 40	57% for girls, BMI > 2 SD	Especially in females. Age-matched controls
Didi et al. *(15)*	ALL, n = 114	46% with BMI > 85th percentile	Especially in females, correlation with chemotherapy, CrXRT 18 vs. 24 Gy no difference. No controls
Craig et al. *(10)*	ALL, n = 298	12% for girls, 10% for boys, BMI z-score > 2	Severe obesity only in females. CrXRT 18–20 Gy worse than 22–24 Gy. Used chemo only as controls
Nysom et al. *(8)*	ALL, n = 95	Direct body fat (BF) measurements. 26% had BF above 90th percentile	Correlated with CrXRT, GH deficiency. Used local controls
Sklar et al. *(9)*	ALL, n = 126	40% with BMI > 85th percentile	CrXRT 24 Gy worse than 18 Gy. Used chemo only as controls

only some of which involve hypothalamic dysfunction. Table 1 recounts the results of these studies. Routinely, ALL patients are treated with long-term high-dose glucocorticoid therapy, which can lead to differentiation of mesenchymal stem cells away from muscle and bone and into adipocytes *(17)*; the adipocytes then accumulate energy, leading to long-term excess adiposity. Furthermore, ALL survivors exhibit less physical activity, which may be due to biochemical, behavioral, or parental factors *(18)*. Thus, the ALL population is at particular risk for increased weight gain after completion of therapy. However, the majority of studies of risk factors for obesity after ALL therapy point to cranial radiation as at least one risk factor.

However, severe, intractable obesity occurs most frequently after direct hypothalamic insult associated with death of VMH neurons. For instance, a frequency of hypothalamic obesity of 30–77% has been documented in survivors after craniopharyngioma treatment *(19–22)* (Fig. 1). It is not clear from these studies whether the hypothalamic damage is due to the tumor, the surgery, or the hypothalamic irradiation that such patients inevitably receive.

We analyzed the BMI curves of 148 children with brain tumors who survived longer than 5 years post-therapy, in order to determine risk factors for the development of obesity *(23)*. We identified four

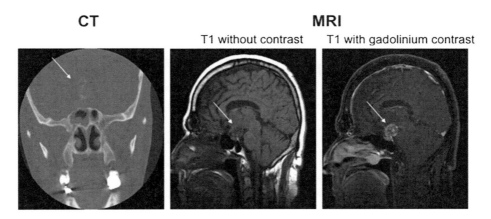

Fig. 1. (a) CT scan (coronal view) showing punctate calcifications within a craniopharyngioma, demonstrating its hypothalamic location. **(b)** Sagittal T1-weighted MRI image without contrast. A multilobulated mass is seen in the suprasellar region. **(c)** Sagittal T1-weighted image following gadolinium. The suprasellar solid component enhances while the cystic areas do not.

parameters as being predictive. First, those with tumors localized to the hypothalamus or thalamus, along with those originating in the temporal lobe (due to stereoscopic position of the hypothalamus during radiation for this area) gained weight much more rapidly than did those with tumors in the posterior fossa or other hemispheric areas. Second, those with tumor histologies prominent in the diencephalon (craniopharyngioma, germinoma, optic glioma, prolactinoma, hypothalamic astrocytoma) also gained weight more rapidly. Third, those with quantitative direct radiation exposure of the hypothalamus of greater than 51 Gy gained excessive weight twice as rapidly after the completion of tumor therapy, even when those with hypothalamic or thalamic locations were removed from the analysis. Lastly, those with some other form of hypothalamic endocrinopathy (i.e., GH deficiency, hypothyroidism, precocious or delayed puberty, ACTH deficiency, diabetes insipidus) exhibited a BMI curve with a steeper upward slope. Thus, each significant risk factor was either linked to hypothalamic location, damage, or dysfunction. Factors not associated with future development of obesity included hydrocephalus, initial high-dose glucocorticoids, and peripheral or intrathecal chemotherapy.

PATHOGENESIS

Hypothalamic obesity results from the inability of leptin to transduce its signal to leptin-receptor positive neurons in the arcuate nucleus, owing to their death. Thus, hypothalamic obesity is an example of "organic" leptin resistance (see Chapter 2).

Rat models of hypothalamic damage, either due to bilateral electrolytic lesions or due to deafferentation of the VMH, lead to intractable weight gain *(24–28)*, even upon food restriction *(29)*. Originally, the obesity was felt to be due to damage to a "satiety" center, which promoted hyperphagia and increased energy storage *(30)*. In the syndrome of "hypothalamic obesity," hypothalamic insult prevents integration of peripheral energy and adiposity signals; the VMH cannot transduce these signals into a sense of energy sufficiency and a subjective state of satiety *(5,6,26,31)*.

Children with hypothalamic obesity exhibit weight gain, even in response to forced caloric restriction to the tune of 500 kcal/day *(5,32)*. This seems paradoxical, as one would expect that if hyperphagia were the reason for the obesity, then caloric restriction would be effective in preventing further weight gain. In fact, analysis of energy intake in children with hypothalamic obesity demonstrates no difference versus control patients with simple obesity *(33)*. Instead, both resting energy expenditure *(34)* and voluntary energy expenditure as measured by accelerometry *(33)* are severely compromised in these patients. Thus, defective leptin signal transduction leads to a state of "CNS starvation" that drives decreased peripheral energy utilization. Indeed, the most prominent and concerning complaints in patients with hypothalamic obesity are persistent fatigue, lack of energy, and lack of physical activity. This generalized malaise is not due to hypopituitarism, as it persists even after full hormonal replacement.

Sympathetic Nervous System Hypofunction

The decrease in both resting and voluntary energy expenditure is mediated through suppression of peripheral SNS activity. Recent reports demonstrate an impaired ability of such patients with hypothalamic obesity to mount an epinephrine response to insulin-induced hypoglycemia *(35,36)* and document decreased 24-h epinephrine excretion (although norepinephrine excretion was similar to controls) *(36)*, along with decreased urinary homovanillic acid and vanillylmandelic acid *(37)*. All of these point to decreased SNS tone in subjects with hypothalamic obesity. It is thought that the malaise and decrease in sympathetic tone may account for decreased rates of lipolysis through the adipocyte β_3-adrenergic receptor *(38)*, which results in decreased resting and voluntary energy expenditure *(39)*.

Vagal Hyperfunction

Defective leptin signaling in hypothalamic obesity also results in overactivation of the vagus nerve *(40)*. Vagal activation results in increased appetite, increased pancreatic β-cell insulin secretion, and excessive peripheral energy storage into energy storage.

The hypothalamus sends efferent projections residing in the medial longitudinal fasciculus to the dorsal motor nucleus of the vagus nerve (DMV) *(41)*. The DMV in turn sends efferent projections throughout the alimentary system, including the β-cells of the pancreas *(42)*. This pathway is responsible for the "cephalic" or preabsorptive phase of insulin secretion, which is glucose-independent and can be blocked by atropine *(43)*. VMH lesions damage this pathway, leading to an increase in vagal firing rate *(44)*. For example, rats with VMH lesions exhibit both increased insulin levels and food intake; however, this can be prevented by pancreatic vagotomy *(27,45,46)*. Increased vagal neurotransmission increases from β-cell insulin secretion through three distinct but overlapping mechanisms *(47)* (see Chapter 2):

1. Vagal firing increases acetylcholine availability and binding to the M_3 muscarinic receptor on the β-cell, which is coupled to a sodium channel within the pancreatic β-cell membrane *(48)*. Under resting conditions, the ATP-dependent potassium channel within the β-cell membrane remains open and leads to a negative β-cell resting membrane potential of approximately -70 mV, with essentially no insulin release. In this state, activation of the sodium channel by acetylcholine only minimally increases β-cell resting membrane potential to -65 mV and has relatively small effects on insulin secretion and peripheral insulin levels. This phenomenon is responsible for the vagally mediated "cephalic" or preabsorptive phase of insulin secretion, which is glucose-independent and can be blocked by atropine *(43)*. As glucose enters the β-cell after ingestion of a meal, the enzyme glucokinase phosphorylates glucose to form glucose-6-phosphate. This increases the generation of intracellular ATP, which induces closure of the β-cell's ATP-dependent potassium channel. Upon channel closure, the β-cell experiences an ATP concentration-dependent β-cell depolarization *(49,50)*, and the opening of a separate voltage-gated calcium channel within the membrane. Intracellular calcium influx increases acutely, which results in rapid insulin vesicular exocytosis. Concomitant opening of the sodium channel by acetylcholine augments the β-cell depolarization, which in turn augments the intracellular calcium influx, and results in insulin hypersecretion *(24,27,51)*. Conversely, knockout of the β-cell M_3 receptor in mice reduces vagal-mediated insulin secretion and results in a hypophagic and lean phenotype *(52)*.

2. Vagally mediated acetylcholine increases phospholipases A_2, C, and D, within the β-cell, which hydrolyze intracellular phosphatidylinositol to diacylglycerol (DAG) and inositol triphosphate (IP_3) *(47)*. DAG is a potent stimulator of protein kinase C (PKC) *(53)* which phosphorylates myristoylated alanine-rich protein kinase C substrate (MARCKS), which then binds actin and calcium-calmodulin, and induces insulin vesicular exocytosis *(54)*. IP_3 potentiates release of calcium within β-cells from intracellular stores, which also promotes insulin secretion *(55)*.

3. The vagus also stimulates the release of glucagon-like peptide-1 (GLP-1) from intestinal L-cells, which circulates and binds to a GLP-1 receptor within the β-cell membrane. Activation of this receptor induces a calcium-calmodulin-sensitive adenyl cyclase, with conversion of intracellular ATP to cAMP, which then activates protein kinase A. PKA causes both the release of intracellular calcium stores and the phosphorylation of vesicular proteins, each contributing to an increase in insulin exocytosis *(56,57)*.

In rodents, the vagus also directly innervates adipocytes to increase energy storage (although confirmation of a similar neural pathway in humans remains elusive). Retrograde tracing of white adipose tissue reveals efferent neurons whose perikarya originating in the DMV *(58)*. These efferents synapse on the M_1 muscarinic receptor on the adipocyte, which increases insulin sensitivity of the adipocyte. Denervation of white adipose tissue results in reduction of glucose and FFA uptake in response to a euglycemic hyperinsulinemic clamp and also results in the induction of HSL, which promotes lipolysis; in concert, these reduce the efficiency of insulin-induced energy storage. Thus, vagal modulation of the adipocyte augments storage of both glucose and FFAs by improving adipose insulin sensitivity *(59)*. Furthermore, the amplitude and duration of pancreatic insulin secretion, and the activity of the insulin molecule at the adipose insulin receptor, play integral roles in the genesis of lipogenesis and weight gain. Within the adipocyte, insulin increases (a) Glut4 expression; (b) acetyl-CoA carboxylase; (c) fatty acid synthase; and (d) lipoprotein lipase *(60)*. Thus, between the direct effect of the vagus on the adipocyte and the indirect effects of the vagus through insulin secretion, rapid and excessive clearance and storage of circulating glucose and lipid promote intractable obesity.

Thus, hypothalamic obesity due to VMH damage from the tumor or trauma, surgery, or radiation results in death of VMH neurons, with resultant "organic" leptin resistance. The brain cannot transduce the peripheral leptin signal, thus activating the "starvation response" (see Chapter 2). The result is decreased sympathetic tone, with energy conservation, and increased vagal tone, with energy storage; in concert, these result in intractable weight gain.

PRESENTATION

Patients with hypothalamic obesity often manifest other cranial endocrinopathies *(61)*. Hypothalamic tumors or their therapy can affect virtually all pituitary hormones, including growth hormone (75%), luteinizing hormone (LH) or follicle stimulating hormone (FSH) (40–44%), and thyroid stimulating hormone (TSH) (25–64%). Growth hormone (GH) deficiency can lead to fatigue, muscle wasting, and excess adiposity, while gonadotropin deficiency can lead to loss of libido or secondary amenorrhea. Subtle endocrinopathies often escape clinical detection for long periods of time and are apparent only in hindsight. Despite the high incidence of GH deficiency, some of these patients continue to exhibit normal linear growth. While some have postulated the existence of an endogenous factor that maintains linear growth in the absence of growth hormone *(62)*, a role for obesity per se or for hyperleptinemia, hyperinsulinemia, or increases in free IGF-1 levels has not been excluded *(21,63)*. It should be noted that patients with combined GH deficiency and tumor- or treatment-induced precocious puberty may have "normal" rates of linear growth. Hyperprolactinemia occurs in approximately 20% of cases from impingement on the pituitary stalk (also known as the "stalk effect"), due to reduced amounts of prolactin inhibitory factor (mainly dopamine) reaching the lactotrophs of the anterior pituitary. Diabetes insipidus occurs in approximately 16% of patients prior to surgery *(64,65)* and is even more common (70–95%) postoperatively. The immediate postoperative course may also be complicated by excess secretion of vasopressin (SIADH) or cerebral salt wasting (CSW) syndrome. Diabetes insipidus is particularly problematic when complicated by thirst dysregulation or complete adipsia (66). Lastly, adrenocorticotropic hormone (ACTH) deficiency manifests in 25–56% of subjects after therapy (67).

Aside from the symptoms of tumor-induced increased intracranial pressure, patients with hypothalamic obesity may exhibit signs of limbic system involvement, such as hypogonadism, somnolence, rage, and hyperphagia (68). However, the majority of patients actually exhibit normal or only slightly increased daily caloric intake. Indeed, caloric restriction of either VMH-lesioned animals or humans with hypothalamic obesity rarely attenuates the weight gain, suggesting a critical role for reduced energy expenditure in disease pathogenesis (69).

Although occasional patients with hypothalamic obesity are already clinically obese upon presentation, most have a milder initial phenotype, with increased body mass index (BMI) at presentation, due to continued weight gain in the presence of attenuated growth (70). The latter may reflect GH and/or thyroid hormone deficiencies. However, the obesity is likely to worsen post-therapy due to VMH damage; the first 6 months appears to accrue the greatest increases in adiposity (71). Rates of weight gain can range from 12 to 20 kg/year, and obesity often becomes the most debilitating aspect of the postoperative course. Patients with hypothalamic obesity also exhibit a high prevalence of obstructive sleep apnea (72). Metabolic complications of the obesity are frequent and can manifest early (73,74). In some cases, lack of appreciation of the syndrome of hypothalamic obesity by physicians has led them to incorrectly deduce that the hydrocortisone dosage is contributing to the patient's weight gain, leading to well meaning but potentially dangerous reductions of hydrocortisone dosage below 10 mg/m^2/day. This accentuates the symptoms of malaise and lethargy.

DIAGNOSIS

A retrospective analysis of growth records of children with craniopharyngioma (70) indicates that increased weight and BMI gain is evident even before the diagnosis of the tumor. However, after surgery or radiotherapy, the weight gain is immediate and rapid. Evidence of aberrant energy deposition is obvious within the first month, although physicians sometimes confuse this weight gain with the pharmacologic effects of glucocorticoids. Children with hypothalamic obesity frequently have normal fasting insulin levels, but on oral glucose tolerance testing (OGTT) demonstrate insulin hypersecretion (as measured by an increased corrected insulin response, or CIR (75)); particularly notable is a marked increase in the 15 min insulin response on the OGTT, suggesting a neural etiology for the early rise in insulin. Patients with hypothalamic obesity tend to manifest increased insulin sensitivity (as measured by an increased composite insulin sensitivity index, or CISI (76)) as compared with BMI-matched otherwise healthy obese children (77) (Fig. 2a, b). However, other studies suggest that some hypothalamic obesity patients may also manifest signs of metabolic syndrome (73,74).

TREATMENT

Bray first demonstrated the futility of lifestyle intervention by noting weight gain even with severe caloric restriction (32). Thus, treatment needs to be early and intensive to have any chance at success. Perhaps the best treatment is prevention. The hypothalamus is extremely sensitive to both surgical intervention and/or external beam radiation. Rather than employing gross total or subtotal resection as a primary therapy for some supra/parasellar tumors, newer strategies have been developed which treat them more conservatively, using stereotactic biopsy and conformal irradiation (78–80). Recently, Hamilton has instituted a strict lifestyle regimen for patients with hypothalamic obesity, with some cases demonstrating successful weight stabilization (personal communication).

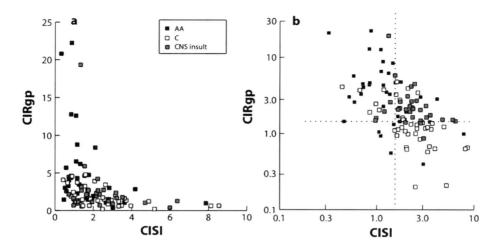

Fig. 2. Scatterplots of insulin secretion (CIRgp) vs. sensitivity (CISI) in 113 obese non-diabetic children. (**a**) CIRgp vs. CISI. (**b**) CIRgp vs. CISI plotted logarithmically. Different racial and etiopathogenic groups tended to plot in different areas. Arbitrary cutoffs (*dashed lines*) for CIRgp (1.5) and CISI (1.7) divide the plot into four quadrants. The majority of Caucasian children (*open squares*) plotted in the *lower right quadrant*, with a CIRgp less than 1.5 and a CISI greater than 1.7, indicating lower insulin secretion and better insulin sensitivity. The preponderance of children with hypothalamic obesity (*gray squares*) plotted in the *upper right quadrant*, with a CIRgp of greater than 1.5, and with a CISI of greater than 1.7, indicating insulin hypersecretion with better insulin sensitivity. Finally the majority of African-American children (*filled squares*) plotted in the upper left quadrant, with a CIRgp of greater than 1.5 and a CISI of less than 1.7, indicating both insulin hypersecretion and resistance (*77*). From Elsevier, with permission.

Pharmacotherapy

Since the hypothalamus is not amenable to therapy, and afferent leptin signal transduction cannot be corrected, pharmacotherapy must instead address the dysfunction in the efferent pathways. Several attempts to use serotonin or norepinephrine reuptake inhibitors (e.g., phen-fen, fluoxetine, and sibu-tramine) have been met with only salutary efficacy. These medications work centrally and do not increase energy expenditure. Mason et al. used dextroamphetamine 5 mg PO bid (*81*), which acts both centrally and peripherally, and achieved weight stability. We have also seen improvement in affect and alertness in treated patients, which is a major benefit. Side effects of dextroamphetamine include tachycardia, hypertension, anxiety, and decreased sleep; however, in low dosage, these effects are less common.

The voltage-gated calcium channel of the β-cell is coupled to a somatostatin (SSTR$_5$) recep-tor (*82,83*). In order to reduce insulin hypersecretion, we examined the effects of the somatostatin analogue octreotide, which limits the opening of this channel, and the amount of insulin released acutely for any specific amount of glucose (*84*). In a pilot trial (*63*), eight patients received subcuta-neously administered octreotide for 6 months, at a dose of 5 μg/kg/day ÷ tid, escalating in monthly 5 μg/kg/day increments to a maximum of 15 μg/kg/day ÷ tid by the third month. Insulin responses to glucose were normalized over 6 months. Of the eight patients, three lost substantial weight, two lost moderate amounts of weight, and three stabilized their weight. The degree of weight loss corre-lated both with changes in insulin response and with changes in leptin levels. The weight loss also appeared to correlate with decreases in appetite, and caloric intake in this cohort decreased by approx-imately 700 kcal/day. Interestingly, an unexpected but welcome side effect of the treatment was the resumption of normal physical activity by four patients, including vigorous exercise. A double-blind, placebo-controlled, 6-month trial of octreotide in 18 subjects with hypothalamic obesity followed (*85*).

Before treatment, annualized weight gain in this population was 16 kg/year. Although the weight loss in this trial was not as pronounced as in the pilot (probably due to a delay in achieving maximum dosage until the fifth month), octreotide was effective in stabilizing weight and BMI as compared to placebo. Insulin secretion during the first 60 min was clearly suppressed by octreotide. Finally, treated children demonstrated marked improvements in physical activity as compared with those treated with placebo, and the improvement in quality of life correlated with the degree of insulin suppression. These findings suggested that insulin hypersecretion may be responsible for lack of physical activity as well as weight gain, which can be improved by normalizing their insulin responses. A retrospective analysis demonstrated that octreotide was most effective in those patients who exhibited both insulin hypersecretion with continued insulin sensitivity *(86)*.

Surgery

The severity and co-morbidities of patients with hypothalamic obesity, and the relative lack of alternatives, have led to various attempts at bariatric surgery. Inge et al. *(87)* reported a 25 kg weight loss after Roux-en-Y gastric bypass in one subject, but whose weight stabilized at an unacceptable level. Recently, Muller et al. reported his experience with four subjects who underwent laparoscopic adjustable gastric banding, with reductions in food intake and slow reductions in BMI *(88)*. The appreciation of the role of dysfunctional vagal tone and insulin hypersecretion in the pathogenesis of hypothalamic obesity originally led to anecdotal case reports of successful treatment with pancreatic vagotomy *(89)*. However, subsequent experience with the procedure was inconsistent *(90)* and it fell out of favor. We have recently resurrected this procedure and have performed laparoscopic truncal vagotomy without pyloromyotomy in four subjects with hypothalamic obesity, with early results being supportive of this procedure, and with relatively few complications or side effects *(91)*.

SUMMARY

In this review, we elaborate the role of the VMH in interpreting energy balance afferent signals and their transduction into autonomic efferent signals to either expend or store energy. When this negative feedback system breaks down, hypothalamic obesity ensues. While this disorder is a defect in the afferent pathway, treatment focuses on the efferent pathway, as it is modulable with currently available drugs and surgical techniques. Physicians need to explain the risks of this disorder to patients prior to tumor therapy and must be willing to act quickly and decisively once intractable weight gain is noted.

ACKNOWLEDGMENTS

The author would like to thank all of the patients with hypothalamic obesity whom he has treated, for their understanding and patience in the face of an incessant disease process, and for their participation in research to understand this disorder more fully.

Editor's Questions and Author's Response

- **Children with hypothalamic obesity are predisposed to fatty liver disease, which may progress to cirrhosis. How common is this in your experience? Does the pathogenesis of fatty liver disease in children with hypothalamic obesity differ from that in other obese children?**

- Most children early in the course of hypothalamic obesity maintain insulin sensitivity during the period of rapid weight gain, as shown in Fig. 2. However, eventually, their degree of adiposity and hyperinsulinemia generates significant insulin resistance. Some may develop metabolic syndrome, of which fatty liver disease is a possible marker, but in our experience it is less frequent in hypothalamic obesity than in the general obese population.

- **I have taken to recommending that children with craniopharyngiomas or other hypothalamic tumors begin caloric restriction *prior to* surgery to prepare them for continuing the diet after they leave the hospital. This approach has proved somewhat successful in limiting postop weight gain in a minority of subjects. We also have anecdotal evidence that metformin, which reduces insulin secretion, may limit the progression of weight gain in post-surgical patients. What is your opinion of these approaches?**

- Dr. Jill Hamilton in Toronto has a cohort of patients with hypothalamic obesity that she is treating with super-intensive lifestyle intervention. The rate of weight gain seems to be lower, but the patients gain weight nonetheless. She has also tried a combination of metformin (to improve insulin sensitivity) and diazoxide (to reduce insulin secretion and mimicking octreotide). These maneuvers seem to slow the rate of weight gain as well, but do not stop the process. We have tried metformin in combination with octreotide in a few patients in a non-protocolized fashion and have sometimes seen a salutary additive effect on weight loss or stability.

REFERENCES

1. Babinski MJ. Tumeur du corps pituitaire san acromegalie et avec arret de developpement des organes genitaux. Rev Neurol. 1900;8:531–3.
2. Frohlich A. Ein fall von tumor der hypophysis cerebri ohne akromegalie. Weiner Klin Rdsch. 1901;15:883–6.
3. Lustig RH. Hypothalamic obesity: the sixth cranial endocrinopathy. Endocrinologist. 2002;12:210–7.
4. Pinkney J, Wilding J, Williams G, MacFarlane I. Hypothalamic obesity in humans: what do we know and what can be done? Obes Rev. 2002;3:27–34.
5. Bray GA. Syndromes of hypothalamic obesity in man. Pediatr Ann. 1984;13:525–36.
6. Daousi C, Dunn AJ, Foy PM, MacFarlane IA, Pinkney JH. Endocrine and neuroanatomic predictors of weight gain and obesity in adult patients with hypothalamic damage. Am J Med. 2005;118:45–50.
7. Rogers PC, Meacham LR, Oeffinger KC, Henry DW, Lange BJ. Obesity in pediatric oncology. Pediatr Blood Cancer. 2005;45:881–91.
8. Nysom K, Holm K, Michaelsen KF, Hertz H, Müller J, Mølgaard C. Degree of fatness after treatment for acute lymphoblastic leukemia in childhood. J Clin Endocrinol Metab. 1999;84:4591–6.
9. Sklar CA, Mertens AC, Walter A, Mitchell D, Nesbit M, O'Leary M, Hutchinson R, Meadows AT, Robison LL. Changes in body mass index and prevalence of overweight in survivors of childhood acute lymphoblastic leukemia: role of cranial irradiation. Med Pediatr Oncol. 2000;35:91–5.
10. Craig F, Leiper AD, Stanhope R, Brain C, Meller ST, Nussey SS. Sexually dimorphic and radiation dose dependent effect of cranial irradiation on body mass index. Arch Dis Child. 1999;81:500–4.
11. Odame I, Reilly JJ, Gibson BES, Donaldson MDC. Patterns of obesity in boys and girls after treatment for acute lymphoblastic leukaemia. Arch Dis Child. 1994;71:147–9.
12. Schell MJ, Ochs JJ, Schriock EA, Carter M. A method of predicting adult height and obesity in long-term survivors of childhood acute lymphoblastic leukemia. J Clin Oncol. 1992;10:128–33.
13. Zee P, Chen CH. Prevalence of obesity in children after therapy for acute lymphoblastic leukemia. Am J Pediatr Hematol/Oncol. 1986;8:294–9.
14. Sainsbury CPQ, Newcombe RG, Hughes IA. Weight gain and height velocity during prolonged first remission from acute lymphoblastic leukaemia. Arch Dis Child. 1985;60:832–6.
15. Didi M, Didcock E, Davies HA, Oligvy-Stuart AL, Wales JKH, Shalet SM. High incidence of obesity in young adults after treatment of acute lymphoblastic leukemia of childhood. J Pediatr. 1995;127:63–7.
16. Reilly JJ. Obesity during and after treatment for childhood cancer. Endocr Dev. 2009;15:40–58.
17. Feldman BJ. Is your metabolism determined by your (cell) fate? Pediatr Res. 2007;61:636–9.
18. Warner JT, Bell W, Webb DK, Gregory JW. Daily energy expenditure and physical activity in survivors of childhood malignancy. Pediatr Res. 1998;43:607–13.

19. Stahnke N, Grubel G, Lagenstein I, Willig RP. Long-term follow-up of children with craniopharyngioma. Eur J Pediatr. 1984;142:179–85.

20. Sorva R. Children with craniopharyngioma: early growth failure and rapid post-operative weight gain. Acta Pediatr Scand. 1988;77:587–92.

21. Pinto G, Bussieres L, Recasens C, Souberbielle JC, Zerah M, Brauner R. Hormonal factors influencing weight and growth pattern in craniopharyngioma. Horm Res. 2000;53:163–9.

22. Vinchon M, Weill J, Delestret I, Dhellemmes P. Craniopharyngioma and hypothalamic obesity in children. Child Nerv Syst. 2009;25:347–52.

23. Lustig RH, Post SM, Srivannaboon K, Rose SR, Danish RK, Burghen GA, Wu S, Xiong X, Merchant TE. Risk factors for the development of obesity in children surviving brain tumors. J Clin Endocrinol Metab. 2003;88:611–6.

24. Rohner-Jeanrenaud F, Jeanrenaud B. Consequences of ventromedial hypothalamic lesions upon insulin and glucagon secretion by subsequently isolated perfused pancreases in the rat. J Clin Invest. 1980;65:902–10.

25. Bray GA, Inoue S, Nishizawa Y. Hypothalamic obesity. Diabetologia. 1981;20:366–77.

26. Satoh N, Ogawa Y, Katsura G, Tsuji T, Masuzaki H, Hiraoka J, Okazaki T, Tamaki M, Hayase M, Yoshimasa Y, Nishi S, Hosoda K, Nakao K. Pathophysiological significance of the *obese* gene product, leptin in ventromedial hypothalamus (VMH)-lesioned rats: evidence for loss of its satiety effect in VMH-lesioned rats. Endocrinology. 1997;138:947–54.

27. Berthoud HR, Jeanrenaud B. Acute hyperinsulinemia and its reversal by vagotomy following lesions of the ventromedial hypothalamus in anesthetized rats. Endocrinology. 1979;105:146–51.

28. Jeanrenaud B. An hypothesis on the aetiology of obesity: dysfunction of the central nervous system as a primary cause. Diabetologia. 1985;28:502–13.

29. Bray GA, Nishizawa Y. Ventromedial hypothalamus modulates fat mobilization during fasting. Nature. 1978;274:900–2.

30. Sklar CA. Craniopharyngioma: endocrine sequalae of treatment. Pediatr Neurosurg. 1994;21:120–3.

31. Thornton JE, Cheung CC, Clifton DK, Steiner RA. Regulation of hypothalamic proopiomelanocortin mRNA by leptin in *ob/ob* mice. Endocrinology. 1997;138:5063–6.

32. Bray GA, Gallagher TF. Manifestations of hypothalamic obesity in man: a comprehensive investigation of eight patients and a review of the literature. Medicine. 1975;54:301–33.

33. Harz KJ, Muller HL, Waldeck E, Pudel V, Roth C. Obesity in patients with craniopharyngioma: assessment of food intake and movement counts indicating physical activity. J Clin Endocrinol Metab. 2003;88:5227–31.

34. Shaikh MG, Grundy RG, Kirk JM. Reductions in basal metabolic rate and physical activity contribute to hypothalamic obesity. J Clin Endocrinol Metab. 2008;93:2588–93.

35. Schofl C, Schleth A, Berger D, Terkamp C, Von Zur Muhlen A, Brabant G. Sympathoadrenal counterregulation in patients with hypothalamic craniopharyngioma. J Clin Endocrinol Metab. 2002;87:624–9.

36. Coutant R, Maurey H, Rouleau S, Mathieu E, Mercier P, Limal JM, Le Bouil A. Defect in epinephrine production in children with craniopharyngioma: functional or organic origin? J Clin Endocrinol Metab. 2003;88:5969–75.

37. Roth CL, Hunneman DH, Gebhardt U, Stoffel-Wagner B, Reinehr T, Muller HL. Reduced sympathetic metabolites in urine of obese patients with craniopharyngioma. Pediatr Res. 2007;61:496–501.

38. al-Adsani H, Hoffer LJ, Silva JE. Resting energy expenditure is sensitive to small dose changes in patients on chronic thyroid hormone replacement. J Clin Endocrinol Metab. 1997;82:1118–25.

39. Lowell BB, Spiegelman BM. Towards a molecular understanding of adaptive thermogenesis. Nature. 2000;404:652–60.

40. Lustig RH. The efferent arm of the energy balance regulatory pathway: neuroendocrinology and pathology. In: Donahoue PA, editor. Obesity and energy metabolism: research and clinical applications. Totowa, NJ: Humana; 2007. pp. 69–86.

41. Powley TL, Laughton W. Neural pathways involved in the hypothalamic integration of autonomic responses. Diabetologia. 1981;20:378–87.

42. D'Alessio DA, Kieffer TJ, Taborsky GJ, Havel PJ. Activation of the parasympathetic nervous system is necessary for normal meal induced-insulin secretion in rhesus macaques. J Clin Endocrinol Metab. 2001;86:1253–9.

43. Ahren B, Holst JJ. The cephalic insulin response to meal ingestion in humans is dependent on both cholinergic and noncholinergic mechanisms and is important for postprandial glycemia. Diabetes. 2001;50:1030–8.

44. Lee HC, Curry DL, Stern JS. Direct effect of CNS on insulin hypersecretion in obese Zucker rats: involvement of vagus nerve. Am J Physiol. 1989;256:E439–44.

45. Tokunaga K, Fukushima M, Kemnitz JW, Bray GA. Effect of vagotomy on serum insulin in rats with paraventricular or ventromedial hypothalamic lesions. Endocrinology. 1986;119:1708–11.

46. Inoue S, Bray GA. The effect of subdiaphragmatic vagotomy in rats with ventromedial hypothalamic lesions. Endocrinology. 1977;100:108–14.

47. Gilon P, Henquin JC. Mechanisms and physiological significance of the cholinergic control of pancreatic β-cell function. Endocr Rev. 2001;22:565–604.

48. Miura Y, Gilon P, Henquin JC. Muscarinic stimulation increases Na^+ entry in pancreatic β-cells by a mechanism other than the emptying of intracellular Ca^{2+} pools. Biochem Biophys Res Commun. 1996;224:67–73.

49. Zawalich WS, Zawalich KC, Rasmussen H. Cholinergic agonists prime the β-cell to glucose stimulation. Endocrinology. 1989;125:2400–6.

50. Nishi S, Seino Y, Ishida H, Seno M, Taminato T, Sakurai H, Imura H. Vagal regulation of insulin, glucagon, and somatostatin secretion in vitro in the rat. J Clin Invest. 1987;79:1191–6.

51. Komeda K, Yokote M, Oki Y. Diabetic syndrome in the Chinese hamster induced with monosodium glutamate. Experientia. 1980;36:232–4.

52. Yamada M, Miyakawa T, Duttaroy A, Yamanaka A, Moriguchi T, Makita R, Ogawa M, Chou CJ, Xia B, Crawley JN, Felder CC, Deng CX, Wess J. Mice lacking the M3 muscarinic acetylcholine receptor are hypophagic and lean. Nature. 2001;410:207–12.

53. Tian YM, Urquidi V, Ashcroft SJH. Protein kinase C in β-cells: expression of multiple isoforms and involvement in cholinergic stimulation of insulin secretion. Mol Cell Endocrinol. 1996;119:185–93.

54. Arbuzova A, Murray D, McLaughlin S. MARCKS, membranes, and calmodulin: kinetics of their interaction. Biochim Biophys Acta. 1998;1376:369–79.

55. Blondel O, Bell GI, Moody M, Miller RJ, Gibbons SJ. Creation of an inositol 1,4,5-triphosphate-sensitive Ca^{2+} store in secretory granules of insulin-producing cells. J Biol Chem. 1994;269:27167–70.

56. Rocca AS, Brubaker PL. Role of the vagus nerve in mediating proximal nutrient-induced glucagon-like peptide-1 secretion. Endocrinology. 1999;140:1687–94.

57. Kiefer TJ, Habener JF. The glucagon-like peptides. Endocr Rev. 1999;20:876–913.

58. Kreier F, Fliers E, Voshol PJ, Van Eden CG, Havekes LM, Kalsbeek A, Van Heijningen CL, Sluiter AA, Mettenleiter TC, Romijn JA, Sauerwein HP, Buijs RM. Selective parasympathetic innervation of subcutaneous and intra-abdominal fat-functional implications. J Clin Invest. 2002;110:1243–50.

59. Boden G, Hoeldtke RD. Nerves, fat, and insulin resistance. N Engl J Med. 2003;349:1966–7.

60. Ramsay TG. Fat cells. Endocrinol Metab Clin North Am. 1996;25:847–70.

61. Sughrue M, Fisch B, Lustig RH, McDermott MW. Craniopharyngioma. In: Gupta N, Banerjee A, Haas-Kogan D, editors. Pediatric CNS tumors. New York, NY: Springer; 2009;135–58.

62. Geffner ME. The growth without growth hormone syndrome. Endocrinol Metab Clin North Am. 1996;25:649–63.

63. Lustig RH, Rose SR, Burghen GA, Velasquez-Mieyer P, Broome DC, Smith K, Li H, Hudson MM, Heideman RL, Kun LE. Hypothalamic obesity in children caused by cranial insult: altered glucose and insulin dynamics, and reversal by a somatostatin agonist. J Pediatr. 1999;135:162–8.

64. Honneger J, Buchfelder M, Fahlbusch R. Surgical treatment of craniopharyngiomas: endocrinological results. J Neurosurg. 1999;90:251–7.

65. de Vries L, Lazar L, Phillip M. Craniopharyngioma: presentation and endocrine sequelae in 36 children. J Pediatr Endocrinol Metab. 2003;16:703–10.

66. Smith D, Finucane F, Phillips J, Baylis PH, Finucane J, Tormey W, Thompson CJ. Abnormal regulation of thirst and vasopressin secretion following surgery for craniopharyngioma. Clin Endocrinol. 2004;61:273–9.

67. Rose SR, Danish RK, Kearney NS, Schreiber RE, Lustig RH, Burghen GA, Hudson MM. ACTH deficiency in childhood cancer survivors. Pediatr Blood Cancer. 2005;45:808–13.

68. Reeves AG, Plum F. Hyperphagia, rage, and dementia accompanying a ventromedial hypothalamic neoplasm. Arch Neurol. 1972;20:616–24.

69. Bray GA, York DA. Hypothalamic and genetic obesity in experimental animals: an autonomic and endocrine hypothesis. Physiol Rev. 1979;59:719–809.

70. Muller HL, Emser A, Faldum A, Bruhnken G, Etavard-Gorris N, Gebhardt U, Oeverink R, Kolb R, Sorenson N. Longitudinal study of growth and body mass index before and after diagnosis of childhood craniopharyngioma. J Clin Endocrinol Metab. 2004;89:3298–305.

71. Ahmet A, Blaser S, Stephens D, Guger S, Rutkas JT, Hamilton J. Weight gain in craniopharyngioma – a model for hypothalamic obesity. J Ped Endocr Metab. 2006;19:121–27.

72. O'Gorman CS, Simoneau-Roy J, MacFarlane J, MacLusky I, Hamilton JK. Sleep disordered breathing in patients with craniopharyngioma and hypothalamic obesity. Baltimore, MD: Pediatric Academic Societies; 2009.

73. Tiosano D, Eisenstein I, Militianu D, Chrousos GP, Hochberg Z. 11β–hydroxysteroid dehydrogenase activity in hypothalamic obesity. J Clin Endocrinol Metab. 2003;88:384.

74. Srinivasan S, Ogle GD, Garnett SP, Briody JN, Lee JW, Cowell CT. Features of the metabolic syndrome after craniopharyngioma. J Clin Endocrinol Metab. 2004;89:81–6.

75. Sluiter WJ, Erkelens DW, Terpstra P, Reitsma WD, Doorendos H. Glucose intolerance and insulin release, a mathematical approach 1. Assay of the beta cell response after glucose loading. Diabetes. 1976;25:241–4.

76. Matsuda M, DeFronzo RA. Insulin sensitivity indices obtained from oral glucose tolerance testing: comparison with the euglycemic insulin clamp. Diabetes Care. 1999;22:1462–70.

77. Preeyasombat C, Bacchetti P, Lazar AA, Lustig RH. Racial and etiopathologic dichotomies in insulin secretion and resistance in obese children. J Pediatr. 2005;146:474–81.

78. Merchant TE, Kienha EN, Sanford RA, Mulhern RK, Thompson SJ, Wilson MW, Lustig RH, Kun LE. Craniopharyngioma: the St. Jude Children's Research Hospital experience 1984–2001. Int J Radiat Oncol Biol Phys. 2002;53:533–42.

79. Spoudeas HA, Saran F, Pizer B. A multimodality approach to the treatment of craniopharyngiomas avoiding hypothalamic morbidity: a UK perspective. J Pediatr Endocrinol Metab. 2006;19:447–51.

80. Karavitaki N, Cudlip S, Adams CB, Wass JA. Craniopharyngiomas. Endocr Rev. 2006;27:371–97.

81. Mason PW, Krawiecki N, Meacham LR. The use of dextroamphetamine to treat obesity and hyperphagia in children treated for craniopharyngioma. Arch Pediatr Adolesc Med. 2002;156:887–92.

82. Mitra SW, Mezey E, Hunyady B, Chamberlain L, Hayes E, Foor F, Wang Y, Schonbrunn A, Schaeffer JM. Colocalization of somatostatin receptor sst5 and insulin in rat pancreatic β-cells. Endocrinology. 1999;140:3790–6.

83. Hsu WH, Xiang HD, Rajan AS, Kunze DL, Boyd AE. Somatostatin inhibits insulin secretion by a G-protein-mediated decrease in Ca^{2+} entry through voltage-dependent Ca^{2+} channels in the beta-cell. J Biol Chem. 1991;266:837–43.

84. Lunetta M, Di Mauro M, Le Moli R, Burrafato S. Long-term octreotide treatment reduced hyperinsulinemia, excess body weight and skin lesions in severe obesity with Acanthosis nigricans. J Endocrinol Invest. 1996;19:699–703.

85. Lustig RH, Hinds PS, Ringwald-Smith K, Christensen RK, Kaste SC, Schreiber RE, Rai SN, Lensing SY, Wu S, Xiong X. Octreotide therapy of pediatric hypothalamic obesity: a double-blind, placebo-controlled trial. J Clin Endocrinol Metab. 2003;88:2586–92.

86. Lustig RH, Mietus-Snyder ML, Bacchetti P, Lazar AA, Velasquez-Mieyer PA, Christensen ML. Insulin dynamics predict BMI and z-score response to insulin suppression or sensitization pharmacotherapy in obese children. J Pediatr. 2006;148:23–9.

87. Inge TH, Pfluger P, Zeller M, Rose SR, Burget L, Sundararajan S, Daniels SR, Tschöp MH. Gastric bypass surgery for treatment of hypothalamic obesity after craniopharyngioma therapy. Nat Clin Pract Endo Metab. 2007;3:606–9.

88. Muller H, Gebhardt U, Wessel V, Schroder S, Kolb R, Sorensen N, Maroske J, Hanisch E. First experiences with laparoscopic adjustable gastric banding for the treatment of morbid obesity in patients with childhood craniopharyngioma. Chicago, IL: The International Society of Pediatric Neuro-Oncology; 2008.

89. Smith DK, Sarfeh J, Howard L. Truncal vagotomy in hypothalmic obesity. Lancet. 1983;1:1330–1.

90. Fobi MA. Operations that are questionable for the control of obesity. Obes Surg. 1993;3:197–200.

91. Lustig RH, Tsai P, Hirose S, Farmer DL. Treatment of hypothalamic obesity by laparoscopic truncal vagotomy: early experience. 8th Lawson Wilkins/European Pediatric Endocrine Society meeting. New York, NY; 2009.

27 Bariatric Surgery in Adolescents

Basil M. Yurcisin and Eric J. DeMaria

CONTENTS

INTRODUCTION
PATIENT/PROCEDURE SELECTION
SURGICAL APPROACHES
PRE-OPERATIVE CONSIDERATIONS
OUTCOMES, COMPLICATIONS, AND POST-OPERATIVE CONSIDERATIONS
SUMMARY
REFERENCES

Key Words: Roux-en-Y, lap band, gastric band, sleeve gastrectomy, ghrelin, peptide YY, type 2 diabetes, vitamin deficiency

INTRODUCTION

It is estimated that 18% of children and adolescents in the United States are now obese *(1)*. According to the NHANES surveys of 1976–1980 and 2003–2006, the prevalence of obesity has risen from 5 to 12.4% in 2–5-year-old children, from 6.5 to 17% in children aged 6–11 years, and from 5 to 17.6% in teenagers *(2)*. The implications are serious and have both immediate and long-term effects. Childhood obesity increases the incidence of hypertension, hyperinsulinemia, and dyslipidemia, which raise the risks of cardiovascular disease. A cross-sectional and longitudinal study of more than 6,000 Louisiana children found that 39% of obese subjects (BMI >95th percentile) had two or more cardio-vascular risk factors; cardiovascular risk was even higher in those with BMI at the 99th percentile *(3)*. A major epidemiologic investigation suggested that obesity may reduce life expectancy by as much as 8 years; more importantly, for any given level of overweight, younger adults have greater reduction in life expectancy than older adults *(4)*. Obese children become obese adults *(3,5,6)*, and as many as a quarter of obese adults were overweight as children *(3)*. The earlier in life a person becomes over-weight, and the more severe his or her obesity, the more likely he or she is to remain obese as an adult *(3)*. Metabolic disturbances in adolescence seem to have a shorter latency period and younger onset, and are more virulent *(7,8)*.

From: *Contemporary Endocrinology: Pediatric Obesity: Etiology, Pathogenesis, and Treatment*
Edited by: M. Freemark, DOI 10.1007/978-1-60327-874-4_27,
© Springer Science+Business Media, LLC 2010

Prevention remains an important strategy for weight management in the pediatric population. Treatment options to be considered once a child becomes obese are behavior modification, pharmacotherapy, and weight loss surgery (WLS). Behavioral modification incorporates increased activity and decreased caloric intake. This approach is time intensive, yielding unexceptional and short-lived results *(9–12)*. When directly compared, Roux-en-Y gastric bypass (RYGB) was shown to be more effective in reducing BMI than a 1-year family-based pediatric behavioral treatment program *(13)*. In combination with behavioral modification, pharmacotherapy with orlistat or sibutramine is moderately effective (see Chapter 23). However, any benefit gained is often reversed when the drug is stopped either voluntarily or because of side effects *(14,15)*. Unfortunately, the drugs may be less effective in those with higher BMI and more co-morbidities *(11,16)*. Bariatric surgery has been shown to cause more significant and durable weight loss than diet/exercise and pharmacotherapy regimens *(11,13,16)*. Indeed, WLS is the most effective means for reducing obesity-related co-morbidities among adults *(17,18)* and adolescents *(10)*.

A variety of co-morbidities are associated with overweight and obesity in the children; among the most notable are type 2 diabetes mellitus, dyslipidemia, metabolic syndrome, hypertension, pseudotumor cerebri, steatohepatitis, obstructive sleep apnea, depression, and low self-esteem. Early retrospective study results for WLS in pediatric patients have demonstrated a co-morbidity and weight loss impact that is at least similar to, if not better than, that seen in adults *(19)*. Increasing length of exposure and severity of disease decrease the likelihood that WLS will lead to resolution of co-morbidities *(20–22)*. Key considerations in safety and patient selection include timing of the intervention in relationship to physical development/maturation; method of consent/assent; surgical approach; pre-operative work-up; and post-operative compliance.

PATIENT/PROCEDURE SELECTION

Expert committees comprised of pediatric surgeons, endocrinologists, and psychiatrists have recently updated practice guidelines for weight loss surgery in adolescents *(23,24)*. Criteria for patient selection emphasize the importance of obesity-related co-morbidities. Published guidelines propose that candidates for WLS include those with (a) BMI > 35 and serious co-morbidities such as type 2 diabetes mellitus, moderate or severe obstructive sleep apnea, pseudotumor cerebri, and/or severe steatohepatitis; or (b) BMI $\geq$ 40 with other co-morbidities such as mild obstructive sleep apnea, hypertension, insulin resistance, glucose intolerance, dyslipidemia, and/or impaired quality of life or activities of daily living. Surgical candidates must have achieved 95% of estimated final height (especially prior to malabsorptive procedures) and sexual maturity (Tanner stage IV or V). In theory, they must have the capacity for mature decision-making and the ability to comply with dietary and physical activity changes needed post-operatively. There should be no untreated or poorly controlled psychiatric disorder and the home environment should be stable and supportive (Table 1). Children with genetic obesity disorders with insatiable appetite and obstreperous behavior are rarely suitable for weight loss surgery *(25)*.

SURGICAL APPROACHES

There is a paucity of data supporting the superiority of any one surgical approach to weight loss in obese patients under 18 years of age; multiple studies provide evidence that both the adjustable gastric band (AGB) and Roux-en-y gastric bypass (RYGB) are safe and efficacious *(23)*. Currently, the only bariatric procedure that should be performed outside of IRB-approved protocols is the RYGB. The use of AGB devices in adolescents requires off-label use of the implant. The sleeve gastrectomy (SG) is being studied as a possible stand-alone procedure in this population, with favorable early results

Table 1
Candidates for adolescent obesity surgery[a]

BMI > 35 kg/m² with severe co-morbidity
– Type 2 diabetes mellitus
– Moderate or severe obstructive sleep apnea
– Pseudotumor cerebri
– Severe steatohepatitis

BMI ≥ 40 kg/m² with other co-morbidity
– Mild obstructive sleep apnea
– Hypertension
– Insulin resistance/glucose intolerance
– Dyslipidemia
– Steatohepatitis
– Venous stasis
– Panniculitis
– Urinary incontinence
– Gastroesophageal reflux
– Weight-related arthropathies
– Severe psychosocial distress
– Impaired quality of life/activities of daily living

Candidates should also (must satisfy all)
– Have attained ≥95% of adult stature
– Failed previous organized weight loss attempts
– Commit to psychological pre- and post-operative evaluation
– If psychiatric condition present, it is under treatment
– Agree to avoid pregnancy for *at least* 1 year post-operatively
– Commit to nutritional guidelines post-operatively
– Demonstrate decisional capacity to give informed assent
– Have a stable and supportive home environment

[a]All candidates should be evaluated on a case-by-case basis.

(26,27). The biliopancreatic diversion and duodenal switch procedures are not recommended in the adolescent population due to the risks of long-term vitamin deficiencies and poor compliance, which create unacceptable risks.

AGB. In 2001, the Food and Drug Administration approved the AGB for use in the United States in adults. The AGB represents a solely restrictive procedure; it causes weight loss by physically limiting the ability to digest calories. Two approved band systems exist (Lap-Band, Allergan, Irvine, CA and Realize, Ethicon Endosurgery, Cincinnati, OH). The AGB is placed around the proximal stomach. Post-operatively the circumference of the band can be changed by altering the amount of saline in the bladder via a subcutaneous port (Fig. 1).

Weight loss following AGB in adults has been reported to range from 56 to 59% of excess body weight (EBW) *(28,29)*; American trials, however, have yielded varied results *(30,31)*. Studies in

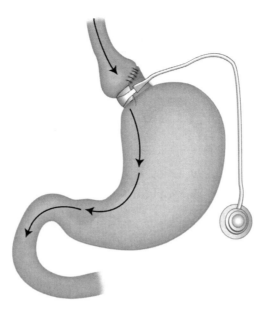

Fig. 1. Adjustable gastric banding (AGB).

pediatric patients have demonstrated reductions of 37–63% EBW after AGB *(32–35)*. The re-operative rate for AGB, however, is not insignificant (8–10%) *(32,33,35)*. Early post-operative complications include gastric or esophageal perforation and bleeding. Late complications include band slippage, gastric obstruction, port malfunction or infection, and band erosion.

A major theoretical advantage of AGB for adolescents is its reversibility. Moreover, surgical complications and vitamin deficiencies are less frequent and less severe than those observed after RYGB (see "Outcomes, Complications, and Post-operative Considerations"). Nevertheless, more long-term investigations are needed to fully assess the role of AGB in children.

RYGB is the most common bariatric surgical procedure performed in the United States. RYGB is a technically demanding procedure *(36)* that combines restriction and malabsorption to assist weight loss. A small, 15- to 30-ml gastric pouch is created along the lesser curve of the stomach near the gastro-espophageal junction, followed by construction of a gastrojejunostomy with a 1-cm stoma to drain the pouch (Fig. 2). A 50-cm jejunal limb provides moderate malabsorption and limits bile reflux. This alimentary limb can be tunneled through the mesocolon (retro-colic) or allowed to pass anterior to the colon and stomach (ante-colic).

Significant weight loss has been achieved in the super-obese population (BMI $\geq$ 50 kg/m^2) with a 150-cm Roux limb, referred to as long-limb gastric bypass *(37)*. At 2 years, adults undergoing successful gastric bypass can expect between 69 and 82% EBW loss *(38,39)*. Similarly, adolescents undergoing RYGB can exhibit ∼60% EBW reduction after RYGB (18,23).

Surgical complications of RYGB include leak, internal hernia, marginal ulceration, and a dumping-like syndrome with postprandial hyperinsulinemia and hypoglycemia (see Post-op Complications, below).

Sleeve Gastrectomy (SG). Originally a component of the biliopancreatic diversion with duodenal switch, the sleeve has evolved from use as a staged procedure for super-obese or high-risk patients to a stand-alone operation. During SG the stomach is freed from its lateral attachments and the greater curvature of the stomach is removed. This effectively creates a tubular "sleeve" of remaining gastric tissue (Fig. 3). The attractiveness of this procedure is based on significant initial weight loss and the suggestion that peri-operative risk is reduced for some high-risk patients when compared to

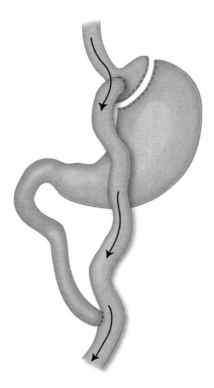

Fig. 2. Roux-en-Y gastric bypass (RYGB).

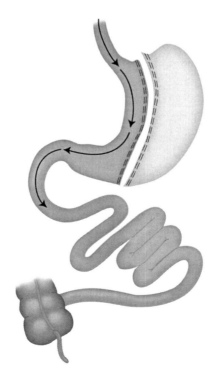

Fig. 3. Sleeve gastrectomy (SG).

gastric bypass. Nevertheless, complications of SG may include leak, stricture, nausea and vomiting, pulmonary embolism, and hemorrhage.

Loss of 59% EBW has been reported in adults 1 year after surgery *(40)*. Long-term results for this procedure are pending, but a growing body of evidence suggests 3–5-year weight loss results similar to other bariatric procedures. Pediatric studies have shown that the SG may be safe with less chance of nutritional deficiencies than the RYGB *(26,27,35)*.

PRE-OPERATIVE CONSIDERATIONS

The Operative Team

Surgeons and institutions that have low operative volumes often have less favorable patient outcomes after WLS *(41,42)*. The American Society of Metabolic and Bariatric Surgery (ASMBS) has recommended that bariatric surgery should be performed at Surgical Review Committee (SRC) centers of excellence (COE). Adolescent WLS requires knowledge of both pediatric medicine and bariatric surgery. Thus, pediatric surgeons performing WLS can find great benefit by integrating their efforts with an adult WLS program *(23)*. Combining of resources, including equipment, nursing, and institutional expertise, can improve outcomes, reduce costs, and facilitate the transition into an adult follow-up program (since these surgeries require life-long monitoring). In order to obtain the COE designation, an institution and its surgeons must adhere to specific safety and volume guidelines established by the SRC. Centers performing adolescent bariatric surgery should also participate in prospective data collection into large multicenter databases. For pediatric patients, the Teen-Longitudinal Assessment of Bariatric Surgery (Teen-LABS) represents such a database *(43)*. SRC mandates that all WLS data from COE be reported in their central data system called BOLD (Bariatric Outcomes Longitudinal Database).

It stands to reason that availability of an organized multi-disciplinary care team trained to evaluate bariatric adolescent patients will allow for appropriate patient selection. The current standard of care requires primary evaluations of the potential patient by a bariatric surgeon, pediatric obesity specialist, dietitian, exercise physiologist, and mental health specialist *(44,45)*. Sub-specialists in pediatric pulmonology, gynecology, endocrinology, and gastroenterology should be available for consultation. The ultimate goal of the pre-operative work-up is to identify modifiable risk factors and incorporate appropriate treatment strategies to reduce peri-operative adverse events. Despite the aforementioned criteria for surgery, the pediatric candidate for bariatric surgery should be assessed on a case-by-case basis taking into account obesity-related co-morbidities, physiologic and psychologic maturity, and the family support system *(23)*.

Pre-op Assessment

The pre-operative evaluation begins with the identification and management of secondary causes of obesity including genetic, neurologic, psychological, drug-induced, and endocrine disorders. The physician should focus on co-morbidities of obesity including but not limited to type 2 diabetes mellitus, hypertension, hyperlipidemia, sleep apnea, orthopedic complaints, and psychiatric sequelae. Significant findings during this evaluation should trigger sub-specialty evaluation and treatment.

Laboratory studies used to identify co-morbidities include echocardiogram, complete blood count, fasting and postprandial glucose levels and HbA1c, lipid panel, urinary assessment, and liver function tests. The serum β-human chorionic gonadotropin should be measured in females. Additional tests to rule out hypothyroidism, Cushing's syndrome, and gall bladder disease are obtained on an as needed basis. An endocrinologist should be consulted in cases of impaired fasting glucose (100–125 mg%), impaired glucose tolerance (2 h glucose 140–199), or frank diabetes. Elevated fasting total triglycerides (> 200 mg/dl) or low levels of HDL may herald metabolic syndrome. Transaminase levels exceeding twice normal require an evaluation by a gastroenterologist.

Questions Regarding Patient Age and Informed Consent

The mortality risk of bariatric surgery increases with increasing BMI and number of co-morbidities (46,47). WLS performed at an earlier time point in disease progression may reduce the risk during and after the surgical procedure (19). Belle et al. performed a longitudinal study comparing mortality rates between groups of extremely obese adults less than 40 years of age. One group underwent WLS; the other did not. The WLS group had 3% mortality over the 13-year follow-up while the non-operated group had a mortality of 13.8% (48). Although this study does not directly demonstrate the benefit of WLS in adolescents as compared with young adults, it does suggest that earlier intervention may have better long-term outcomes.

A recent study (49) of 61 consecutive RYGB procedures in obese adolescents (BMI 40–95) showed that pre-operative BMI served as an accurate predictor of nadir BMI 1 year post-operatively. Interestingly, BMI decreased by 37% irrespective of baseline BMI; consequently; 1 year after surgery, only 17% of patients achieved a BMI in the non-obese range (<30 kg/m^2). The authors concluded that "late" referral for bariatric surgery may preclude reversal of obesity and co-morbidities. Bariatric surgeons treating obese pediatric patients have long called for WLS to be performed earlier in life at a lower BMI, in order to achieve long-term benefit (19,50).

The problem of obtaining informed consent in this patient population is repeatedly noted in the literature. The guardian of the obese child should be counseled as to the risks of persistent (or progressive) obesity: parental obesity, length of exposure to a high BMI in childhood, and increasing age increase the risks of adult obesity (23). The surgical options (as noted above) should be discussed in detail, with full consideration given to the pros and cons of each in relation to peri-operative risks, co-morbidity resolution, and weight loss. There should be congruent perceptions on the part of the family and adolescent as to the desire for WLS and the expected outcomes; quite often this is not the case (11,51). The multidisciplinary team should be attuned to any signs of coercion on the part of the family. Parents are asked to give consent for the procedure; however, the patient should be assessed for the capacity to make an informed decision and given every opportunity to do so. Under nearly all circumstances, the patient, although a minor and therefore unable to give legally appropriate consent, should give his or her assent to the procedure (52).

OUTCOMES, COMPLICATIONS, AND POST-OPERATIVE CONSIDERATIONS

BMI and Co-morbidities

As noted previously, bariatric surgery can reduce excess body weight by 50–80% in adolescents, at least in the short-term (18,23,28–40). Preliminary studies suggest that weight loss surgery may also reverse or reduce the severity of co-morbidities associated with severe obesity. For example, Inge et al. (49) reported significant reductions in systolic (–8.8%) and diastolic (–13.5%) blood pressure, fasting insulin (–75.8%), total cholesterol (–16.8%), LDL (–17.7%), and triglyceride (–37.3%) levels in 61 obese adolescents (mean BMI 51) who underwent RYGB. Moreover, HbA1c was normalized (from 7.3 to 5.6%) in 10 of 11 patients with pre-surgical type 2 diabetes (53). Similar findings have been recorded in other studies (23,54). Sleep apnea resolves or may improve significantly; left ventricular mass decreases and diastolic function may improve (55). Short-term data demonstrate improvements in depression, eating disturbances, and quality of life (10,23,56).

It should be noted that available studies in adolescents are underpowered; larger numbers are required to confirm actual resolution rates of co-morbidities. The inclusion of outcomes data into large databases (teen-LABS) will help to answer these questions.

Mechanisms of Weight Loss

Restriction of caloric intake and (in the case of RYGB and SG) malabsorption of nutrients clearly contribute to weight loss and subsequent increases in insulin sensitivity and improvement or resolution of co-morbidities. However, changes in secretion of gastrointestinal hormones may also play roles in the metabolic adaptation to surgery. A review *(57)* of studies suggests that diversion of nutrients from, or resection of large parts of, the stomach, may blunt the rise in ghrelin that would normally be expected after caloric restriction or weight loss. Moreover, postprandial levels of peptide YY levels are increased following RYGB. Since ghrelin simulates food intake and PYY inhibits appetite, the relative decrease in ghrelin and increase in PYY may facilitate long-term weight loss.

Glycemic control in glucose-intolerant subjects can improve significantly following RYGB even before weight loss is demonstrable. Possible explanations include the catabolic state associated with caloric deprivation and/or an increase in post-prandial levels of glucagon-like peptide 1 (GLP-1) *(57)*, which promotes glucose-stimulated insulin secretion and decreases food intake. The rise in GLP-1 may derive from delivery of nutrients to the GLP-1-secreting L cells in the distal ileum and proximal ascending colon.

Complications

A recent LABS consortium study reported that the 30-day operative mortality rate post-bariatric surgery has been reduced to ∼0.3%, which is equal to or less than that of cholecystectomy. Extremes of BMI, a history of or factors that increase the risk of deep-vein thrombosis or pulmonary embolus, a diagnosis of obstructive sleep apnea, and/or impaired functional status are each independently associated with an increased risk morbidity and mortality *(58)*. The two most common causes of post-operative mortality are leak (either at the gastro-jejunal or jejuno-jejunal anastomoses, or divided stomach staple line) and peritonitis and lethal pulmonary embolus (PE) *(59)*. It is recommended that patients receive prophylaxis for deep vein thrombosis (DVT) and PE with either heparin or enoxaparin peri-operatively. No optimal regimen has been adopted by consensus at this time, but the ASMBS recommends the use of sequential compression stockings and chemical prophylaxis when no contraindication exists.

As noted previously, patients undergoing RYGB can develop postprandial hypoglycemia associated with hyperinsulinemia *(60)*. The latter may respond to a low carbohydrate diet and/or an inhibitor of alpha-glucosidase like Acarbose *(60)*. Rapid and dramatic weight loss following bariatric surgery has also been associated with the development of cholecystitis *(61)*. Post-operative vitamin deficiencies are more common after malabsorptive procedures than with AGB: a university-based study *(62)* of 366 adults revealed deficiencies of vitamins A (11%), C (34.6%), 25OH D (7%), B1 (18.3%), B2 (13.6%), B6 (17.6%), and B12 (3.6%) 12–24 months after RYGB. Some patients have developed beriberi *(63)* with peripheral polyneuropathy or Wernicke's encephalopathy; others have bone demineralization and are at risk for osteoporosis *(64)*. Iron and zinc deficiencies are common. Nearly all patients undergoing malabsorptive surgery will require standard multivitamin preparations *as well as* specific supplements of vitamin B12, iron, calcium/vitamin D, and folic acid. This highlights the need for vigilance in managing patients post-operatively *(65)*. Non-compliance with preventative nutritional supplementation regimens is of particular concern in the adolescent population *(10,23)*; strict adherence to supplementation protocols is important to prevent complications.

Pregnancy is safe after RYGB and AGB *(66–68)*, provided the patient delays conception until at least 18 months after surgery when body weight typically stabilizes. There is a significant rate of teen pregnancy in young female post-operative RYGB patients; whether this is due to increased self-esteem, increased number of sexual encounters, poor contraceptive compliance, or increased fertility due to a weight loss effect is unclear *(23)*.

Follow-Up

Life-long follow-up with a bariatric surgery program is necessary to optimize outcomes. The first post-operative visit for adolescents should occur during the first month, then monthly over the first 3 months, followed by quarterly visits thereafter.

Bariatric surgery as a specialty has been troubled with high rates of medicolegal liability actions; this is believed to be even more of an issue when bad outcomes occur in adolescents undergoing WLS. The three most common issues underlying bariatric surgery litigation are death, post-operative complications, and failure to obtain informed consent. The team dealing with the adolescent bariatric patient and his/her family is advised to thoroughly document each interaction *(23,52)*. The importance of diligent follow-up for prevention and detection of vitamin deficiencies and for monitoring of dietary compliance in this population cannot be overstated *(23,62–65)*.

SUMMARY

WLS has emerged as the most effective and durable method to achieve weight loss and resolution of co-morbidities of obesity. RYGB, AGB, and SG are safe and provide significant resolution of co-morbidities. Many clinicians are enthusiastic about the AGB procedure for obese adolescents because it has lower risks of life-threatening complications and nutritional deficiencies, and is reversible. The obese pediatric patient considered for WLS should be evaluated by a multidisciplinary team; surgery should be performed in a registered bariatric surgery COE with significant experience with bariatric surgery and appropriate non-surgical specialists available for the care of adolescents. Post-operative follow-up is of great importance as adolescents are at risk for sequelae of poor compliance post-operatively. The inclusion of patient data in large, multicenter, national databases will likely provide important information going forward to answer many of the questions facing those who provide both WLS care and non-surgical care for obese children.

Editor's Questions and Authors' Response

- **The decision to consider bariatric surgery revolves in large part around the question of co-morbidities. Do we have evidence that bariatric surgery can reverse or reduce the severity of atherosclerotic lesions in adults or children? Such evidence would provide even stronger support for surgical intervention in teenagers or young adults.**

- There have been many reports linking weight loss with reduction of cardiovascular risk factors and atherosclerosis in adults (Droyvold et al., 2005; Huang et al., 1998; Moore et al., 2005; Stevens et al., 2001; Truesdale et al., 2008). Meta-analysis demonstrated the reduction or elimination of hypertension (62%), diabetes (82%), and hyperlipidemia (70%) following bariatric surgery (Buchwald et al., 2004). Weight loss surgery as a mechanism to reduce body mass index (BMI) and the aforementioned factors was evaluated in 500 patients after roux-en-Y gastric bypass (RYGB). After 1 year, the absolute risk reduction of cardiac events was a mean of 63% in diabetics and 56% in men (Torquati et al., 2007). Another study to evaluate the impact of bariatric surgery on carotid artery atherosclerosis measured by ultrasound imaged carotid bulb intima-media thickness (IMT) compared lean controls to obese patients undergoing gastroplasty and those receiving only dietary management. At 3–4 years, obese patients who had surgery had progression of their IMT equal to lean controls while the IMT progression rate in obese, diet-controlled individuals was three times higher (Karason et al., 1999). In a recent prospective study evaluating 50 consecutive patients undergoing RYGB, subjects were followed for markers of coronary atherosclerosis pre-operatively and 6, 12, and 24 months post-operatively. At 2 years, reductions were noted in BMI (47–29.5 kg/m^2), carotid IMT (0.84–0.50 mm), and C-reactive protein (1.23–0.35 mg/dl); mean brachial artery flow-mediated dilation favorably increased (6.0–14.9%) (Habib et al., 2009). The impact of weight loss surgery on atherosclerosis has yet to be fully elucidated, but the available data indicate an improvement of risk factors of cardiovascular disease and progression of atherosclerosis.

Buchwald H, Avidor Y, Braunwald E, et al. Bariatric surgery: a systematic review and meta-analysis. JAMA. 2004;292(14):1724–37.

Droyvold WB, Midthjell K, Nilsen TI, Holmen J. Change in body mass index and its impact on blood pressure: a prospective population study. Int J Obes (Lond). 2005;29(6):650–5.

Habib P, Scrocco JD, Terek M, et al. Effects of bariatric surgery on inflammatory, functional and structural markers of coronary atherosclerosis. Am J Cardiol. 2009;104(9):1251–5.

Huang Z, Willett WC, Manson JE, et al. Body weight, weight change, and risk for hypertension in women. Ann Intern Med. 1998;128(2):81–8.

Karason K, Wikstrand J, Sjostrom L, Wendelhag I. Weight loss and progression of early atherosclerosis in the carotid artery: a 4-year controlled study of obese subjects. Int J Obes Relat Metab Disord. 1999;23(9):948–56.

Moore LL, Visioni AJ, Qureshi MM, et al. Weight loss in overweight adults and the long-term risk of hypertension: the Framingham study. Arch Intern Med. 2005;165(11):1298–303.

Stevens VJ, Obarzanek E, Cook NR, et al. Long-term weight loss and changes in blood pressure: results of the Trials of Hypertension Prevention, phase II. Ann Intern Med. 2001;134(1):1–11.

Torquati A, Wright K, Melvin W, Richards W. Effect of gastric bypass operation on Framingham and actual risk of cardiovascular events in class II to III obesity. J Am Coll Surg. 2007;204(5):776–82; discussion 782–3.

Truesdale KP, Stevens J, Cai J. Effect of 3-year weight history on blood pressure: the atherosclerosis risk in communities study. Obesity (Silver Spring). 2008;16(5):1112–9.

- **In theory, a candidate for bariatric surgery should have the capacity for mature decision-making and the ability to comply with dietary and physical activity changes needed post-operatively. There should be no untreated or poorly controlled psychiatric disorder, and the home environment should be stable and supportive. After surgery, the child must be available for regular clinic visits, and in the case of a malabsorptive procedure will likely have to take a minimum of 3–4 vitamin supplements to prevent critical nutrient deficits, even if there are no major surgical complications.**

- **Admittedly this is a tall order for a teenager who presumably has made some errors in judgment in becoming severely obese in the first place. Compliance with recommendations is often a major and longstanding problem in this age group. In your experience or in the experience of others, what makes it likely that teenagers (and families) in a real-world setting (outside a clinical research unit) will change their eating behaviors and comply with complicated medication regimens and regular post-op clinic visits following surgery?**

- Compliance assessment is an important component of the evaluation for bariatric surgical treatment in patients of all ages, but is of particular importance in the adolescent patient. Many adolescents exhibit non-compliance with healthy behaviors recommended by both their parents and other adult authorities. When confronted by life-altering major GI surgery, the potential consequences of non-compliance increase exponentially and include vitamin and essential nutrient deficiencies, weight loss failure or weight regain, etc. Assessment of an individual adolescent patient's ability to understand and comply with treatment recommendations after bariatric surgery therefore becomes a key issue with great potential impact on the safety of surgical treatment.

- The best estimate of an individual patient's potential for adherence to treatment recommendations comes from evaluating the individual's history of compliant behavior rather than simply asking the individual to understand or describe the desired behaviors. Non-compliance is typically a chronic condition rather than one which develops suddenly. Patients who can be predicted to demonstrate non-compliance after bariatric surgery typically demonstrate a chronic history of missed office appointments, failure to take recommended medications, etc. They may also exhibit failure in other venues such as skipping school or failing to do homework resulting in failing grades.

- Verbalization of understanding the consequences of non-compliance should generally not reassure the multidisciplinary bariatric care team that an individual will comply with recommendations. Emotional maturity should be assessed by confronting adolescent patients when they deviate from expected behaviors. Oppositional defiance when confronted with irresponsible behavior is a particularly worrisome response from an adolescent candidate for bariatric surgery and should raise significant concerns about the individual's maturity. Of course, in the setting of an underage patient, unreliability of the parents becomes a complicating factor in assessing the adolescent's ability to attend appointments, fill prescriptions, etc. However one might logically argue that whether blame rests with the adolescent patient or the unreliable guardian(s) does not alter the end product result and raises concerns regarding the patient's ability to adhere to treatment recommendations no matter the cause.

- Many adolescent patients, particularly in the late teen years, are highly motivated to do well and can be expected to comply with treatment recommendations following bariatric surgery (Nadler et al., 2008). However, those candidates with a track record of non-compliance should be required to prove their adherence to treatment recommendations before proceeding with life-altering surgery.

Nadler EP, Youn HA, Ren CJ, Fielding GA. An update on 73 US obese pediatric patients treated with laparoscopic adjustable gastric banding: comorbidity resolution and compliance data. J Pediatr Surg. 2008;43(1):141–6.

Editor's Comments

- Meta-analyses [e.g. *(10,23)* in the text and (Dixon et al., 2009)] demonstrate that bariatric surgery reduces BMI in adolescents as well as adults and can revere or reduce the severity of metabolic complications including type 2 diabetes, dyslipidemia, hypertension, sleep apnea, and steatohepatitis. RYGB appears to be more potent than AGB in reducing BMI but is associated with higher rates of serious complications such as pulmonary embolus, shock, intestinal obstruction, bleeding, and profound vitamin and nutrient deficiencies. Nevertheless, data from the Swedish obesity study (Sjostrom et al., 2007) and the Utah gastric bypass study (Adams et al., 2007) suggest that long-term mortality rates are lower in surgically treated than in non-surgically treated obese adults. Reductions in mortality were ascribed to reductions in deaths from cardiovascular disease, cancer, and diabetes.

- Proponents of surgical intervention in obese adolescents often argue that obesity co-morbidities such as type 2 diabetes may become irreversible if we do not intervene aggressively at an early age. This may be true, but it is difficult to reconcile that hypothesis with the surgical data that shows apparent reversal of longstanding type 2 diabetes in young and middle-aged adults. The development of cardiovascular disease might follow a course similar to that of type 2 diabetes, with a long prodrome (beginning in childhood or adolescence) terminating in major clinical illness. The rationale for early surgical intervention would be strengthened by demonstrating that bariatric surgery is more effective than lifestyle intervention and pharmacotherapy in reversing or preventing progression of atherosclerotic lesions. As noted by Drs. Yurcisin and Demaria, recent studies in adults show that bariatric surgery can reduce carotid intimal medial thickness and brachial artery flow-mediated vasodilation (see references above and Habib et al., 2009; Sturm et al., 2009); similar findings in adolescents would provide even stronger support for early surgical intervention.

- The authors of this chapter take a balanced and reasonable approach that reserves surgical intervention for obese adolescents with serious co-morbidities. *Careful selection of surgical candidates and availability of multidisciplinary teams of experts in centers of excellence are essential components of success in the pediatric population.*

Adams TD, et al. Long-term mortality after gastric bypass surgery. N Engl J Med. 2007;357:753–61.

Dixon JB, Jones K, Dixon M. Medical versus surgical interventions for the metabolic complications of obesity in children. Semin Pediatr Surg. 2009 Aug;18(3):168–75.

Habib P, Scrocco JD, Terek M, Vanek V, Mikolich JR. Effects of bariatric surgery on inflammatory, functional and structural markers of coronary atherosclerosis. Am J Cardiol. 2009 Nov 1;104(9):1251–5.

Sjostrom L, et al. Effects of bariatric surgery on mortality in Swedish obese subjects. N Engl J Med. 2007;357: 741–52.

Sturm W, et al. Effect of bariatric surgery on both functional and structural measures of premature atherosclerosis. Eur Heart J. 2009;30:2038–43.

REFERENCES

1. Ogden CL, Carroll MD, Curtin LR, et al. Prevalence of overweight and obesity in the United States, 1999–2004. JAMA. 2006;295(13):1549–55.
2. Ogden CL, Carroll MD, Flegal KM. High body mass index for age among US children and adolescents, 2003–2006. JAMA. 2008;299(20):2401–5.
3. Freedman DS, Mei Z, Srinivasan SR, et al. Cardiovascular risk factors and excess adiposity among overweight children and adolescents: the Bogalusa Heart Study. J Pediatr. 2007;150(1):12–7.
4. Fontaine KR, Redden DT, Wang C, et al. Years of life lost due to obesity. JAMA. 2003;289(2):187–93.
5. Serdula MK, Ivery D, Coates RJ, et al. Do obese children become obese adults? A review of the literature. Prev Med. 1993;22(2):167–77.
6. Whitaker RC, Wright JA, Pepe MS, et al. Predicting obesity in young adulthood from childhood and parental obesity. N Engl J Med. 1997;337(13):869–73.
7. Young-Hyman D, Schlundt DG, Herman L, et al. Evaluation of the insulin resistance syndrome in 5- to 10-year-old overweight/obese African-American children. Diabetes Care. 2001;24(8):1359–64.
8. Levin PD, Weissman C. Obesity, metabolic syndrome, and the surgical patient. Med Clin North Am. 2009;93(5):1049–63.
9. Yanovski JA, Yanovski SZ. Treatment of pediatric and adolescent obesity. JAMA. 2003;289(14):1851–3.
10. Treadwell JR, Sun F, Schoelles K. Systematic review and meta-analysis of bariatric surgery for pediatric obesity. Ann Surg. 2008;248(5):763–76.
11. Levine MD, Ringham RM, Kalarchian MA, et al. Is family-based behavioral weight control appropriate for severe pediatric obesity? Int J Eat Disord. 2001;30(3):318–28.
12. Epstein LH, Valoski A, Wing RR, McCurley J. Ten-year follow-up of behavioral, family-based treatment for obese children. JAMA. 1990;264(19):2519–23.
13. Lawson ML, Kirk S, Mitchell T, et al. One-year outcomes of Roux-en-Y gastric bypass for morbidly obese adolescents: a multicenter study from the Pediatric Bariatric Study Group. J Pediatr Surg. 2006;41(1):137–43; discussion 137–43.
14. Chanoine JP, Hampl S, Jensen C, et al. Effect of orlistat on weight and body composition in obese adolescents: a randomized controlled trial. JAMA. 2005;293(23):2873–83.
15. Berkowitz RI, Wadden TA, Tershakovec AM, Cronquist JL. Behavior therapy and sibutramine for the treatment of adolescent obesity: a randomized controlled trial. JAMA. 2003;289(14):1805–12.
16. Zeller M, Kirk S, Claytor R, et al. Predictors of attrition from a pediatric weight management program. J Pediatr. 2004;144(4):466–70.

17. Sjostrom L, Lindroos AK, Peltonen M, et al. Lifestyle, diabetes, and cardiovascular risk factors 10 years after bariatric surgery. N Engl J Med. 2004;351(26):2683–93.

18. Buchwald H, Avidor Y, Braunwald E, et al. Bariatric surgery: a systematic review and meta-analysis. JAMA. 2004;292(14):1724–37.

19. Garcia VF, DeMaria EJ. Adolescent bariatric surgery: treatment delayed, treatment denied, a crisis invited. Obes Surg. 2006;16(1):1–4.

20. Schauer PR, Burguera B, Ikramuddin S, et al. Effect of laparoscopic Roux-en Y gastric bypass on type 2 diabetes mellitus. Ann Surg. 2003;238(4):467–84; discussion 84–5.

21. Dixon JB, O'Brien PE. Changes in comorbidities and improvements in quality of life after LAP-BAND placement. Am J Surg. 2002;184(6B):51S–4S.

22. Breaux CW. Obesity surgery in children. Obes Surg. 1995;5(3):279–84.

23. Pratt JS, Lenders CM, Dionne EA, et al. Best practice updates for pediatric/adolescent weight loss surgery. Obesity (Silver Spring). 2009;17(5):901–10.

24. August GP, Caprio S, Fennoy I, Freemark M, Kaufman FR, Lustig RH, Silverstein JH, Speiser PW, Styne DM, Montori VM. Prevention and treatment of pediatric obesity: an endocrine society clinical practice guideline based on expert opinion. J Clin Endocrinol Metab. 2008;93:4576–99.

25. Scheimann AO, Butler MG, Gourash L, Cuffari C, Klish W. Critical analysis of bariatric procedures in Prader-Willi syndrome. J Pediatr Gastroenterol Nutr. 2008;46(1):80–3.

26. Aggarwal S, Kini SU, Herron DM. Laparoscopic sleeve gastrectomy for morbid obesity: a review. Surg Obes Relat Dis. 2007;3(2):189–94.

27. Cottam D, Qureshi FG, Mattar SG, et al. Laparoscopic sleeve gastrectomy as an initial weight-loss procedure for high-risk patients with morbid obesity. Surg Endosc. 2006;20(6):859–63.

28. Ceelen W, Walder J, Cardon A, et al. Surgical treatment of severe obesity with a low-pressure adjustable gastric band: experimental data and clinical results in 625 patients. Ann Surg. 2003;237(1):10–6.

29. Dargent J. Laparoscopic adjustable gastric banding: lessons from the first 500 patients in a single institution. Obes Surg. 1999;9(5):446–52.

30. DeMaria EJ, Sugerman HJ, Meador JG, et al. High failure rate after laparoscopic adjustable silicone gastric banding for treatment of morbid obesity. Ann Surg. 2001;233(6):809–18.

31. Ren CJ, Weiner M, Allen JW. Favorable early results of gastric banding for morbid obesity: the American experience. Surg Endosc. 2004;18(3):543–6.

32. Angrisani L, Favretti F, Furbetta F, et al. Obese teenagers treated by Lap-Band System: the Italian experience. Surgery. 2005;138(5):877–81.

33. Nadler EP, Youn HA, Ginsburg HB, et al. Short-term results in 53 US obese pediatric patients treated with laparoscopic adjustable gastric banding. J Pediatr Surg. 2007;42(1):137–41; discussion 141–2.

34. Silberhumer GR, Miller K, Kriwanek S, et al. Laparoscopic adjustable gastric banding in adolescents: the Austrian experience. Obes Surg. 2006;16(8):1062–7.

35. Yitzhak A, Mizrahi S, Avinoach E. Laparoscopic gastric banding in adolescents. Obes Surg. 2006;16(10):1318–22.

36. Schauer P, Ikramuddin S, Hamad G, Gourash W. The learning curve for laparoscopic Roux-en-Y gastric bypass is 100 cases. Surg Endosc. 2003;17(2):212–5.

37. Brolin RE, Kenler HA, Gorman JH, Cody RP. Long-limb gastric bypass in the superobese. A prospective randomized study. Ann Surg. 1992;215(4):387–95.

38. Wittgrove AC, Clark GW. Laparoscopic gastric bypass, Roux-en-Y-500 patients: technique and results, with 3–60 month follow-up. Obes Surg. 2000;10(3):233–9.

39. Schauer PR, Ikramuddin S, Gourash W, et al. Outcomes after laparoscopic Roux-en-Y gastric bypass for morbid obesity. Ann Surg. 2000;232(4):515–29.

40. Lee CM, Cirangle PT, Jossart GH. Vertical gastrectomy for morbid obesity in 216 patients: report of 2-year results. Surg Endosc. 2007;21(10):1810–6.

41. Oliak D, Owens M, Schmidt HJ. Impact of fellowship training on the learning curve for laparoscopic gastric bypass. Obes Surg. 2004;14(2):197–200.

42. Schirmer BD, Schauer PR, Flum DR, et al. Bariatric surgery training: getting your ticket punched. J Gastrointest Surg. 2007;11(7):807–12.

43. Inge TH, Zeller M, Harmon C, et al. Teen-Longitudinal Assessment of Bariatric Surgery: methodological features of the first prospective multicenter study of adolescent bariatric surgery. J Pediatr Surg. 2007;42(11):1969–71.

44. Gastrointestinal surgery for severe obesity: National Institutes of Health Consensus Development Conference Statement. Am J Clin Nutr. 1992;55(2 Suppl):615S–9S.

45. Inge TH, Garcia V, Daniels S, et al. A multidisciplinary approach to the adolescent bariatric surgical patient. J Pediatr Surg. 2004;39(3):442–7; discussion 446–7.

46. DeMaria EJ, Murr M, Byrne TK, et al. Validation of the obesity surgery mortality risk score in a multicenter study proves it stratifies mortality risk in patients undergoing gastric bypass for morbid obesity. Ann Surg. 2007;246(4):578–82; discussion 583–4.

47. DeMaria EJ, Portenier D, Wolfe L. Obesity surgery mortality risk score: proposal for a clinically useful score to predict mortality risk in patients undergoing gastric bypass. Surg Obes Relat Dis. 2007;3(2):134–40.

48. Belle SH, Berk PD, Courcoulas AP, et al. Safety and efficacy of bariatric surgery: Longitudinal Assessment of Bariatric Surgery. Surg Obes Relat Dis. 2007;3(2):116–26.

49. Inge TH, Jenkins TM, Zeller M, et al. Baseline BMI is a strong predictor of Nadir BMI after Adolescent Gastric Bypass. J Pediatr. 2010;156(1):103–8.

50. Inge TH, Xanthakos SA, Zeller MH. Bariatric surgery for pediatric extreme obesity: now or later? Int J Obes (Lond). 2007;31(1):1–14.

51. Zeller MH, Modi AC. Predictors of health-related quality of life in obese youth. Obesity (Silver Spring). 2006;14(1):122–30.

52. Wilde ML. Bioethical and legal implications of pediatric gastric bypass. Willamette Law Rev. 2004;40(3):575–625.

53. Inge TH, Miyano G, Bean J, Helmrath M, Courcoulas A, Harmon CM, Chen MK, Wilson K, Daniels SR, Garcia VF, Brandt ML, Dolan LM. Reversal of type 2 diabetes mellitus and improvements in cardiovascular risk factors after surgical weight loss in adolescents. Pediatrics. 2009;123(1):214–22.

54. Xanthakos SA, Inge TH. Extreme pediatric obesity: weighing the health dangers. J Pediatr. 2007;150(1):3–5.

55. Ippisch HM, Inge TH, Daniels SR, Wang B, Khoury PR, Witt SA, Glascock BJ, Garcia VF, Kimball TR. Reversibility of cardiac abnormalities in morbidly obese adolescents. J Am Coll Cardiol. 2008;51(14):1342–8.

56. Zeller MH, Modi AC, Noll JG, Long JD, Inge TH. Psychosocial functioning improves following adolescent bariatric surgery. Obesity (Silver Spring). 2009;17(5):985–90.

57. Saliba J, Wattacheril J, Abumrad NN. Endocrine and metabolic response to gastric bypass. Curr Opin Clin Nutr Metab Care. 2009;12(5):515–21.

58. Flum DR, Belle SH, King WC, et al. Perioperative safety in the longitudinal assessment of bariatric surgery. N Engl J Med. 2009;361(5):445–54.

59. Podnos YD, Jimenez JC, Wilson SE, et al. Complications after laparoscopic gastric bypass: a review of 3464 cases. Arch Surg. 2003;138(9):957–61.

60. Kellogg TA, Bantle JP, Leslie DB, Redmond JB, Slusarek B, Swan T, Buchwald H, Ikramuddin S. Postgastric bypass hyperinsulinemic hypoglycemia syndrome: characterization and response to a modified diet. Surg Obes Relat Dis. Jul–Aug 2008;4(4):492–9.

61. Li VK, Pulido N, Fajnwaks P, Szomstein S, Rosenthal R, Martinez-Duartez P. Predictors of gallstone formation after bariatric surgery: a multivariate analysis of risk factors comparing gastric bypass, gastric banding, and sleeve gastrectomy. Surg Endosc. 2009;23(7):1640–4.

62. Clements RH, Katasani VG, Palepu R, Leeth RR, Leath TD, Roy BP, Vickers SM. Incidence of vitamin deficiency after laparoscopic Roux-en-Y gastric bypass in a university hospital setting. Am Surg. 2006;72(12):1196–202.

63. Towbin A, Inge TH, Garcia VF, et al. Beriberi after gastric bypass surgery in adolescence. J Pediatr. 2004;145(2):263–7.

64. Coates PS, Fernstrom JD, Fernstrom MH, et al. Gastric bypass surgery for morbid obesity leads to an increase in bone turnover and a decrease in bone mass. J Clin Endocrinol Metab. 2004;89(3):1061–5.

65. Alvarez-Leite JI. Nutrient deficiencies secondary to bariatric surgery. Curr Opin Clin Nutr Metab Care. 2004;7(5):569–75.

66. Woodard CB. Pregnancy following bariatric surgery. J Perinat Neonatal Nurs. 2004;18(4):329–40.

67. Wittgrove AC, Jester L, Wittgrove P, Clark GW. Pregnancy following gastric bypass for morbid obesity. Obes Surg. 1998;8(4):461–4; discussion 465–6.

68. Dao T, Kuhn J, Ehmer D, et al. Pregnancy outcomes after gastric-bypass surgery. Am J Surg. 2006;192(6):762–6.

IX CHALLENGES TO LONG-TERM SUCCESS

28 Neuroendocrine and Metabolic Adaptations in the Central Nervous System That Facilitate Weight Regain

Ronald M. Lechan and Csaba Fekete

CONTENTS

Key Words: Leptin, arcuate nucleus, melanocortin, thyroid hormone, insulin, adiponectin, ghrelin, endocannabinoid, nutrient sensing

INTRODUCTION

Obesity is reaching epidemic proportions, yet short of surgical approaches, other modalities of treatment, in particular dietary restriction and behavioral modification, have been largely unsuccessful *(1)*. At best, only ~20% of overweight individuals are able to maintain at least a 10% weight reduction with diet for more than 1 year *(2)*. The explanation for this largely dismal outlook is the remarkable nature of potent, compensatory, homeostatic systems in the brain that function to maintain body weight, uncoupling energy intake and output by increasing appetite, reducing energy expenditure, and promoting the hedonistic aspects of feeding behavior. As shown in studies by Rosenbaum et al. *(3)*, maintaining a 10% reduced weight in men or women is accompanied by a reduction in resting and non-resting energy expenditure out of proportion to changes in body composition, decreases in sympathetic

From: *Contemporary Endocrinology: Pediatric Obesity: Etiology, Pathogenesis, and Treatment*
Edited by: M. Freemark, DOI 10.1007/978-1-60327-874-4_28,
© Springer Science+Business Media, LLC 2010

nervous activity as measured by heart rate analysis and urinary catecholamine excretion, a reduction in circulating levels of thyroid hormones (T3 and T4), and an increase in skeletal muscle work efficiency. In addition, functional MRI in obese subjects shows that maintenance of reduced body weight activates regions of the brain associated with hedonic aspects of energy homeostasis (4). Presumably, these biologic responses are evolutionarily conserved survival mechanisms, intended to allow energy conservation and promote food-seeking behavior at times of nutrient insufficiency. While the central mechanisms involved in these biologic responses are complex and involve a number of different regulatory pathways which will be described below, it has become clear that at the crux of this homeostatic response is the circulating, largely white adipose tissue-derived hormone, leptin. Indeed, humans with mutations of the leptin gene resulting in leptin deficiency, or with mutations of the leptin receptor, are markedly obese as a result of intense hyperphagia with food-seeking behavior, abnormalities in sympathetic nervous function, alteration in thyroid function, and reduced ability to discriminate between the rewarding properties of food (5). Furthermore, exogenous administration of leptin to obese subjects maintaining a 10% weight loss can reverse neuroendocrine, autonomic, skeletal muscle, and neural activity responses back to pre-weight loss levels (3,4).

LEPTIN–BRAIN INTERACTIONS DURING FASTING/CALORIC RESTRICTION

The discovery of leptin in 1994 (6) revolutionized thinking on the mechanisms governing appetite and satiety. Leptin serves as an important humoral signal that reflects body fat stores and, by acting on discrete regions in the hypothalamus, brainstem and perhaps other regions of the brain (7), orchestrates metabolic, neuroendocrine, and behavioral adaptations to nutrient availability. Thus, during nutrient abundance, leptin secretion is increased, leading to decreased appetite and increased caloric disposal. Flier and Ahima (8), however, proposed that the decline in leptin associated with fasting or nutrient insufficiency (such as dieting) is the most important function of this hormone, increasing appetite and energy conservation and shifting to a neuroendocrine profile that facilitates metabolic adaptation to maintain body weight.

Leptin Signaling

A major site of leptin action is the mediobasal hypothalamus, primarily the hypothalamic arcuate nucleus, where it binds to specific receptors (Ob-Rb) that influence the activities of two separate groups of neurons with opposing functions: α-MSH-producing neurons that co-express CART and AGRP neurons that co-express NPY (9). When circulating leptin levels decline, the expression of genes that promote weight loss and energy expenditure, including α-MSH and CART, is suppressed; simultaneously there is a marked increase in the expression of genes that promote weight gain and reduce energy expenditure, including AGRP and NPY.

After binding to Ob-Rb, leptin induces activation of the JAK/STAT and phosphoinositide-3 kinase (PI3-K) signaling pathways. STAT3 signaling is of particular importance in α-MSH/CART neurons since POMC-specific STAT3-deficient mice develop obesity (10), whereas leptin signaling through PI3-K may be of critical importance for both α-MSH/CART and AGRP/NPY neuronal populations (11). PI3-K activation results in Akt-mediated phosphorylation of the transcription factor, FoxO1, and the shuttling of FoxO1 out of the nucleus and into the cytoplasm (12). When leptin levels decline during fasting, FoxO1 is dephosphorylated in the cytoplasm of both α-MSH/CART and AGRP/NPY neurons and then translocates back to the nucleus where it inhibits POMC transcription (13,14) and induces transcription of both the AGRP and NPY genes (12,13). Reduced circulating levels of leptin also increase AMP-activated protein kinase (AMPK) activity in arcuate nucleus neurons and, by suppressing mammalian target of rapamycin complex (mTOR), similarly lead to inhibition of POMC while activating AGRP and NPY gene expression (15).

Leptin also affects synaptic remodeling of α-MSH/CART and AGRP/NPY neurons, providing yet another mechanism whereby POMC-expressing neurons are suppressed and AGRP/NPY neurons activated during fasting. Thus, when leptin levels decline, there are significantly greater numbers of excitatory postsynaptic currents (EPSCs) and an increased ratio of excitatory *vs* inhibitory synapses on AGRP/NPY neurons, but a greater number of inhibitory postsynaptic currents (IPSCs) on α-MSH/CART neurons *(16)*.

Effects of Leptin on Appetite, Energy Homeostasis, and Behavior

Leptin-responsive arcuate nucleus neurons send monosynaptic projections to identical targets within discrete regions of the hypothalamus where the signals are integrated and then relayed by independent pathways to regions of the brain governing appetite, hypophysiotropic function, and energy expenditure. NPY is a potent orexigen and when injected into the brain rapidly increases body weight as a result of increased food consumption and a simultaneous decrease in energy expenditure, the latter mediated through effects on the sympathetic nervous system and the hypothalamic-pituitary-thyroid axis *(17)*. By inhibiting the sympathetic nervous system, NPY not only decreases heat production by brown adipose tissue *(18)* but also stimulates insulin secretion *(19)* and increases the respiratory quotient (VCO_2/VO_2). These actions promote catabolism of carbohydrate in favor of fat synthesis and lipid deposition in white adipose tissue *(20)*. The effects of NPY on the hypothalamic pituitary-thyroid axis are described in detail below.

It is becoming increasingly apparent, however, that the melanocortin signaling system may be the predominant regulatory system governing appetite and energy expenditure. Whereas animals with targeted deficiency of NPY or AGRP have an essentially normal phenotype and intact responses to fasting *(21,22)*, animal models with targeted deletion of the melanocortin 4 receptor (MC4R) and humans bearing mutations that interfere with the function of the MC4R, POMC gene, or processing enzymes necessary to generate a fully mature α-MSH develop a severe obesity syndrome *(23–25)*. Down-regulation of α-MSH is of major importance in the drive to feed as indicated by the loss of typical compensatory feeding responses following a fast in animals with selective inactivation of STAT3 in POMC neurons *(10)*. In addition, selective ablation of POMC-expressing cells is sufficient to produce obesity and reduce energy expenditure *(26)*. As AGRP functions as both a competitive antagonist and an inverse agonist at the MC4R *(27)*, the rise in AGRP during fasting or caloric deprivation cooperates in down-regulation of melanocortin signaling by antagonizing the action of α-MSH concurrently with inhibition of the POMC gene. Direct, synaptic connections between the arcuate nucleus NPY/AGRP neurons and α-MSH/CART neurons also are present *(28)*, further contributing to the suppression of POMC gene expression with fasting.

CNS Targets for Leptin-Regulated Neurons in the Arcuate Nucleus

A. Hypothalamic Paraventricular Nucleus

One of the main output targets of leptin-responsive arcuate nucleus neurons is the hypothalamic paraventricular nucleus (PVN), a major hypothalamic center where integration of neuroendocrine and autonomic information takes place *(29)*. The PVN consists of two major parts: a magnocellular and a parvocellular division. Neurons in the magnocellular division project to the posterior pituitary and release vasopressin and oxytocin. The parvocellular division is more complicated and contains anterior, periventricular, medial, ventral, dorsal, and lateral parvocellular subdivisions. These neurons are involved in regulating the anterior pituitary and mediating a number of neuroendocrine and autonomic functions. The importance of the PVN in the regulation of body weight is implicit in the observations by Kablaoui et al. *(30)* and Michaud et al. *(31)* that disruption of the Sim1 gene, which is essential for the normal development of the PVN, causes severe obesity in both man and experimental animals. Both melanocortin (MC3R and MC4R) and NPY (Y1 and Y5) receptors are present in the PVN *(32,33)*, establishing the significance of the melanocortin and AGRP/NPY signaling systems in the regulation of the PVN.

The PVN has a particularly important role in mediating the actions of melanocortin signaling on food intake. If the MC4R is reintroduced into the PVN of the MC4R knockout mouse but excluded from other hypothalamic or brainstem nuclei, control of food intake can be completely restored to normal *(34)*. A particularly attractive locus for the regulation of food intake in the PVN is the ventral parvocellular subdivision (PVNv), which is densely innervated by α-MSH- and AGRP-containing axons and shows a marked increase in c-fos activity 2 h after fasting animals have been refed; c-fos induction can be prevented by intracerebroventricular administration of AGRP *(35)*. The PVN is also involved in the regulation of the autonomic nervous system through descending projections to brainstem and spinal cord targets *(36)*, contributing to the regulation of energy disposal by controlling heat loss from brown adipose tissue through effects on uncoupling protein-1 (UCP-1) and by affecting lipolysis and proteolysis in white fat and muscle *(37,38)*. Nevertheless, in contrast, to the effect on food intake, restoring the MC4R in the PVN of MC4R knockout mice has no effect on their reduced energy expenditure, suggesting that other brain targets are involved.

In addition to the PVN, leptin-responsive α-MSH/CART and AGRP/NPY arcuate nucleus neurons project to the hypothalamic dorsomedial nucleus (DMN), ventromedial nucleus (VMN), and lateral hypothalamus (LH) *(39)*. Each of these regions also expresses leptin receptors *(40)*, indicating that leptin can influence the activity of VMN, DMN, and LH neurons by both indirect and direct pathways. In fact, the demonstration that selective disruption of leptin receptors in either POMC or AGRP/NPY arcuate nucleus neurons results in only a modest obesity syndrome (compared to that of animals with complete leptin receptor deficiency) suggests that leptin signaling must be mediated by both indirect and direct pathways. In contrast, the PVN expresses few to no leptin receptors, indicative of its complete dependence on leptin actions exerted in other regions of the brain.

B. Hypothalamic Dorsomedial Nucleus

The hypothalamic DMN is well known to be involved in the regulation of food intake *(41)* that can be altered by its disconnection from the arcuate nucleus *(42)*. In addition, both dorsal and ventral subdivisions of the DMN show c-fos activation following the refeeding of fasting animals that can be diminished by pretreatment with AGRP *(35)*. This supports a role for DMN neurons in mediating the effects of melanocortin signaling, presumably by way of their extensive projections to the PVN *(43)* and/or descending projections to brainstem autonomic centers *(41)*. The DMN may also participate in the regulation of thermogenesis in brown adipose tissue *(44,45)*, recently demonstrated to be present in adult humans *(46,47)*. Brown adipose tissue has an important role in the regulation of energy expenditure by short circuiting the proton gradient across the inner mitochondrial membrane through the activation of UCP-1, which uncouples fuel oxidation from the synthesis of ATP to generate heat *(48)*. As UCP-1 is regulated by leptin in experimental animal models and reduced by fasting *(49)*, a reduction in the efficiency of mitochondrial respiration may contribute to weight regain following caloric restriction.

C. Ventromedial Nucleus

The VMN has long been implicated in the regulation of feeding behavior as lesions of the VMN produce hyperphagia *(50)*, but these observations were likely due to transection of surrounding fiber pathways. Recent studies in transgenic animals in which the leptin receptor is selectively removed from VMN neurons, however, reveal that these animals develop obesity *(51)* and have defective adaptive thermogenic responses to a high-fat diet, gaining weight, and increasing oxygen consumption only

~50% of that of wild-type mice *(52)*. Relatively little is known, however, about the factors that mediate the effects of leptin signaling in the VMN and the precise mechanisms involved in its regulation of energy balance.

One potential VMN mediator is brain-derived neurotrophic factor (BDNF), an anorectic peptide that is highly concentrated in the dorsomedial part of the VMN *(53)*. Conditional mutants in which BDNF is removed in the post-neonatal brain *(54)* or mutations of its receptor in animals or humans *(55,56)* result in a severe obese phenotype due to hyperphagia and reduced energy expenditure, suggesting an important role in the regulation of body weight. BDNF-expressing neurons in the VMN are inversely regulated by leptin *(53)* such that with fasting or caloric restriction, BDNF mRNA is markedly suppressed *(56)*. Evidence that BDNF may be regulated by melanocortin signaling is shown by a reduction in BDNF gene expression in mice overexpressing the MC4R antagonist, agouti, and its increase following the intraventricular administration of the MC4R agonist, MTII, to fasting animals *(56)*.

d. Lateral Hypothalamus

Both α-MSH/CART and AGRP/NPY neurons from the arcuate nucleus have extensive neuronal connections with the lateral hypothalamus and innervate two groups of leptin-responsive neurons that produce either melanin-concentrating hormone (MCH) or orexin *(57)*. Both neuronal populations are inversely regulated by leptin. MCH acts as an endogenous stimulator of food intake and its mRNA is increased during fasting *(58)*, whereas orexin promotes arousal responses, contributing to food-seeking behavior during periods of nutrient deficiency *(59)*. While both neuronal populations project to a number of different regions of the brain including the cerebral cortex and brainstem, MCH-producing neurons also project to the nucleus accumbens *(60)* and orexin-producing neurons project to the ventral tegmental area (VTA) *(61)*, well-recognized reward centers involved in hedonic eating and addiction. Orexin also increases gastric contractility through projections to the dorsal vagal complex and, by reducing gastric distension, suppresses satiety signals carried by the vagus nerve *(62)*. Thus, during caloric restriction, activation of orexin- and MCH-producing LH neurons would have several actions to promote increased food ingestion and promote weight gain through effects on appetite, behavior, and the incentive to feed. Leptin signaling may also have direct effects on neurons in the VTA itself *(63)*, contributing to the regulation of food-associated reward by regulating the content of dopamine in the striatum, amygdala, and prefrontal cortex *(64)*. Dopamine has a major role in the regulation of reward processing including the desire for sweet foods and drugs of abuse *(65)*. In concert with animal studies, human studies using functional MRI have shown leptin deficiency to be associated with increased neuronal activation in the nucleus accumbens when subjects are exposed to food images; this is abolished following leptin treatment *(66)*.

Effects of Leptin on Thyroid Hormone Regulation

The leptin-responsive, arcuate-PVN projection pathway has a particularly important role in the regulation of the hypothalamic-pituitary-thyroid axis by influencing the set point for feedback regulation by thyroid hormone *(67)*. Fasting and caloric restriction reduce circulating thyroid hormone levels in both experimental animals and man; these can be restored to normal by the administration of leptin *(67,68)*. Since thyroid hormone has an important role in the regulation of energy expenditure by affecting obligatory thermogenesis (energy expenditure necessary to sustain basal homeostatic functions) and adaptive thermogenesis (additional heat produced in response to triggering signals to sustain core temperature), a decline in circulating thyroid hormone levels would serve to conserve calories. Indeed, basal metabolic rate can be reduced by as much as 30% in the absence of thyroid hormone and adaptive thermogenesis in cold exposed animals is markedly impaired *(69)*. Although the molecular mechanisms are not precisely known, thyroid hormone has an important role in activation of UCP-1 in brown adipose tissue *(70)* and may also influence thermogenesis by acting on uncoupling proteins in muscle *(71)*.

The effects of leptin on the hypothalamic-pituitary-thyroid axis are mediated through the α-MSH/CART- and AGRP/NPY-producing arcuate nucleus neurons *(72)*. Both α-MSH and CART have activating effects on hypophysiotropic TRH neurons and when administered intracerebroventricularly to fasting animals restore TRH mRNA to levels in ad lib feeding animals *(73)*. The mechanism involves the phosphorylation of the transcription factor CREB, as shown by the ability of α-MSH to increase the number of phospho-CREB-containing TRH neurons in the PVN when given to fasting animals *(74)* and by the loss of TRH promoter activation by α-MSH in vitro in the presence of a dominant-negative inhibitor of CREB that cannot be phosphorylated *(75)*. The mechanism by which CART activates TRH neurons in the PVN remains unknown.

Conversely, both NPY and AGRP have profound inhibitory effects on TRH gene expression in hypophysiotropic neurons. When administered intracerebroventricularly to ad lib feeding animals, a state of central hypothyroidism is created that closely compares to that observed in fasting animals *(76,77)*. The inhibitory effects of AGRP on TRH gene expression are the result of antagonizing the activating effects of α-MSH at MC4Rs and/or by suppressing constitutively active melanocortin receptors by functioning as an inverse agonist *(73)*. While NPY and the melanocortins act through different receptors, the two peptidergic systems can interact at a post-receptor level and, by inhibiting cAMP production, attenuate α-MSH-induced CREB-phosphorylation in the nucleus of TRH neurons *(78)*.

Thus during fasting or caloric restriction, when circulating leptin levels decline, the simultaneous inhibition of α-MSH production and increase in AGRP and NPY production in arcuate nucleus neurons reduce the availability of phospho-CREB for binding to the TRH promoter. Since liganded thyroid hormone receptor may interact with phospho-CREB at the TRH promoter *(79)*, the inhibitory feedback effects of thyroid hormone bound to its receptor on the TRH promoter may become enhanced due to reduced competition by lower intranuclear concentrations of pCREB, lowering the set point for feedback inhibition of the TRH gene by thyroid hormone. A direct action of leptin signaling on hypophysiotropic TRH neurons has been proposed *(75)* but is less likely due to the paucity of leptin receptors in the PVN *(40)*.

Thyroid hormone may also contribute to weight gain by direct effects on the hypothalamic arcuate and ventromedial nuclei. Although caloric restriction leads to a decline in circulating thyroid hormone levels, tissue levels of thyroid hormone in the mediobasal hypothalamus may increase *(80)*. It is proposed that this increase is secondary to a modest increase in type 2 iodothyronine deiodinase (D2) in tanycytes *(81)*, specialized ependymal cells lining the walls of the third ventricle *(82)*. The major function of D2 is to regulate local bioavailability of tri-iodothyronine (T3) in tissue by converting thyroxine (T4) to its more potent biologically active metabolite. As tanycytes lie at the interface of the blood/CSF–brain barrier, they are capable of extracting T4 from the bloodstream or CSF, converting T4 to T3, and then releasing T3 into the adjacent hypothalamic neuropil through long cytoplasmic projections that extend into the adjacent arcuate and ventromedial nuclei. Thyroid hormone-induced hyperphagia may arise as a result of a T3-mediated increase in NPY in the arcuate nucleus *(80,83)* or through direct effects on the hypothalamic ventromedial nucleus (VMN) *(84)*.

INSULIN–BRAIN INTERACTIONS DURING FASTING/CALORIC RESTRICTION

Prior to the discovery of leptin, insulin was believed to be the major effector of energy homeostasis (see Niswender et al. *(85)* for review). When infused into the brain, insulin reduces food intake; conversely, eradication of insulin signaling, achieved by central administration of insulin antibodies *(86)* or a reduction in hypothalamic insulin receptors *(87)*, causes hyperphagia and weight gain. Leptin has more profound effects on the central nervous system than insulin, as demonstrated by a less severe obesity phenotype in brain-specific knockouts of the insulin receptor as compared to the leptin receptor *(88,89)*. However, circulating levels of insulin, like those of leptin, decline with fasting. In addition, like leptin, insulin is capable of regulating PI3-K in both α-MSH/CART and AGRP/NPY neurons *(12,14)*, such that a decline in insulin levels might be expected to reduce POMC and activate AGRP/NPY in arcuate nucleus neurons. Indeed, decreasing hypothalamic insulin receptors using antisense RNA has been shown to increase the expression of both NPY and AGRP *(87)*.

There is also a substantial literature implicating a role for insulin in the modulation of food reward *(90)*. Insulin receptors have been identified in the VTA and on dopamine neurons *(91)*, suggesting the VTA as yet another site where leptin and insulin signaling could converge. Insulin, however, is believed to regulate dopamine secretion by increasing the expression and activity of the dopamine uptake transporter (DAT), rapidly clearing dopamine from the synapse *(90)*. Thus, when insulin levels decline in association with fasting or caloric restriction, the resulting down-regulation of DAT may promote increased dopamine signaling at synapses, thereby contributing to hedonic eating.

ADIPONECTIN–BRAIN INTERACTIONS DURING FASTING/CALORIC RESTRICTION

Adiponectin is also believed to have an important role in the regulation of appetite and energy expenditure and has been proposed to serve as a starvation signal to preserve fat reserves *(92)*. Like leptin, adiponectin is a white adipose tissue-derived adipokine but exists as multimeric forms and enters the CNS from the circulation as both trimers and hexamers *(92)*. In contrast to leptin, however, adiponectin increases in the plasma with fasting, thereby functioning inversely to leptin in the brain *(92)*. Adiponectin binds to the adiponectin receptor 1 (AdipoR1) in the arcuate nucleus where AGRP/NPY neurons reside (see previously) and activates AMPK *(93)*. This results in an increase in food intake that can be prevented by overexpression of a dominant-negative AMPK selectively in the arcuate nucleus, as well as a reduction in energy expenditure by suppressing UCP-1 in brown adipose tissue *(93)*.

GHRELIN–BRAIN INTERACTIONS DURING FASTING/CALORIC RESTRICTION

In addition to leptin and insulin, a number of gut peptides contribute to the central regulation of appetite and satiety (Table 1), either by acting directly on the hypothalamic arcuate nucleus or by transmitting information to the dorsal vagal complex, an important relay center in the brainstem for visceral sensory information carried by the vagus nerve (see *(94,95)* for recent reviews). While a fasting-induced decline in any of these anorexic peptides could contribute to increased eating, the associated rise in ghrelin, the only gut peptide with known orexigenic activity, has generated particular interest.

Ghrelin is a 28 amino acid octanoylated peptide (acyl ghrelin) synthesized primarily by the stomach *(96)*. In a variety of animal models, systemic or intracerebroventricular administration of ghrelin increases feeding and decreases energy expenditure through effects on the sympathetic nervous system and brown adipose tissue, ultimately increasing fat mass and reducing the use of lipids for generation of energy *(97–99)*. These actions are mediated by direct binding of ghrelin to receptors (GHS-R) expressed on arcuate AGRP/NPY neurons and its activation of AMPK *(100,101)*, through effects on endocannabinoids within the PVN (see below), and through effects on vagal afferents to the dorsal vagal complex in the brainstem *(102)*. Like leptin, ghrelin contributes to synaptic remodeling in the arcuate nucleus; but in contrast to leptin, ghrelin increases the number of excitatory inputs and decreases inhibitory inputs on AGRP/NPY neurons *(16)*.

Table 1
Gut Peptides Affecting Appetite and Satiety

Peptide	Origin	Action
Ghrelin	Gastric X/A-like cells	O
Amylin	Pancreatic β cells	A
CCK	Intestinal I cells	A
GLP-1	Intestinal L cells, DVC	A
Insulin	Pancreatic β cells	A
Nesfatin-1	Gastric X/A-like cells	A
Obestatin	Gastric X/A-like cells	A
Oxyntomodulin	Intestinal L cells	A
Pancreatic polypeptide	Pancreatic F cells	A
PYY_{3-36}	Intestinal L cells	A

A = anorexigenic, O = orexigenic.

Ghrelin also has effects on reward centers in the mesolimbic system, contributing to food intake through activation of dopaminergic neurons in the VTA or through effects on orexin-producing neurons in the lateral hypothalamus [103,104]. Conversely, when ghrelin receptor-null mice are fed a high-fat diet, they accumulate less body fat than controls and preferentially use fat as an energy substrate [105]. In addition, central administration of the ghrelin receptor antagonist BIM28163 attenuates the refeeding response following fasting [103].

In humans, ghrelin has a similar potent effect on appetite and increases just prior to meals, supporting its role in the initiation of feeding [106]. In addition, plasma ghrelin levels rise with caloric deprivation [107]. Thus energy deficit and weight loss are accompanied by a fall in plasma leptin and insulin and a rise in ghrelin, which in concert hinder or prevent further weight loss and promote weight regain.

ENDOCANNABINOID–BRAIN INTERACTIONS

The endocannabinoid system, a relatively recently discovered signaling system of the brain, has also been implicated in the regulation of energy homeostasis and may play a role in the desire to eat during fasting and caloric deprivation [108,109]. Of the two known cannabinoid receptors, type 1 (CB1) and type 2 (CB2), CB1 is the primary cannabinoid receptor in the central nervous system [110]. CB1 has a widespread distribution in most areas of the brain including the hypothalamus and limbic structures and localizes to presynaptic axons [111,112]. Endogenous ligands for CB1 include anandamide (AEA) and 2-arachidonoyl glycerol (2-AG) [108,110]. These arachidonic acid derivatives inhibit the synaptic release of transmitters in both excitatory and inhibitory terminals [111]. Since the endocannabinoids are synthesized by neurons postsynaptic to axon terminals containing CB1 receptors, the endocannabinoid system is actually a retrograde signaling system [111]. Neuronal release of endocannabinoids, therefore, regulates the activity of the cells' own CB1-containing innervation.

The importance of cannabinoids in the regulation of the energy homeostasis was well known even before the discovery of the endocannabinoid system. Low doses of exogenously administered Δ^9-tetrahidrocannabinol (Δ^9-THC) increase food intake and, if administered chronically, increase body weight [113]. Conversely, decreased CB1 receptor function reduces food intake and results in weight loss *(108)*. In humans, the CB1 antagonist, rimonabant (SR141716), causes clinically significant weight loss and reduces waist circumference *(114)*.

The main action of the central endocannabinoid system to control energy homeostasis is mediated through axons and neuronal groups in the hypothalamus and the reward circuitry of the mesolimbic system *(109)*. Feeding-related nuclei in the hypothalamus, like arcuate, ventromedial, and paraventricular nuclei, synthesize endocannabinoids and are innervated by CB1-containing axon terminals *(112,115,116)*. Indeed, injection of cannabinoid agonists directly into the ventromedial nucleus, lateral hypothalamus, or PVN results in increased food intake, indicating that endocannabinoids can exert orexigenic effects at multiple sites of the hypothalamus *(117–119)*. The activity of the hypothalamic endocannabinoid system correlates negatively with the status of peripheral energy stores such that fasting increases endocannabinoid levels in the hypothalamus, while refeeding decreases it *(108)*. These changes may be mediated by both leptin and ghrelin, as leptin decreases, while ghrelin increases, hypothalamic levels of endocannabinoids *(115)*. In addition, loss of CB1 in CB1 KO mice completely prevents orexigenic effects of ghrelin *(115)*, suggesting that the endocannabinoid system may play crucial role in mediating the action of peripheral hormones on energy homeostasis. Furthermore, in accord with the retrograde signaling nature of the endocannabinoid system, endocannabinoids block the inhibitory input to orexigenic MCH neurons in the lateral hypothalamus *(120)* and attenuate the excitatory input of the anorexigenic parvocellular neurons in the PVN *(115)*.

Endocannabinoids also activate the mesolimbic dopamine system: CB1 receptors are expressed in both the VTA and nucleus accumbens *(109)*, and rimonabant reduces intake of sweet food in non-food-deprived animals *(121)* and prevents novel palatable food-induced dopamine release in the accumbens shell *(122)*. Furthermore, microinjection of anandamide into the nucleus accumbens increases licking behavior induced by the intraoral administration of sucrose *(109)*. Thus, in addition to contributing to orexigenic drive through action on the hypothalamus during periods of caloric restriction, the endocannabinoid signaling system may also make it more difficult to lose weight by increasing the rewarding properties of food.

ROLE OF NUTRIENT SENSING DURING FASTING/CALORIC RESTRICTION

Nutrient sensing of glucose, fatty acids, and the amino acid, L-leucine, by the brain also contributes to the regulation of appetite and satiety. When injected into the cerebral ventricles, each of these substances induces anorexia *(123)*. Depending on the type of diet, therefore, reduction in delivery of one or more nutrients to the brain might be expected to trigger hypothalamic responses that favor weight maintenance.

Hypoglycemia or interference with glucose transport or phosphorylation in neurons increases feeding, presumably through brainstem neurons in the dorsal vagal complex that project to the hypothalamus (PVN and arcuate nucleus) to regulate NPY gene expression *(124)*. Since intracerebroventricular administration of glucose to fasting animals reduces NPY mRNA in arcuate nucleus neurons *(125)*, the fasting-associated decline in glucose is presumably a necessary step to permit proper signaling in NPY neurons by other mediators such as leptin and insulin. AMPK activation would appear to be the main mechanism by which hypoglycemia increases gene expression of AGRP/NPY in arcuate nucleus neurons *(126)*, since mice lacking the AMPK α2-subunit selectively in AGRP/NPY neurons lose normal electrophysiological responses to low glucose levels *(127)*. Increased AMPK may also reduce malonyl-CoA levels in the cytoplasm of neurons to affect lipid signaling (see below) and causes cell depolarization by inactivating plasma membrane ion channels *(128,129)*. Direct effects of hypoglycemia on hypothalamic AGRP/NPY- and orexin-producing neurons may also occur *(129,130)*.

Long chain fatty acids (LCFAs) also affect food intake by regulating AGRP and NPY in arcuate nucleus neurons *(131,132)*. As a result of AMPK-induced inhibition of acetyl-CoA carboxylase during fasting, malonyl-CoA is reduced in arcuate nucleus neurons. This prevents LCFAs from entering mitochondria for oxidation. Since lowering malonyl-CoA by overexpressing malonyl-CoA decarboxylase causes hyperphagia and weight gain *(133)*, the entry of LCFA into the mitochondria would appear to be an important step in the regulation of AGRP and NPY gene expression.

Following a mixed meal, L-leucine increases in the cerebrospinal fluid and hypothalamus *(134)* and reduces food intake without affecting energy expenditure *(135)*. The ability to block the anorexic effects of leucine by pretreatment with the MC4R antagonist, SHU9119 *(135)*, indicates an effect on POMC neurons, although leucine-induced activation of the mTOR pathway simultaneously reduces AGRP and NPY in arcuate nucleus neurons *(136)*. Presumably, therefore, a reduction in tissue levels of leucine in the brain may contribute to activation of AGRP/NPY neurons and may explain the observation that a diet reduced in protein increases daily cumulative food intake and increases both AGRP and NPY gene expression in the arcuate nucleus *(137,138)*.

INTEGRATION: THE NEUROENDOCRINE RESPONSE TO CALORIC DEPRIVATION AND WEIGHT LOSS

Attempts to lose weight by caloric restriction are met with a series of potent counter-regulatory responses mediated by humoral and neuronal signals that act in concert to prevent weight loss and promote weight regain. These are summarized in Fig. 1. While these systems are homeostatic and

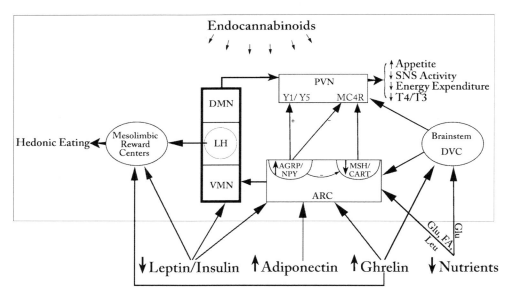

Fig. 1. Simplified schematic representation of some of the regulatory factors and pathways involved in neuroendocrine and metabolic adaptations to weight loss and their response to fasting or caloric restriction. Circulating factors derived from fat, pancreas, liver, and the gastrointestinal tract converge on the hypothalamus and/or brainstem to orchestrate a series of responses that promote increased appetite, decreased energy expenditure, activation of mesolimbic reward centers, and reduce circulating thyroid hormone levels. Note similarities of target regions in the brain by several regulatory factors, particularly for AGRP/NPY and α-MSH/CART neurons in the hypothalamic arcuate nucleus. The endocannabinoid system exerts regulatory effects on neurons in multiple regions of the brain. ARC = arcuate nucleus, DMN = dorsomedial nucleus, DVC = dorsal vagal complex, LH = lateral hypothalamus, PVN = paraventricular nucleus, SNS = sympathetic nervous system, VMN = ventromedial nucleus (Courtesy, Dr. Praful Singru).

beneficial for survival when food sources are scarce, they present a formidable problem for any individual who wishes to reduce his/her weight by dietary restriction alone. The counter-regulatory systems responding to weight loss are redundant; it is therefore not surprising that anti-obesity therapies using pharmacologic agents that target only one part of the regulatory system are largely unsuccessful in the long term.

Restoration of circulating levels of leptin or induction of leptin receptor signaling would seem an essential component of therapy, given the central role of the hormone in decreasing appetite, increasing energy expenditure, and reducing hedonic patterns of eating. Yet, obesity is associated with leptin resistance (139). Thus combination therapy using agents that potentiate leptin signaling, target receptors downstream of leptin signaling, and/or target other regulatory mechanisms may be required to completely override the compensatory responses of caloric restriction. One such approach using a long acting leptin preparation together with a GLP-1 agonist with known anorexigenic activity has already been shown effective in experimental models (140) and is currently entering clinical trials (141). Ghrelin receptor antagonists and drugs that prevent the acylation of ghrelin by inhibiting gastric O-acyl transferase (GOAT) are also under development, allowing targeting of a separate regulatory pathway. CB1 receptor antagonists would seem to be particularly attractive although its prototype, rimonabant, was removed from the commercial market in the USA due to behavioral side effects. It is anticipated that as a result of rapidly advancing knowledge about the mechanisms involved in the regulation of body weight, however, new, safe, and effective combination treatments that overcome compensatory responses will soon be forthcoming, allowing more promising approaches to weight control.

Editor's Question and Authors' Response

- **How do you think the contrasting peripheral and central actions of insulin are balanced to achieve weight homeostasis?**

- During fasting, plasma levels of insulin fall, allowing for the release of glucose from peripheral stores. This action is critical to assure that adequate amounts of glucose are available for the brain. Nevertheless, despite depletion of energy stores that contribute to weight loss, the simultaneous effect of low insulin levels on the brain increases appetite and reduces energy expenditure, diminishing the severity of weight loss during fasting or caloric restriction as part of an important survival mechanism. With continued fasting, however, the weight-sustaining central effects of low insulin levels will eventually be overcome. In contrast, obese patients have both peripheral and central insulin resistance, which in the fed state, may promote weight gain by activating similar pathways as observed during fasting.

- **Do you think that circulating endogenous ligands for cannabinoid receptors play a physiologic role in the brain?**

- Circulating levels of endocannabinoids in plasma are very low compared to concentrations in the brain. In addition, 2-AG and anandamide are rapidly cleared in the brain due to the widespread expression of cannabinoid metabolizing enzymes. Furthermore, peripheral administration of even large pharmacological doses of anandamide results in only a minimal increase in brain endocannabinoid levels. Accordingly, it is unlikely that plasma endocannabinoids exert much of an effect, if any, in the brain.

REFERENCES

1. Mark AL. Dietary therapy for obesity: an emperor with no clothes. Hypertension. Jun 2008;51(6):1426–34; discussion 34.
2. Wing RR, Phelan S. Long-term weight loss maintenance. Am J Clin Nutr. Jul 2005;82(1 Suppl):222S–5S.
3. Rosenbaum M, Goldsmith R, Bloomfield D, et al. Low-dose leptin reverses skeletal muscle, autonomic, and neuroendocrine adaptations to maintenance of reduced weight. J Clin Invest. 2005 Dec;115(12):3579–86.
4. Rosenbaum M, Sy M, Pavlovich K, Leibel RL, Hirsch J. Leptin reverses weight loss-induced changes in regional neural activity responses to visual food stimuli. J Clin Invest. 2008 Jul;118(7):2583–91.
5. Farooqi IS, O'Rahilly S. Leptin: a pivotal regulator of human energy homeostasis. Am J Clin Nutr. 2009 Mar;89(3):980S–4S.
6. Zhang Y, Proenca R, Maffei M, Barone M, Leopold L, Friedman JM. Positional cloning of the mouse obese gene and its human homologue. Nature. 1 Dec 1994;372(6505):425–32.
7. Myers MG Jr, Munzberg H, Leinninger GM, Leshan RL. The geometry of leptin action in the brain: more complicated than a simple ARC. Cell Metab. Feb 2009;9(2):117–23.
8. Ahima RS, Prabakaran D, Mantzoros C, et al. Role of leptin in the neuroendocrine response to fasting. Nature. 18 Jul 1996;382(6588):250–52.
9. Ahima RS, Saper CB, Flier JS, Elmquist JK. Leptin regulation of neuroendocrine systems. Front Neuroendocrinol. Jul 2000;21(3):263–307.
10. Xu AW, Ste-Marie L, Kaelin CB, Barsh GS. Inactivation of signal transducer and activator of transcription 3 in proopiomelanocortin (Pomc) neurons causes decreased pomc expression, mild obesity, and defects in compensatory refeeding. Endocrinology. Jan 2007;148(1):72–80.
11. Konner AC, Klockener T, Bruning JC. Control of energy homeostasis by insulin and leptin: targeting the arcuate nucleus and beyond. Physiol Behav. 14 Jul 2009;97(5):632–8.
12. Fukuda M, Jones JE, Olson D, et al. Monitoring FoxO1 localization in chemically identified neurons. J Neurosci. 10 Dec 2008;28(50):13640–8.
13. Kitamura T, Feng Y, Kitamura YI, et al. Forkhead protein FoxO1 mediates Agrp-dependent effects of leptin on food intake. Nat Med. May 2006;12(5):534–40.
14. Plum L, Belgardt BF, Bruning JC. Central insulin action in energy and glucose homeostasis. J Clin Invest. Jul 2006;116(7):1761–6.
15. Minokoshi Y, Shiuchi T, Lee S, Suzuki A, Okamoto S. Role of hypothalamic AMP-kinase in food intake regulation. Nutrition. Sept 2008;24(9):786–90.
16. Pinto S, Roseberry AG, Liu H, et al. Rapid rewiring of arcuate nucleus feeding circuits by leptin. Science. 2 Apr 2004;304(5667):110–5.
17. Morton GJ, Schwartz MW. The NPY/AgRP neuron and energy homeostasis. Int J Obes Relat Metab Disord. Dec 2001;25(Suppl 5):S56–62.
18. Egawa M, Yoshimatsu H, Bray GA. Effect of corticotropin releasing hormone and neuropeptide Y on electrophysiological activity of sympathetic nerves to interscapular brown adipose tissue. Neuroscience. 1990;34(3):771–5.
19. Vettor R, Zarjevski N, Cusin I, Rohner-Jeanrenaud F, Jeanrenaud B. Induction and reversibility of an obesity syndrome by intracerebroventricular neuropeptide Y administration to normal rats. Diabetologia. Dec 1994;37(12):1202–8.
20. Ong JM, Kirchgessner TG, Schotz MC, Kern PA. Insulin increases the synthetic rate and messenger RNA level of lipoprotein lipase in isolated rat adipocytes. J Biol Chem. 15 Sept 1988;263(26):12933–8.
21. Qian S, Chen H, Weingarth D, et al. Neither agouti-related protein nor neuropeptide Y is critically required for the regulation of energy homeostasis in mice. Mol Cell Biol. Jul 2002;22(14):5027–35.
22. Erickson JC, Clegg KE, Palmiter RD. Sensitivity to leptin and susceptibility to seizures of mice lacking neuropeptide Y. Nature. 30 May 1996;381(6581):415–21.
23. Huszar D, Lynch CA, Fairchild-Huntress V, et al. Targeted disruption of the melanocortin-4 receptor results in obesity in mice. Cell. 10 Jan 1997;88(1):131–41.
24. Krude H, Biebermann H, Luck W, Horn R, Brabant G, Gruters A. Severe early-onset obesity, adrenal insufficiency and red hair pigmentation caused by POMC mutations in humans. Nat Genet. Jun 1998;19(2):155–7.
25. Farooqi IS, Yeo GS, Keogh JM, et al. Dominant and recessive inheritance of morbid obesity associated with melanocortin 4 receptor deficiency. J Clin Invest. Jul 2000;106(2):271–9.
26. Xu AW, Kaelin CB, Morton GJ, et al. Effects of hypothalamic neurodegeneration on energy balance. PLoS Biol. Dec 2005;3(12):e415.
27. Tolle V, Low MJ. In vivo evidence for inverse agonism of Agouti-related peptide in the central nervous system of proopiomelanocortin-deficient mice. Diabetes. Jan 2008;57(1):86–94.
28. Cowley MA, Smart JL, Rubinstein M, et al. Leptin activates anorexigenic POMC neurons through a neural network in the arcuate nucleus. Nature. 24 May 2001;411(6836):480–4.

29. Swanson LW, Sawchenko PE. Paraventricular nucleus: a site for the integration of neuroendocrine and autonomic mechanisms. Neuroendocrinology. Dec 1980;31(6):410–7.

30. Kublaoui BM, Gemelli T, Tolson KP, Wang Y, Zinn AR. Oxytocin deficiency mediates hyperphagic obesity of Sim1 haploinsufficient mice. Mol Endocrinol. Jul 2008;22(7):1723–34.

31. Michaud JL, Boucher F, Melnyk A, et al. Sim1 haploinsufficiency causes hyperphagia, obesity and reduction of the paraventricular nucleus of the hypothalamus. Hum Mol Genet. 1 Jul 2001;10(14):1465–73.

32. Liu H, Kishi T, Roseberry AG, et al. Transgenic mice expressing green fluorescent protein under the control of the melanocortin-4 receptor promoter. J Neurosci. 6 Aug 2003;23(18):7143–54.

33. Wolak ML, DeJoseph MR, Cator AD, Mokashi AS, Brownfield MS, Urban JH. Comparative distribution of neuropeptide Y Y1 and Y5 receptors in the rat brain by using immunohistochemistry. J Comp Neurol. 22 Sept 2003;464(3):285–311.

34. Balthasar N, Dalgaard LT, Lee CE, et al. Divergence of melanocortin pathways in the control of food intake and energy expenditure. Cell. 4 Nov 2005;123(3):493–505.

35. Singru PS, Sanchez E, Fekete C, Lechan RM. Importance of melanocortin signaling in refeeding-induced neuronal activation and satiety. Endocrinology. Feb 2007;148(2):638–46.

36. Sawchenko PE, Swanson LW. Immunohistochemical identification of neurons in the paraventricular nucleus of the hypothalamus that project to the medulla or to the spinal cord in the rat. J Comp Neurol. 1 Mar 1982;205(3):260–72.

37. Haynes WG, Morgan DA, Djalali A, Sivitz WI, Mark AL. Interactions between the melanocortin system and leptin in control of sympathetic nerve traffic. Hypertension. Jan 1999;33(1 Pt 2):542–47.

38. Bamshad M, Aoki VT, Adkison MG, Warren WS, Bartness TJ. Central nervous system origins of the sympathetic nervous system outflow to white adipose tissue. Am J Physiol. Jul 1998;275(1 Pt 2):R291–9.

39. Elmquist JK. Hypothalamic pathways underlying the endocrine, autonomic, and behavioral effects of leptin. Int J Obes Relat Metab Disord. 2001 Dec;25(Suppl 5):S78–82.

40. Scott MM, Lachey JL, Sternson SM, et al. Leptin targets in the mouse brain. J Comp Neurol. 10 Jun 2009;514(5):518–32.

41. Bellinger LL, Bernardis LL. The dorsomedial hypothalamic nucleus and its role in ingestive behavior and body weight regulation: lessons learned from lesioning studies. Physiol Behav. Jul 2002;76(3):431–42.

42. Evans SA, Messina MM, Knight WD, Parsons AD, Overton JM. Long-Evans and Sprague-Dawley rats exhibit divergent responses to refeeding after caloric restriction. Am J Physiol Regul Integr Comp Physiol. Jun 2005;288(6):R1468–76.

43. Singru PS, Fekete C, Lechan RM. Neuroanatomical evidence for participation of the hypothalamic dorsomedial nucleus (DMN) in regulation of the hypothalamic paraventricular nucleus (PVN) by alpha-melanocyte stimulating hormone. Brain Res. 7 Dec 2005;1064(1–2):42–51.

44. Oldfield BJ, Giles ME, Watson A, Anderson C, Colvill LM, McKinley MJ. The neurochemical characterisation of hypothalamic pathways projecting polysynaptically to brown adipose tissue in the rat. Neuroscience. 2002;110(3):515–26.

45. Dimicco JA, Zaretsky DV. The dorsomedial hypothalamus: a new player in thermoregulation. Am J Physiol Regul Integr Comp Physiol. Jan 2007;292(1):R47–63.

46. Cypess AM, Lehman S, Williams G, et al. Identification and importance of brown adipose tissue in adult humans. N Engl J Med. 9 Apr 2009;360(15):1509–17.

47. van Marken Lichtenbelt WD, Vanhommerig JW, Smulders NM, et al. Cold-activated brown adipose tissue in healthy men. N Engl J Med. 9 Apr 2009;360(15):1500–8.

48. Jezek P. Possible physiological roles of mitochondrial uncoupling proteins–UCPn. Int J Biochem Cell Biol. Oct 2002;34(10):1190–206.

49. Sivitz WI, Fink BD, Donohoue PA. Fasting and leptin modulate adipose and muscle uncoupling protein: divergent effects between messenger ribonucleic acid and protein expression. Endocrinology. Apr 1999;140(4):1511–9.

50. Hetherington AW, Ranson SW. The relation of various hypothalamic lesions to adiposity in the rat. J Comp Neurol. 1942 1942;76:475–99.

51. Dhillon H, Zigman JM, Ye C, et al. Leptin directly activates SF1 neurons in the VMH, and this action by leptin is required for normal body-weight homeostasis. Neuron. 19 Jan 2006;49(2):191–203.

52. Bingham NC, Anderson KK, Reuter AL, Stallings NR, Parker KL. Selective loss of leptin receptors in the ventromedial hypothalamic nucleus results in increased adiposity and a metabolic syndrome. Endocrinology. May 2008;149(5):2138–48.

53. Komori T, Morikawa Y, Nanjo K, Senba E. Induction of brain-derived neurotrophic factor by leptin in the ventromedial hypothalamus. Neuroscience. 2006;139(3):1107–15.

54. Lebrun B, Bariohay B, Moyse E, Jean A. Brain-derived neurotrophic factor (BDNF) and food intake regulation: a minireview. Auton Neurosci. Jun 2006;30(126–127):30–38.

55. Yeo GS, Connie Hung CC, Rochford J, et al. A de novo mutation affecting human TrkB associated with severe obesity and developmental delay. Nat Neurosci. Nov 2004;7(11):1187–9.

56. Xu B, Goulding EH, Zang K, et al. Brain-derived neurotrophic factor regulates energy balance downstream of melanocortin-4 receptor. Nat Neurosci. Jul 2003;6(7):736–42.

57. Elias CF, Saper CB, Maratos-Flier E, et al. Chemically defined projections linking the mediobasal hypothalamus and the lateral hypothalamic area. J Comp Neurol. 28 Dec 1998;402(4):442–59.

58. Qu D, Ludwig DS, Gammeltoft S, et al. A role for melanin-concentrating hormone in the central regulation of feeding behaviour. Nature. 21 Mar 1996;380(6571):243–7.

59. Sakurai T. Roles of orexins in regulation of feeding and wakefulness. NeuroReport. 12 Jun 2002;13(8):987–95.

60. Georgescu D, Sears RM, Hommel JD, et al. The hypothalamic neuropeptide melanin-concentrating hormone acts in the nucleus accumbens to modulate feeding behavior and forced-swim performance. J Neurosci. 16 Mar 2005;25(11):2933–40.

61. Harris GC, Wimmer M, Aston-Jones G. A role for lateral hypothalamic orexin neurons in reward seeking. Nature. 22 Sept 2005;437(7058):556–9.

62. Krowicki ZK, Burmeister MA, Berthoud HR, Scullion RT, Fuchs K, Hornby PJ. Orexins in rat dorsal motor nucleus of the vagus potently stimulate gastric motor function. Am J Physiol Gastrointest Liver Physiol. Aug 2002;283(2): G465–72.

63. Fulton S, Pissios P, Manchon RP, et al. Leptin regulation of the mesoaccumbens dopamine pathway. Neuron. 21 Sept 2006;51(6):811–22.

64. Leininger GM, Jo YH, Leshan RL, et al. Leptin acts via leptin receptor-expressing lateral hypothalamic neurons to modulate the mesolimbic dopamine system and suppress feeding. Cell Metab. Aug 2009;10(2):89–98.

65. Kelley AE, Berridge KC. The neuroscience of natural rewards: relevance to addictive drugs. J Neurosci. 1 May 2002;22(9):3306–11.

66. Farooqi IS, Bullmore E, Keogh J, Gillard J, O'Rahilly S, Fletcher PC. Leptin regulates striatal regions and human eating behavior. Science. 7 Sept 2007;317(5843):1355.

67. Lechan RM. The dilemma of the nonthyroidal illness syndrome. Acta Biomed. Dec 2008;79(3):165–71.

68. Rosenbaum M, Murphy EM, Heymsfield SB, Matthews DE, Leibel RL. Low dose leptin administration reverses effects of sustained weight-reduction on energy expenditure and circulating concentrations of thyroid hormones. J Clin Endocrinol Metab. May 2002;87(5):2391–4.

69. Silva JE. The thermogenic effect of thyroid hormone and its clinical implications. Ann Intern Med. 5 Aug 2003;139(3):205–13.

70. Ribeiro MO, Carvalho SD, Schultz JJ, et al. Thyroid hormone–sympathetic interaction and adaptive thermogenesis are thyroid hormone receptor isoform–specific. J Clin Invest. Jul 2001;108(1):97–105.

71. Collin A, Cassy S, Buyse J, Decuypere E, Damon M. Potential involvement of mammalian and avian uncoupling proteins in the thermogenic effect of thyroid hormones. Domest Anim Endocrinol. Jul 2005;29(1):78–87.

72. Fekete C, Lechan RM. Negative feedback regulation of hypophysiotropic thyrotropin-releasing hormone (TRH) synthesizing neurons: role of neuronal afferents and type 2 deiodinase. Front Neuroendocrinol. Aug–Sept 2007;28 (2–3):97–114.

73. Lechan RM, Fekete C. Role of melanocortin signaling in the regulation of the hypothalamic-pituitary-thyroid (HPT) axis. Peptides. Feb 2006;27(2):310–25.

74. Sarkar S, Legradi G, Lechan RM. Intracerebroventricular administration of alpha-melanocyte stimulating hormone increases phosphorylation of CREB in TRH- and CRH-producing neurons of the hypothalamic paraventricular nucleus. Brain Res. 26 Jul 2002;945(1):50–59.

75. Harris M, Aschkenasi C, Elias CF, et al. Transcriptional regulation of the thyrotropin-releasing hormone gene by leptin and melanocortin signaling. J Clin Invest. Jan 2001;107(1):111–20.

76. Fekete C, Kelly J, Mihaly E, et al. Neuropeptide Y has a central inhibitory action on the hypothalamic-pituitary-thyroid axis. Endocrinology. Jun 2001;142(6):2606–13.

77. Fekete C, Marks DL, Sarkar S, et al. Effect of Agouti-related protein (Agrp) in regulation of the Hypothalamic-pituitary-thyroid (Hpt) axis in the Mc4-R Ko mouse. Endocrinology. 15 Jul 2004;145(11):4816–21.

78. Sarkar S, Lechan RM. Central administration of neuropeptide Y reduces alpha-melanocyte-stimulating hormone-induced cyclic adenosine 5′-monophosphate response element binding protein (CREB) phosphorylation in pro-thyrotropin-releasing hormone neurons and increases CREB phosphorylation in corticotropin-releasing hormone neurons in the hypothalamic paraventricular nucleus. Endocrinology. Jan 2003;144(1):281–91.

79. Lechan RM, Hollenberg A, Fekete C. Hypothalamic-pituitary-thyroid axis: organization, neural/endocrine control of TRH. In: Squire LR, editor. Encyclopedia of neuroscience. 3rd ed. Oxford: Academic Press; 2009. pp. 75–87.

80. Coppola A, Liu ZW, Andrews ZB, et al. A central thermogenic-like mechanism in feeding regulation: an interplay between arcuate nucleus T3 and UCP2. Cell Metab. Jan 2007;5(1):21–33.

81. Coppola A, Meli R, Diano S. Inverse shift in circulating corticosterone and leptin levels elevates hypothalamic deiodinase type 2 in fasted rats. Endocrinology. Jun 2005;146(6):2827–33.

82. Lechan RM, Fekete C. Infundibular tanycytes as modulators of neuroendocrine function: hypothetical role in the regulation of the thyroid and gonadal axis. Acta Biomed. 2007;78(Suppl 1):84–98.

83. Ishii S, Kamegai J, Tamura H, Shimizu T, Sugihara H, Oikawa S. Hypothalamic neuropeptide Y/Y1 receptor pathway activated by a reduction in circulating leptin, but not by an increase in circulating ghrelin, contributes to hyperphagia associated with triiodothyronine-induced thyrotoxicosis. Neuroendocrinology. Dec 2003;78(6):321–30.

84. Kong WM, Martin NM, Smith KL, et al. Triiodothyronine stimulates food intake via the hypothalamic ventromedial nucleus independent of changes in energy expenditure. Endocrinology. Nov 2004;145(11):5252–8.

85. Niswender KD, Baskin DG, Schwartz MW. Insulin and its evolving partnership with leptin in the hypothalamic control of energy homeostasis. Trends Endocrinol Metab. Oct 2004;15(8):362–9.

86. McGowan MK, Andrews KM, Grossman SP. Chronic intrahypothalamic infusions of insulin or insulin antibodies alter body weight and food intake in the rat. Physiol Behav. Apr 1992;51(4):753–66.

87. Obici S, Feng Z, Karkanias G, Baskin DG, Rossetti L. Decreasing hypothalamic insulin receptors causes hyperphagia and insulin resistance in rats. Nat Neurosci. Jun 2002;5(6):566–72.

88. Bruning JC, Gautam D, Burks DJ, et al. Role of brain insulin receptor in control of body weight and reproduction. Science. 22 Sept 2000;289(5487):2122–5.

89. de Luca C, Kowalski TJ, Zhang Y, et al. Complete rescue of obesity, diabetes, and infertility in db/db mice by neuron-specific LEPR-B transgenes. J Clin Invest. Dec 2005;115(12):3484–93.

90. Figlewicz DP, Benoit SC. Insulin, leptin, and food reward: update 2008. Am J Physiol Regul Integr Comp Physiol. Jan 2009;296(1):R9–19.

91. Figlewicz DP, Evans SB, Murphy J, Hoen M, Baskin DG. Expression of receptors for insulin and leptin in the ventral tegmental area/substantia nigra (VTA/SN) of the rat. Brain Res. 21 Feb 2003;964(1):107–15.

92. Kadowaki T, Yamauchi T, Kubota N. The physiological and pathophysiological role of adiponectin and adiponectin receptors in the peripheral tissues and CNS. FEBS Lett. 9 Jan 2008;582(1):74–80.

93. Kubota N, Yano W, Kubota T, et al. Adiponectin stimulates AMP-activated protein kinase in the hypothalamus and increases food intake. Cell Metab. Jul 2007;6(1):55–68.

94. Jayasena CN, Bloom SR. Role of gut hormones in obesity. Endocrinol Metab Clin North Am. Sept 2008;37(3):769–87.

95. Karra E, Batterham RL. The role of gut hormones in the regulation of body weight and energy homeostasis. Mol Cell Endocrinol. 27 Jun 2009;316(2):120–8.

96. Kojima M, Hosoda H, Date Y, Nakazato M, Matsuo H, Kangawa K. Ghrelin is a growth-hormone-releasing acylated peptide from stomach. Nature. 9 Dec 1999;402(6762):656–60.

97. Nakazato M, Murakami N, Date Y, et al. A role for ghrelin in the central regulation of feeding. Nature. 11 Jan 2001;409(6817):194–8.

98. Theander-Carrillo C, Wiedmer P, Cettour-Rose P, et al. Ghrelin action in the brain controls adipocyte metabolism. J Clin Invest. Jul 2006;116(7):1983–93.

99. Tschop M, Smiley DL, Heiman ML. Ghrelin induces adiposity in rodents. Nature. 19 Oct 2000;407(6806):908–13.

100. Willesen MG, Kristensen P, Romer J. Co-localization of growth hormone secretagogue receptor and NPY mRNA in the arcuate nucleus of the rat. Neuroendocrinology. Nov 1999;70(5):306–16.

101. Kola B, Hubina E, Tucci SA, et al. Cannabinoids and ghrelin have both central and peripheral metabolic and cardiac effects via AMP-activated protein kinase. J Biol Chem. 1 Jul 2005;280(26):25196–201.

102. Date Y, Shimbara T, Koda S, et al. Peripheral ghrelin transmits orexigenic signals through the noradrenergic pathway from the hindbrain to the hypothalamus. Cell Metab. Oct 2006;4(4):323–31.

103. Abizaid A, Liu ZW, Andrews ZB, et al. Ghrelin modulates the activity and synaptic input organization of midbrain dopamine neurons while promoting appetite. J Clin Invest. Dec 2006;116(12):3229–39.

104. Toshinai K, Date Y, Murakami N, et al. Ghrelin-induced food intake is mediated via the orexin pathway. Endocrinology. Apr 2003;144(4):1506–12.

105. Zigman JM, Nakano Y, Coppari R, et al. Mice lacking ghrelin receptors resist the development of diet-induced obesity. J Clin Invest. Dec 2005;115(12):3564–72.

106. Shiiya T, Nakazato M, Mizuta M, et al. Plasma ghrelin levels in lean and obese humans and the effect of glucose on ghrelin secretion. J Clin Endocrinol Metab. Jan 2002;87(1):240–4.

107. Cummings DE, Weigle DS, Frayo RS, et al. Plasma ghrelin levels after diet-induced weight loss or gastric bypass surgery. N Engl J Med. 23 May 2002;346(21):1623–30.

108. Pagotto U, Marsicano G, Cota D, Lutz B, Pasquali R. The emerging role of the endocannabinoid system in endocrine regulation and energy balance. Endocr Rev. Feb 2006;27(1):73–100.

109. Di Marzo V, Ligresti A, Cristino L. The endocannabinoid system as a link between homoeostatic and hedonic pathways involved in energy balance regulation. Int J Obes (Lond). Jun 2009;33(Suppl 2):S18–24.

110. Piomelli D. The molecular logic of endocannabinoid signalling. Nat Rev Neurosci. Nov 2003;4(11):873–84.

111. Freund TF, Katona I, Piomelli D. Role of endogenous cannabinoids in synaptic signaling. Physiol Rev. Jul 2003;83(3):1017–66.

112. Wittmann G, Deli L, Kallo I, et al. Distribution of type 1 cannabinoid receptor (CB1)-immunoreactive axons in the mouse hypothalamus. J Comp Neurol. 10 Jul 2007;503(2):270–9.

113. Greenberg I, Kuehnle J, Mendelson JH, Bernstein JG. Effects of marihuana use on body weight and caloric intake in humans. Psychopharmacology (Berl). 26 Aug 1976;49(1):79–84.

114. Despres JP, Golay A, Sjostrom L. Effects of rimonabant on metabolic risk factors in overweight patients with dyslipidemia. N Engl J Med. 17 Nov 2005;353(20):2121–34.

115. Kola B, Farkas I, Christ-Crain M, et al. The orexigenic effect of ghrelin is mediated through central activation of the endogenous cannabinoid system. PLoS One. 2008;3(3):e1797.

116. Hentges ST, Low MJ, Williams JT. Differential regulation of synaptic inputs by constitutively released endocannabinoids and exogenous cannabinoids. J Neurosci. 19 Oct 2005;25(42):9746–51.

117. Anderson-Baker WC, McLaughlin CL, Baile CA. Oral and hypothalamic injections of barbiturates, benzodiazepines and cannabinoids and food intake in rats. Pharmacol Biochem Behav. Nov 1979;11(5):487–91.

118. Jamshidi N, Taylor DA. Anandamide administration into the ventromedial hypothalamus stimulates appetite in rats. Br J Pharmacol. Nov 2001;134(6):1151–4.

119. Verty AN, McGregor IS, Mallet PE. Paraventricular hypothalamic CB(1) cannabinoid receptors are involved in the feeding stimulatory effects of Delta(9)-tetrahydrocannabinol. Neuropharmacology. Dec 2005;49(8):1101–9.

120. Jo YH, Chen YJ, Chua SC Jr., Talmage DA, Role LW. Integration of endocannabinoid and leptin signaling in an appetite-related neural circuit. Neuron. 22 Dec 2005;48(6):1055–66.

121. Simiand J, Keane M, Keane PE, Soubrie P. SR 141716, a CB1 cannabinoid receptor antagonist, selectively reduces sweet food intake in marmoset. Behav Pharmacol. Mar 1998;9(2):179–81.

122. Melis T, Succu S, Sanna F, Boi A, Argiolas A, Melis MR. The cannabinoid antagonist SR 141716A (Rimonabant) reduces the increase of extra-cellular dopamine release in the rat nucleus accumbens induced by a novel high palatable food. Neurosci Lett. 4 Jun 2007;419(3):231–5.

123. Obici S. Minireview: Molecular targets for obesity therapy in the brain. Endocrinology. Jun 2009;150(6):2512–7.

124. Ritter S, Dinh TT, Li AJ. Hindbrain catecholamine neurons control multiple glucoregulatory responses. Physiol Behav. 30 Nov 2006;89(4):490–500.

125. Fekete C, Singru PS, Sanchez E, et al. Differential effects of central leptin, insulin, or glucose administration during fasting on the hypothalamic-pituitary-thyroid axis and feeding-related neurons in the arcuate nucleus. Endocrinology. Jan 2006;147(1):520–9.

126. Xue B, Kahn BB. AMPK integrates nutrient and hormonal signals to regulate food intake and energy balance through effects in the hypothalamus and peripheral tissues. J Physiol. 1 Jul 2006;574(Pt 1):73–83.

127. Claret M, Smith MA, Batterham RL, et al. AMPK is essential for energy homeostasis regulation and glucose sensing by POMC and AgRP neurons. J Clin Invest. Aug 2007;117(8):2325–36.

128. Han SM, Namkoong C, Jang PG, et al. Hypothalamic AMP-activated protein kinase mediates counter-regulatory responses to hypoglycaemia in rats. Diabetologia. Oct 2005;48(10):2170–8.

129. Mountjoy PD, Rutter GA. Glucose sensing by hypothalamic neurons and pancreatic islet cells: AMPle evidence for common mechanisms? Exp Physiol. Mar 2007;92(2):311–9.

130. Marty N, Dallaporta M, Thorens B. Brain glucose sensing, counterregulation, and energy homeostasis. Physiology (Bethesda). Aug 2007;22:241–51.

131. Lane MD, Wolfgang M, Cha SH, Dai Y. Regulation of food intake and energy expenditure by hypothalamic malonyl-CoA. Int J Obes (Lond). Sept 2008;32(Suppl 4):S49–54.

132. Lopez M, Tovar S, Vazquez MJ, Nogueiras R, Senaris R, Dieguez C. Sensing the fat: fatty acid metabolism in the hypothalamus and the melanocortin system. Peptides. Oct 2005;26(10):1753–8.

133. Hu Z, Dai Y, Prentki M, Chohnan S, Lane MD. A role for hypothalamic malonyl-CoA in the control of food intake. J Biol Chem. 2 Dec 2005;280(48):39681–3.

134. Choi YH, Fletcher PJ, Anderson GH. Extracellular amino acid profiles in the paraventricular nucleus of the rat hypothalamus are influenced by diet composition. Brain Res. 23 Feb 2001;892(2):320–8.

135. Blouet C, Jo YH, Li X, Schwartz GJ. Mediobasal hypothalamic leucine sensing regulates food intake through activation of a hypothalamus-brainstem circuit. J Neurosci. 1 Jul 2009;29(26):8302–11.

136. Cota D, Proulx K, Smith KA, et al. Hypothalamic mTOR signaling regulates food intake. Science. 12 May 2006;312(5775):927–30.

137. White BD, He B, Dean RG, Martin RJ. Low protein diets increase neuropeptide Y gene expression in the basomedial hypothalamus of rats. J Nutr. Aug 1994;124(8):1152–60.

138. Morrison CD, Xi X, White CL, Ye J, Martin RJ. Amino acids inhibit Agrp gene expression via an mTOR-dependent mechanism. Am J Physiol Endocrinol Metab. Jul 2007;293(1):E165–71.
139. Howard JK, Flier JS. Attenuation of leptin and insulin signaling by SOCS proteins. Trends Endocrinol Metab. Nov 2006;17(9):365–71.
140. Roth JD, Roland BL, Cole RL, et al. Leptin responsiveness restored by amylin agonism in diet-induced obesity: evidence from nonclinical and clinical studies. Proc Natl Acad Sci USA. 20 May 2008;105(20):7257–62.
141. Ravussin E, Smith SR, Mitchell JA, et al. Enhanced weight loss with pramlintide/metreleptin: an integrated neurohormonal approach to obesity pharmacotherapy. Obesity (Silver Spring). 11 Jun 2009;17(9):1736–43.

29 The Socio-cultural Context for Obesity Prevention and Treatment in Children and Adolescents: Influences of Ethnicity and Gender

Shiriki Kumanyika, Joanna Holsten, and Elizabeth Prout Parks

CONTENTS

Key Words: Race, ethnicity, socioeconomic status, neighborhood, school, home, advertising, breast feeding, family, body image

INTRODUCTION

Obesity prevention and treatment programs in children and adolescents attempt to establish and reinforce eating and physical activity behaviors that foster healthy growth and development for both physical and mental health *(1,2)*. Long-term effectiveness requires that contextual influences on food and eating, and physical activity and sedentary behavior, in the child's immediate and surrounding environments be recognized and, where possible, accounted for in interventions. These influences include behaviors of family caregivers, school personnel, and day care providers. Particularly for younger children, these caregivers make decisions about what foods and physical activity options are available to children and which behaviors are encouraged, discouraged, allowed, modeled, or restricted. Eating and physical activity behaviors are strongly influenced by socio-cultural variables (i.e., norms, values, and beliefs) and social structural contexts (i.e., physical and economic characteristics, policies, and practices) in homes, neighborhoods, schools, and media environments. This chapter

From: *Contemporary Endocrinology: Pediatric Obesity: Etiology, Pathogenesis, and Treatment*
Edited by: M. Freemark, DOI 10.1007/978-1-60327-874-4_29,
© Springer Science+Business Media, LLC 2010

will consider the interactions of socio-cultural/environmental factors with race/ethnicity (referred to as "ethnicity") and gender and will discuss their impacts on obesity risk in children. The chapter concludes with a discussion of the need to account for socio-cultural and environmental variables in efforts to improve the effectiveness of interventions.

BACKGROUND

The context for pediatric obesity prevention and treatment has changed in recent decades due to major societal trends associated with increases in children's caloric consumption: increases in food and beverage portion sizes, total energy intake from foods obtained away-from-home, the intake of added sugars, and consumption of sweetened beverages *(1,3)*. These trends have emerged against a background of inadequate levels of physical activity, declines in the numbers of children enrolled in physical education classes and walking to school, and dramatic increases in the amount of time spent on sedentary entertainment *(1,4)*. This scenario, which has also occurred in other countries *(3,5,6)*, paints a challenging picture for achieving obesity prevention and treatment goals. Contexts for eating and physical activity are now overwhelmingly "obesogenic," meaning that the default choices, that is, what people do without thinking, and the most heavily promoted lifestyles are conducive to overeating and inactivity. These pervasive socio-cultural and environmental influences on obesity development are difficult to overcome even with deliberate actions by those so motivated *(6)*. Human regulatory systems for appetite control and the achievement of energy balance are simply no match for current environmental challenges to achieving energy balance. Thus, obesity prevention and treatment – which were never considered easy for either patient or provider – have become even more difficult. It is doubtful that long-term success in obesity treatment will be achieved without interventions that directly address this added difficulty *(1,7)*.

Addressing contextual issues that may complicate or limit the effectiveness of obesity prevention and treatment will be critical for eliminating ethnic disparities in obesity and related health risk factors and outcomes. Obesity levels are higher in black/African-American, Hispanic/Latino, American Indian, and Pacific Islander children and adolescents compared to white children and adolescents *(8–10)*. US National Health and Nutrition Examination Survey (NHANES) estimates of obesity prevalence rates for non-Hispanic white, non-Hispanic black, and Mexican American children are shown in Table 1 *(8)*. The effect of gender differs by ethnicity. Obesity prevalence is notably higher in non-Hispanic black girls than in non-Hispanic white girls and non-Hispanic black boys. By contrast, in Mexican Americans, obesity prevalence is notably higher in boys than in girls; and Mexican American boys have the highest obesity prevalence among all boys. More non-Hispanic black and Mexican American children are in families with incomes below the federal poverty level: 43 and 40%, respectively, compared with 16% of non-Hispanic white children *(11)*. The ethnic disparity (higher obesity levels in non-Hispanic black and Mexican American than in non-Hispanic white children) is evident at nearly all income levels (Table 2). However, in these data with ages and sexes combined, the inverse gradient in obesity prevalence among non-Hispanic white and to some extent in Mexican American children is not evident among non-Hispanic black children. In fact, obesity prevalence in non-Hispanic black children, particularly girls, is highest among children in families with incomes three to four times the poverty level. In data for 4-year-old children in the Early Childhood Longitudinal Study, 22.2 and 21.8% of Hispanic boys and girls, respectively, had body mass index (BMI) levels in the obese range, compared to 17.4 and 14.3% of non-Hispanic whites of the same sex *(10)*. Among American Indian/Alaska Native children, obesity prevalence was 37% for boys and 25.8% for girls. Asian American children had a lower percentage of obesity (15.8% in boys and 10.0% in girls) than the non-Hispanic white children. However, based on data for adults, BMI-related risks

Table 1
Obesity Prevalence Among US Children by Age, Ethnicity, and Gender, 2003–2006

Age group	Ethnic subgroup					
	Males			Females		
	Non-Hispanic white (%)	Non-Hispanic black (%)	Mexican American (%)	Non-Hispanic white (%)	Non-Hispanic black (%)	Mexican American (%)
Children aged 2–5 years	11.1	13.3	18.8	10.2	16.6	14.5
Children aged 6–11 years	15.5	18.6	27.5	14.4	24.0	19.7
Children aged 12–19 years	17.3	18.5	22.1	14.5	27.7	19.9

– Based on height and weight measurements of child respondents in the National Health and Nutrition Examination Survey.
– Obesity is defined as ≥95th percentiles of the sex- and age-specific BMI charts of the CDC Growth Charts.
Source: Ogden et al. *(8)*.

Table 2
Obesity Prevalence in Children Age 2–19 Years by Ethnicity and Income Level, 1999–2004

Poverty income ratio	Non-Hispanic white(%)	Non-Hispanic black(%)	Mexican American(%)
Less than 100%	17	18	22
100–199%	15	19	18
200–299%	15	17	21
300–399%	14	27	21
400% or more	11	21	12

The poverty income ratio expresses family income as a ratio of the federal poverty level for a family of that size.
Source: Freedman et al. *(11)*.

may be higher among people of Asian descent than would be expected based on data for European descent populations, for example *(12)*.

While there are clear differences in individuals' biological predispositions to obesity, ethnic disparities and to some extent gender differences reflect differences in the socio-cultural, environmental, and behavioral rather than genetic determinants of weight gain and obesity *(6)*. This is reflected in relatively steep trends of increasing obesity within the same ethnic group, for example, in African-American girls *(13)*. Although high levels of obesity have been observed in black women for several decades *(14)*, higher than average levels of obesity in African-American girls are a relatively recent phenomenon. Also suggesting environmental influences, obesity prevalence in people of the same ethnic group is higher in environments where the average overall level of obesity is higher. For example, data for people of African descent indicate that obesity prevalence is progressively higher, when comparing those living in West Africa, the Caribbean, the United Kingdom, and the United States *(15)*. Obesity levels of immigrants of diverse backgrounds increase with increasing duration of US residence

(16). The opposite directions of the gender difference in black compared to Mexican American children and the relatively small gender differences in obesity among white children suggest that gender differences, when observed, are environmentally or culturally mediated.

PHYSICAL ENVIRONMENTS

The environmental exposures in the neighborhood, school, home, and media environments may contribute to the ethnic disparities or gender differences in obesity risk or prevention and treatment contexts. In addition, male and female children may generally experience the same environments differently with respect to physical, social, or cultural influences on eating and physical activity behaviors. Some examples of these differences follow. Also, even where obesity prevalence is similar by ethnicity and gender, different approaches may be needed for successful prevention or treatment because of the different environments or responses of children in different ethnic, gender, and socioeconomic status (SES) groups.

Neighborhood and Community Environments

Neighborhood food and fitness resources vary greatly in communities of different ethnic and socioeconomic composition; these may foster disparities in obesity *(17)*. With respect to food availability and access, studies have demonstrated that ethnic minority neighborhoods had more than double the number of grocery stores, half the number of supermarkets *(18)*, and almost two-thirds more fast-food restaurants per square mile *(19)* compared to predominantly white neighborhoods. Studies have shown a significant inverse association between supermarket availability and BMI in adolescents, especially for African-Americans *(20)*, and of the number of residents per fast-food restaurant with obesity prevalence *(21)*. In addition, a systematic review *(22)* concluded that availability of food stores, products within stores, and food promotions within stores in communities with high proportions of African-American residents were consistently less conducive to healthful eating compared to those in predominantly white neighborhoods.

Both gender and ethnic differences have been reported regarding aspects of or responses to the neighborhood environment in relation to outdoor physical activity, including walkability, recreational facilities, and crime. Studies have found sex-specific effects for neighborhood design, with preschool girls less likely to be overweight or obese in "walkable" neighborhoods with a greater number of intersections *(23)*. In a different study, adolescent girls made more active trips per week in communities with more traffic lights; boys were more active if living on a cul-de-sac rather than off a main road and in neighborhoods with more speed bumps *(24)*. With respect to the availability of recreational facilities, data from the National Longitudinal Study of Adolescent Health reveal less access in neighborhood block groups with high proportions of minority or low SES residents *(25)*. Crime is another key factor in neighborhood environments; youth in high crime areas may be less likely to walk to the store or play outside. Areas around schools with greater poverty and Hispanic student populations have been shown to have higher crime rates *(26)*. A meta-analysis of environmental factors that affect obesity found that crime was inversely associated with adolescent physical activity in two out of three studies *(27)*.

School Environments

Food and activity options available in schools impact the weight status of children and adolescents. In the large, nationally representative Monitoring the Future annual survey of 8th, 10th, and 12th grade students, African-American students were found to have less availability of healthier sweet and savory snacks, and Hispanic students had greater availability of ice cream, fruit, and vegetables *(28)*. While almost all students had access to soft drinks in schools, Hispanic youth were most likely to have access to them at school during the entire school day *(29)*. Competitive foods and drinks sold outside of meals were most often high-calorie and low-nutrient density *(30)* and are relatively more available in low SES schools *(28)*. With respect to school physical activity, physical education requirements and participation decrease from middle to high school, and only a small sub-sample of students participate in sports, with lower participation among African-American and Hispanic students compared to white students *(31)*.

Home Environments

The home is a critical environment for children, since the food and activity options in the home not only affect behaviors in the setting but also serve as the context for learning behaviors from a young age *(32)*. Fruit and vegetable intake, considered to be obesity protective, serves as a prime example of socio-cultural variation in the interface between dietary behaviors and the home environment. The Project EAT data demonstrated that household availability was positively associated with fruit and vegetable intake for girls, but not boys, suggesting a gender difference in the way children relate to the food environment *(33)*. In the High 5 Intervention to increase fruit and vegetable intake, girls were more likely than boys to have fruits and vegetables at home *(34)*. African-American children not only had *increased* odds of having several fruits and vegetables in the home compared to white children but also had a higher prevalence of obesity, which is contrary to expectation. This suggests a need to investigate variables such as food preparation styles and other potential covariates of BMI within the relevant socio-cultural context *(34)*.

Resources and cues for physical activity or inactivity at home, such as television and computer screens, play equipment, and outdoor space, are also important environmental considerations related to child obesity, but influences may differ by gender. For example, a longitudinal study of 10 to 12-year-olds found that access to video games and television was associated with subsequent higher BMI for boys; greater access to physical activity equipment was associated with decreased BMI in girls *(35)*. In a study of preschool children, outdoor play equipment and back yard size were positively associated with outdoor playtime with no gender difference *(36)*. Ethnic differences in television availability and use are frequently reported, in a direction less favorable for African-American and Hispanic children, as discussed below.

Technology, Media, and Advertising Environments

The effects of technology and information are pervasive in all of the settings reviewed above. Marketing of products that encourage unhealthy eating and activity behaviors persists in neighborhoods, schools, and homes. The Institute of Medicine confirmed the effects of food advertising on children's food preferences and food intake *(37)*. Children of different socio-cultural backgrounds have different exposures to advertising and experience different effects based on those exposures *(38)*. A Kaiser Family Foundation survey found that among children and adolescents age 8 to 18, African-Americans, Latinos, and children with lower family incomes or lower parental education were more likely to have one or more of the following: television constantly on; television in their bedroom; or meals in front of the television *(4)*. Taveras et al. reported that African-American and Hispanic children between 2 and 13 years were over three times more likely (70%/74% vs. 22%) to have a television in their bedroom compared to white children. Reviews by Grier and Kumanyika *(22)* and Grier *(39)* found consistent evidence of greater than average frequency and intensity of advertisements for less healthful foods and beverages in television and digital media markets that reach African-Americans. Television advertising exposures of Latino children appear to be similarly adverse *(40,41)*.

Outdoor and in-school advertising reflect additional exposures that may contribute to disparities. Yancey and colleagues *(42)* reported that African-American neighborhoods had the highest densities of obesity-promoting outdoor advertisements (i.e., fast food and sedentary entertainment), closely followed by Latino neighborhoods. Hillier et al. (43) found disproportionate clustering of outdoor advertisements for less healthful products around schools in black neighborhoods in Philadelphia. The Monitoring the Future survey reported an inverse relationship between the SES of the school and the amount of advertising and promotion of soft drinks (29).

SOCIO-CULTURAL VARIATION

US ethnic minority populations have different socio-political and ethnocultural histories and influences, related to factors such as region or neighborhood of residence, food culture, family and intergenerational relationships, social institutions, language, and media exposures, with varying gender dimensions. Some potentially important influences on excessive weight gain and obesity are highlighted below.

Infant Feeding

Obesity development may be influenced by breastfeeding and by the timing of formula feeding and introduction of other foods. Exclusive breastfeeding for 6 months is recommended by the American Academy of Pediatrics (44), There is consistent evidence of ethnic differences in prevalence and duration of breastfeeding. African-American mothers are less likely to initiate and continue breastfeeding compared with white mothers (45). By contrast, Mexican American mothers are more likely than non-Hispanic white mothers to initiate breastfeeding and continue for longer periods of time (46). Teen mothers, i.e., women who are under age 20 years at the time of the baby's birth, are the least likely to breastfeed for 3 months or more. About twice as many African-American and Latino mothers give birth before age 20 years compared with white or Asian American mothers (47).

Supplementing breastfeeding with formula early on has been linked to less successful breastfeeding and early discontinuation of breastfeeding (48). Among low-income women who participate in the Supplemental Nutrition program for Women, Infants, and Children (WIC), the African-American and Hispanic participants who breastfeed are more likely to take the supplemental formula package than the supplemental food package (48). Employment considerations, e.g., the need to return to work and a lack of breastfeeding support in the workplace, may also discourage low-income mothers from breastfeeding. Full-time employment and earlier return to work have also been noted as a factor associated with shorter breastfeeding duration in African-American women (49).

Caregiver, Family, and Peer Influences

The behavior of caregivers influences children's food intake and food habit development during infancy, throughout the preschool and school age years and even in adolescence. In addition to breastfeeding, behaviors of interest for child weight status may include those that encourage receptivity to and consumption of healthful foods and discourage frequent consumption of energy-dense foods and sweetened beverages. "Non-responsive parenting" has been associated with indulgent feeding and overfeeding as well as excessive restriction and with child overweight (32,50). This type of parenting is controlling, insensitive to the child's behavioral cues, and/or developmentally inappropriate. Available studies do not clearly identify parenting styles that may be associated with child obesity development in African-American and Latino families (51). Based on studies in WIC participants, low-income mothers may be more concerned about hunger and underweight than about childhood overweight, leading to the types of feeding practices that are associated with child overweight (52).

Early involvement of caregivers other than parents is associated with a lesser tendency to initiate and continue breastfeeding (53). Involvement of non-parental or multiple caregivers may be associated with single parenthood and sole wage earner status, which is more common among African-American mothers (53). Intergenerational caregiving may result in a clash of cultural norms or inconsistencies in infant and child feeding practices; for example, grandparents or older relatives may have beliefs about infant feeding that differ from those of parents and from recommendations made by health-care providers. Bentley *(54)* reported that in a sample of teen mothers, the infant's grandmother often controlled decisions about infant feeding; this may perpetuate cultural norms such as the addition of cereal in the infant's bottle as early as 1–2 weeks of age and the introduction of semisolid foods within the first month of life.

As youth move into and through the stage of adolescence their interactions with both family and friends evolve, creating dynamics that affect weight status. Although the role of peers in their lives increases, research has demonstrated that interactions with family members, particularly parents, remain paramount. Parents serve as gatekeepers, role models, and sources of social support. In many qualitative studies, youth identify mothers as gatekeepers of food in the home. Focus groups with low-income, African-American youth revealed that children identified an "external locus of control at home" in food choices at home, with a mother or grandmother mentioned most often as decision makers *(55, p. 249)*. Social support and healthy role modeling from family members have been found to correlate positively with healthful food choices *(56)* and activity *(35)*. However, interviews with low-income parents revealed a stressful work–family balance that constrained healthy family food choices *(57)*, highlighting an important socio-cultural consideration. In contrast to the supportive role of parents, peers may contribute negative support for making healthy food choices *(55)*. While weight-related teasing from both family and peers is a problem for youth of all ethnicities and genders, girls are socially marginalized and teased more often than boys regarding weight issues *(58)*.

Gender differences also emerge as adolescent girls play a greater role in shopping and food preparation, which in turn affects their food choices and weight status. Cross-sectional data from 4,764 adolescents demonstrate that female adolescents helped with both food shopping and preparation more than males; preparation was associated with more healthful food choices, whereas food shopping was associated with some less healthful food choices *(59)*.

A socio-cultural influence on obesity that may be shared by children in several ethnic groups is maternal or female caregiver obesity. Although levels of obesity are high among adults in the US population as a whole, obesity prevalence among women in non-Hispanic black, Mexican American, and American Indian and Pacific populations is substantially above that in non-Hispanic white populations *(9)*. Prevalent maternal obesity indicates that many children will have been exposed to obesogenic environments during gestation *(60)*. It also means that excess weight gain and obesity are normative among children's female caregivers and role models. Effective obesity prevention and treatment interventions for children may, therefore, require that we address the problem of adult (particularly maternal) obesity.

Food Intake and Physical Activity

Key dietary behaviors as youth age include breakfast consumption, fast food intake, and sugar-sweetened beverage intake. Many studies show that skipping breakfast increases as children age and correlates with obesity in females and males *(61,62)*. Breakfast skipping may differ by ethnicity and SES. A longitudinal study following 2,216 adolescents over a 5-year period found that breakfast consumption was more common among white and higher SES youth *(63)*. Intake of fast foods and sugar-sweetened beverages rises during late childhood and puberty, with relatively greater increases in ethnic minority youth *(64,65)*.

Activity levels of children are lower than recommended in all ethnic and gender groups and environmental influences supportive of physical activity are less common, on average, in ethnic minority and low-income communities *(1,17)*. Gender and ethnic differences in patterns of physical activity in children and adolescents become prominent during the transition into adolescence. Decreases in physical activity have been linked with increases in BMI, especially for girls *(66)*, and more so for

African-American than white girls. Following a cohort of girls over 10 years, the National Heart, Lung, and Blood Institute Growth and Health study revealed that activity decreased over time for all girls; nevertheless, white girls were more active at the beginning and throughout the 10-year study compared to African-American girls (67). In addition to activity, decreases in sedentary behaviors such as screen time correlated with lower prevalence of obesity (68) only for girls – suggesting a possibly important focal point for gender-specific intervention.

Body Image and Weight Concern

Weight concerns may emerge very early in childhood (69) and become particularly important during the pubertal transition. Both gender and ethnic differences in body image have received significant attention in the obesity literature. For example, among adolescents in Project EAT (58), body satisfaction was highest among African-American girls and boys and lowest among Hispanic girls and Asian American boys. African-American girls and boys had the highest prevalence of desire to *gain* weight, while current attempts at weight loss were most prevalent in Hispanic girls and boys. Unhealthy weight control behaviors (i.e., fasting, skipping meals, smoking cigarettes) were most common in Native American girls and Asian American boys. Overall for weight-related concerns and behaviors, African-American girls had fewer and girls of all other ethnicities had greater concerns compared to white girls, while boys from all other ethnicities had equal or greater concerns compared to white boys. These differences between girls and boys of different socio-cultural backgrounds illustrate the need for an understanding of the complex, multi-ethnic picture of social norms regarding weight and body size. This will permit development of acceptable measures to address weight issues. Since social constructs of body size are associated with overweight status and mental health in adolescence, they are crucial in designing appropriate interventions. Potential aggravation of inappropriate weight concern or dieting behaviors is a key reason that obesity interventions for children and adolescents tend to focus on developing positive eating and physical activity behaviors rather than on weight per se.

ADDRESSING SOCIO-CULTURAL AND CONTEXTUAL INFLUENCES IN INTERVENTIONS

Obesity prevention and treatment programs may focus on high-risk children for individually oriented or group counseling programs or may attempt to reach all children in the community by changing the aforementioned environmental determinants of excessive weight gain. Elements of behavioral change theories that are commonly used to inform the development of interventions make explicit reference to the reciprocity of individual behaviors and environmental influences and the need to consider multilevel influences and the interactions across levels (70,71). The socio-ecological model conceptualizes five levels of influence: *intrapersonal* level (taste preferences, habits, and nutritional knowledge and skills); *interpersonal level/social environment* (processes whereby culture, social traditions, and role expectations impact eating practices and patterns within peer groups, friends, and family); and *organizational, community, and public policy levels/physical environment* (environmental factors that affect food access and availability) (72). Interventions that address multiple levels of intervention and person–environment interactions are particularly important for effective intervention with ethnic minority and low SES populations, because – as described above – these populations are more likely to confront environmental challenges, e.g., targeted marketing of unhealthful foods and limited options for safe outdoor activity (7,17,25). Addressing behavior at the individual or family level alone may be inadequate and even unethical if the environmental supports for the desired behaviors are not improved.

Both prevention and treatment programs for children and adolescents are more likely than those in adults to include family members; in some cases programs may work directly with family caregivers and only indirectly with the children themselves *(73)*. This potentially provides opportunities to address family context variables that are particularly salient in ethnic or socioeconomic status groups, including gender-related influences. As already noted, a high proportion of caregivers and role models of children in ethnic minority populations may be obese, and their concerns about child overweight may be relatively low *(69)*. On the other hand, it may be possible to leverage the strong familial orientation in some ethnic groups to improve intervention effectiveness. For example, although a prior study in whites indicated that treating obese adolescent girls and their mothers together in group sessions was less effective than treating them in separate groups *(74)*, treating girls and mothers together was *more* effective when a similar study was conducted with African-Americans *(75)*.

The concepts of cultural targeting and cultural tailoring refer to deliberate attempts to account for ethnocultural variables in program design and implementation. The distinction made by Kreuter *(76)* of *targeting* as addressing cultural variables at the group level and *tailoring* as addressing cultural variables at the individual level is a useful one. Targeting recognizes the commonalities of ethnocultural groups and the possible advantages of culture-specific programming and intra-group support. Tailoring recognizes the individual heterogeneity within groups, including individual differences in the ways that socio-cultural contextual variables affect attitudes and behaviors. Also implicit in tailoring is the reality that individuals function simultaneously in several cultures defined, for example, by age or developmental stage as well as gender and ethnicity. Both targeting and tailoring may be useful for maximizing and sustaining intervention effects.

What constitutes cultural targeting and tailoring has been described by Resnicow *(77)* and Kreuter *(76)*. Distinctions are made between accounting for surface or peripheral influences to increase familiarity, salience, or accessibility of an intervention and accounting for deeper cultural constructs in ways that may invoke different paradigms. That is, interventions that attempt to work with cultural "deep structure," to use Resnicow's terminology, frame or re-frame intervention concepts, processes, and desired outcomes to align with the ethos of the group in question and attempt to leverage cultural assets and strengths to facilitate positive outcomes. However, these approaches may be underspecified if culture is defined too narrowly to refer only to attitudes, beliefs, and values without acknowledging the extent to which culture interacts with the relevant social and environmental contexts.

It is necessary to identify nutritional, physical activity, and other obesity interventions that are effective with children and adolescents (as well as adults) in ethnic minority and low-income populations; this effort must determine how cultural adaptations add value to theoretically sound intervention approaches *(78–80)*. Some evidence suggests that trade-offs made in attempts to culturally adapt programs may inadvertently have an unfavorable effect on the strength of intervention in other respects. Promising models for interventions targeted or tailored for ethnic minority populations in afterschool, preschool, or school settings include Dance for Health in 8-to-10-year-old African-American and Latino children *(81)*; the Girls Health Enrichment Multi-site Studies (GEMS) pilot studies for obesity prevention in pre-adolescent girls *(82–85)*; the Hip Hop to Health program with African-American and Latino children in Head Start *(86)*; Planet Health, a school-based study in 11-to-13-year-old predominantly African-American boys and girls *(87)*; Eat Well and Keep Moving in 4th and 5th grade African-American students *(88)*; Pathways – an obesity prevention program in 8-to-11-year-old American Indians *(89)*; and the El Paso Child and Adolescent Trial for Cardiovascular Health in 3rd grade, low-income Latinos *(90)*. Two examples of models for working with parents of infants or toddlers at home may also be of interest: a mother–child intervention for reducing obesity prevalence in toddlers in a Native American community *(91)* and a model that incorporates nutrition education into the Parents as Teachers program, a general parent education program offered free to parents of children between birth and age 3 *(92)*.

With respect to gender, group level interventions that reach both sexes may have differential effectiveness with girls and boys. For example, in the Planet Health study with 6th and 7th grade students *(87)*, reductions in obesity and improvements in fruit and vegetable consumption were observed in girls but not in boys; reductions in hours of TV viewing were observed in both sexes. Whether gender-specific interventions are feasible and superior to gender-nonspecific approaches depends on the setting and other factors. What specific approaches work better in boys vs. girls is uncertain and should be considered by developmental stage. The GEMS studies cited above were all specific to African-American girls. The Trial of Adolescent Activity in Girls study (TAAG) was also gender specific, motivated by the lower levels of physical activity in girls *(93)*. Modest improvements in physical activity were observed, but were somewhat less notable in the African-American and Hispanic girls.

CONCLUSION

This chapter has highlighted ethnic, gender, and SES differences in obesity prevalence. These differences reflect variation in environmental contexts and socio-cultural aspects of eating, physical activity, and weight gain that have important influences on the design and outcomes of obesity prevention and treatment programs. Recognizing the greater challenges posed by the physical contexts of children in ethnic minority populations and for children and families in low SES groups is important for setting realistic expectations of what can be accomplished by counseling individual children or family members and for identifying needs and opportunities for intervention at the community level. Group-targeted programs, particularly those that are community based and community partnered, offer opportunities to influence environmental context variables, e.g., to change food availability or physical activity options and to shift social norms away from those that promote overeating and inactivity. Gender variation within and across ethnic groups argues for paying close attention to differences in responses to physical environments. In addition, differences in socio-cultural expectations, roles, and concerns for male and female children and adolescents appear to have important implications for weight status, particularly during the pubertal transition and in adolescence. Examples of intervention approaches relevant for addressing these variables have been cited, although research related to how best to use knowledge of environmental and socio-cultural variations in obesity influences is very limited. Greater emphasis in this area of clinical and public health practice and research will improve the long-term effectiveness of obesity prevention and treatment programs during childhood and adolescence and will have the potential to reduce the numbers of children who become or remain obese during adulthood.

REFERENCES

1. Koplan JP, Liverman CT, Kraak VI, editors. Preventing childhood obesity: health in the balance. Washington, DC: National Academies Press; 2005.
2. Daniels SR, Arnett DK, Eckel RH, et al. Overweight in children and adolescents: pathophysiology, consequences, prevention, and treatment. Circulation. 19 Apr 2005;111 15:1999–2012.
3. Ebbeling CB, Pawlak DB, Ludwig DS. Childhood obesity: public-health crisis, common sense cure. Lancet. 10 Aug 2002;360(9331):473–82.
4. Rideout V, Roberts DF, Foehr UG, Generation M. Media in the lives of 8–18 year olds. Washington, DC: Kaiser Family Foundation; 2005.
5. Lobstein T, Baur L, Uauy R, TaskForce IIO. Obesity in children and young people: a crisis in public health. Obes Rev. May 2004;5(Suppl 1):4–104.
6. Obesity: Preventing and Managing the Global Epidemic. Report of a WHO consultation. World Health Organ Tech Rep Ser. 2000;894:i–xii, 1–253.
7. Kumanyika SK. Environmental influences on childhood obesity: ethnic and cultural influences in context. Physiol Behav. 2008;94(1):61–70.

8. Ogden CL, Carroll MD, Flegal KM. High body mass index for age among US children and adolescents, 2003–2006. J Am Med Assoc. 28 May 2008;299(20):2401–5.

9. Wang Y, Beydoun MA. The obesity epidemic in the United States – gender, age, socioeconomic, racial/ethnic, and geographic characteristics: a systematic review and meta-regression analysis. Epidemiol Rev. 2007;29:6–28.

10. Anderson SE, Whitaker RC. Prevalence of obesity among US preschool children in different racial and ethnic groups. Arch Pediatr Adolesc Med. Apr 2009;163(4):344–8.

11. Freedman DS, Ogden CL, Flegal KM, Khan LK, Serdula MK, Dietz WH. Childhood overweight and family income. MedGenMed. 2007;9(2):26.

12. WHO Expert Consultation. Appropriate body-mass index for Asian populations and its implications for policy and intervention strategies. Lancet. 10 Jan 2004;363(9403):157–63.

13. Freedman DS, Khan LK, Serdula MK, Ogden CL, Dietz WH. Racial and ethnic differences in secular trends for childhood BMI, weight, and height. Obesity (Silver Spring). Feb 2006;14 2:301–8.

14. Kumanyika S. Obesity in black women. Epidemiol Rev. 1987;9:31–50.

15. Luke A, Cooper RS, Prewitt TE, Adeyemo AA, Forrester TE. Nutritional consequences of the African diaspora. Annu Rev Nutr. 2001;21:47–71.

16. Oza-Frank R, Cunningham SA. The weight of US residence among immigrants: a systematic review. Obes Rev. 15 Jun 2009.

17. Taylor WC, Poston WSC, Jones L, Kraft MK. Environmental justice: obesity, physical activity, and healthy eating. J Phys Activity Health. Feb 2006;3(Suppl 1):30–54.

18. Moore LV, Diez Roux AV. Associations of neighborhood characteristics with the location and type of food stores. Am J Publ Health. Feb 2006;96(2):325–31.

19. Block JP, Scribner RA, DeSalvo KB. Fast food, race/ethnicity, and income: a geographic analysis. Am J Prev Med. Oct 2004;27 3:211–7.

20. Powell LM, Auld MC, Chaloupka FJ, O'Malley PM, Johnston LD. Associations between access to food stores and adolescent body mass index. Am J Prev Med. 2007;33(4 Suppl):S301–7.

21. Maddock J. The relationship between obesity and the prevalence of fast food restaurants: state-level analysis. Am J Health Promot. Nov–Dec 2004;19(2):137–43.

22. Grier SA, Kumanyika SK. The context for choice: health implications of targeted food and beverage marketing to African Americans. Am J Publ Health. 2008;98(9):1616–29.

23. Spence JC, Cutumisu N, Edwards J, Evans J. Influence of neighbourhood design and access to facilities on overweight among preschool children. Int J Pediatr Obes (An Official Journal of the International Association for the Study of Obesity). 2008;3(2):109–16.

24. Carver A, Timperio AF, Crawford DA. Neighborhood road environments and physical activity among youth: the CLAN study. J Urban Health Bull NY Acad Med. 2008;85(4):532–44.

25. Gordon-Larsen P, Nelson MC, Page P, Popkin BM. Inequality in the built environment underlies key health disparities in physical activity and obesity. Pediatrics. Feb 2006;117(2):417–24.

26. Zhu X, Lee C. Walkability and safety around elementary schools economic and ethnic disparities. Am J Prev Med. Apr 2008;34(4):282–90.

27. Ferreira I, van der Horst K, Wendel-Vos W, Kremers S, van Lenthe FJ, Brug J. Environmental correlates of physical activity in youth – a review and update. Obes Rev. 2007;8(2):129–54.

28. Delva J, O'Malley PM, Johnston LD. Availability of more-healthy and less-healthy food choices in American schools – a national study of grade, racial/ethnic, and socioeconomic differences. Am J Prev Med. 2007;33:S226–39.

29. Johnston LD, Delva J, O'Malley PM. Soft drink availability, contracts, and revenues in American secondary schools. Bridging the Gap – Research Informing Practice and Policy for Healthy Youth Behavior. Am J Prev Med 2007;33(4 Suppl 1):S209–25.

30. Fox MK, Gordon A, Nogales Re, Wilson A. Availability and consumption of competitive foods in US public schools. The School Food Environment, Children's Diets, and Obesity – Findings from the Third School Nutrition Dietary Assessment Study. J Am Diet Assoc 2009;109(2 Suppl 1):S57–66.

31. Johnston LD, Delva J, Malley PM. Sports participation and physical education in American secondary schools: current levels and racial/ethnic and socioeconomic disparities. Bridging the Gap – Research Informing Practice and Policy for Healthy Youth Behavior. Am J Prev Med 2007;33(4 Suppl 1):S195–208.

32. Birch LL, Davison KK. Family environmental factors influencing the developing behavioral controls of food intake and childhood overweight. Pediatr Clin N Am. Aug 2001;48(4):893–907.

33. Hanson NI, NeumarkSztainer D, Eisenberg ME, Story M, Wall M. Associations between parental report of the home food environment and adolescent intakes of fruits, vegetables and dairy foods. Publ Health Nutr. Feb 2005;8(1): 77–85.

34. Ard JD, Fitzpatrick S, Desmond RA, et al. The impact of cost on the availability of fruits and vegetables in the homes of schoolchildren in Birmingham, Alabama. Am J Publ Health. 2007;97(2):367–72.

35. Timperio A, Salmon J, Ball K, et al. Family physical activity and sedentary environments and weight change in children. Int J Pediatr Obes (IJPO: An Official Journal of the International Association for the Study of Obesity). 2008;3(3):160–7.

36. Spurrier NJ, Magarey AA, Golley R, Curnow F, Sawyer MG. Relationships between the home environment and physical activity and dietary patterns of preschool children: a cross-sectional study. Int J Behav Nutr Phys Act. 30 May 2008;5:31.

37. McGinnis JM, Gootman JA, Kraak VI, editors. Food marketing to children and youth: threat or opportunity? Washington, DC: National Academies Press; 2006.

38. Kumanyika S, Grier S. Targeting interventions for ethnic minority and low-income populations. Future Child. 2006;16(1):187–207.

39. Grier S. African American and Hispanic youth vulnerability to target marketing: implications for understanding the effects of digital marketing. Paper presented at 2nd NPLAN/BMSG meeting on Digital Media and Marketing to Children, 29–30 Jun 2009. Berkeley, CA: Berkeley Media Studies Group.

40. Thompson DA, Flores G, Ebel BE, Christakis DA. Comida en venta: after-school advertising on Spanish-language television in the United States. J Pediatr. Apr 2008;152(4):576–81.

41. Bell RA, Cassady D, Culp J, Alcalay R. Frequency and types of foods advertised on Saturday morning and weekday afternoon English- and Spanish-language American television programs. J Nutr Educ Behav. Nov–Dec 2009;41(6): 406–13.

42. Yancey AK, Cole BL, Brown R, et al. A cross-sectional prevalence study of ethnically targeted and general audience outdoor obesity-related advertising. Milbank Q. Mar 2009;87(1):155–84.

43. Hillier A, Cole BL, Smith TE, et al. Clustering of unhealthy outdoor advertisements around child-serving institutions: a comparison of three cities. Health Place. 2009;15(4):935–45.

44. Gartner LM, Morton J, Lawrence RA, et al. Breastfeeding and the use of human milk. Pediatrics. Feb 2005;115(2): 496–506.

45. Forste R, Hoffmann JP. Are US mothers meeting the Healthy People 2010 breastfeeding targets for initiation, duration, and exclusivity? The 2003 and 2004 National Immunization Surveys. J Hum Lact. Aug 2008;24(3):278–88.

46. McDowell MM, Wang CY, Kennedy-Stephenson J. Breastfeeding in the United States: findings from the national health and nutrition examination surveys, 1999–2006. NCHS Data Brief. Apr 2008;5:1–8.

47. Andrulis DP. Moving beyond the status quo in reducing racial and ethnic disparities in children's health. Public Health Rep. Jul–Aug 2005;120(4):370–7.

48. Rose D, Bodor JN, Chilton M. Has the WIC incentive to formula-feed led to an increase in overweight children? J Nutr. Apr 2006;136(4):1086–90.

49. Ryan AS, Zhou W, Arensberg MB. The effect of employment status on breastfeeding in the United States. Women's Health Issues. Sept–Oct 2006;16(5):243–51.

50. Luther B. Looking at childhood obesity through the lens of Baumrind's parenting typologies. Orthop Nurs. 2007;26(5):270–8.

51. Hughes SO, Anderson CB, Power TG, Micheli N, Jaramillo S, Nicklas TA. Measuring feeding in low-income African-American and Hispanic parents. Appetite. Mar 2006;46(2):215–23.

52. Baughcum AE, Burklow KA, Deeks CM, Powers SW, Whitaker RC. Maternal feeding practices and childhood obesity: a focus group study of low-income mothers. Arch Pediatr Adolesc Med. Oct 1998;152(10):1010–4.

53. Kim J, Peterson KE. Association of infant child care with infant feeding practices and weight gain among US infants. Arch Pediatr Adolesc Med. Jul 2008;162(7):627–33.

54. Bentley M, Gavin L, Black MM, Teti L. Infant feeding practices of low-income, African-American, adolescent mothers: an ecological, multigenerational perspective. Soc Sci Med. Oct 1999;49(8):1085–100.

55. Molaison EF, Connell CL, Stuff JE, Yadrick MK, Bogle M. Influences on fruit and vegetable consumption by low-income black American adolescents. J Nutr Educ Behav. Sept–Oct 2005;37(5):246–51.

56. Arcan C, Neumark-Sztainer D, Hannan P, van den Berg P, Story M, Larson N. Parental eating behaviours, home food environment and adolescent intakes of fruits, vegetables and dairy foods: longitudinal findings from Project EAT. Publ Health Nutr. Nov 2007;10(11):1257–65.

57. Devine CM, Jastran M, Jabs J, Wethington E, Farell TJ, Bisogni CA. "A lot of sacrifices:" work-family spillover and the food choice coping strategies of low-wage employed parents. Soc Sci Med. Nov 2006;63(10):2591–603.

58. Neumark-Sztainer D, Croll J, Story M, Hannan PJ, French SA, Perry C. Ethnic/racial differences in weight-related concerns and behaviors among adolescent girls and boys: findings from Project EAT. J Psychosom Res. Nov 2002;53(5):963–74.

59. Larson NI, Story M, Eisenberg ME, Neumark-Sztainer D. Food preparation and purchasing roles among adolescents: associations with sociodemographic characteristics and diet quality. J Am Diet Assoc. Feb 2006;106(2):211–8.

60. Leddy MA, Power ML, Schulkin J. The impact of maternal obesity on maternal and fetal health. Rev Obstet Gynecol. Fall 2008;1(4):170–8.

61. Haines J, Neumark-Sztainer D, Wall M, Story M. Personal, behavioral, and environmental risk and protective factors for adolescent overweight. Obesity (Silver Spring, Md.). Nov 2007;15(11):2748–60.

62. Niemeier HM, Raynor HA, Lloyd-Richardson EE, Rogers ML, Wing RR. Fast food consumption and breakfast skipping: predictors of weight gain from adolescence to adulthood in a nationally representative sample. J Adolesc Health (Official publication of the Society for Adolescent Medicine). Dec 2006;39(6):842–9.

63. Timlin MT, Pereira MA, Story M, Neumark-Sztainer D. Breakfast eating and weight change in a 5-year prospective analysis of adolescents: project EAT (Eating Among Teens). Pediatrics. Mar 2008;121(3):e638–45.

64. Arcan C, Kubik MY, Fulkerson JA, Story M. Sociodemographic differences in selected eating practices among alternative high school students. J Am Diet Assoc. May 2009;109(5):823–9.

65. Wang YC, Bleich SN, Gortmaker SL. Increasing caloric contribution from sugar-sweetened beverages and 100% fruit juices among US children and adolescents, 1988–2004. Pediatrics. Jun 2008;121(6):e1604–14.

66. Berkey CS, Rockett HRH, Gillman MW, Colditz GA. One-year changes in activity and in inactivity among 10-to 15-year-old boys and girls: relationship to change in body mass index. Pediatrics. 2003;111(4):836–43.

67. Kimm SY, Glynn NW, Kriska AM, et al. Decline in physical activity in black girls and white girls during adolescence. N Engl J Med. 5 Sept 2002;347(10):709–15.

68. Boone JE, Gordon-Larsen P, Adair LS, Popkin BM. Screen time and physical activity during adolescence: longitudinal effects on obesity in young adulthood. Int J Behav Nutr Phys Act. 2007;4:26.

69. Adams K, Sargent RG, Thompson SH, Richter D, Corwin SJ, Rogan TJ. A study of body weight concerns and weight control practices of 4th and 7th grade adolescents. Ethn Health. 2000;5(1):79–94.

70. Baranowski T, Cullen KW, Nicklas T, Thompson D, Baranowski J. Are current health behavioral change models helpful in guiding prevention of weight gain efforts? Obes Res. Oct 2003;11 Suppl:23S–43S.

71. Bandura A. Self-efficacy: toward a unifying theory of behavioral change. Psychol Rev. Mar 1977;84(2):191–215.

72. Robinson T. Applying the socio-ecological model to improving fruit and vegetable intake among low-income African Americans. J Commun Health. Dec 2008;33 6:395–406.

73. Golan M, Crow S. Targeting parents exclusively in the treatment of childhood obesity: long-term results. Obes Res. Feb 2004;12(2):357–61.

74. Brownell KD, Kelman JH, Stunkard AJ. Treatment of obese children with and without their mothers: changes in weight and blood pressure. Pediatrics. Apr 1983;71(4):515–23.

75. Wadden TA, Stunkard AJ, Rich L, Rubin CJ, Sweidel G, McKinney S. Obesity in black adolescent girls: a controlled clinical trial of treatment by diet, behavior modification, and parental support. Pediatrics. Mar 1990;85(3):345–52.

76. Kreuter MW, Lukwago SN, Bucholtz RD, Clark EM, Sanders-Thompson V. Achieving cultural appropriateness in health promotion programs: targeted and tailored approaches. Health Educ Behav. Apr 2003;30(2):133–46.

77. Resnicow K, Baranowski T, Ahluwalia JS, Braithwaite RL. Cultural sensitivity in public health: defined and demystified. Ethn Dis. Winter 1999;9(1):10–21.

78. Whitt-Glover MC, Kumanyika SK. Systematic review of interventions to increase physical activity and physical fitness in African-Americans. Am J Health Promot. 2009;23(6):S33–56.

79. Teufel-Shone NI, Fitzgerald C, Teufel-Shone L, Gamber M. Systematic review of physical activity interventions implemented with American Indian and Alaska native populations in the United States and Canada. Am J Health Promot. 2009;23(6):S8–32.

80. Wilson DK. New perspectives on health disparities and obesity interventions in youth. J Pediatr Psychol. Apr 2009;34(3):231–44.

81. Flores G, Tomany-Korman SC. Racial and ethnic disparities in medical and dental health, access to care, and use of services in US children. Pediatrics. Feb 2008;121(2):e286–98.

82. Baranowski T, Baranowski JC, Cullen KW, et al. The Fun, Food, and Fitness Project (FFFP): the Baylor GEMS pilot study. Ethn Dis. Winter 2003;13(1 Suppl 1):S30–9.

83. Beech BM, Klesges RC, Kumanyika SK, et al. Child- and parent-targeted interventions: the Memphis GEMS pilot study. Ethn Dis. Winter 2003;13(1 Suppl 1):S40–53.

84. Robinson TN, Killen JD, Kraemer HC, et al. Dance and reducing television viewing to prevent weight gain in African-American girls: the Stanford GEMS pilot study. Ethn Dis. Winter 2003;13(1 Suppl 1):S65–77.

85. Story M, Sherwood NE, Himes JH, et al. An after-school obesity prevention program for African-American girls: the Minnesota GEMS pilot study. Ethn Dis. Winter 2003;13(1 Suppl 1):S54–64.

86. Fitzgibbon ML, Stolley MR, Schiffer L, Van Horn L, KauferChristoffel K, Dyer A. Two-year follow-up results for Hip-Hop to Health Jr.: a randomized controlled trial for overweight prevention in preschool minority children. J Pediatr. May 2005;146(5):618–25.

87. Gortmaker SL, Peterson K, Wiecha J, et al. Reducing obesity via a school-based interdisciplinary intervention among youth: planet health. Arch Pediatr Adolesc Med. Apr 1999;153(4):409–18.

88. Gortmaker SL, Cheung LW, Peterson KE, et al. Impact of a school-based interdisciplinary intervention on diet and physical activity among urban primary school children: eat well and keep moving. Arch Pediatr Adolesc Med. Sept 1999;153(9):975–83.

89. Caballero B, Clay T, Davis SM, et al. Pathways: a school-based, randomized controlled trial for the prevention of obesity in American Indian schoolchildren. Am J Clin Nutr. Nov 2003;78(5):1030–8.

90. Coleman KJ, Tiller CL, Sanchez J, et al. Prevention of the epidemic increase in child risk of overweight in low-income schools: the El Paso coordinated approach to child health. Arch Pediatr Adolesc Med. Mar 2005;159(3):217–24.

91. Harvey-Berino J, Wellman A, Hood V, Rourke J, Secker-Walker R. Preventing obesity in American Indian children: when to begin. J Am Diet Assoc. May 2000;100(5):564–6.

92. Haire-Joshu D, Brownson RC, Nanney MS, et al. Improving dietary behavior in African Americans: the parents as teachers high 5, low fat program. Prev Med. Jun 2003;36(6):684–91.

93. Webber LS, Catellier DJ, Lytle LA, et al. Promoting physical activity in middle school girls: trial of Activity for Adolescent Girls. Am J Prev Med. Mar 2008;34(3):173–84.

X THE FUTURE OF CHILDHOOD OBESITY IN THE GLOBAL MARKETPLACE

30 The Marketing and Distribution of Fast Food

Michelle Christian and Gary Gereffi

CONTENTS

Key Words: Social context, global food chain, global value chain, transnational corporation, fast food, marketing

INTRODUCTION

Today childhood obesity is widely recognized as a global health crisis; obesity rates in children have risen dramatically in developed countries since the 1960s and in developing countries since the 1980s. Recent conferences, NGO initiatives, and academic publications testify to increasing awareness of the problem. There is an emerging consensus that the study of childhood obesity should go beyond the medical interventionist model and incorporate multiple levels of analysis. Investigators from diverse social and scientific backgrounds now argue that "obesity should be framed as a complex system in which behavior is affected by multiple individual-level and socioenvironmental factors *(1, p. 1)*," rather than solely by individual choice.

Glass and McAtee *(2)* were among the first to call for an integration of the natural, behavioral, and social sciences to study childhood obesity. They argue that individual behavior choices are embedded within a social context that places "constraints," "inducements," and "pressures" upon their environment and their ability to act independently. They propose a "stream of causation" model of nested levels of analysis that highlight different social factors that induce and constrain health-related behaviors for all individuals. Glass and McAtee's original thesis was bolstered by a series of articles in the July 2009 edition of *Preventing Chronic Diseases* (see, *1*) that incorporates a systems-based analysis.

This chapter seeks to advance the multilevel approach to studying childhood obesity by focusing on the "macro" level of corporations in the global economy. We use a global value chains (GVC) framework to explain how the structure of food and agricultural value chains, with an emphasis on

From: *Contemporary Endocrinology: Pediatric Obesity: Etiology, Pathogenesis, and Treatment*
Edited by: M. Freemark, DOI 10.1007/978-1-60327-874-4_30,
© Springer Science+Business Media, LLC 2010

the fast-food segment, affects individual consumption choices. Food value chains shape consumption habits in various ways: they have a direct impact on the availability of foods; they foster the international dissemination of consumption patterns through the interplay between global and local food chains; they highlight the key role of transnational corporations (TNCs) in using marketing to define the consumer's perceptions of food; and they show where leverage can be exercised throughout the chain to push for change. (For a more detailed analysis of GVC methodology and its linkage to consumption see *(3)*.)

The GVC model is based on a series of steps that can be applied to any global industry to understand how it is organized and evolves *(4)*. First, we identify the lead firms in the industry, and how their strategies and roles are changing. Second, we show the linkages between economic activities that constitute the input–output structure of the chain, from raw materials to the production, distribution, and sale of the final product, which helps us understand how value is distributed across the chain and who captures value at each stage. Third, we reveal the governance structure that dictates how the chain operates and who controls the diffusion of technology, standards, and business practices within the chain. Lastly, we analyze the institutions (i.e., governments, unions, non-governmental organizations, and multilateral agencies) that establish the rules, incentives, and norms that guide the behavior of firms in the chain.

The global value chain for food operates at both the global and the local levels. In Fig. 1, we highlight the interaction of global and local food value chains between developed and developing countries. There are different types of lead firms at the global level, including the fast-food franchises that are household brand names in the United States (e.g., McDonald's, KFC, Wendy's, and Pizza Hut), the TNC food and beverage manufacturers (e.g., Kraft, PepsiCo, Coca Cola, Nestlé), and large supermarkets and food retailers (e.g., Kroger, Costco, and Wal-Mart). These corporations develop elaborate global sourcing and production networks to procure agricultural and food inputs from around the world that go into their final products.

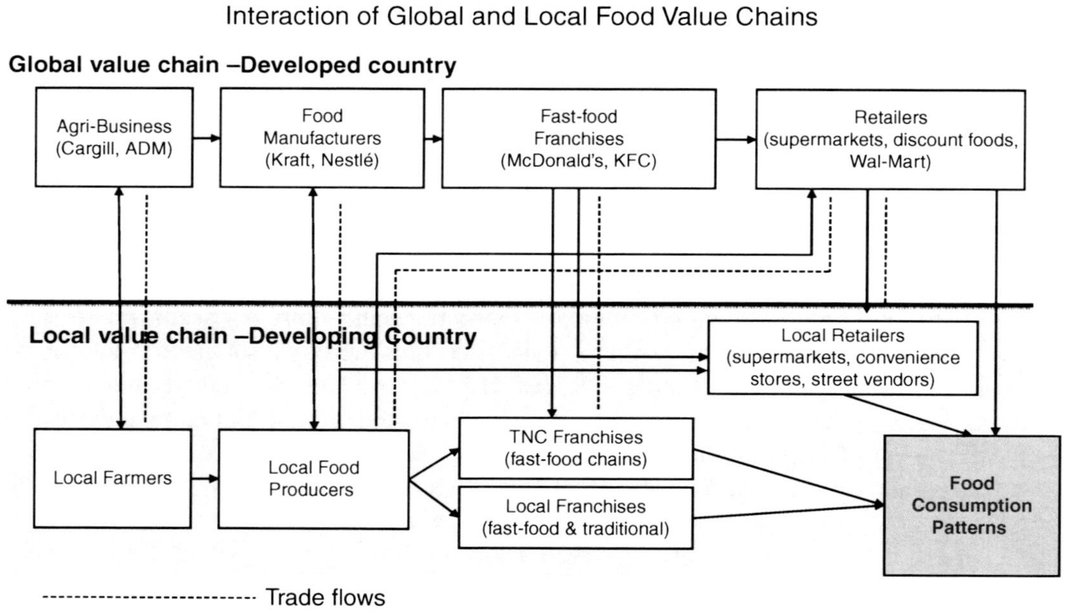

Interaction of Global and Local Food Value Chains

Fig. 1. Global and local food value chains.

The retail end of the chain includes fast-food chains and retailers that sell directly to consumers. Within the food and agricultural GVC, we focus on the organization of the fast-food segment because of the concerns often raised about the industry's impact on childhood obesity. Researchers have correlated the rise of fast food over the past couple of decades to the growth in high-caloric, energy-dense consumption and eating away from home, which has paralleled the rise in obesity rates. Survey results from the United States Department of Agriculture (USDA) chronicle how the proportion of total calories consumed in the United States that comes from fast-food has quadrupled from 3 to 12% from 1977 to 1995 (5). In another USDA survey, away-from-home consumption for children aged 2–19 averaged around 26% between 1994 and 1996, accounting for 32% of total daily energy, with researchers suggesting that children eat bigger proportions with higher caloric intake of fat and saturated fat away from home (6).

In the remainder of the chapter, we highlight four areas of the fast-food industry that exhibit the influence and power of large branded fast-food firms in shaping food production, distribution, and consumption. First, we document the rise of the industry in the United States and explain the linkages between the firms along the chain. Second, we address the international expansion of leading fast-food companies and the imitation effects that followed their global rise. Third, we chronicle how the marketing strategies of fast-food firms helped to expedite the growth of the industry and its direct relationship to children. Lastly, we discuss recent initiatives by the fast-food industry to provide healthier food options due to the public outcry that fast food is unhealthy. We focus on two companies (McDonald's and KFC) to show how fast food has revolutionized consumption, and also how societies, institutions, and consumers can have an impact on some of the world's largest companies.

THE RISE OF FAST FOOD IN THE UNITED STATES

According to Austin et al., fast-food sales soared 900% from US $16 billion in 1975 to US $153 billion by the mid-2000s (7). In 2007, the value of US fast-food sales grew by 5% to reach $179 million with restaurants totaling 248,400 units (8). Since 2002, the chained fast-food subsector, which includes top brands such as McDonald's, Yum! Brands (KFC, Taco Bell, Pizza Hut), and Burger King, represented over 60% of fast-food units and total sales (see Figs. 2 and 3). McDonald's is the clear leader in chained fast food in its percentage of global brand owner shares, followed by Yum! Brands (see Fig. 4).

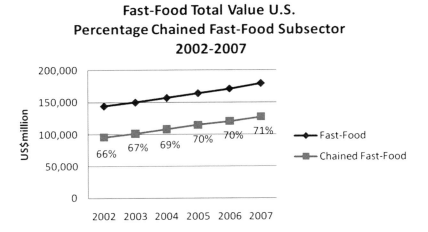

Fig. 2. Fast food by subsector, foodservice value 2002–2007, US$ million.
Source: Euromonitor International 2008.

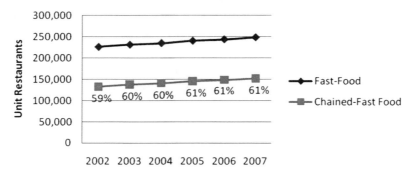

Fig. 3. Fast food by subsector, unit restaurants 2002–2007.
Source: Euromonitor International 2008.

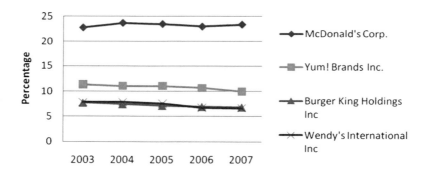

Fig. 4. Global brand owner shares of chained fast food in the United States.
Source: Euromonitor International 2008.

The top fast-food chains influence and shape the manufacturing segments that support their huge demand for staple products like processed French fries, chicken, and hamburger patties. Lead firms in the fast-food sector have dominant shares of the market, which gives them the power to set the performance standards for other firms along the chain. While purchasing power is key *(9)*, the strength of lead firms also comes from their direct and/or indirect control of production, market concentration, brand recognition, and technological innovation *(10)*. Multidimensional control of market forces is integral to lead firm status.

The origin of fast-food chains began with the franchising of McDonald's in the 1960s, and since then the strength of fast-food brands has grown at a meteoric rate. The largest fast-food chains (such as McDonald's and Yum! Brands) brought the mass production concept to foodservice, and in the process, changed how food is produced, distributed, and marketed. The activities of each segment of the chain are determined by the specifications of the lead firms, the branded fast-food restaurants, and their suppliers. The fast-food brands determine the production of food through their requirements for how food products should be cultivated, manufactured, packaged, distributed, and displayed. They work directly with food processors, who in turn work with farmers (see Fig. 1).

The stringent standards placed on farmers and food suppliers spearheaded the rise of industrialized agriculture and food processing. The industrial uses of corn are a good example of food technology conforming to buyer demands. Refining corn into corn meal, corn starch, or corn sweetener by companies like ConAgra has bolstered corn sales, with 530 million bushels every year going into high fructose corn syrup alone. Furthermore, 60% of corn production goes into feed for beef, cattle and chicken, which caters to the needs of the food service industry, particularly fast food *(11)*.

KFC is an example of a fast-food brand impacting the entire chicken supply chain configuration. Because KFC is one of the largest buyers of chicken in the world, it specifies what type of chickens it expects farmers to raise, and manufacturers to process, under exacting quality and safety standards. Because these standards require a high level of technological sophistication and efficiency, only the largest food processors (known in industry jargon as "integrators"), such as Tyson's and Pilgrim's Pride, can compete as a global supplier for KFC. Due to the scientific management required by modern chicken breeding, hatching, growing, and processing, the largest integrators handle most segments of the chain in-house and require the agricultural industry (like corn growers and processors) to meet their quantity and quality standards for chicken feed.

The demands of fast-food brands on their suppliers facilitated the further concentration of giant firms throughout the chain (a process known as "co-evolution"). French fries are a good example. The French fries served by fast-food chains (e.g., McDonald's, Burger King, and Wendy's) are supplied by a few very large manufacturers of French fries (e.g., McCain Foods and J.R. Simplot), which purchase russet potatoes from big growers/shippers (e.g., United Fresh Potato Growers of Idaho) that receive seeds, herbicides, and pesticides from a specialized corps of crop science firms (e.g., Bayer Crop Science and Monsanto). McDonald's is the largest purchaser of potatoes in the United States, with McCain Foods being its biggest supplier followed by J.R. Simplot. These two potato processors have globally expanded to meet McDonald's exacting standards as they enter new markets.

Another by-product of concentration is that the food varieties that manufacturers are producing and the fast-food that restaurants are selling spur imitation by competitors. Therefore, the rise of fast-food created a platform for the proliferation of processed food varieties that typically are higher in saturated fats and sodium, and lower in fiber, iron and other nutrients *(6)*. Highly processed inputs are attractive to fast-food chains because they have longer shelf life, can travel further distances without degradation, can be produced in large scale, and yield higher profit margins. Processed chicken (i.e., patties, breaded strips, and nuggets) is emblematic of the shift from whole foods toward processed varieties channeled through fast-food venues. Chicken fast food represents 55% of all chicken consumed outside of the home *(12)*.

INTERNATIONAL EXPANSION OF FAST FOOD

Fast-food chains have fueled their rapid growth through global expansion. This pace has increased exponentially in developing economies since the 1990s, where the gradual removal of market barriers and trade restrictions made the process of internationalization smoother for leading companies. Yum! Brands is a conglomerate that includes KFC, Pizza Hut, Taco Bell, Long John Silver, and A&W. In 2008 the company boasted 36,000 units in more than 110 countries and territories. KFC is the company's strongest brand with 5,253 units in the United States and 10,327 internationally, including 2,497 in Mainland China alone *(13)*. However, McDonald's is by far the global fast-food brand leader. In 2008 the company's total system units were 31,967, with 56% of those units being internationally based *(14)* (see Fig. 5). Like KFC, China leads the international market for McDonald's with 1,021 units in 2008, doubling since 2003.

System Unit Restaurants by Region

1994-2008

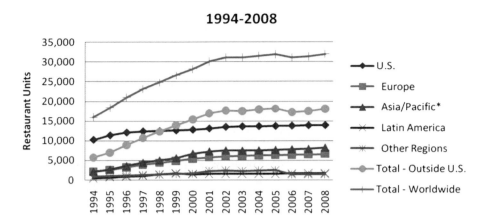

Fig. 5. McDonald's global operations.
Source: McDonald's Annual Reports 1994–2008.

Other countries like Mexico, Brazil, India, Vietnam, and the Philippines have quickly adopted the fast-food revolution. McDonald's operates 379 units in Mexico and 562 in Brazil. India, a country with a rich spice tradition and many varieties of local cuisine, is experiencing a "fascination" with fast food *(15)*. Since 2006, KFC has opened more than 45 restaurants with projections to surpass 120 by 2010. Pizza Hut operates 120 stores in 34 cities and McDonald's 132 stores, with further expansion planned in the coming years *(16)*. Entrepreneurs in Vietnam, now a member of the World Trade Organization, are trying to push forward franchise agreements with Carl's Jr. and Round Table Pizza *(17)*, while by the year 2000, the Philippines had 2,000 national and global brand chained fast-food restaurants *(18)*.

When fast-food firms enter emerging markets, they have the strength, technological prowess, and modern Western image to impact local food production in various ways. Matejowsky claims that the "efficiency and regimentation" of fast-food production styles reinforce the idea that fast food is often superior to local food because it is "scientifically designed" *(18)*.

Interaction effects between global and local fast-food value chains are seen in the global agro-businesses that buy products from local farms around the world or else they set up their own farms where they lease out plots to local growers to cultivate the crops the agro-businesses want. These local farms may supply internationally based fast-food units, local food manufacturers, or transnational corporations that have set up operations in developing countries in order to serve the domestic market. In developing economies, TNCs are certainly not the only actors that are practicing industrialized farming, making processed foods, and setting-up fast-food restaurants. Domestic companies do this as well. However, the global and local food chains are connected because the standards, practices, and technological achievements that local farmers, manufacturers, and fast-food companies are using were generally adopted from Western firms. Thus, there is an interaction effect. Schlosser argues that McDonald's and other fast-food chains impart to developing countries new systems of agriculture and food production, which reorient local food systems from staple domestic crops to externally induced needs *(19)*.

For example, when J.R. Simplot entered China in 1993 and created the first commercial French fry for the Chinese market, agricultural producers began cultivating potatoes to meet this new demand for processed food *(20)*. Similarly in India, after importing processed French fries for several years, by 2010 each McDonald's French fry is expected to come from Indian soil but processed by McCain Foods. McCain worked with Indian growers for 9 years to change their potato crop to the Shepody variety to meet McDonald's exacting standards *(21)*. This is a switch from the typical Indian potato varieties that are low in solids and high in water. Both companies see emerging economies as cornerstones for the frozen food market.

The dissemination of global fast-food production and consumption through local imitators is evident in the rapid growth of local fast-food brands in developing countries, as well. Jollibee, southeast Asia's version of McDonald's, is considered one of the region's most profitable corporations with over 1,655 franchises, branches, and subsidiaries across Asia-Pacific *(18)*.

China symbolizes the penetration of fast foods in developing countries and the interaction between global and local dynamics. KFC is one of the most successful fast-food chains in China. As of 2008, there were over 2,497 restaurants in Mainland China. Five hundred or more restaurants are planned for 2009. The emergence of KFC and other leading fast-food chains in China is shaping local food systems in lasting ways. Agricultural imports have increased because foreign firms are demanding particular commodities as key ingredients for their fast-food staples. The food-processing industry in China has grown at high double digits over the past 5 years. Large foreign food manufacturers have continued to set up facilities and expand their Chinese operations to cater to the demand from both global and local firms in China. For example, Tyson's, a top supplier to KFC, had two acquisitions in 2008. As with poultry farmers in the United States, Tyson pushes standards onto Chinese poultry farmers (e.g., types of feed and antibiotics used) and in the process impacts local agricultural suppliers (e.g., farmers switching to soy bean cultivation which is used as feed for poultry).

THE POWER OF MARKETING

What has spurred the meteoric rise of fast-food chains and allowed them to solidify their market power while not being food producers themselves is the role of marketing and brands. For the past 50 years, the fast-food revolution was buoyed by the top brands' ability to mold marketing messages in multiple media that impacted how consumers perceived fast-food. Corporations like McDonald's and KFC expanded their brand image with extensive marketing and advertising.

Image creation for food products and brands, domestically and internationally, is one of the most powerful tools that affect food choices. In 2001 the global advertising budget for food products was around $40 billion, with confectionary, sweetened breakfast cereals, and fast-food restaurants representing the most frequently advertised food options *(22)*. Lang and Millstone argue that selective advertising of foods high in fat, sugar, and salt undermines the ability of individuals to make healthy food choices.

Rather than being passive consumers subject to adult wishes, children are often the target in the messaging and creation of fast-food brand identities. They are also more vulnerable to the marketing messages being transmitted. Story and French document how fast-food companies influence purchasing behavior through television advertisements and school marketing programs. Food advertisers are second only to automakers in television advertising expenditures, with campaigns targeted toward children estimated to cost $1 billion *(23)*. Ninety-five percent of US fast-food restaurants' budgets are allocated to television placements with children typically viewing one food commercial every 5 min. According to TNS Media Intelligence, in 2007 overall TV spending by McDonald's, Kellogg, General Mills, and Campbell Soup rose to $1.7 billion; 12% ($204 million) of this was spent for advertisements on children's television channels like Nickelodeon and the Cartoon Network *(24)*. Furthermore, children are inundated with food marketing at schools through product placements, soft drink pouring rights, and sole vendor contracts.

Fast-food marketing campaigns oriented toward children remain strong, particularly within the realm of movies. McDonald's 2008 total marketing budget was $1.7 billion and in 2009 they launched a major promotional campaign linked to the blockbuster movie Avatar (25). Since 1997, McDonald's has had a global alliance with the Walt Disney Co. whereby they shared exclusive marketing rights for films like Toy Story and A Bug's Life. As children enjoyed their Chicken McNugget Happy Meals, they also were able to play with toys of Buzz Lightyear. McDonald's moved their partnership to DreamWorks studios in 2007 to take advantage of the immense popularity of the Shrek movie franchise (26). Thus, children associate fun and exciting entertainment with particular brands and food choices.

Strong marketing and promotional initiatives in the United States by the largest fast-food companies parallel the marketing campaigns that follow a fast-food company's entry into foreign markets. These companies have continued to target children in their global operations. The marketing strategy "think global, act local" has become the rallying cry of global marketing campaigns (27) with children and youth representing a key part of this "glocalisation." Both McDonald's and KFC have marketing campaigns, particularly in East Asia, that appeal to children and teenagers through the use of Internet texting, in-store prizes inspired by the summer Olympics, and the marketing of "cool." Li highlights how KFC marketing strategies in China have a dual strategy that keeps KFC "hip" for young consumers who want a Western brand experience and culturally sensitive for adults who appreciate the Chinese-style menu items like the Old Beijing Chicken Roll (28).

FAST-FOOD COMPANIES ON THE DEFENSIVE

During the past decade, consumer and public health advocates and government bodies have begun to highlight the health dangers of excessive consumption of fast foods and the irresponsibility of fast-food marketing campaigns oriented toward children. This public outcry has spurred an attempt by fast-food firms to "rebrand" themselves by offering healthier food options. These shifts could lead to significant changes along the value chain if fast-food buyers begin to demand healthier products (including additives and other inputs) from their suppliers, but many are skeptical that these "healthy choice" changes are in fact superficial.

The launching of health-conscious initiatives by fast-food firms followed a series of well-publicized reports and lawsuits criticizing the marketing practices of the top firms and the lack of nutritional value in their food options. In 2008 the Center for Science in the Public Interest and the California Center for Public Health Advocacy released a study that concluded that most of the kids' options at venues such as McDonald's, KFC, and Wendy's are too high in calories (29). In addition, in 2004 the World Health Organization launched its Global Strategy on Diet, Physical Activity, and Health that called on governments and private industry to curb the marketing of unhealthy dietary practices. However, most actions by the industry regarding standards for marketing practices are merely voluntary. The Children's Advertising Review Unit (CARU) of the National Council of Better Business Bureaus sets guidelines for policies and standards for food advertisers in the United States, but it has no enforcement authority.

The most visible government actions to change fast-food industry practices have involved the regulation of *trans*-fats, a common component of fast-food products, and required nutritional labeling. This has mainly been handled on a state-by-state basis. California, New York City, and Texas have already enacted or put forward legislation banning *trans*-fats in chained restaurants. In addition, the Labeling Education and Nutrition (LEAN) Act, a recent 2008 federal legislation that would create one standard for disclosing information in chain restaurants nationwide, is garnering some industry support, but many companies still oppose detailed labeling such as listing grams of saturated and *trans*-fats and sodium levels as menu items *(30)*. With greater public awareness about fast-food health issues and the push for government regulation, the industry has sought to deflect this new market pressure. As of 2008, according to Euromonitor International, almost all the leading fast-food chains have either eliminated or are attempting to eliminate *trans*-fat *(31)*.

Both McDonald's and KFC have begun new marketing campaigns to highlight their moves toward more nutritious meals. Fast-food brands still struggle, however, between new healthier claims and the core brand messaging of their classic meals, while trying to avoid formal regulation. Yum! Brands, KFC's parent company, leads the industry in putting forward calorie count menu boards, and KFC touts their *trans*-fat-free chicken items. KFC has also created new healthier items, such as boneless and grilled chicken options, salads, and wraps. These initiatives have accelerated since 2003 when the company began to push the idea that chicken is part of a healthy diet, particularly in comparison to the offerings of their fast-food competitors. Marketing analysts have praised the effectiveness of this strategy, since consumers now think that fast-food chicken is better than fast-food beef *(32)*.

McDonald's, more than any fast-food company, was subject to harsh criticism for the low nutritional value of its food. Public exposes with lawsuits, the 2004 documentary "Supersize Me," and bestseller books and documentaries that excoriate the economic and social abuses of our industrialized fast-food culture and the agricultural systems that support it (e.g., Food Inc., *Fast Food Nation, Omnivore's Dilemma,* and *In Defense of Food*) have all spotlighted the fast-food industry and its top representative, McDonald's. Originally McDonald's went on the defensive, but in the last few years the company has attempted to rebrand itself as a restaurant that offers food options for a balanced diet. They started educational campaigns in 2004 where Ronald McDonald touted four key messages that range from making balanced food choices to embracing an active lifestyle *(33)*. Diverse salad menu options, new forms of wraps, and fruit options for kids' Happy Meals are also part of the rebranding effort. Similar to KFC, McDonald's has used its Web site as a medium to push its initiatives, such as providing nutritional facts of meals and recommending to customers "simple steps to trim fat," "save on sodium," or "cut calories."

The initiatives from KFC and McDonald's demonstrate how lead firms can be pressured to modify some of their business practices. Nevertheless, many questions remain regarding the significance of these changes. Are these initiatives merely part of what Simon labels "nutriwashing" *(34)* or attempts to cover up what Brownell calls the epidemic of a "toxic food environment" *(35)*. Euromonitor International points out that most of the growth and profits of fast-food firms are still generated by sales of fatty food options. Moreover, McDonald's executives are quick to highlight personal responsibility and choice as the reasons why individuals make bad dietary decisions and to assert that "advertising is not the issue" in influencing food choices *(36)*. These statements seem to contradict the value McDonald's puts on marketing and advertising, as witnessed by its nearly $2 billion marketing budget, revitalized campaigns for the classic McDonald's Big Mac, its dollar menu, and its global brand positioning. Critics argue McDonald's products are not as healthy as claimed and that calorie counts are an inadequate basis to determine the nutritional quality of food *(37)*.

The US fast-food industry's attempts to counter criticism need to be placed in a global perspective. The chains' practice of opening up restaurants abroad, particularly in developing countries, brings fast-food menu items to new markets but changes local food production systems through global–local interaction effects. At the beginning of the twenty-first century a new McDonald's was opening somewhere in the world every 8 h *(19)*. The size, influence, and modern image of fast-food business practices change how local foods are produced, marketed, and distributed, with long-term effects for food and agriculture systems beyond the fast-food industry in these countries. The lax regulatory environment in many developing countries and the value placed on economic development, often to the detriment of social and environmental protection, underscore the multiple dimensions of fast food's meteoric rise.

CONCLUSION

The severity of the global childhood obesity pandemic calls for new theoretical frameworks and research agendas that take into account the broad factors that affect consumption patterns and behavioral choices related to public health crises. The GVC paradigm gives us a foundation to examine how some of the main corporate strategies and international processes relating to the production, distribution, and the marketing of fast-food companies are linked to consumption patterns around the world and to childhood obesity as a health problem.

The rise of the fast-food industry has influenced the social conditions of life in developed and developing countries in ways that can contribute to childhood obesity. Many fast-food companies have already been compelled to change certain practices within the fast-food global value chain, but research is still needed to assess whether the health-related initiatives of top firms are merely superficial. The structural environment that these companies shape, nationally and globally, continues to constrain, induce, and pressure how individuals, and especially children, make food choices that can adversely affect their health.

ACKNOWLEDGMENTS

The authors gratefully acknowledge the valuable research assistance they received in preparing this paper from Joonkoo Lee, Kim Rogers, Yisel Valdes, and Aileen Zhang.

Editor's Question and Authors' Response

- **Global corporations wield enormous power over the worldwide production, distribution, and consumption of food. You have argued that corporate decisions and practice promote the dissemination and consumption of fast food and thereby contribute to the epidemic of childhood and adult obesity. A growing movement now focuses on support of local producers of fresh fruits, vegetables, and meats. Do you think that this "locavore" movement can compete effectively with global corporations for a share in the global food market?**

- The "go local" approach to food consumption has gained a lot of momentum with the publication of books like Eric Schlosser's *Fast Food Nation* (2001) and Michael Pollan's *The Omnivore's Dilemma* (2006), and Robert Kenner's newly released film, "Food, Inc." (2009). These materials highlight the vast power of contemporary food and agricultural multinational companies and the growing health, safety, and environmental concerns that our mechanized, highly concentrated, and increasingly global agricultural and food production systems have generated. While the "locavore" movement is a welcome countertrend to the commodification of our food choices, it is by itself inadequate to address the larger issues at hand.

- For all the criticisms that can be made of our industrialized food system, it has one big advantage: it has staved off (at least for the time being) the earlier and dire Malthusian fears of an inadequate food supply. The scientific advancements that have led to improved seed varieties for staple crops like rice, corn, and wheat and the manufacturing and logistical advances in producing and distributing food to reach both urban and rural population centers around the world mean that a small fraction of our workforce (less than 1% of the US population of 285 million are farmers) *(39)* is producing vast quantities of relatively inexpensive food accessible to everyone.

- A major value of the "locavore" movement is that it is making clearer the hidden costs of our industrialized food system. Not only are the low nutritional value and dietary abuses of "cheap calories" in our fast-food culture being critically evaluated but the environmental dangers of this system are also being exposed. Buying local reduces the "food miles" (and thus the carbon footprint) of our food choices, and it also promotes economic diversity and a healthier local ecosystem, which are important steps toward sustainable consumption.

- However, local food systems will not replace globalized food and agriculture for various reasons. There is a scaling up problem, which is also related to costs. To feed the ever larger urban populations of the world, there is no substitute for the concentrated and highly coordinated production and distribution system put in place by global agribusiness companies. Perhaps even more surprising than the "backlash" to these giant firms represented by the locavore movement is the pervasive imitation of modern fast-food concepts in the developing world. Equally distressing is the fact that some of the icons in the healthy food counterculture movement are themselves conglomerates. Whole Foods, Ben & Jerry's, Danone and Starbucks are now transnational firms, not so dissimilar from the fast-food and standardized brands they railed against.

- The locavore movement is a positive trend, but it is more of social movement than an economic counterweight to our global food and agriculture system. The healthy food culture will need to be buttressed by supportive government legislation, which makes healthy diets and preventive health care more affordable and accessible to our entire population, rather than an attractive option for small subsets of our population.

REFERENCES

1. Huang TT, Drewnowski A, Kumanyika SK, Glass TA. A systems-oriented multilevel framework for addressing obesity in the 21st century. Prev Chronic Dis. 2009;6(3):1–10.
2. Glass T, McAtee M. Behavioral science at the crossroads in public health: extending horizons, envisioning the future. Soc Sci Med. 2006;62:1650–71.
3. Gereffi G, Christian M. Trade, transnational corporations and food consumption: a global value chain approach. In: Hawkes C, Bouin C, Henson S, Drager N, Dubé L, editors. Trade, food, diet and health: perspectives and policy options. Oxford: Wiley Blackwell; 2010;91–110.
4. For more information on global value chain analysis, see the Concepts and Tools section of the Global Value Chains website http://www.globalvaluechains.org maintained by the Center on Globalization, Governance & Competitiveness at Duke University.
5. Lin B, Frazao E, Guthrie J. Away-from-home foods increasingly important to quality of American diets. Agricultural Information Bulletin, vol. 33733. Washington, DC: United States Department of Agriculture, Economic Research Service; 1999.
6. Lin B, Guthrie J, Frazao E. Quality of children's diets at and away from home: 1994–1996. Food Rev. United States Department of Agriculture. Economic Research Service. Jan–Apr 1999;22(1):2–10.
7. Austin SB, Melly SJ, Sanchez BN, Patel A, et al. Clustering of fast-food restaurants around schools: a novel application of spatial statistics to the study of food environments. Am J Publ Health. 2005;95(9):1575–82.
8. Fast food – US 2008 Country Sector Briefing. Euromonitor International.
9. Sturgeon T. From commodity chains to value chains: interdisciplinary theory building in an age of globalization. In: Blair J, editor. Frontiers of commodity chain research. Palo Alto, CA: Stanford University Press; 2009;110–35.
10. Gereffi G, Lee J, Christian M. The emergence of governance structures in US-based food and agricultural value chains and their relevance to healthy diets. Paper prepared for the Healthy Eating Research Program, Robert Wood Johnson Foundation. Princeton, NJ; 2008.
11. Pollan M. The omnivore's dilemma: a natural history of four meals. New York, NY: Penguin Books; 2006.
12. Domestic Market Segments. http://www.nationalchickencouncil.com/statistics/stat_detail.cfm?id=6 (2009). Accessed 1 Mar 2009.
13. Yum! Brands Annual Report. 2008.
14. McDonald's Annual Report. 2008.
15. Mitra K. Bon appétit; while most companies have been forced onto the back foot by the slowdown, fast-food companies are doing rollicking business. Business Today. 22 Mar 2009.

16. Block JP, Scribner RA, DeSalvo KB. Fast food, race, ethnicity, and income. Am J Prev Med. 2004;27(3):211–7.
17. Edwards W. Vietnam ready for franchising. Franchising World. 2009;41(3):23–6.
18. Matejowsky T. Fast food and nutritional perceptions in the age of 'globesity': perspectives from the provincial Philippines. Food Foodways. 2009;17:29–49.
19. Schlosser E. Fast food nation: the dark side of the all-American meal. New York, NY: Harper Collins; 2001.
20. Simplot in China. http://www.simplot.com.cn/s2e.html (2009). Accessed 2 Jul 2009.
21. Mitra K. McDonald's: from field to fries. Sify. Mar 2009. http://www.google.com/search?hl=en&q=McCain+foods+mc donalds&sourceid=navclient-ff&rlz=1B3GGGL_enUS332US333&ie=UTF-8&aq=h (2009). Accessed 2 Jul 2009.
22. Lang T, Millstone E. The atlas of food: who eats what, where and why. Berkeley, CA: University of California Press; 2008.
23. Story M, French S. Food advertising and marketing directed at children at adolescents in the US. Int J Behav Nutr Phys Act. 2004;1(3):1–17.
24. York E, Hamp A. Food spend rises despite ad crackdown. Advert Age. 2008;79(8):13.
25. York EB. What new CMO has in store for McDonald's. Advert Age. 2008;79(23):12.
26. Marr M, Gray S. McDonald's signs marketing deal with DreamWorks. Wall Str J. 2005;B3.
27. Vignali C. McDonald's: 'think global, act local' – the marketing mix. Br Food J. 2001;103:2.
28. Li D. Do in China as the Chinese do: an overview of KFC's localization strategies in China. 2004. http:blog.lidan.net/2004/04kfcs_localization_strategies_in_china.html. Accessed 15 Aug 2007.
29. Obesityon kids' menus at top chains. Business Wire. 2008. http://proquest.umi.com/pqdweb?index=143&sid=10&srch mode=1&vi. Accessed 15 Apr 2009.
30. Jennings L. Industry calls for national standards. Nation's Restaurant News. 2008;42(40):90–2.
31. St-Onge MP, Keller K, Heymsfield SB. Changes in childhood food consumption patterns: a cause for concern in light of increasing body weights. Am J Clin Nutr. 2003;78:1068–73.
32. Fernandez J. KFC: marching on our stomachs. Marketing Week. 2009;25.
33. Rogers E. McDonald's ads answer anti-obesity challenge. Marketing. 2004.
34. Simon M. Appetite for profit how the food industry undermines our health and how to fight back. New York, NY: Nation Books; 2006.
35. Brownell KD, Horgen KB. Food fight: the inside story of the food industry, America's obesity crisis, and what we can do about it. Columbus, OH: McGraw-Hill; 2003.
36. Gray S, Adamy J. McDonald's gets healthier – but burgers still rule. Wall Str J. 23 Feb 2005;B7. Campaign. Message from McDonald's. Campaign. 26 Apr 2007;9.
37. McDonald's Corp. amended suit claims food fare is less healthful than billed. Wall Str J. 2003;B8.
38. Leung S. Experts differ on healthiness of 'fast' salad. Wall Str J. 2003;B1.
39. See US Environmental Protection Agency, "Ag 101" http://www.epa.gov/oecaagct/ag101/demographics.html

31 Local and National Policy-Based Interventions: To Improve Children's Nutrition

Marlene B. Schwartz and Kelly D. Brownell

CONTENTS

Key Words: Food policy, WIC, federal feeding programs, school lunch, food industry, marketing

Government agencies have great power to improve public health through federal, state, and local policies. Many examples illustrate how government involvement can help protect or improve the public's health, including mandated car seats for children, child immunizations, smoking bans in public places, and high tobacco taxes.

Among the most pressing health issues today is the rise in childhood obesity, and again, public health experts are looking to government policies as a means to promote better nutrition for children *(1)*. Because of the multiple contributors to poor diet and inactivity among children, many policy approaches have been suggested. Some are primarily activity focused (e.g., safe routes to school, mandating recess and gym, keeping schools open for town sports programs) and others emphasize nutrition (e.g., improving school food, increasing access to grocery stores, changing government subsidies). The challenge is to identify policies that will have greatest impact *(2)*.

This chapter reviews key policy options to improve children's nutrition that may be implemented at local, state, and federal levels. We discuss: (a) why policy change may be more cost-effective and have a greater impact than programs aimed at individuals; (b) how federal feeding programs can be strengthened; and (c) which policies have potential to change the food industry's behavior.

From: *Contemporary Endocrinology: Pediatric Obesity: Etiology, Pathogenesis, and Treatment*
Edited by: M. Freemark, DOI 10.1007/978-1-60327-874-4_31,
© Springer Science+Business Media, LLC 2010

WHY CHANGE FOOD POLICIES?

A common belief is that eating behavior is driven by personal and individual factors, such as emotional experiences with food, flavor preferences, nutrition knowledge, and plain old willpower. Overweight people, the assumption goes, do not know the proper way to eat or have no self-discipline. The resulting approach to reducing obesity involves educating and imploring people to change, partly through a vast array of diets. Even the best of these that deal with systematic behavior change have disappointing long-term results (3). In the absence of some pharmacologic miracle, it will never be possible to affect prevalence rates through treatment because the small number of successes is offset by the vast number of people in the population becoming overweight.

Many health professionals and organizations have called for a shift away from the medical model of treating obesity to a public health approach for preventing obesity (4,5). Policy then becomes an important tool. Public health approaches often use the strategy of changing the environment so healthy behavior becomes more likely, even the default (6). Fluoride in the water creates better defaults and does not rely on educating people about fluoride use. Educating and motivating people to improve eating behavior may be desirable, even necessary, but is clearly insufficient or obesity rates would have been reversed by now. It is essential to create environmental conditions that make healthy eating an easy behavior (7).

Many studies document how default environments have a powerful impact on behavior. A striking example is the case of organ donor rates across countries. In some European countries, people must opt in to become organ donors, while in others they are automatically considered donors unless they opt out. Even though the choices are the same in both conditions, about 15% become donors when the default is not to be a donor, compared to approximately 98% with the opposite default (8,9). It is unlikely that any amount of education about the importance or desirability of becoming an organ donor could ever approach the impact of simply changing the default. Furthermore, education costs money and in many cases, changing the default does not. Indeed, it can even raise revenue; one example would be a tax on sugar-sweetened beverages (10,11).

The default nutrition environment has a substantial impact on children. One key venue is the school environment; there is strong evidence that children's diets are influenced by the foods served and sold in school cafeterias and vending machines, the schools' nutrition policies, and the availability of unhealthy snacks in the area surrounding schools (12–16). Changing what is sold may be more effective than nutrition education, or at the very least, must be a necessary companion to education. The following sections examine the actions that federal, state, and local governments can take to improve children's nutrition.

STRENGTHENING FEDERAL FEEDING PROGRAMS

The federal government has several programs designed to ensure adequate nutrition for American children. Most noteworthy are: (a) the Women Infants and Children Program (WIC), (b) the Child and Adult Care Feeding Program (CACFP), and (c) the National School Lunch Program (NSLP) and Breakfast Program (NSBP). These are federal programs but are administered by the states, typically through the state departments of health or education. Depending on the assignment of regulatory authority within a state, some state or city agencies will have authority to strengthen the nutrition standards of each program. For school food in particular, individual school districts have the authority to set their own nutrition standards through local school wellness policies. Opportunities to improve nutrition through each of these programs are described below.

Women, Infants, and Children Program

The mission of the WIC program is to provide nutritious foods to supplement the diets of low-income, nutritionally at-risk women, infants, and children up to age 5. In addition to providing food, the program delivers information on healthy eating, conducts screenings, and makes referrals to health, welfare, and social services *(9)*. WIC has tremendous reach, currently serving 45% of all infants born in the United States *(9)*.

The WIC food package was originally designed to supplement diets of the participants with foods rich in five target nutrients: vitamins A and C, calcium, iron, and protein. These nutrients had been identified as key dietary deficiencies in the target populations; therefore, the specific foods promoted through the WIC food packages were infant formula, juice, cereal, milk, cheese, eggs, dried beans/peas and/or peanut butter, tuna, and carrots. Undernutrition was the chief concern.

The WIC program has been successful in meeting its initial goals. WIC participation improves children's general health status, decreases the likelihood of anemia, and increases rates of consuming a nutrient-rich diet *(17,18)*. Yet, obesity rates among children participating in WIC are alarmingly high. A 2004 study in New York found that 40% of children aged 2–5 were overweight or obese *(19)*. A 2008 government report found that WIC children take in more nutrients than eligible non-participants, but also consume more high-fat and high-sugar foods, and have lower intakes of whole grains and produce.

At USDA's request in 2003, the Institute of Medicine reviewed nutritional needs of the WIC population and developed scientifically based, cost-neutral recommendations for WIC food packages *(20)*. A primary goal was to reduce excessive and inadequate nutrient intakes among WIC participants and improve overall diet to be consistent with the Dietary Guidelines for Americans. In December 2007, the USDA announced an interim final rule that revised WIC food packages. Only 2% or lower fat milk is authorized for children aged 2 and older and a number of foods have been added to the package including fruit and vegetables, whole grains, and milk alternatives (e.g., soy-based beverages and tofu). Whole grain options include a variety of nutritious foods such as whole wheat or whole grain bread, soft corn and whole grain tortillas, brown rice, oatmeal, bulgur, and barley. Fruit and vegetables are specifically encouraged through cash-value vouchers ($6, $8, and $10 per month depending on a participant's category) that can be used to purchase a wide variety of fresh, canned, or frozen products.

States may use the WIC requirements as a minimum standard and promote even better nutrition. In some cases, states are able to pilot innovative strategies that later inspire federal policy change. For example, in 1988 New York State conducted a pilot program to allow WIC coupons to be used at farmer's markets *(21)*. By 1992 Congress had established and funded a USDA farmer's market nutrition program that today funds 38 states to allow WIC vouchers at farmer's markets *(22)*.

The reformulation of the WIC food package represents a significant step in improving the diets of WIC participants and will hopefully provide inspiration for other federal feeding programs to improve nutrition standards. It is also important to test for spillover effects in communities. For instance, compared with stores in higher income areas, those in low-income neighborhoods are less likely to have low-fat dairy, whole wheat bread, and high-quality produce *(23)*; the new guidelines may improve the food landscape in low-income neighborhoods as WIC participating stores are required to carry these foods. Research is underway to evaluate the effect of these changes, but the WIC program leads the way in promoting better nutrition by changing defaults *(24)*.

Child and Adult Care Feeding Program

The CACFP supports foodservice operations for child-care centers enrolling at least 25% of children from low-income families *(17)*. CACFP nutrition standards require centers to provide adequately sized servings of four food groups at each meal: (a) meat/meat substitute, (b) dairy, (c) fruit/vegetable, and (d) grain. For snacks, two of these components must be served. While these standards ensure some variety in the children's meals and snacks, they are not specific enough to guarantee that menus meet current dietary recommendations. For example, Oakley and colleagues surveyed 92 child-care centers in Mississippi and found that almost all center menus met these requirements, but the mean amount of energy and some nutrients were lower than recommended and the percent calories from fat was significantly higher than recommended (40.8% instead 30%) by the Dietary Guidelines for Americans *(25)*.

CACFP standards could be improved in a number of ways. Current guidelines list the foods that must be available but do not address the importance of excluding additional high-calorie, low-nutrient foods. Hence, centers can serve calorie-dense snacks such as chips and donuts that compete with the CACFP foods and may thereby decrease consumption of healthier options. Second, CACFP requirements are inconsistent with the Dietary Guidelines for Americans *(26)* and the National Health and Safety Performance Standards *(27)*, which recommend that at least half of all grains consumed be whole grains and that children aged 2–8 years should consume only fat-free or low-fat dairy products. CACFP also does not address the problem of serving milks or yogurts flavored with added sugars. Finally, juice can be served instead of whole fruit as a fruit serving, and there is no clear limit to the amount of juice served. The American Academy of Pediatrics currently recommends a maximum of 4–6 ounces per day based on the age of the child *(28)*. This weak juice policy warrants particular attention due to research examining the links among juice consumption, overall dietary quality, and overweight in children *(29–34)*.

CACFP is under the umbrella of the Federal WIC Reauthorization Act. Federal programs have the opportunity to set minimum national nutrition standards, which is the most efficient way to have a large impact on children's health. At the same time, this program is administered at the state level, typically through the Department of Health or the Department of Education. Therefore, a faster and potentially more politically feasible avenue to create very strong nutrition standards may be to write state regulations.

There are two current examples of activities to strengthen CACFP guidelines in states. The California Food Policy Advocates released recommendations in January 2009 for state legislation to strengthen CACFP standards, focusing on limiting juice, sugared cereals, fried potatoes, and sweet grains and increasing low-fat milk and vegetable servings *(35)*. In New York, regulations adopted in October 2009 by the Department of Health strengthened CACFP requirements and made additional recommendations. Notably, flavored milk is not allowed for children 5 and under, all milk for children over 2 years of age must be skimmed or 1%, juice is limited to 1 serving per day, sweet grain products and sweet cereals may not be served at lunch or supper (and are limited to two per week), and yogurt must be low-fat or fat-free and made without artificial sweeteners *(36)*. Some of the additional recommendations include having three or more servings of fresh fruit and vegetables per week, serving only whole grain breads and cereals, and limiting processed and high-fat meat to only once per week *(36)*.

National School Breakfast and Lunch Programs

Thirty million children per day participate in the National School Lunch Program (NSLP) and 10 million participate in the National School Breakfast Program (NSBP). The meals served in each of these programs have always been required to meet federal nutrition standards, and since 1995 must be consistent with the Dietary Guidelines for Americans. Recent research from the School Nutrition Dietary Assessment-III study, however, found that meals typically met the standards for protein, vitamin A, vitamin C, calcium, and iron, but exceeded the limits on fat and saturated fat *(37)*. At the present time, the USDA has sponsored the Institute of Medicine to update the meal patterns and nutrition standards for the NSLP and NSBP *(38)*.

In addition to the reimbursable breakfast and lunch in these programs, nearly all school districts sell additional foods, termed "competitive foods." These are sold in many ways, including a la carte sales in lunch lines, vending machines, school stores, and fundraisers. Competitive foods are virtually unregulated, which has allowed foods like ice cream, potato chips, baked goods, and sports drinks to be sold in competition with the school lunch. The only foods excluded from sale during the lunch period are those defined as foods of minimal nutritional value (FMNV), which were identified over 30 years ago and are limited to four categories: soda water, water ices, chewing gum, and certain candies (39).

Much needs to be done to remedy the problematic nutrition environment in schools. The definition of FMNV must be updated and expanded to include the array of nutritionally poor foods that currently compete with school lunches. In 2007, the Institute of Medicine released a report with specific recommendations for competitive foods in elementary, middle, and high schools (40), but these guidelines have not been adopted by the USDA.

While waiting for the federal government to update its nutrition standards for the NSLP, NSBP, and FMNV, states are free to create stronger regulations, and in the last 6 years many have. According to the 2009 Trust for America's Health "F as in Fat" report, nineteen states now have stricter NSLP and NSBP standards than the USDA requires, and 27 states have set standards for competitive foods and beverages sold in schools (41).

School Wellness Policies. Beyond state regulation, a unique opportunity has emerged to use local policies to improve the school environment. In 2004, Section 204 of the Child Nutrition and WIC Reauthorization Act required all school districts participating in federally funded school meal programs to create a school wellness policy (SWP) by the start of the 2006–2007 school year (42). The federal law required policies to have five features: (1) goals for nutrition education, physical activity, and other school-based activities; (2) nutrition guidelines for all foods available on each school campus during the school day; (3) an assurance that guidelines for reimbursable school meals shall not be less restrictive than federal regulations and guidance; (4) a plan for measuring implementation of the local wellness policy, including designation of one or more responsible persons; and (5) the involvement of parents, students, and representatives of the school food authority, the school board, school administrators, and the public in the development of the school wellness policy (43).

The strategy of placing the responsibility on school districts to establish their own policies has both benefits and risks. On the positive side, part of the federal mandate is that the policies must be written by a committee that includes representatives from many stakeholders, including parents, students, the public, school administrators, the board of education, and the food service. This sets the stage for each district to hear viewpoints from relevant parties and achieve buy-in, cooperation, and better compliance with implementation. On the other hand, there are no minimum national standards for the nutritional value of competitive foods or the amount of time devoted to physical activity, which enables the creation of some weak policies and creates a national landscape with considerable variability among districts (44).

The impact of requiring local districts to write their own policies is still unknown. Research to date suggests that districts have been able to meet the minimum requirements in their policies. The strongest parts of the policies tended to be the sections on school meals (44), likely because the mandate came through the USDA and the food service director was ultimately responsible for the policy. A comprehensive review of the policies from a national sample of approximately 600 school districts concluded that the quality of policies varied, and many were underdeveloped, fragmented, and lacked sufficient plans for implementation and monitoring (45). There is substantial opportunity for local districts to strengthen the policies and for states to require such action. However, in order for these changes to be consistent throughout the country, it will likely require adequate funding and a revision to the federal mandate that includes minimum nutrition standards for meals and snacks, minimum standards for physical education and opportunities for physical activity, and a standard mechanism for oversight and evaluation.

One idea is to manage the oversight of local wellness policies at the state level. Models of this exist because some states have taken additional steps to encourage compliance and stronger policies from their districts (46). Pennsylvania required all districts to submit their policies to the Department of Education for review (47). Florida posted all policies on a central website to ensure transparency (48). The most involved state may be Connecticut, which collected and coded all policies on compliance and strength using a validated evaluation tool then sent reports back to the districts with directions on how they can improve their policies (49).

POLICY INTERVENTIONS DESIGNED TO CHANGE FOOD INDUSTRY ACTIONS

Much of the work to address obesity has focused on changing the behavior of individuals. It is also important to change behavior of the food industry. The industry states that it responds to consumer demand, but there are instances where consumers have requested changes but the industry has refused to comply. Two examples are menu labeling and marketing to children.

Menu labeling. The issue of chain restaurant menu labeling has received a substantial amount of attention by policy makers and the restaurant industry (50). In 2006, the City of New York broke new ground by requiring chain restaurants to provide calories on their menus and menu boards. A flurry of litigation followed, with the restaurant industry twice suing the city to block the regulation, but the city prevailed and the regulation was enforced in July 2007.

Other states and localities have followed suit, and at the present time, menu labeling is enacted in California, Massachusetts, Maine, and Oregon, as well as four New York counties (Ulster, Suffolk, Westchester, and Albany), Nashville, Philadelphia, and King County (Seattle) Washington. Connecticut also introduced menu labeling bills in 2007 and 2009. The 2009 Connecticut bill passed the House and Senate, but was vetoed by the Governor. These successes may motivate other states and cities to pursue menu labeling legislation.

The restaurant industry notes that different menu labeling laws throughout the country leads to confusion and expense (as there are different requirements for menus and menu boards), the ostensible reason it sought federal legislation that would create a national standard. An alternative explanation is that the industry predicted a wave of action at state and local levels and therefore lobbied for federal legislation to lock in a weak national standard that would preempt non-federal action. In early 2009, the industry worked with federal legislators to create a unified federal law. Initially two competing bills were introduced; one sponsored by Rep. Rosa DeLauro (D-CT) and Senator Tom Harkin (D-IA), called the Menu Education and Labeling (MEAL) Act, and an industry-supported bill sponsored by Rep. Jim Matheson (D-UT) and Senator Thomas Carper (D-DE), called the Labeling Education and Nutrition (LEAN) Act. Later in the session in 2009, the sponsors of the competing bills announced that a compromise had been reached and the new language was attached to health-care reform legislation. The national health care reform law passed in late 2009 – officially called The Patient Protection and Affordable Care Act – contains a section (4205) that requires all chain restaurants with 20 or more locations to provide clear labeling of the calories counts of their standard menu items by March 2011. Restaurants must also display a statement that the average individual should consume 2000 calories per day. Other information such as fat, cholesterol, sodium, carbohydrates, sugars, fiber, and protein must be provided upon request. Further, vending machines from companies that operate 20 or more machines will be required to display the calories per item in a way that the prospective buyer can read the information prior to purchase (51).

Food marketing to youth. The food industry spends enormous sums to market its products; in 2006 they spent $870 million marketing to children aged 2–11 and $1.05 billion marketing to adolescents aged 12–17 *(52)*. Food marketing is often cited as a contributing factor to childhood obesity *(53–56)*. The research tracking the prevalence and impact of marketing has grown, but scientists must chase a moving target because marketing has evolved with the quickly growing world of web-based entertainment, social networking, and cell phone text communications *(57,58)*. There is more food marketing than ever through media that parents do not monitor or control (such as website game sites) and subtle methods that individuals may not recognize as marketing (such as product placements in popular television shows, movies, and video games).

Industry has responded in a number of ways to increasing public disapproval of marketing unhealthy foods to children. Food companies focused on the importance of physical activity and invested in promoting more activity for children by sponsoring events and putting branded playgrounds in schools *(59)*. In 2007, a group of food companies appeared to acknowledge that marketing unhealthy foods to children is a problem and announced through the Council of Better Business Bureaus that child marketing practices would change *(60,61)*. Evaluation of the impact of this effort is needed.

Local, state, and the federal governments can and must take action to protect children from food marketing. A series of reports from the Education and the Public Interest Center and Commercialism in Education Research Unit has documented the vast branded marketing that occurs inside school buildings and on school grounds *(62)*. Locally, school wellness policies can include language that prohibits branding on the school grounds (e.g., branded score boards, books that teach counting through branded candy, "free" book covers that contain food company logos, and nutrition education materials that contain food company logos). Districts can also set policies to disallow commercial television in school (such as Channel One) and targeted commercial radio programs on school buses (such as Bus Radio).

At the state or city level, school-based policies such as those described above may be established as law. States may also broaden marketing regulations to apply to other sites that serve children and receive government funding, such as child-care programs, after school programs, and community centers. Some other ideas that have been put forward include local ordinances to restrict mobile vending of unhealthy foods near playgrounds and schools, zoning regulations to limit the density of fast food restaurants, and incentive programs to encourage retail outlets to reduce point-of-sale marketing of unhealthy foods (e.g., candy-free check out aisles) *(1)*.

CONCLUSIONS

The early history of using public policy for the prevention of obesity is being written now. Until recently, the nation focused decades of effort on treating obesity and on various approaches to individual behavior change. Research monies went to basic research on genetics, pathophysiology, and pharmacology on one hand, and treatment research on the other, with little attention paid to changing conditions that drive obesity.

This picture began to change as prevalence statistics soared and realization set in that existing approaches were not working. Especially since the turn of the century, there has been growing conceptualization of obesity as a public health matter, greater emphasis on prevention, and vitally needed discussions of public policy. A public health approach has begun to dominate.

Obesity does not represent a biological abnormality nor a failure of personal will – neither can explain rapidly rising prevalence in every corner of the world. Food and physical activity environments have changed dramatically with rampant obesity, an understandable consequence. Changing these environments must be the top priority if prevalence is to decrease.

We believe that public policy must be placed at the heart of a national (and global) effort to prevent obesity and that policies should strive to create better defaults. The person who eats the recommended diet and/or has the recommended levels of physical activity is now the exception because modern food and activity conditions make healthy behavior difficult and encourage unhealthy choices. Portions are too large, food prices promote overconsumption, a tidal wave of marketing overwhelms good judgment, schools sell unhealthy foods, and have subtracted activity from the curriculum, just to begin the list of toxic influences.

A number of public policy options have been discussed in this chapter, and our coverage is not exhaustive. A key question is what will be most effective and what approaches will produce greatest benefit at lowest cost. Sadly guesswork is more plentiful than data. There are clear gaps in knowledge that must be addressed with an aggressive funding strategy by government that produces research on the factors contributing to obesity at the population level, models for policies that change these factors, and immediate and thorough evaluation of policies once implemented.

It is essential that science and policy work together. Demanding perfect science before implementing policy change, and yielding to arguments that many factors contribute to obesity and hence no single policy will solve the problem, will permit paralysis to prevail over invention, lock in the status quo, and let death and disability continue unabated. On the other hand, science should be an ally to policy and stronger connections between the scientific community and elected leaders will be necessary. We feel encouraged by signs that this is happening.

Editor's Comment

- A campaign ("Let's Move") to target childhood obesity has recently been initiated by the White House under the direction of First Lady Michelle Obama. In March, 2010, a White House Task Force on Childhood Obesity issued a comprehensive report that recommends a variety of federal, state, and local policy changes that may be helpful in reversing the obesity epidemic and improving child health. The Task Force Report (called Solving the Problem of Childhood Obesity Within a Generation) can be accessed online at http://www.letsmove.gov/taskforce_childhoodobesityrpt.html

---

REFERENCES

1. Institute of Medicine. Local government actions to prevent childhood obesity. Washington, DC: National Academy of Sciences; 2009.
2. Brescoll VL, Kersh R, Brownell KD. Assessing the feasibility and impact of federal childhood obesity policies. Ann Am Acad Pol Soc Sci. 2008;615:178–94.
3. Jeffery RW, Drewnowski A, Epstein LH, et al. Long-term maintenance of weight loss: current status. Health Psychol. 2000;19:S5–16.
4. Story M, Kaphingst KM, Robinson- O'Brien R, Glanz K. Creating healthy food and eating environments: policy and environmental approaches. Annu Rev Publ Health. 2008;29:253–72.
5. Obesity-related legislation action in states. 2007. http://www.fns.usda.gov/fns/nutrition.htm. Accessed 2007.
6. Brownell KD, Kersh R, Ludwig DS, et al. Personal responsibility and obesity: a constructive approach to a controversial issue. Health Aff. 2010;29:379–87.
7. Wansink B. Mindless eating: why we eat more than we think. New York, NY: Bantam Books; 2006.
8. Johnson J, Goldstein D. Do defaults save lives? Sci Justice. 2003;302:1338–9.
9. About WIC. 2009. http://www.fns.usda.gov/wic/aboutwic/mission.htm. Accessed 25 Aug 2009.
10. Brownell KD, Farley T, Willett WC, et al. The public health and economic benefits of taxing sugar-sweetened beverages. N Engl J Med. 2009 (in press online).
11. Brownell KD, Frieden TR. Ounces of prevention – the public policy case for taxes on sugared beverages. N Engl J Med. 2009;360:1805–8.
12. Cullen KW, Zakeri I. Fruits, vegetables, milk, and sweetened beverages consumption and access to a la carte/snack bar meals at school. Am J Public Health. 2004;94:463–7.

13. Kubik MY, Lytle LA, Hannan PJ, Perry CL, Story M. The association of the school food environment with dietary behaviors of young adolescents. Am J Publ Health. 2003;93:1168–72.

14. Kubik MY, Lytle LA, Story M. Schoolwide food practices are associated with body mass index in middle school students. Arch Pediatr Adolesc Med. 2005;159:1111–4.

15. Schwartz MB. The influence of a verbal prompt on school lunch fruit consumption: a pilot study. Int J Behav Nutr Phys Act. 2007;4:6.

16. Schwartz MB, Novak SA, Fiore SS. The impact of removing snacks of low nutritional value from middle schools. Health Educ Behav. 2009;36:999–1011.

17. Fox MK, Hamilton W, Biing-Hwan L. Effects of food assistance and nutrition programs on nutrition and health: executive summary of the literature review, vol. 4. Washington, DC: United States Department of Agriculture, Rural Economics Division, Economic Research Service Abt Associates Inc; 2004.

18. Cole N, Fox MK. Nutrient intake and diet quality of WIC participants and nonparticipants. Food and Nutrition Service. Washington, DC: US Department of Agriculture ed.; 2008.

19. Nelson JA, Chiasson MA, Ford V. Childhood overweight in a New York City WIC population. Am J Public Health. 2004;94:458–62.

20. Institute of Medicine. WIC food packages: time for a change. Washington, DC: National Academy of Sciences; 2005.

21. Farmer's Market Nutrition Program. 2009. http://www.nyswica.org/php/prog/farmer.php. Accessed 25 Sept 2009.

22. WIC Farmer's Market Nutrition Program. 2009. http://www.fns.usda.gov/wic/fmnp/FMNPfaqs.htm. Accessed 25 Sept 2009.

23. Andreyeva T, Blumenthal DM, Schwartz MB, Long MW, Brownell KD. Availability and prices of foods across stores and neighborhoods: the case of New Haven, Connecticut. Health Aff (Millwood). 2008;27:1381–8.

24. Oliveira V, Frazao E. The WIC program: background, trends, and economic issues. Economic Research Service. Washington, DC: Department of Agriculture ed.; 2009.

25. Oakley CB, Bomba AK, Knight KB, Byrd SH. Evaluation of menus planned in Mississippi child-care centers participating in the Child and Adult Care Food Program. J Am Diet Assoc. 1995;95:765–8.

26. Services USDoHaH, Agriculture USDo. Dietary guidelines for Americans. 6th ed. Washington, DC: Government Printing Office; 2005.

27. American Academy of Pediatrics APHA, and National Resource Center for Health and Safety in Child Care. Caring for our children: national health and safety performance standards: guidelines for out-of-home child care programs. 2nd ed. Elk Grove Village, IL: American Academy of Pediatrics and Washington, DC: American Public Health Association; 2002.

28. American Academy of Pediatrics. The use and misuse of fruit juice in pediatrics. Pediatrics. 2001;107:1210–3.

29. Dennison BA, Rockwell HL, Baker SL. Fruit and vegetable intake in young children. J Am Coll Nutr. 1998;17:371–8.

30. O'Connor TM, Yang SJ, Nicklas TA. Beverage intake among preschool children and its effect on weight status. Pediatrics. 2006;118:e1010–8.

31. Welsh JA, Cogswell ME, Rogers S, Rockett H, Mei Z, Grummer-Strawn LM. Overweight among low-income preschool children associated with the consumption of sweet drinks: Missouri, 1999–2002. Pediatrics. 2005;115:e223–9.

32. Faith MS, Dennison BA, Edmunds LS, Stratton HH. Fruit juice intake predicts increased adiposity gain in children from low-income families: weight status-by-environment interaction. Pediatrics. 2006;118:2066–75.

33. Newby PK, Peterson KE, Berkey CS, Leppert J, Willett WC, Colditz GA. Beverage consumption is not associated with changes in weight and body mass index among low-income preschool children in North Dakota. J Am Diet Assoc. 2004;104:1086–94.

34. Fox MK, Reidy K, Novak T, Ziegler P. Sources of energy and nutrients in the diets of infants and toddlers. J Am Diet Assoc. 2006;106:S28–42.

35. California Food Policy Advocates. Recommendations on child care nutrition. Oakland, CA; 2009.

36. CACFP Healthy Child Meal Pattern (CACFP-102). In: State of New York Department of Health, ed. Number 132C (05/09); 2009.

37. Gordon AR, Crepinsek MK, Briefel RR, Clark MA, Fox MK. The third School Nutrition Dietary Assessment Study: summary and implications. J Am Diet Assoc. 2009;109:S129–35.

38. Story M, Nanney MS, Schwartz MB. Schools and obesity prevention: creating school environments and policies to promote healthy eating and physical activity. Milbank Q. 2009;87:71–100.

39. School Meals: Foods of Minimal Nutrition Value. http://www.fns.usda.gov/cnd/menu/fmnv.htm. Accessed 16 Sept 2009.

40. Institute of Medicine. Nutrition standards for foods in schools: leading the way toward healthier youth. Washington, DC: National Academies Press; Apr 2007.

41. Trust for America's Health. Washington, DC. http://healthyamericans.org/reports/obesity2009. Accessible 2009.

42. Smith R. Passing an effective obesity bill. J Am Diet Assoc. 2006;106:1349–50, 52–3.

43. The Child Nutrition and WIC Reauthorization Act. Public Law 108–265—June 30, 2004.

44. Belansky E, Chriqui JF, Schwartz MB. Local School Wellness Policies: how are schools implementing the congressional mandate? Washington, DC: RWJF Research Brief, Robert Wood Johnson Foundation; 2009.

45. Chriqui J, Schneider L, Chaloupka F, Ide K, Pugach O. Local Wellness Policies: assessing school district strategies for improving children's health. School years 2006–2007 and 2007–2008. Chicago, IL: Healthy Policy Center, Institute for Health Research and Policy, University of Illinois at Chicago; 2009.

46. Pekruhn CE, Bogden JF. State strategies to support local wellness policies. Alexandria: National Association of State Boards of Education; 2007.

47. Probart C, McDonnell E, Weirich JE, Schilling L, Fekete V. Statewide assessment of local wellness policies in Pennsylvania public school districts. J Am Diet Assoc. 2008;108:1497–502.

48. Florida Links to Local Wellness Policies. 2006. http://www.fldoe.org/FNM/wellness/localpolicies.asp. Accessed 17 Sept 2009.

49. Schwartz MB, Lund AE, Grow HM, et al. A comprehensive coding system to measure the quality of school wellness policies. J Am Diet Assoc. 2009;109:1256–62.

50. Ludwig DS, Brownell KD. Public health action amid scientific uncertainty: the case of restaurant calorie labeling regulations. J Am Med Assoc. 2009;302:434–5.

51. Whelan EM, Russell L, Sekhar, S. Confronting America's childhood obesity epidemic: how the health care reform law will help prevent and reduce obesity. Center for American Progress. 2010 May. Available online at: www.americanprogress.org

52. Marketing Food to Children and Adolescents. A review of industry expenditures, activities, and self-regulation. 2008. www.ftc.gov. Accessed 20 Sept 2008.

53. Borzekowski D, Robinson T. The 30-second effect: an experiment revealing the impact of television commercials on food preferences of preschoolers. J Am Diet Assoc. 2001;101:42–6.

54. Harris JL, Pomeranz JL, Lobstein T, Brownell KD. A crisis in the marketplace: how food marketing contributes to childhood obesity and what can be done. Annu Rev Publ Health. 2009;30:211–25.

55. Powell L, Szczypka G, Chaloupka F, Braunschweig C. Nutritional content of television food advertisements seen by children and adolescents in the United States. Pediatrics. 2007;120:576–83.

56. Batada A, Seitz M, Wootan M, Story M. Nine out of 10 food advertisements shown during Saturday morning children's television programming are for foods high in fat, sodium, or added sugars, or low in nutrients. J Am Diet Assoc. 2008;108:673–8.

57. Roberts DF, Foehr UG, Rideout V. Generation M: media in the lives of 8–18 year olds. Menlo Park, CA: Kaiser Family Foundation Study; 2005.

58. Alvy L, Calvert S. Food marketing on popular children's web sites: a content analysis. J Am Diet Assoc. 2008;108:710–3.

59. Mayer CE. Work off those cheetos! Snack-food makers promote exercise, healthful diets for kids. Washington Post 2005.

60. Changing the Landscape of Food & Beverage Advertising. The children's food and beverage advertising initiative in action. 2008. http://us.bbb.org/WWWRoot/storage/16/documents/CFBAI/ChildrenF&BInit_Sept21.pdf. Accessed 10 Jul 2008.

61. Children's Food and Beverage Advertising Initiative. 2008. http://www.bbb.org/us/WWWRoot/storage/16/documents/InitiativeProgramDocument.pdf. Accessed 10 Jun 2008.

62. Molnar A, Boninger F, Wilkinson G, Fogarty J. At Sea in a Marketing-Saturated World: The Eleventh Annual Report on Schoolhouse Commercialism Trends: 2007–2008. Boulder, CO and Tempe, AZ: Education and the Public Interest Center & Commercialism in Education Research Unit; 2008.

Appendix

From: *Contemporary Endocrinology: Pediatric Obesity: Etiology, Pathogenesis, and Treatment*
Edited by: M. Freemark, DOI 10.1007/978-1-60327-874-4,
© Springer Science+Business Media, LLC 2010

Table 1
Valuable Reference Sites

CDC growth charts

– http://www.cdc.gov/growthcharts/

BMI and BMI *z*-calculations

– http://stokes.chop.edu/web/zscore/

Obesity gene databases

–http://www.ncbi.nlm.nih.gov/projects/mapview/ map_ search.cgi?
taxid=9606&query=obesity&qchr=&strain=All

– Hofker M, Wijmenga C. Nat Genet. 2009;41(2):139–40

Estimates of risks of type 2 diabetes and metabolic syndrome in obese
adolescents and adults

– Narayan KM, et al. Diabetes Care. 2007;30(6):1562–6

– Hariri S, et al. Genet Med. 2006;8(2):102–8

– Schubert CM, et al. J Pediatr. 2009;155(3):S6.e9–13

Tables of glycemic index and glycemic load of foods

– Atkinson FS, et al. Diabetes Care. 2008;31(12):2281–3

White House Task Force Report on Childhood Obesity ("Solving the
Problem of Childhood Obesity Within a Generation")

– http://www.letsmove.gov/taskforce_childhoodobesityrpt.html

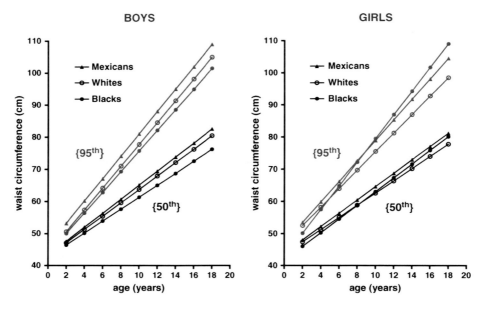

Fig. 1. Waist circumference in children of varying ethnicities. Adapted from Fernandez JR, et al. J Pediatr. 2004; 145:439–44.

Table 2
Energy Equivalents of Some Daily Activities
(Approximate)

Activity	Met
Sleeping	0.9
Watching television	1.0
Sitting quietly	1.0
Desk work	1.8
Walking <2 mph	2.0
Housework	2.5–3.5
Home exercises	3.6
Lifting continuously	4.0
Biking <10 mph	3–6
Walking 3–5 mph	4–8
Hiking cross-country	6
Swimming	6–10
Jogging	7
Tennis, soccer	6–10
Biking >10 mph	8–12
Vigorous calisthenics	8
Aerobic step, 10–12 in.	7–10
Running	8–18

MET (metabolic equivalent) = multiple of resting metabolic rate (~ 1 kcal (4.184 kJ)/kg/h).

Adapted from Ainsworth BE, et al. Med Sci Sports Exerc. 2000;32(9 Suppl):S498–516.

Table 3
Medications That Can Alter Triglyceride and HDL Levels

Medication	Triglycerides	HDL
Estrogens	Increased	Increased
Androgens	Increased	Decreased
Progestins	Decreased	Decreased
Glucocorticoids	Increased	Increased
Thiazides	Increased	Decreased
Beta-blockers	Increased	Decreased
Valproic acid	Increased	Decreased
Isotretinoin	Increased	Decreased
Cyclosporin	Increased	Increased
Tacrolimus	Increased	Increased
Protease inhibitors	Increased	–

Adapted from Brunzell JD. Hypertriglyceridemia. N Engl J Med. 2007;357:1009–17.

SUBJECT INDEX

Note: The letters 'f', and 't' following locators refer to figures and tables respectively.